T0251562

Antibiotic Therapy for Geriatric Patients

Antibiotic Therapy for Geriatric Patients

Edited by

THOMAS T. YOSHIKAWA
Charles R. Drew University of Medicine and Science
Martin Luther King, Jr.–Charles R. Drew Medical Center
Los Angeles, California, U.S.A.

SHOBITA RAJAGOPALAN
Charles R. Drew University of Medicine and Science
Martin Luther King, Jr.–Charles R. Drew Medical Center
Los Angeles, California, U.S.A.

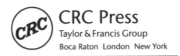

CRC Press
Taylor & Francis Group
Boca Raton London New York

CRC Press is an imprint of the
Taylor & Francis Group, an **informa** business

Preface

Infections are major causes of morbidity and mortality in older adults. The diagnosis of infections in the elderly patient may be difficult and often delayed. Thus, life-saving treatments may be omitted or initiated late in the course of the illness, resulting in poor outcomes. Diagnostic procedures to facilitate a more specific microbiological diagnosis are often not performed in elderly patients because of potentially greater complication rates, difficulty in obtaining cooperation from cognitively impaired or physically disabled patients, or failure to understand the importance of elucidating a specific microbiological diagnosis. Consequently, empirical antibiotic therapy with broad-spectrum drugs is frequently prescribed. Not surprisingly, there is an increasing prevalence of antibiotic-resistant pathogens, especially in the institutional setting and among frail, debilitated elderly persons. To combat these resistant organisms, newer and more potent antibiotics are being constantly manufactured. The number and types of newer antimicrobial agents can become overwhelming and impossible to comprehend for the clinician who cares for older patients. Moreover, new and emerging infectious agents (e.g., West Nile virus, severe acute respiratory syndrome) often attack the elderly population with greater frequency and/or severity. A current knowledge of effective treatments (if any) for these pathogens is imperative.

Most clinicians caring for a large number of geriatric patients have little time for in-depth reading on topics that are relevant to their day-to-day care of patients. Thus, any reference source should be clinically relevant, easy to read, accurate, current, and relatively inexpensive. It should also provide quick access to the essential or core information about a clinical issue or topic.

Antibiotic Therapy for Geriatric Patients is such a book. It is written by the foremost authorities in the area of infection and aging. The book is divided into five major sections: I. Important Principles and Concepts of Infections and Aging; II. Specific Important Antibiotics; III. Major Clinical Infections; IV. Selected Pathogens; and V. Infections in Long-Term Care. Section I summarizes many of the unique and important aspects and concepts of infectious diseases in older adults, such as epidemiology, clinical manifestations, altered host resistance, and pharmacology. Section II provides all of the key and necessary information regarding the most important and clinically relevant antibiotics prescribed for elderly patients. The information is organized in a consistent, concise, and clear manner so that the reader can quickly access and review the information. Pharmacokinetic and pharmacodynamic information, indications, dosage, precautions, and adverse effects relevant to older patients are presented. Section III describes in a concise manner the diagnosis and treatment of major infections in the elderly with emphasis on key features that are specific or relevant to elderly patients. Section IV discusses select and common pathogens associated with infections encountered in aging adults. Section V is devoted to the special problems of infections in long-term care facilities such as a nursing home. References are provided with each chapter. Each chapter is summarized with "key points" that highlight important and practical aspects of the specific topic.

Antibiotic Therapy for Geriatric Patients is an ideal and authoritative resource for practicing clinicians including geriatricians, infectious disease specialists, gerontologists, primary care physicians, internists, pharmacists, nursing home directors and administrators, infection control practitioners, and upper-level undergraduate and graduate students in these disciplines.

Thomas T. Yoshikawa, M.D.
Shobita Rajagopalan, M.D.

Contents

Contributors

Abbasi J. Akhtar   Department of Internal Medicine, Division of Infectious Diseases, Charles R. Drew University of Medicine and Science, Martin Luther King, Jr.–Charles R. Drew Medical Center, Los Angeles, California, U.S.A.

Richard S. Baker   Charles R. Drew University of Medicine and Science, Los Angeles, California, U.S.A.

Steven L. Berk   Texas Tech University Health Sciences Center School of Medicine, Amarillo, Texas, U.S.A.

Robert A. Bonomo   Section of Infectious Diseases, Department of Medicine, Louis Stokes Veterans Affairs Medical Center, Cleveland, Ohio, U.S.A.

Suzanne F. Bradley   Geriatric Research Education and Clinical Center, Veterans Affairs Ann Arbor Healthcare System, and Divisions of Infectious Diseases and Geriatric Medicine, University of Michigan Medical School, Ann Arbor, Michigan, U.S.A.

John G. Carson   Department of Surgery, University of California, Irvine, California, U.S.A.

Richard Casey   Charles R. Drew University of Medicine and Science, Los Angeles, California, U.S.A.

Steven C. Castle   Veterans Affairs, Greater Los Angeles Healthcare System, UCLA School of Medicine, Los Angeles, California, U.S.A.

Chester Choi   Department of Medicine, St. Mary Medical Center, Long Beach, California, U.S.A. and David Geffen School of Medicine, University of California at Los Angeles, Los Angeles, California, U.S.A.

Anthony W. Chow   Division of Infectious Diseases, Department of Medicine, University of British Columbia and Vancouver Hospital Health Sciences Center, Vancouver, British Columbia, Canada

Burke A. Cunha   Infectious Disease Division, Winthrop-University Hospital, Mineola and Department of Medicine, State University of New York School of Medicine, Stony Brook, New York, U.S.A.

Sanjeet Dadwal   City of Hope Medical Center, Duarte, California, U.S.A.

Vinod K. Dhawan   Charles R. Drew University of Medicine and Science, Martin Luther King, Jr.–Charles R. Drew Medical Center, UCLA School of Medicine, Los Angeles, California, U.S.A.

Ghinwa Dumyati   University of Rochester, Rochester General Hospital, Rochester, New York, U.S.A.

Ronan Factora   Section of Geriatric Medicine, Department of General Internal Medicine, Cleveland Clinic Foundation, Cleveland, Ohio, U.S.A.

Ann R. Falsey   University of Rochester School of Medicine and Dentistry, Department of Medicine, Rochester General Hospital, Rochester, New York, U.S.A.

Charles W. Flowers, Jr.   Charles R. Drew University of Medicine and Science, Los Angeles, California, U.S.A.

Susan Fryters   Department of Regional Pharmacy Services, Capital Health, Edmonton, Alberta, Canada

Allen S. Funnyé   Divisions of General Internal Medicine and Geriatrics, Department of Internal Medicine, Charles R. Drew University of Medicine and Science, Martin Luther King, Jr.–Charles R. Drew Medical Center, Los Angeles, California, U.S.A.

David R. P. Guay   Department of Experimental and Clinical Pharmacology and Institute for the Study of Geriatric Pharmacotherapy, University of Minnesota, College of Pharmacy and Division of Geriatrics, HealthPartners Inc., Minneapolis, Minnesota, U.S.A.

Nancy Hanna   Department of Internal Medicine, Charles R. Drew University of Medicine and Science, Martin Luther King, Jr.–Charles R. Drew Medical Center, Los Angeles, California, U.S.A.

Kevin P. High   Sections of Infectious Diseases and Hematology/Oncology, Wake Forest University School of Medicine, Winston-Salem, North Carolina, U.S.A.

Charles Huynh   Department of Internal Medicine, Division of Infectious Diseases, Charles R. Drew University of Medicine and Science, Martin Luther King, Jr.–Charles R. Drew Medical Center, Los Angeles, California, U.S.A.

Carol A. Kauffman   Division of Infectious Diseases, University of Michigan Medical School, Infectious Diseases Section, Veterans Affairs Ann Arbor Healthcare System, Ann Arbor, Michigan, U.S.A.

Jiwon Kim University of Southern California, Los Angeles, California, U.S.A.

Anh Le Department of Oral and Maxillofacial Surgery, Charles R. Drew University of Medicine and Science, Los Angeles, California, U.S.A.

Mark Loeb Departments of Pathology and Molecular Medicine and Clinical Epidemiology and Biostatistics, McMaster University, Hamilton, Ontario, Canada

Takashi Makinodan Veterans Affairs, Greater Los Angeles Healthcare System, UCLA School of Medicine, Los Angeles, California, U.S.A.

Stephen Marer Department of Internal Medicine, Division of Infectious Diseases, Charles R. Drew University of Medicine and Science, Martin Luther King, Jr.–Charles R. Drew Medical Center, Los Angeles, California, U.S.A.

Thomas J. Marrie Department of Medicine, University of Alberta, Edmonton, Alberta, Canada

Glenn E. Mathisen Division of Infectious Diseases, UCLA School of Medicine, Olive View–UCLA Medical Center, Sylmar, California, U.S.A.

Jack D. McCue University of Maryland School of Medicine, Franklin Square Hospital Center, Baltimore, Maryland, U.S.A.

Joseph L. McQuirter Department of Oral and Maxillofacial Surgery, Charles R. Drew University of Medicine and Science, Los Angeles, California, U.S.A.

Lona Mody Division of Geriatric Medicine, University of Michigan Medical School and Veterans Affairs Ann Arbor Healthcare System, Ann Arbor, Michigan, U.S.A.

Deborah Moran Department of Internal Medicine, Charles R. Drew University of Medicine and Science, Martin Luther King, Jr.–Charles R. Drew Medical Center, Los Angeles, California, U.S.A.

L. E. Nicolle Departments of Internal Medicine and Medical Microbiology, University of Manitoba, Health Sciences Centre, Winnipeg, Manitoba, Canada

Dean C. Norman UCLA Geffen School of Medicine, Veterans Affairs Greater Los Angeles Healthcare System, Los Angeles, California, U.S.A.

Ryan F. Osborne Head and Neck Oncology, Cedars Sinai Medical Center, Otolaryngology/Head and Neck Surgery, Charles R. Drew University of Medicine and Science, Los Angeles, California, U.S.A.

Joseph G. Ouslander Geriatric Research, Education, and Clinical Center (GRECC), Atlanta, Georgia, U.S.A.

Robert M. Palmer Section of Geriatric Medicine, Department of General Internal Medicine, Cleveland Clinic Foundation, Cleveland, Ohio, U.S.A.

Ryan W. Patterson   Department of Surgery, University of California, Irvine, California, U.S.A.

Parmis Pouya   Department of Internal Medicine, Charles R. Drew University of Medicine and Science, Martin Luther King, Jr.–Charles R. Drew Medical Center, Los Angeles, California, U.S.A.

Asif Rafi   Veterans Affairs, Greater Los Angeles Healthcare System, UCLA School of Medicine, Los Angeles, California, U.S.A.

Shobita Rajagopalan   Department of Internal Medicine, Division of Infectious Diseases, Charles R. Drew University of Medicine and Science, Martin Luther King, Jr.–Charles R. Drew Medical Center, Los Angeles, California, U.S.A.

Jay P. Rho   Kaiser Foundation Hospital, Los Angeles, California, U.S.A.

Chesley L. Richards, Jr.   Division of Healthcare Quality Promotion, National Center for Infectious Diseases, Centers for Disease Control and Prevention, Atlanta, Georgia, U.S.A. and Division of Geriatric Medicine and Gerontology, Department of Medicine, Emory University School of Medicine, Atlanta, Georgia, U.S.A.

Hidetada Sasaki   Department of Geriatric and Respiratory Medicine, Tohoku University School of Medicine, Sendai, Japan

Kenneth E. Schmader   Center for the Study of Aging and Human Development, Duke University and Durham Veterans Affairs Medical Centers, Durham, North Carolina, U.S.A.

Sunil Singhania   Department of Internal Medicine, Charles R. Drew University of Medicine and Science, Martin Luther King, Jr.–Charles R. Drew Medical Center, Los Angeles, California, U.S.A.

Lorraine M. Smith   Otolaryngology/Head and Neck Surgery, Charles R. Drew University of Medicine and Science, Los Angeles, California, U.S.A.

Made Sutjita   Department of Internal Medicine, Division of Infectious Diseases, Charles R. Drew University of Medicine and Science, Martin Luther King, Jr.–Charles R. Drew Medical Center, Los Angeles, California, U.S.A.

Robert S. Urban   Texas Tech University Health Sciences Center School of Medicine, Amarillo, Texas, U.S.A.

Koichi Uyemura   Veterans Affairs, Greater Los Angeles Healthcare System, UCLA School of Medicine, Los Angeles, California, U.S.A.

Samuel Eric Wilson   Department of Surgery, University of California, Irvine, California, U.S.A.

Jack Wu   Division of Infectious Diseases, Department of Medicine, University of British Columbia and Vancouver Hospital Health Sciences Center, Vancouver, British Columbia, Canada

Mutsuo Yamaya   Department of Geriatric and Respiratory Medicine, Tohoku University School of Medicine, Sendai, Japan

Thomas T. Yoshikawa   Department of Internal Medicine, Charles R. Drew University of Medicine and Science, Martin Luther King, Jr.–Charles R. Drew Medical Center, Los Angeles, California, U.S.A.

1

Epidemiology and Unique Aspects of Infections

Deborah Moran and Thomas T. Yoshikawa

Department of Internal Medicine, Charles R. Drew University of Medicine and Science, Martin Luther King, Jr.–Charles R. Drew Medical Center, Los Angeles, California, U.S.A.

Key Points:

- Life expectancy in the United States has dramatically increased (secondary to medical advances in public health), which has resulted in a large population of elderly persons.
- The elderly are now encountering infections as a major health care problem.
- Older persons commonly present with significant infection in the absence of classic signs.
- The microbiology of select infections in the elderly may be more diverse compared with younger adults.
- Infection remains the cause of death for many elders, with ethical care centering on the principles of autonomy, beneficence, and nonmaleficence.

1. INTRODUCTION

The word *epidemiology* derives from *epidemic* and originates from the Greek words *epi* (upon) + *demos* (people) + *logy* (study of). Epidemiology is an interdisciplinary field that draws from biostatistics, social and behavioral sciences, as well as from clinical medicine (1). In 1979, Terris wrote that epidemiology "must draw upon and synthesize knowledge from the biological sciences of man and of his parasites, from the numerous sciences of the physical environment, and from the sciences concerned with human society" (2).

An understanding of infectious disease epidemiology should not be simply a discussion of an infectious agent inflicting disease upon a host. This cannot be done since a person's state of health represents a dynamic equilibrium—a balance of forces—between host factors, characteristics of the infectious agent, and environmental influences (3).

Infectious disease epidemiology in the elderly, therefore, is unique compared with that of younger persons given the dynamic equilibrium inherent in the elderly "host."

In 1846 during the measles epidemic on the Faroe Islands, Peter Ludwig Panum made the following observations, "when a physician is called to work in a place, his first problem is to study the hygienic potentialities which affect the state of health of the inhabitants. It is, in fact, these hygienic conditions which contribute toward the development and frequency of some diseases and the improbability and rarity of others, and which more or less modify the symptoms of every disease" (3).

Controlling infectious diseases is an example of epidemiology at work in the community. Although there have been many advances in the prevention and treatment of infectious diseases, there remain significant causes of morbidity and mortality for the world's population in developed as well as developing countries. Until the mid-20th century, infectious diseases were the major causes of death and disability in the United States. Major outbreak of diseases such as smallpox, diphtheria, cholera, typhoid fever, typhus, plague, and tuberculosis accounted for the deaths of millions of people worldwide. In addition, diseases such as scarlet fever, rheumatic fever, mumps, measles, pertussis, syphilis, and poliomyelitis caused not only death but also severe disabilities, deformities, functional incapacity, and social rejection (4).

Infectious diseases today are responsible for one-third of all deaths in the world. The World Health Organization (WHO) estimates that nearly 50,000 people die each day from an infectious disease (5). This is ironic, since, in the second half of the 20th century, there was a substantial reduction in deaths and morbidity related to infectious diseases in industrialized nations. This reduction in deaths and morbidity was significantly influenced by the development of "the germ theory of disease." Louis Pasteur and Robert Koch, in 1876, postulated that "a specific disease is caused by a specific type of microorganism." (6). This revolutionary way of thinking led to major advances in sanitation, public health measures, antisepsis, antibiotics, and vaccination.

2. LIFE EXPECTANCY

In the United States today, the average life expectancy at birth is 75 years with some variations depending on ethnic or racial background (7). In contrast, the average life expectancy in this country in 1900, when infections were the leading cause of death, was approximately 47 years (7). At that time, only 4% of the entire population was 65 years of age or older (8). Currently, it is estimated that the U.S. population in this age group is 13% and it is expected that by the year 2030, one out of every five Americans (21%) will be 65 years or older (8).

It is also expected that the composition and characteristics of the elderly population will change, with the greatest growth in the "old-old," defined as those persons aged 85 years and older (9). This demographic trend will change the epidemiology of many diseases, including infections. The old-old subgroup of the elderly is relevant clinically because they are the most vulnerable to infectious diseases and their sequelae. Associated factors, such as malnutrition, alcoholism, immobility, institutionalization, and urinary incontinence, superimposed on underlying illness (e.g., diabetes mellitus, cerebrovascular accidents, and malignancies), and altered immune function with senescence further contribute to this enhanced risk for severe infections with aging (10).

As observed, the life expectancy in the United States has dramatically increased (secondary to medical advances in public health), which has resulted in a large population of elderly persons. The major causes of death through the early 20th century were related to infectious diseases. Though the top causes for death in the general population currently are heart diseases, cancers, and strokes, persons in the older age group are now encountering infections as a major health care problem, with pneumonia and influenza being the fourth most common cause of death in the elderly. Additionally, complications from diabetes mellitus (including infections) and complications from bacteremia are the sixth and ninth most frequent causes of death in this age group (11). It is paradoxical that our life expectancy has increased secondary to medical advances (which reduced death and complications related to infections), while the elderly again are encountering infection as a major health care problem.

3. THE EPIDEMIOLOGIC TRIANGLE

The pathogenesis of disease may be represented epidemiologically as a triangle that recognizes three major factors: host, agent, and the environment (12). Though the etiology of infectious diseases involves more complex multivariate causality as well, this section will discuss each of these three areas of the "triangle" as it relates to the elderly: the older host, the infectious agent, (diverse microbial causes), and environmental influences (altered clinical manifestations).

3.1. The Older Host

Changes in the aging immune system represent a permissive factor for the frequent occurrence and the severity of disease in older persons compared with younger adults (13). The major features of immune senescence are depressed T-cell responses and T-cell-macrophage interactions. Immunosenescence is the state of dysregulated immune function that contributes to the increased susceptibility to infection of the elderly (14).

In addition to immunosenescence, elderly persons also suffer from a variety of chronic disorders, both physiologic and pathologic, which affect the host resistance to infection. There are also multiple stresses, polypharmacy (and altered pharmacokinetics), and limited reserve capacity, which add to an increased complexity for diagnosis and treatment of infectious disease in the elderly (see also Chapter 2). Table 1 outlines the factors thought to contribute to a mortality/morbidity rate three times (3×) higher among elderly patients as compared with younger adults (15).

Also contributing to the complexity involved in the evaluation of an elderly host is the understanding that variability increases among individuals as age

Table 1 Factors Contributing to Increased Morbidity and Mortality of Infectious Disease in the Elderly

---

Age-related reduced physiologic reserve capacity
Chronic underlying diseases
Decreased host resistance
Delayed or poor response to antimicrobial therapy
Delays in diagnosis and therapy
Greater risk and incidence of nosocomial infections
Higher rates of adverse reactions to drugs
Poor tolerance to invasive diagnostic and therapeutic procedures

---

Source: Adapted from Ref. 15.

Table 2 Infections in the Elderly According to Functional Status

Functional status	Common (decreasing frequency)
Frail, disabled, nursing home resident	Pneumonia
	UTI
	Skin/soft tissue
	Gastroenteritis
	Tuberculosis
Bedridden, hospitalized	UTI
	Aspiration pneumonia
	Skin/soft tissue
	Septic thrombophlebitis
Healthy, independent	Pneumonia, bronchitis
	UTI
	Cholecystitis, diverticulitis, or appendicitis
	Tuberculosis
	Septic arthritis
	Bacterial meningitis
	Infective endocarditis

Abbreviation: UTI, urinary tract infection.
Source: Adapted from Ref. 16.

increases, since the elderly are not a homogenous group. Actually, heterogeneity is characteristic of the physiology of aging: individuals vary widely and the rate of aging of each function also varies widely. These changes and their interrelation may explain some differences in the incidence or severity of disease. The diagnostic approach to infections can be simplified by determining the health and functional status of the patient and the environment in which the person resides. Table 2 outlines common infections according to functional status in the elderly (16).

3.2. Diverse Microbiology

Infections in the older patient may be caused by more diverse pathogens than infections in young adults. Though commonly encountered organisms in younger adults also cause infection in the elderly, more diverse organisms may be found (Table 3). Additionally, infections with higher predilection for the elderly may be seen (Table 4). Several studies have shown that certain infections occur more often in elderly persons; and, as mentioned before, morbidity and mortality from infections are also higher than among younger adults (15).

3.3. Altered Clinical Manifestations

It has long been recognized that older persons commonly present with significant infection in the absence of classic signs. Definitions used in infectious disease epidemiology change secondary to differences in disease presentation of the elderly, and therefore knowledge of age-specific differences in presentation is essential to avoid selection and misclassification bias (17). Fever, the cardinal sign of infection, may be absent or blunted 20% to 30% of the time (18). Castle et al. suggest that lowering the temperature criterion improves detection of infections in nursing home residents (Table 5) and that as many as 25% of elderly patients with infections may fail to demonstrate a febrile response (19) (see also Chapter 2).

Table 3 Common Organisms Causing Infection in Young and Older Adults

Infection	Organism(s): Young adult	Organism(s): Elderly
Urinary tract infection	*Escherichia coli* *Staphylococcus saprophyticus*	*E. coli* *Proteus* spp. *Klebsiella* spp. *Enterobacter* spp. *Pseudomonas aeruginosa*
Bacteria meningitis	*Streptococcus pneumoniae*	*S. pneumoniae* *Listeria monocytogenes* Gram-negative bacilli
Infective endocarditis	Staphylococci and streptococci	Staphylococci and streptococci *Streptococcus bovis* Enterococci

Source: Adapted from Ref. 15.

Table 4 Infections with Higher Predilection for the Elderly

Urinary tract infections
Lower respiratory tract infections
Skin and soft tissue infections
Intra-abdominal infections, especially:
    Cholecystitis
    Diverticulosis
    Appendicitis
    Abscesses
Infective endocarditis
Bacterial meningitis
Tuberculosis
Herpes zoster

Source: Adapted from Ref. 15.

Fever (and lack thereof) in elderly persons is only one clinical presentation that can be used when suspecting a serious disease. The presence of fever in an elderly person is generally associated with a serious underlying infection (most often of bacterial origin). Infections, like all other illnesses in the geriatric patient, may occur with a variety of presentations. The clinical findings presented are often nonspecific, atypical, or nonclassic. Unexplained change in functional capacity or mental status, weight loss/failure to thrive, and falls are only some of the clues that may aid the clinician in considering infection in the elderly patient (20). Such atypical clinical

Table 5 Defining Fever in Frail Long-Term Care Residents

Temperature, T	Sensitivity (%)	Specificity (%)
> 99°F [37.2°C]	82.5	89.9
> 100°F [37.7°C]	70.0	98.3
> 101°F [38.3°C]	40.0	99.7

Source: Adapted from Ref. 19.

presentations of infections delay and complicate diagnosis and early treatment in this age group.

4. UNIQUE ETHICAL CONSIDERATIONS

Ethical care for the elderly centers around the principles of autonomy, beneficence, and nonmaleficence (21,22). The challenge of healthcare providers is to balance compassionate and appropriate care with respect for the patient's choice while safeguarding professional standards and ethical integrity (23). Today, infection remains the cause of death for many elders (24,25). In the postantibiotic era, the ethical issues concerning the use of antibiotics are discussed much less frequently compared with the issues of resuscitation and the use of high technology (26). Often, antibiotics are the treatment that patients and family members are least willing to forgo (26). Similarly, physicians may find the administration of antibiotics "routine" and feel more comfortable attempting to correct a theoretically reversible condition (26). Ethical principles may address and be applied to the concerns of futility, public health issues, the individual patient, and health care resources as they relate to antimicrobial therapy.

Of course, ethical principles cannot be used as straightforward guides for making clinical decisions; however, they form a framework for discussing ethical issues (27). As the population of older persons in this country soars, the vast majority of serious infectious diseases will be seen in this population. Clinicians must become well versed in the biology of aging and the unique aspects of infections in the elderly. It is by accomplishing these goals that medical care of the older adult will be improved and sculpted to the "uniqueness" of each older individual.

REFERENCES

1. Friis RH, Sellers TA. The history and scope of epidemiology. In: Friis RH, Sellers TA, eds. Epidemiology for Public Health Practice. Maryland: Aspen, 1999:1–32.
2. Terris M. The epidemiologic tradition. Publ Health Rep 1979; 94:203–209.
3. Weber DJ, Rutala WA. Biological basis of infectious disease epidemiology. In: Thomas JC, Weber DJ, eds. Epidemiologic Methods for the Study of Infectious Diseases. New York: Oxford University Press, 2001:3–27.
4. Lyons AS, Petrucelli RJ. Medicine: An Illustrated History. New York: Harry N. Abrams, 1978.
5. Kupersmith C. Three Centuries of Infectious Disease: An Illustrated History of Research and Treatment. Greenwich, Connecticut: Greenwich Press, 1998.
6. Pasteur L. Germ theory and its applications to medicine and surgery, 1878. In: Eliot CW, ed. Modern History Sourcebook: Scientific Papers; Physiology, Medicine, Surgery, Geology, with Introductions, Notes and Illustrations. The Harvard Classics. Vol. 38. New York: P.F. Collier and Son, 1910.
7. U.S. Department of Health and Human Services (DHHS), Public Health Service, National Center for Health Statistics: Health United States 1985. D.H.H.S. Publication No. (P.H.S.) 86–1232. Hyattsville, MD: DHHS, 1986.
8. U.S. Bureau of the Census. Decennial censuses of population, 1900–1980 and projections of the population of the United States: 1985–2050 (advance report). Current Population Reports Series P-25, No. 922. Washington, DC; Bureau of the Census, October 1982.
9. Rajagopalan S, Moran D. Infectious disease emergencies. In: Yoshikawa TT, Norman DC, eds. Acute Emergencies and Critical Care of the Geriatric Patient. New York: Marcel Dekker, 2000:337–355.

10. Rhyne RL, Roche RJ. Infection in the elderly. In: Brillman JC, Quenzer RW, eds. Infectious Disease in Emergency Medicine. Philadelphia: Lippincot-Raven, 1997: 291–316.

11. National Center for Health Statistics. Leading causes of death and number of deaths according to age: United States, 1980 and 1993. In: Health United States, 1995. Department of Health and Human Services (DHHS) Publication No. (P.H.S.) 96–1232. Hyattsville, MD: DHHS, 1996.

12. Friis RH, Sellers TA. Epidemiology of infectious diseases. In: Friis RH, Sellers TA, eds. Epidemiology for Public Health Practice. Maryland: Aspen, 1999:333–375.

13. Grubeck-Loebenstein B. Changes in the aging immune system. Biologicals 1997; 25(2):205–208.

14. Castle SC. Clinical relevance of age-related immune dysfunction. Clin Infect Dis 2000; 31(2):578–585.

15. Yoshikawa TT. Epidemiology and unique aspects of aging and infectious diseases. Clin Infect Dis 2000; 30:931–933.

16. Yoshikawa TT. Perspective: aging and infectious diseases: past, present and future. J Infect Dis 1997; 176:1053–1057.

17. Hanson LC. Infections among the elderly. In: Thomas JC, Webew DJ, eds. Epidemiologic Methods for the Study of Infectious Diseases. New York: Oxford University Press, 2001:394–403.

18. Norman DC. Fever in the elderly. Clin Infect Dis 2000; 31(1):148–151.

19. Castle SC, Yeh M, Toledo S, Yoshikawa TT, Norman DC. Lowering the temperature criterion improves detection of infections in nursing home residents. Aging Immunol Infect Dis 1993; 4(2):67–76.

20. Norman DC, Yoshikawa TT. Fever in the elderly. Infect Dis North Am 1996; 10(1): 93–99.

21. Engelhardt HT. Principles of Bioethics. Oxford: Oxford University Press, 1986.

22. Beauchamp TL, Childress JF. Principles of Biomedical Ethics. 4th ed. New York: Oxford University Press, 1994.

23. Gee WM. Causes of death in a hospitalized geriatric population:autopsy study of 3000 patients. Virchows Arch Pathol Anat Histopathol 1993; 423:343–349.

24. Gordon M. Ethical challenges in end-of-life therapies in the elderly. Drugs Aging 2002; 19(5):321–329.

25. Miller DK. Withholding antibiotics as a form of care: an ethical perspective. In: Powers DC, Morley JE, Coe RM, eds. Aging, Immunity, and Infection. New York: Springer, 1994: 283–298.

26. Marcus EL, Clarfield AM, Moses AE. Ethical issues relating to the use of antimicrobial therapy in older adults. Clin Infect Dis 2001; 33(10):1697–1705.

27. Storey P, Knight CF. American Academy of Hospice and Palliative Medicine's Self Study Program: UNIPAC 6. Larchmont, New York: Mary Ann Liebert Publishing Inc, 2003.

SUGGESTED READING

Gavazzi G, Krause K. Ageing and infection. Lancet Infect Dis 2002; 2:659–666.

High KP. Nutritional strategies to boost immunity and prevent infection in elderly individuals. Clin Infect Dis 2001; 33:1892–1900.

Nicolle LE. Infection control in long-term care facilities. Clin Infect Dis 2000; 31:752–756.

Norman DC. Fever in the elderly. Clin Infect Dis 2000; 31(1):148–151.

Yoshikawa TT. Epidemiology and unique aspects of aging and infectious diseases. Clin Infect Dis 2000; 30:931–933.

2

Clinical Manifestations of Infections

Nancy Hanna and Thomas T. Yoshikawa
Department of Internal Medicine, Charles R. Drew University of Medicine and Science, Martin Luther King, Jr.–Charles R. Drew Medical Center, Los Angeles, California, U.S.A.

Key Points:

- Typical symptoms and signs of infection may be delayed in onset, atypical, or absent.
- Fever may be normal or low in the presence of serious infection.
- The finding of fever generally indicates the presence of an active, serious infection.
- Delirium, functional incapacity, falls, anorexia, or fatigue may be the initial manifestations of infection.
- A complete blood count, chest radiograph, urinalysis, arterial blood gas, and serum chemistry panel are recommended for all patients suspected of a serious infection.

1. INTRODUCTION

Infections are the fourth leading cause of death in the elderly, becoming increasingly common as immunity and general resistance wane with age. The clinical presentation of common infectious diseases in the very old patient differs markedly from presentation in a younger patient (1). Some of the factors that contribute to the increased severity of infections in the elderly include the anatomical and physiological changes that occur with aging, impaired immune response, presence of coexisting diseases, increased hospitalization that lead to nosocomial exposure to drug-resistant pathogens, and increased use of catheters.

Severe acute illness in older individuals often presents with vague, nonspecific, or trivial symptoms. Typical symptoms and signs of infection may be absent or delayed in older patients, which leads to delay in the diagnosis and initiation of therapy. A change in mental status or decline in function may be the only presenting problem in an older patient with infection. Moreover, both morbidity and mortality for many infections may be several-fold higher in the old compared with the young. Although prevention is the optimal method for reducing morbidity, mortality, the early recognition and initiation of appropriate supportive and antimicrobial therapy are also critical strategy for managing infections in older persons.

Table 1 Age-Related Immune System Changes

Granulocytes (PMN)	Neutrophilia with possibly some decrease in phagocytosis
Monocytes/macrophages/cytokines	Alterations in cytokine secretion
Natural killer cells	Increase in number with decreased response to cytokines
T and B lymphocytes	Involution of thymus; impaired T cell; decreased generation of B lymphocytes leads to decreased specific antibodies, and increased autoantibodies

2. IMMUNOSENESCENCE

Immunosenescence usually refers to the notion that there is an age-related dysfunction of the immune system which leads to enhanced risk of infection. There is no doubt that decreased immune function in the elderly does exist (See also chapter, "Impact of Age and Chronic Illness-related Immune Dysfunction on Risk of Infection"). Two examples, both with respect to antibody production and T-cell proliferative responses, are reactivation of tuberculosis in the elderly population (2) and the decreased effectiveness of influenza vaccination in the elderly (3). Total lymphocyte count remains unchanged with aging, but certain lymphocyte subpopulations are altered (Table 1), leading to reductions in cell-mediated immunity. Although it is convenient to ascribe these changes to the increased risk of infections in older persons, they have thus far only been proven to be important for the excess incidence in certain viral diseases, such as influenza or varicella zoster infection, and tuberculosis (4).

3. HISTORY

Evaluation of the elderly patient can be frustrating and difficult, as underlying illness may complicate the evaluation. A survey found that many emergency medicine physicians are uncomfortable evaluating elderly patients because it is more difficult to evaluate and manage this population (5). Obtaining a medical history from an elderly patient can require long and meticulous efforts because cognitive deficits may compromise the elderly patient's recall of recent and past medical problems. Physical deficits may also impede the history-taking process; often, elderly patients have difficulty hearing, which impairs communication and can lead to misunderstanding and misinformation.

Instead of a typical constellation of several specific symptoms of an infectious disease as seen in younger adults, infections in the elderly may have fewer and nonspecific symptoms. Typical nonspecific symptoms and signs that may represent infection in old age are summarized in Table 2. Besides fever, the most common general manifestations of infection in the elderly are falls, delirium, anorexia, or generalized weakness (6,7). It should be mentioned that similar clinical presentations are also commonly seen in geriatric patients with noninfectious diseases, which make infectious diseases all that more difficult to diagnose (7). The onset of such symptoms, either abruptly or over a matter of days, should alert the physician to the possibility of an underlying acute infection.

Table 2   Nonspecific Symptoms That May Represent Specific Illness

Confusion/delirium
Apathy
Falling
Incontinence
Self-neglect
Anorexia
Fatigue
Unexplained change in functional status

3.1. Cognitive Changes

The brain is a vulnerable organ, so that a change in mental status is one of the most common presenting symptoms of acute infection in older patients. Abnormalities of mental status may occur with severe infection without the presence of an infectious agent in the central nervous system. These include anxiety, confusion, delirium, stupor, convulsions, and coma, with the clinical features of encephalopathy. Delirium is one of the most common mental disorders encountered in elderly with acute medical illness; it may be the only finding, suggesting acute infection in older patients. Frank, delirium occurs in 50% of older adults with infections. In population studies, the conditions noted most commonly associated with delirium are fluid and electrolyte disturbances (dehydration) and infections.

3.2. Falls

Falls could be the initial and only presentation of acute infection. Falls usually occur when a threat (e.g., infection, fever, and/or dehydration) to the normal homeostatic mechanisms that maintain postural stability is superimposed upon underlying age-related declines. The elderly person is unable to compensate for the additional stress (acute infection) because of age-related changes in function. The regulation of systemic blood pressure is another important physiologic contributor to the successful maintenance of upright posture. Hypotension may lead to failure to perfuse the brain, thereby increasing the risk of a fall.

3.3. Urinary Incontinence

Transient or reversible urinary incontinence could be the sole presentation of an otherwise asymptomatic urinary tract infection and/or other acute infections. Delirium associated with infection could lead to impaired ability or willingness to go to the toilet and thus cause functional urinary or fecal incontinence.

3.4. Pain

The absence of pain in older adults with infectious diseases may be multifactorial including cognitive impairment, or other unknown factors. In a very large study ($n = 704$), pressure pain threshold was shown to increase by about 15% in older adults, although the effect was considerably stronger in females (8).

4. PHYSICAL EXAMINATION

The clinician must be aware that the physical examination findings may be mis-
leadingly benign in an elderly patient, despite the presence of a potentially lethal
infection. A complete physical examination is often difficult or impossible in the
confused or uncooperative ill elderly patient. Under these circumstances, clinicians
should instead perform a focused assessment, concentrating upon vital signs, the
state of hydration, skin condition, and the potential site of infection. False-positive
findings may occur as well as false-negative manifestation (e.g., nuchal rigidity may
not be due to meningitis).

4.1. Temperature

Fever is the cardinal manifestation of infection, but this important diagnostic sign may
be absent or blunted in a significant number of the elderly patients with infectious
diseases. Thermoregulatory responses may be inappropriate, leading to increased
incidence of hypothermia in the presence of an infection. Absence of fever in the face
of bacterial infection is not unusual in older patients, with up to 30% of elderly patients
with serious infection presenting with a blunted or absent fever response (9). For example, Finkelstein et al. (10) studied 187 adults with community-acquired pneumo-
coccemia and found that those 65 years of age or older had an average admission
temperature of 100.8°F; 29% were afebrile or hypothermic. In comparison, subjects
aged 20–49 years had an average admission temperature of 102.5°F; only 9% were
afebrile.

Persistent elevation of body temperature of at least 2°F over baseline values in
an elderly patient regardless of baseline body temperature should also raise the suspicion of an infectious process. In a retrospective study of 111 nursing home patients, it
has been suggested that much of the decreased fever response in this population was
because of a low basal temperature (11). In a prospective study by Castle et al. (12)
over a 6-month period, at least 1300 temperature measurements were recorded and
44 infectious processes were identified. Of the 1300 readings of temperature, the sensitivity and specificity of a temperature of 101°F or more as a predictor of infection
were 40% and 99.7%, respectively; for a temperature of 100°F or more, they were
70% and 98.3%; and for a temperature of 99°F or more, they were 83% and 89%,
respectively. These findings would suggest that elderly nursing home residents with
a temperature of more than 99°F or 100°F or a rise in body temperature of at least
2°F or more from baseline should be evaluated for the presence of infection.

Furthermore, the temperature measurements must be accurate; oral temperatures may be spuriously low in elderly patients, so rectal temperatures should be
taken whenever an infectious disease is suspected. Varney et al. (13) compared oral,
tympanic, and rectal temperature measurements in the elderly. They enrolled 95
elderly patients (>60 year old) in a cross-sectional study to determine if rectal
temperatures could identify fevers more often than oral or tympanic temperatures
when the chief compliant suggested an infection. Rectal thermometry identified a
fever in 14 of 95 (14.7%) patients who were afebrile by both oral and tympanic
measures. Five of 90 (5.6%) patients who were afebrile rectally were febrile by both
oral and tympanic thermometry. Thus, rectal thermometry more often identified
fevers missed by oral and tympanic thermometry in the elderly patients. When
fever is present, elderly patients are much more likely to have a serious bacterial
or fungal infection than younger patients. Of all febrile elderly patients presenting

to an emergency room, 89% prove to have an infectious disease (4). Clearly, fever in an elderly patient must be taken seriously, with rapid and appropriate evaluation. However, a lack of fever does not exclude infection in an elderly patient with vague complaints.

The pathogenesis of a lower febrile response to infection in older persons is not understood. Studies on the febrile response of older rodents to certain pyrogens, such as tumor necrosis factor, interleukin-6, and endotoxin, produced conflicting results (14). Some of these studies may be relevant to human disease, but specific biological confirmation is lacking. Fever is also an important host defense mechanism. Fever may enhance host defense and improve chance of survival; higher temperatures appear to directly inhibit pathogen growth.

Fever of unknown origin (FUO) is not frequent in the elderly but it has its specificities. A cause of FUO is almost invariably found in the elderly (95% of cases compared with only about two-thirds of the cases in younger adults) (15). Thus, FUO in the elderly warrants careful investigation and a high diagnostic yield.

4.2. Blood Pressure

Age leads to a reduction in total body water, which places older individuals at an increased risk of hypovolemia with acute infections. Also, a progressive decrease in basal and stimulated renin levels causing a reduction in aldosterone secretion may promote the development of volume depletion in the face of dehydrating stresses, e.g., high fever. Hypotension also arises from impairment of cardiovascular responses, decreased elasticity of blood vessels, and increased adverse events to medications.

4.3. Heart Rate

Age-related declines in baroreflex sensitivity to hypotensive stimuli are manifested as a failure to increase the heart rate to the usual stimuli (e.g., fever). In addition to physiologic changes that may affect the physical examination, medications may alter the response of elderly patients to physiologic stressors. Antihypertensive drugs in particular may alter the patient's ability to mount a tachycardia in response to hypovolemia or infection (e.g., β-blockers).

4.4. Respiratory Rate

Tachypnea with respiratory rate >20 per minute and tachycardia (>100 per minute) were seen in only two-thirds of elderly people with pneumonia (16) and may precede other clinical findings by 3–4 days. The typical triad of cough, fever, and dyspnea was present in only 56% of 48 elderly patients admitted for community-acquired pneumonia, and 10% of patients had none of these symptoms (17).

5. DIAGNOSTIC PROCEDURES

Investigative procedures may be less well tolerated by older people. Thus, the investigative pathway is more complex, with decision making dependent on clinical presentation, sensitivity and specificity of tests, risks and discomfort of the test, hazards of "blind" treatment or "watchful waiting," and the wishes of the patient. A given diagnostic procedure may not have sufficient yield in the elderly. A good example of this is transthoracic echocardiography; its sensitivity is 75% in the younger adult, but drops to 45% in the elderly due to interference from echogenic calcifications (18). Only when an additional transesophageal echocardiography is done will there be a good diagnostic sensitivity (90%) in the elderly (18). Many other diagnostic procedures may have similar low yield, but more studies are needed to address this question.

5.1. White Blood Cell Count

As seen with younger patients, the triad of leukocytosis, neutrophilia, and left shift strongly suggests the presence of a bacterial infection although these tests lack sensitivity (19). Infectious diseases commonly evoke leukocytosis, with an increased number of neutrophils and immature circulating neutrophils (bands). The neutrophils released result from the direct action of interleukin-1 on bone marrow neutrophil stores, although early changes in white blood cell count reflect demargination and release of less mature granulocytes from the marrow storage pool. While 60% of older adults with serious infections develop leukocytosis, its absence does not exclude an infectious process (20).

5.2. Radiology

Although they are often difficult to perform under optimum conditions, plain chest radiographs are important for confirming the clinical suspicion of pneumonia; assessing extension of the disease; detecting potential complications such as cavitations, parapneumonic effusion, or empyema; and documenting signs of preexisting pulmonary disorder. Initially, chest x-ray examination in elderly patients with pneumonia may be normal; many clinicians believe that the radiologic changes are delayed in old age and in part may be related to dehydration.

5.3. Urinalysis

Urinary tract infections (UTI) are the most common bacterial infections in the elderly population. However, a substantial proportion of the elderly have asymptomatic bacteriuria. This age-dependent increase in asymptomatic bacteruria is paralleled by an increase in symptomatic UTI. Factors contributing to bacterial colonization and infection of the urinary tract of the elderly include mechanical changes (reduction in bladder capacity, decreased urinary flow rate, incomplete emptying of bladder), uroepithetial changes that increase bacterial adherence, prostatic hypertrophy in men, and hormonal changes in women. Attempts to prevent progression from asymptomatic bacteriuria to symptomatic UTI have been disappointing and, accordingly, asymptomatic bacteriuria in the elderly should not be treated, even if accompanied by leukocytouria (21) (see also the chapter "Urinary Tract Infection").

5.4. Arterial Blood Gas

The American Thoracic Society guidelines recommend that arterial blood gas be obtained on admission in patients who are hospitalized with severe illness, not only for detection of hypoxemia (for which pulse oximetry is sufficient), but also for that of hypercapnia, which occurs at a much higher frequency in the very old because of lower pulmonary functional reserve and presence of chronic obstructive pulmonary disease (22,23).

5.5. Blood Chemistry

Hyponatremia and elevations of hepatic enzymes (alanine aminotransferase and aspartate aminotransferase) occur often and are nonspecific but are not reported as adverse prognostic factors for acute infectious diseases. However, low serum albumin and renal failure are associated with an increased mortality and poor functional outcome in the elderly (23).

5.6. Lumbar Puncture

Older patients with bacterial meningitis are more likely to present with delirium rather than the classic triad of fever, headache, and meningismus. Nevertheless, bacterial meningitis is a relatively uncommon disorder in the elderly and routine cerebrospinal fluid evaluation is usually not necessary in febrile or septic-appearing older patients with delirium as long as another primary infectious focus has been identified. This was illustrated in a retrospective study of elderly patients who were admitted to the hospital for evaluation of fever and mental status changes (24). Cerebrospinal fluid (CSF) cultures were negative for bacterial growth in 80 out of 81 patients. One case of bacterial meningitis was diagnosed in a 73-year-old alcoholic who was unresponsive in the emergency department. Most hospitalized older patients with fever and delirium have primary causes of the confusion outside the central nervous system and do not necessarily require a routine evaluation of their CSF.

5.7. Microbiology

Microbiology evaluation should include bacterial, fungal, viral, and mycobacterial cultures of blood and other accessible body fluids, as well as serological studies as indicated (e.g., legionellosis). The types of microorganism encountered during a specific type of infection may be different in the elderly in comparison with a younger adult with the same infection (1,25). There are also practical difficulties in achieving a microbiological diagnosis. It is more difficult to obtain appropriate clinical specimens in many older persons. Older patients with pneumonia and other respiratory infections often are unable to cough or cough sufficiently enough to produce sputum. Also, mental status changes may lead to difficulties in cooperation and collection of clinical specimens (26).

5.8. Procalcitonin

Procalcitonin (PCT), a propeptide of calcitonin, is normally produced in the C cells of the thyroid. In healthy individuals, PCT levels are very low (<0.1 ng/mL). In patients with sepsis, however, PCT levels increases dramatically, sometimes to more than several hundred nanograms per milliliter. During severe infections PCT is produced by extra thyroid tissue. The exact site of PCT production during sepsis is unknown; however, mononuclear leukocytes and the liver seem to be the major source of PCT (27). Furthermore, unlike C-reactive protein (CRP), PCT levels reflect the severity of illness, with PCT levels paralleling the severity of illness. It is a relatively specific marker of severe sepsis which has not been yet adequately assessed in the elderly population (28).

5.9. Serum C-Reactive Protein (CRP)

CRP is an acute-phase protein released by the liver after the onset of inflammation or tissue damage. It is a very sensitive marker of infection, but unfortunately lacks specificity, particularly in the elderly population. However, given the absence of a reliable febrile response, CRP measurements are extremely useful in the geriatric setting: a normal CRP concentration allows exclusion of a severe bacterial infection with a high probability; a rapid increase in CRP is highly suggestive of bacterial infection.

REFERENCES

1. Yoshikawa TT. Epidemiology and unique aspects of aging and infectious disease. Clin Infect Dis 2000; 30:291–293.
2. Rajagopalan S. Tuberculosis and aging: a global health problem. Clin Infect Dis 2001; 33:1034–1039.
3. Murasko DM, Bernstein ED, Gardner EM, Gross P, Munk G, Dran S, Abrutyn E. Humoral and cell-mediated immunity in protection from influenza disease after immunization of healthy elderly. Exp Gerontol 2002; 37:427–439.
4. Marco CA, Schoenfeld CN, Hansen KN, Hexter DA, Stearns DA, Kelen GD. Fever in geriatric emergency patients: clinical features associated with serious illness. Ann Emerg Med 1995; 26:18.
5. McNamara RM, Rousseau E, Sanders AB. Geriatric emergency medicine: a survey of practicing emergency physician. Ann Emerg Med 1992; 21:796–801.
6. Chassagne P, Perol MB, Doucet J, Trivalle C, Menard JF, Manchon ND, Maynot Y, Humbert G, Bourreille J, Bercoff E. Is presentation of bacteremia in the elderly the same as younger patients? Am J Med 1996; 100:65–70.
7. Norman DC, Toledo SD. Infections in the elderly persons. An altered clinical presentation. Clin Geriatr Med 1992; 8:713–719.
8. Jensen R, Rasmussen BK, Pedersen B, Lous I, Olesen J. Cephalic muscle tenderness and pressure pain threshold in general population. Pain 1992; 48:197–202.
9. Norman DC, Yoshikawa TT. Fever in the elderly. Infect Dis Clin North Am 1996; 10: 93–99.
10. Finkelstein M, Petkun W, Freedman M, Antopol SC. Pneumococcal bacteremia in adults: age-dependent differences in presentation and in outcome. J Am Geriatr Soc 1983; 31:19–27.
11. Castle SC, Yeh M, Norman DC, Miller D, Yoshikawa TT. Fever response in the elderly: are the older truly colder? J Am Geriatr Soc 1991; 39:853–857.
12. Castle SC, Yeh M, Toledo S. Lowering the temperature criterion improves detection of infections in nursing home residents. Aging Immunol Infect Dis 1993; 4:67–76.
13. Varney SM, Manthey DE, Culpepper VE, Creedon JF Jr. A comparison of oral, tympanic, and rectal temperature measurement in the elderly. J Emerg Med 2002; 22:153–157.
14. Bender BS, Scarpace P. Fever in the elderly. In: Mackowiak P, ed. Fever: Basic Mechanism and Management. Philadelphia, PA: Lippincott-Raven, 1997:363–373.
15. Knockaert DC, Vanneste LJ, Bobbaers HJ. Fever of unknown origin in the elderly patients. J Am Geriatr Soc 1993; 41:1187–1192.
16. Fein AM, Feinsilver SH, Niederman MS. Atypical manifestations of pneumonia in the elderly. Clin Chest Med 1991; 12:319–336.
17. Harper C, Newton P. Clinical aspects of pneumonia in the elderly veteran. J Am Geriatr Soc 1989; 37:867–872.
18. McCusker J, Cole M, Dendukuri N, Belzile E, Primeau F. Delirium in older medical inpatients and subsequent cognitive and functional status: a prospective study. Can Med Assoc J 2001; 165:575–583.

19. Lord JM, Butcher S, Killampali V, Lascelles D, Salmon M. Neutrophil ageing and immunesenescence. Mech Ageing Dev 2001; 122:1521–1535.
20. Yoshikawa TT, Norman DC. Fever in the elderly. Infect Med 1998; 15:704–706.
21. Nicolle LE. Urinary tract infection in geriatric and institutionalized patients. Curr Opin Urol 2002; 12:51–55.
22. Janssens JP, Pache JC, Nicod LP. Physiological changes in respiratory function associated with ageing. Eur Respir J 1999; 13:197–205.
23. Fernandez-Sabe N, Carratala J, Roson B, Dorca J, Verdaguer R, Manrosa F. Community-acquired pneumonia in very elderly patients. Causative organisms, clinical characteristics and outcomes. Medicine (Balt) 2003; 82:159–169.
24. Warshaw G, Tanzer F. The effectiveness of lumbar puncture in the evaluation of delirium and fever in the hospitalized elderly. Arch Fam Med 1993; 2:293–297.
25. Marrie TJ. Community-acquired pneumonia in the elderly. Clin Infect Dis 2000; 31:1066–1078.
26. Nicolle LE. Infection control in long-term care facilities. Clin Infect Dis 2000; 31:752–756.
27. Gramm HJ, Hannemann L. Activity markers for the inflammatory host response and early criteria of sepsis. Clin Intensive Care 1996; 7(suppl 1):1–3.
28. Reinhart K, Karzai W, Meisner M. Procalcitonin as a marker of the systemic inflammatory response to infection. Intensive Care Med 2000; 26:1193–1200.

SUGGESTED READING

Finkelstein M, Petkun W, Freedman M, Antopol SC. Pneumococcal bacteremia in adults: age-dependent differences in presentation and in outcome. J Am Geriatric Soc 1983; 31:19–27.
Norman DC, Toledo SD. Infections in the elderly persons. An altered clinical presentation. Clin Geriatr Med 1992; 8:713–719.
Norman DC, Yoshikawa TT. Fever in the elderly. Infect Dis Clin North Am 1996; 10:93–99.
Yoshikawa TT. Epidemiology and unique aspects of aging and infectious disease. Clin Infect Dis 2000; 30:291–293.

3

Impact of Age and Chronic Illness-Related Immune Dysfunction on Risk of Infections[*]

Steven C. Castle, Asif Rafi, Koichi Uyemura, and Takashi Makinodan
Veterans Affairs, Greater Los Angeles Healthcare System, UCLA School of Medicine, Los Angeles, California, U.S.A.

Key Points:

- The immune response consists of innate or natural immunity (neutrophils, macrophages, eosinophils, basophils, natural killer cells, dendritic cells), which is the first line of defense against many microorganisms, and acquired or adaptive immunity (T and B cells) which is a second line of defense when the innate immune system cannot recognize or eliminate an infectious organism.
- The interaction of age-related changes in immune response and chronic illness adversely impacts the host's risk and severity to infection such as influenza, pneumonia, tuberculosis, and herpes zoster.
- Age-related changes in immune function are complex and involve different sites in the cascade and multiple sites of cellular and biochemical interactions, and are often difficult to separate from the effects of chronic illness.
- Dietary deficiencies may contribute to immune dysregulation. Dietary supplements may have a role in improving immune responses in the elderly.
- Select medications have immunomodulating effects, as do certain hormones.

1. INTRODUCTION

The increased risk and severity of infections in the older adult population are well documented, and immunosenescence, the state of dysregulated immune function associated with aging, is felt to be a significant contributor to this increased risk. This is underscored by the high risk of nosocomial infections in older adults residing in

[*] Sources of financial support: U.S. Department of Veterans Affairs, Geriatric Research, Education and Clinical Center (GRECC) and Research Service, and National Institute of Aging RO3AG18497.

long-term care facilities (LTCF). Of note, in 1999, surveillance of LTCF-acquired infections by the National Nosocomial Infections Surveillance system reported a high incidence of 3.82 infections per 1000 resident-days of care, but with significant variability (1). Data vary widely depending on the type of facility, nature of the residents, definitions used for infections, and type of data analysis. If the goal is to prevent serious infections in older adults, the field of geriatric immunology/ infectious disease is faced with the tremendous challenge of studying a very diverse population of chronically ill older adults, in addition to the study of very healthy older persons. Grouping individuals by disease severity or by level of impairment of specific components of immunity may assist in advancing our ability to improve host defense in an at-risk population (2).

2. IMMUNOSENESCENCE

2.1. Studies of Aging Exclude the Impact of Disease

Immunosenescence is defined as the state of dysregulated immune function that contributes to the increased susceptibility of older adults to infection, and possibly to autoimmune disease and cancer (3). This review will focus on the relevance age-related immune dysregulation has toward susceptibility to infectious disease, though there also is a growing interest in the role dysregulated immunity plays in common age-related illness including atherosclerosis, Alzheimer's dementia, diabetes mellitus, and osteoporosis.

The immune system can be divided into innate and acquired components (Fig. 1), and recent advances in the field have focused attention on the interaction between these two components. Extensive studies in very healthy older adults have identified modest age-related changes in immunity, and furthermore, these studies have been essentially limited to phenotypic and functional changes in T cells of the acquired immune component.

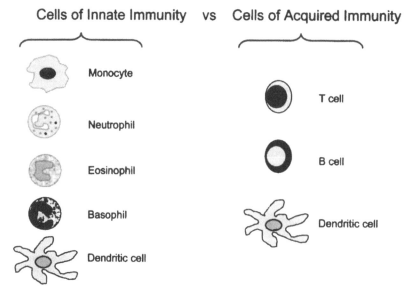

Figure 1   Key effector cells of the innate vs. acquired immune response. Note that dendritic cells play pivotal roles in both innate and acquired immunity.

In an attempt to standardize laboratory methods and isolate age-related changes from external changes of disease and medications, studies over the past 15 years have included only the very healthy older adults. This has been accomplished by the exclusion of subjects with evidence of disease or use of medications, by applying rigorous criteria as defined by the SENIEUR Protocol (4). This concept of distinguishing nature (genetic) vs. nurture (environment) has long been debated, and tends to distinguish the subtle differences in the fields of gerontology (the study of aging) and geriatrics (the care of the aged). The SENIEUR Protocol criteria exclude subjects with unhealthy lifestyle choices; the presence of infection, inflammation, malignancy, or other immune disorders; abnormal organ function; and anyone on medications for treatment of a defined disease. These stringent criteria exclude 90% of subjects aged 65 or older, even 25% of younger subjects, and virtually 100% of the population residing in LTCF (4). Although it would appear that the original intent of the SENIEUR protocol was to develop a reference population, it has been applied to exclude subjects with significant external/environmental exposure, limiting our understanding of mechanisms of vulnerability to infections in the at-risk population with underlying chronic diseases. Yet, despite extensive studies on possible mechanisms for age-related changes in T-cell phenotype and function in a very healthy population, no compelling scientific evidence has shown that these changes have direct relevance to the common infections seen in the aged population (3,5,6).

3. IMPACT OF CHRONIC ILLNESS ON INFECTIONS SEEN IN THE OLDER ADULT

Despite 90% complete involution of the T-cell-generating thymus by age 40, true opportunistic infections are not seen among older adult patients, even those with significant chronic disease. This suggests that there is likely compensation for lost immunological activity of the thymus gland. Infections that are a problem in this population of older adults are well known to the clinician: primarily, bacterial infections (i.e., pneumonia, urinary tract, and skin, and soft tissue infections), some viral infections (i.e., reactivation of herpes zoster, and significantly increased morbidity and mortality associated with influenza virus), and some infections that are related to colonization of severely ill individuals or associated with the use of antibiotics (*Clostridium difficile*, methicillin-resistant *Staphylococcus aureus*). In addition, changes in immunity create difficulty in detecting both active (primary and reactivation) and inactive tuberculosis. Response to vaccination, which requires intact cell-mediated immunity to drive the humoral response, is clearly diminished in many different older adult populations as well as in aged laboratory animals.

3.1. Impact of Age and Chronic Illness on Influenza

Age-related changes in immunity likely have the most clinical relevance toward an impaired response to influenza infection or immunization to influenza. An estimated 90% of the 10,000–40,000 deaths attributed to influenza infections annually in the United States occur in persons 65 years of age or older. The national health objective for the year 2000 was to achieve a >90% coverage rate for influenza vaccination of noninstitutionalized elders, and the 2000 Advisory Committee on Immunization Practices have broadened the recommendation for vaccination to adults 50–64 years of age. In 2002, via a random-digit telephone survey, 36.4% of respondents aged

50–64 years and 66.4% of respondents ≥65 years reported having received the influenza vaccine in the prior 12 months (7). The Centers for Disease Control and Prevention report on the prevention and control of influenza states that when the antigenic match between vaccine and circulating virus is close, infection is prevented in 70–90% of subjects less than 65 years of age, compared with only 30–40% in those 65 years of age or older (8). A past review of studies on antibody response to influenza found that 10 (33%) studies identified a decline in antibody response in an aged population, 16 (53%) studies reported no change, and 4 (13%) showed an increased response. This variability is related to both differences between populations and differences in defining a protective antibody response. For instance, a general medicine outpatient population (mean age 80 years) that (a) did not have any history of major medical illness, (b) did not take immunosuppressive medications, (c) did not smoke or report abuse of alcohol, and (d) reported no hospitalizations or any episode of pneumonia in the past year, was found to have comparable immune cell subsets, response to vaccines (i.e., tetanus, diphtheria, pneumococcal) and proliferative response to a wide range of mitogenic stimulation, in comparison with a young adult population (9). Interpreting the significance of these immune studies in relation to influenza infection is complicated, given the low attack rate and challenge in confirming actual influenza infection, as well as differences in defining an antibody response, since older individuals often have higher prevaccination antibody levels in comparison with younger individuals who have had less exposure to infection and prior vaccination. Even if antibody response was intact, it may not provide the same level of protection as in younger individuals. Thus, for example, in a study reported on 72 vaccinated older adults, who later were confirmed to have influenza infection, 60% had antibody titers ≥1:40, and 31% had titers ≥1:640 4 weeks postvaccination (10). Not only is vaccine response low in this population, even when vaccine response appears adequate, protection from infection is still lower than in younger adults. This is likely related to the quality of the antibody produced in neutralizing viral pathogenesis by older adults. Nevertheless, despite the low efficacy in prevention of infections, it needs to be emphasized that vaccination in people aged 65 years and older has been effective in reducing adverse events. In those 65 years of age or older, vaccination reduced the incidence of hospitalization due to pneumonia by 50–60%, and mortality was reduced by 80%. In a 3-year study on more than 75,000 community dwelling older adults, there was a 46% (range of 39–54%) reduction in all-cause mortality associated with individuals who received influenza vaccination (8). Though antibody response to vaccination (both magnitude and duration) is impaired in those aged 65 years and older, protective benefit to host defense could occur because cytotoxic T-lymphocyte killing efficiency against virally infected cells and the duration of activity were reported to be intact in older subjects in one study (11).

Underlying chronic illness dramatically increases the risk of influenza infection and impairs the response to vaccination. The presence of one or two chronic illnesses (such as emphysema, diabetes mellitus, or chronic renal insufficiency) is associated with a 40–150-fold increase in the incidence rate of influenza pneumonia (12). Whether chronic illnesses, medications, or other related external conditions further compromise immune competence has not been elucidated. One study on vaccine response in nursing home residents demonstrated that only 50% of residents had an adequate response (i.e., a fourfold increase in antibody titers). Furthermore, the response to vaccination did not correlate with nutritional status or dehydroepiandrosterone levels (13). Another study in a nursing home setting reported that only 36% of 137 vaccinated residents demonstrated a rise in antibody titer, and there was no correlation with age, body mass index, or functional status, as measured by the Barthel Index (14).

Conversely, exercise and psychosocial factors have been shown to modulate immune response to influenza vaccine. There was a graded response of peripheral blood mononuclear cells that correlated to the level of exercise. These data suggest that regular and vigorous exercise can improve immune response to influenza vaccine (15).

3.2. Impact of Age and Chronic Illness on Pneumonia

The risk and severity of pneumococcal pneumonia and tuberculosis increase with age. The incidence of pneumococcal infection is high in the first 2 years of life, then declines through adulthood, and finally increases dramatically in people aged 75 years and older. Rates of bacteremia and meningitis from the pneumococcal infection are higher in older adults and mortality rises with advanced age, approaching 80% in those aged 85 years and older. In fact, unlike all other age groups, mortality from pneumococcal pneumonia has actually increased in those over 75 years of age since the antibiotic era (1950 vs. 1985). Clearly, disease burden plays a crucial role in the risk and severity of infection. A 4-year study demonstrated that in adults 65 years or older, death due to pneumonia, influenza, and chronic lung disease was particularly high in nursing home residents (52.1 per 1000), and higher among senior housing residents (4.2 per 1000) than community residents (2.6 per 1000) (18).

Efficacy of the pneumococcal vaccine in preventing infection has been difficult to demonstrate in randomized control trials but has been reported to be 50–80% effective in case series studies. Five years after vaccination, the efficacy remains about 70% for those under 75 years of age, but only 53% in subjects 75–85 years of age, and only 22% in those over 85 years of age (19). Of note, one study found that antibody response to pneumococcal vaccination in preventing pneumonia recurrences, following hospitalization for community-acquired pneumonia in nonimmunocompromised adults (50–85 years of age), correlated inversely with the risk of recurrent pneumonia 32 months after vaccination. A lower risk was seen with a fourfold rise in antibody titers postvaccination (20). An outbreak of multidrug-resistant *Streptococcus pneumoniae* (serotype 23F) occurred in a nursing home in rural Oklahoma in 1996. Risk of infection was associated with the recent use of antibiotics (relative risk, 3.6; 95% CI, 1.2–10.8), and only 4% of residents had received pneumococcal vaccine (21).

The overall case rate for tuberculosis declined 26% in the United States between 1992 and 1997, with the highest number of cases reported in the 25–44-year-old age group, which could reflect the human immunodeficiency virus (HIV) epidemic. Prior to this epidemic, tuberculosis case rates had an upward inflection point at 75 years of age, due to both reactivation and primary cases of residents in institutional settings, while community cases may go undetected (12). The disease in older adults remains largely distinct from tuberculosis associated with HIV infection, and the majority of cases remain isoniazid sensitive. Differences in presentation include more subtle presentation (less pronounced cough, night sweats, or x-ray findings) and skin testing is difficult to interpret due to both a waning of delayed hypersensitivity (i.e., false negative for inactive and active disease) and a more pronounced booster effect (i.e., false positive for conversion).

Mouse studies on tuberculosis show an age-related increase in susceptibility, with minor shifts in the immune response. Briefly, it appears that in older animals there is a delayed recruitment of CD4+ T cells, with less interferon gamma production. Hence, the infection tends to disseminate more and eventual containment is reduced. Adoptive transfer studies show that transfer of young T cells into old animals could reverse much of these changes (22).

3.3. Changes in Immunity in Subjects with Herpes Zoster Infection

The incidence of herpes zoster dramatically increases in individuals aged 75 years and older (see also the chapter on "Herpes Zoster"). While younger individuals who develop active zoster infections have an increased association with immunosuppressive illness, outbreaks are not associated with occult malignancy in older adults. Factors that control or predict reactivation of latent infections are not known. Limited epidemiological studies have shown that blacks have less risk of developing zoster than whites, and measures of stress were not significantly associated with zoster infection. Risk factors associated with the development of postherpetic neuralgia, such as the degree of immunological recall to the virus, have not been studied (23). One study on vaccine response to both live-attenuated and heat-inactivated varicella vaccine showed no difference in antibody production or proliferation of peripheral blood mononuclear cells in response to varicella zoster virus in 167 older subjects (mean age, 66 years) (24). Careful studies of immune changes in subjects who have had an outbreak of acute zoster or postherpetic neuralgia have not been done, nor studies assessing the association of zoster infection with subsequent development of bacterial, tubercular, or influenza infection, or response to vaccination.

3.4. Risk Factors for Colonization with Resistant Bacteria

Colonization of resistant bacteria in residents of LTCF, including methicillin-resistant *S. aureus*, vancomycin-resistant enterococci, aminoglycoside-resistant enterococci, and multidrug-resistant Gram-negative bacilli vary significantly from facility to facility (see also the chapter on "Common Infections in a Nursing Home Setting"). Bacterial colonization may be more common in LTCF than acute care facilities, although infection from these organisms is less common. Epidemiological markers of risk of colonization and infection generally are any indication of end-stage illness and frailty, including prior acute hospitalization, extended stay in an LTCF, recurrent urinary bladder catheterization, urinary incontinence, pressure ulcers, insertion of gastrostomy tubes, and poor functional status. Despite these markers of frailty, studies have not been performed to correlate colonization of resistant bacteria with specific changes in immunity, poor vaccine response, or risk of influenza, or other bacterial infections. Hence, efforts toward prevention of colonization with resistant bacteria have included use of appropriate antibiotics and infection control measures of hand washing and isolation protocols, but efforts to enhance immunity in the frail have not been attempted (25).

4. AGE-RELATED CHANGES OF IMMUNE RESPONSE

Immune response consists of two interactive components, an innate and an acquired response. Innate immunity provides a first line of defense against many common microorganisms. It has a cellular component, made up of macrophages, eosinophils, basophils, natural killer (NK) cells, and dendritic cells (DC). These immune cells detect the presence of foreign protein by several receptors that bind to molecules secreted by or carried on the surface of the pathogen. DCs are the predominant antigen-presenting cells (APCs) involved in the initial innate inflammatory response. In response to the pathogen, DCs produce bursts of inflammatory proteins that not only kill the pathogen but also produce other proteins called cytokines that recruit and promote the further differentiation of other DCs. However, when the innate immune system cannot recognize or eliminate an infectious organism, the acquired immune system provides a resourceful second line of defense.

Acquired immunity utilizes lymphocytes (T and B cells) with specific cell-surface receptors generated by random recombination of gene segments. These recombinations and pairings of different variable chains produce a wide repertoire of lymphocytes with specific unique receptors that can recognize virtually any infectious organism or pathogen. Therefore, acquired immune system has the unique characteristic of specificity of response to a given antigen. Furthermore, another unique feature of acquired immunity is establishment of memory cells, which enables a rapid response upon subsequent rechallenge with the same antigen. The distinctive cells of innate and acquired immunity are shown in Figure 1. Since it is necessary to clonally expand antigen-specific lymphocytes to a novel pathogen, acquired immunity requires 4–7 days to generate appropriate numbers of cells to counter the infection as shown in Figure 2. Yet, cells of the innate immune system interact to play a pivotal role in the initiation and subsequent direction of acquired immune responses.

To initiate an acquired immune response, T cells must be activated by APC. The degree or quality of interaction of lymphocytes and APCs can influence the type and magnitude of immune response. If a foreign or infectious organism is encountered by APCs and presented to a particular T cell bearing the appropriate receptor, the T cells undergo clonal expansion and differentiate into effector cells that can

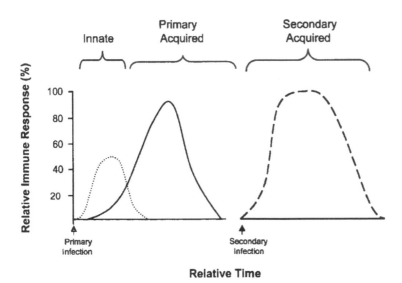

Figure 2 Kinetics of immune response: innate vs. acquired immunity. Innate immune responses occur immediately after the initial encounter with a pathogen. A more vigorous primary acquired immune response follows the innate response. Memory cells, generated by the primary acquired immune response, respond quickly and decisively following a second infection by the same pathogen.

eliminate the infectious organism. However, when APCs present self-antigens to lymphocytes bearing receptors that recognize such self-antigens, these lymphocytes are eliminated through a process called apoptosis (programmed cell death). Hence, it is at this key interface between innate and acquired immunity that regulation of turning on or off of an immune response occurs (3,5,12,26).

Cytokines have been classified as pro- or anti-inflammatory cytokines depending on their effects on immune function (3,12,26). Furthermore, these cytokines often act in networks or cascades to regulate their complex biological activities. Interaction between the different immune constituent cell types of host defense is carried out by the strength and balance of cytokine signals. The ability of effector cells to differentiate or respond to specific signals is likely affected by aging and chronic illness. In general, activation of acquired immunity that involves cell-mediated immune response, which is protective against most infectious agents, is described as a T helper 1 (Th1) response and is associated with production of high levels of the cytokines interleukin-2 (IL-2) and interferon-gamma (IFN-γ). In contrast, a T helper 2 (Th2) response, which is associated with allergic or parasitic infections but not associated with clearance of most bacterial or viral infections, is associated with production of high levels of IL-10, IL-4, and IL-5. The relative concentrations of proinflammatory cytokines, defined as those that upregulate a Th1 response, or anti-inflammatory cytokines that are important in turning off an inflammatory response, are influenced by gene activation of effector immune cells and allows further specificity of the eventual outcome of an inflammatory response.

A recent study has demonstrated that mature DCs are required for efficient activation of influenza-specific cytotoxic T cells (26). Consequently, the differentiation of regulatory APCs at the site of inflammation is important in determining the quality of the subsequent immune response. Hence, aging, and more likely chronic diseases, alter the cytokine mix at the site of inflammation, and adjuvants that may impact on cytokine production affecting DCs to differentiation should be considered in improving the suboptimal vaccine response seen in residents of LTCF (27).

5. SUMMARY OF AGE-RELATED CHANGES IN ACQUIRED IMMUNITY

The overall impact of age on host immunity is thought to occur primarily along two mechanisms. The first is replicative senescence that may limit T-cell clonal expansion (Hayflick phenomenon or loss of telomerase activity/telomere length, and may be more related to exposure to antigen than age). The second is developmental changes associated with involution of the thymus that precedes dysfunction of the T-cell component of adaptive immunity. Studies have shown a decrease in telomere length with age in T cells and B cells; however, it was demonstrated that there is no significant change in telomerase activity (28). While this study may not have included individuals with repeated exposure to antigen (characteristic of chronic illness), it suggests that age-specific changes are more due to developmental changes in T cells. Several recent reviews have summarized extensive studies on changes in T-cell function with aging (29). The age-related decline in T-cell function is preceded by involution of the thymus gland, with dramatic decline in thymic hormone levels. In addition, changes in bone marrow stem cells have also been described which are distinct from thymic changes. These changes are thought to result in a shift in the phenotype of circulating T cells, with a decrease in the number of naive T cells, and a relative accumulation of memory T cells. The memory cells that persist include T cells with impaired proliferative and effector capacity (16,30). At the same time, there appears to be a propensity toward a Th2 anti-inflammatory response, as evidenced by an increase in IL-10 production (3,12,31,32). Although a wide spectrum of findings have been reported, it has been found that the healthier the population, the lesser the impact on changes in T cell function (29).

Significant age-related alteration is more often identified if the assay system requires cell-to-cell interaction. For instance, little age difference is found when T cells are stimulated by fixed anti-CD3 antibody instead of systems that require T-cell stimulation by APC (3). Age-related changes in T-cell cytokines other than IL-2 and IL-10 have demonstrated a much more varied response, especially cytokines IFN-γ and IL-4, which may relate to species differences between human and mouse studies and the type of stimulation (4,30,33). Finally, despite the rather universal changes in T-cell response with age, the relevance is unclear. Though in vitro support of antibody response of T cells has been shown to be impaired with age (11), impaired proliferative response, even to specific antigen and even after adjusting for relative sensitivity to mitogen, failed to correlate with impaired antibody response to influenza immunization (11).

Changes in B cells are much less clear, but appear to have similarities to T-cell age-related changes. B cells from older individuals show impaired activation and proliferation that could also be related to changes in costimulatory molecule expression (12). Both primary and secondary antibody responses to vaccination have been found to be impaired. The specificity and efficacy of antibodies produced in older adults is lower than in younger populations (12,29). One longitudinal study of young and older adults demonstrated that the proliferative responses to influenza antigen upon yearly immunization were lower in older adults, as was the percentage of older adults with protective antibody titers (33).

Furthermore, chronic disease seems to have a significant effect on vaccine response. A study has shown that both aging and increasing serum creatinine reduce the response to hepatitis B vaccine in renal failure patients. The findings showed that 86% of patients with creatinine at or below 4 mg/dL had a protective antibody titer following hepatitis B immunization, in comparison with only 37% of individuals with a serum creatinine above 4 mg/dL. Likewise, age independently was inversely associated with antibody response. Hence, immunization of patients with chronic renal insufficiency before serum creatinine exceeds 4 mg/dL is essential (34).

6. INTERACTION BETWEEN INNATE AND ACQUIRED IMMUNITY

Studies to date have shown that (a) age-related changes in immunity have been largely limited to the T cells of acquired immunity, with intact APC function in healthy older adults and (b) infection rates are increased in chronically ill older adults. It is surmised that chronic illness can impair both innate and acquired immunity. Innate immunity is critical to both the number of immunocompetent units and the magnitude of the immunological burst upon activation, and could very well be the target of chronic illness in reducing immune competence beyond normal age-related changes (2). Evidence for the most part has suggested that innate immunity remains intact or is upregulated with aging. The frequently reported nonspecific increase of proinflammatory substances produced by the innate immune system and downregulation of acquired immunity may reflect a compensatory event by either component, but their causality is unclear (2,12,22).

It has been reported that larger numbers of DCs could be generated in vitro from circulating monocytes of very healthy older adults, in comparison with younger adults, and the DCs generated in vitro from healthy older adults were effective in restoring the proliferative capacity of T cells and in preventing the development of apoptosis in T cells grown to senescence (no longer able to proliferate) in culture (32,33). Likewise, the antigen presentation capacity of circulating APCs (including DCs) is higher in number in healthy older adults in comparison with younger adult controls, and is associated with higher IL-12 and IL-10 levels (31). Preliminary studies in a nursing home population with chronic illness suggest a reversal in APC function, with impaired antigen presentation, impaired DC differentiation, and no increased levels of the proinflammatory cytokine IL-12 (31, unpublished data). Hence, DCs could reflect a physiologic measure of vulnerability due to loss of immune competence, resulting from a threshold of severity or extent of disease burden, especially since the differentiation of DC has been identified as a key variable in the stimulation of effector T cell function. DC are an important target for immunotherapeutic adjuvants to improve antigen delivery to boost immunity in general, and, therefore, it is likely that more focus should be placed on their role as targets for improving vaccination of vulnerable older adults. Hence, a model of how aging and chronic illness impacts specific components of innate and acquired immunity and ultimately the response to infectious exposure is summarized in Figure 3.

The regulation and interaction of cytokines produced by cells of innate immunity are very complex. The relative timing and quantities of the cytokines of innate immunity are crucial to the priming of the acquired immune response.

Studies suggest that there is a nonspecific increase in production of proinflammatory proteins in the aged population (22). Low-level, nonspecific autoimmunity throughout different tissues as well as a nonimmune responsiveness to infectious pathogens are hallmarks of aging. Studies on age-related changes in proinflammatory cytokines have had varied findings, most likely related to the very complex nature of response to cytokine networks. However, most have shown an increase in production of IL-6, IL-8, and tumor necrosis factor-alpha (TNF-α), and a decrease in IL-1 (3,12). Of note, experiments that involve cell-to-cell communication to stimulate cytokine production tend to show much greater effects of aging. A recent review describes 14 studies that report increases in IL-6 with aging (35). IL-6 itself has been shown to be inhibitory to mycobacteriostatic activities in macrophages (36).

Chronic illness likely contributes to further dysregulation of control of immune response. A study comparing IL-2 and IL-6 levels in young adults, healthy older adults, and "almost-healthy" older adults (individuals who did not meet the SENIEUR protocol because of no history of regular exercise, or the use of medications for conditions such as hypertension or osteoarthritis) reported lower levels of IL-2 and higher levels of IL-6 in the "almost-healthy" older adult population (6).

Several papers reported an association of aging and many chronic diseases with elevated serum IL-6 levels, or other so-called "markers" of inflammation, such as TNF-α. Higher circulating levels of IL-6 are associated with and predictive of functional disability, as well as increased mortality in older adults who did not have functional impairment at entry into these longitudinal studies. Associations have also been\found between physical activity and lower levels of serum IL-6 (37). Higher serum IL-6 levels have been reported in many chronic diseases, with slight (27–72% increase in relative risk) but significant increase in coronary heart disease, stroke,

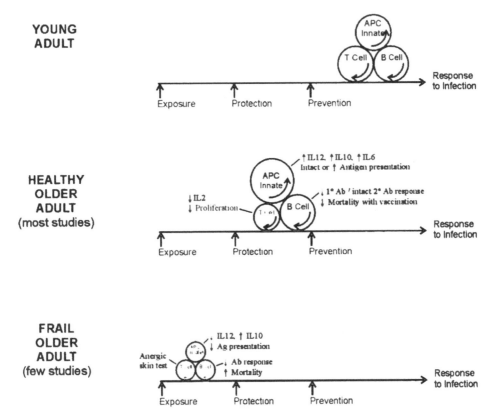

Figure 3 Diagram of response to infection as affected by aging and chronic disease. This model shows the response to infection as the distance driven by the immune "car" with the vigor of the three main immune components represented by size, with the response of younger adults as the standard. In healthy older adults, the immune response drives far enough to provide protection but may not provide prevention of infection, due to a decline in T cell function (accumulation of memory T cells in place of more plastic naive T cells, with a decline in IL-2 and impaired proliferative response to stimulation). B cell function is altered but remains effective with impaired primary antibody (Ab) response but an intact secondary Ab, with a decline in mortality with vaccination. This maintenance of immune competence may be due to enhanced APC function (increased IL-12 and IL-6 despite increased anti-inflammatory IL-10, with enhanced antigen presentation). In frail older adults, the immune "car" does not even provide protection from infection as there is a decline in both innate (increased IL-10, decreased IL-12 and antigen presentation) and acquired immunity (T cell and skin test anergy, impaired antibody response), resulting in loss of immune competence (increased risk and severity of infection, loss of protection from immunization).

and congestive heart failure in subjects 70–79 years of age without evidence of cardiovascular disease at baseline (38). Of note, these inflammatory markers (IL-6, TNF-α, C-reactive protein), especially serum IL-6, demonstrated an equal or higher relative risk than traditional risk factors as predictors of cardiovascular disease. Given this strong epidemiologic data, IL-6 appears to be associated with many chronic diseases, including Alzheimer's disease and emphysema. However, it remains unclear exactly what increased serum IL-6 levels represent. It has been found that high plasma levels of TNF-α and IL-6 in healthy older adults and in patients with type 2 diabetes mellitus are in particular associated with increased truncal fat mass, and that the TNF-α could contribute to sarcopenia, or the loss of muscle mass with age (39). Hence, it is likely that there will be increasing focus on IL-6 and its role as an inflammatory marker. However, the association with disease is more likely from a hormonal effect of IL-6, mediated by catabolic changes in somatic muscle, rather than on immunological basis (40,41). Very few studies have been done comparing how circulating levels of IL-6 or other markers of inflammation correlate with traditional measures of cell-mediated immunity. In one study, only one out of 32 Alzheimer's disease patients demonstrated a decline in production of IL-6 and TNF-α associated with severe dementia, in comparison to IL-6 and TNF-α levels from mild to moderately demented patients (42).

Other confounding medical conditions that may alter immunity include stress and depression, and primary diseases such as heart failure, kidney disease, or liver disease. These conditions make it difficult to identify causation of impaired host defense. Research involving chronically ill individuals is extremely challenging due to the difficulty in studying patients on numerous medications with multiple medical problems. It is difficult to control for specific medications or illnesses, and then deduce that decreased immunity is due to a certain illness or medication. Hence, there is an interaction of aging, chronic illness, and impaired immunity that leads to adverse health effects and subsequent manifestations of chronic disease including sarcopenia, impaired mobility, and malnutrition (Fig. 4), all of which further contribute to adverse health outcomes and further decline in immunity and progression of chronic illness.

7. IMMUNE POTENTIATING EFFECTS OF DIETARY SUPPLEMENTS AND MEDICATIONS

7.1. Modification of Immunity with Nutritional Treatments in the Elderly with Nutritional Deficiencies

See Chapter 5: Assessment of Nutritional Status and Interventions to Reduce Infection Risk in the Elderly.

7.2. Common Medications That Have Significant Immunopotentiation

In addition to immunosuppressive medications such as corticosteroids, nonsteroidal anti-inflammatory agents (including cyclo-oxygenase type 2 inhibitors), and antineoplastic agents, recent research has shown that several common medications have significant effects toward immune potentiation. β-adrenergic receptor antagonists (β-blockers) have been shown to block the immunosuppressive effects of acute stress (43). In a study of patients with dilated cardiomyopathy, those patients receiving β-blockers were found to have a decreased rate of anergy (from 70% down to 20%), and increased percentage of T cells and NK cells, and increased stimulation of IL-2 receptors by conconavalin A. Histamine, a potent mediator of inflammation, has also been found to modulate the immune response. In addition, histamine is associated with promoting allergic reactions, gastric acid secretion, and tumorigenesis (44,45). Histamine modulates the immune response by binding to dendritic cells and promoting a Th2 immune response. DCs are potent APCs and they have histamine type 2 (H_2) receptors on their cell surface. Histamine antagonists, especially type 2, have been shown to enhance the cell-mediated and humoral immune response. Studies have shown that the administration of H2 blockers in rats has improved delayed-type hypersensitivity (DTH) responses and increased antibody titers (44,46). Histamine antagonists have also

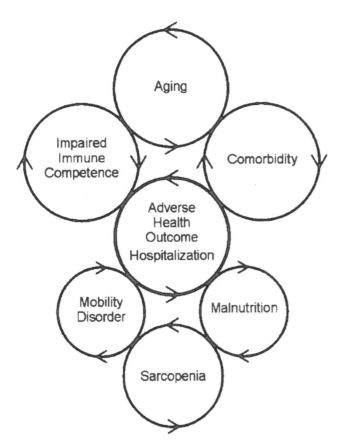

Figure 4 Interdependence of aging, chronic illness, immune dysfunction, and its health consequences. This model shows the interaction of aging, comorbidity, immune dysfunction, and subsequent adverse health outcomes as connected wheels that can accelerate decline to frailty. Aging changes on immunity are primarily altered T-cell function, while increasing comorbidity (certain specific diseases or accumulation of a threshold of multiple diseases) results in more widespread immune dysregulation. This results in both an increased risk and severity of infections and adverse health outcomes including hospitalization, with increasing comorbidity. Decline in muscle mass (sarcopenia), development of malnutrition and subsequent decline in mobility and function are commonly described outcomes of older adults with multiple chronic illnesses following hospitalization. Interventions to improve treatment of chronic illness (disease management), immunomodulation, nutritional supplementation, and improved mobility/function from therapy could be considered as "brakes" to the spinning wheels that could be critical to slowing down the rate of decline commonly seen in older adults with significant underlying chronic illness as they become frail from the interaction of these factors.

been shown to boost the proliferative response of T cells to IL-2, improve healing to herpes zoster infection, and boost DTH reactions in humans (44,47). Other studies have shown increased survival of patients with gastric and colorectal cancer when taking H2 blockers.

Cyclo-oxygenase inhibitors have also been shown to modulate the immune response. Prostaglandins, especially PGE2, have been demonstrated to suppress cell-mediated immunity (Th1 immune response) and enhance humoral immunity

(Th2 immune response). In addition, prostaglandins indirectly downregulates DC function through increased production of IL-10, the major cytokine of the Th2 response (48–51). The critical step in the production of prostaglandins is the oxygenation of arachidonic acid by cyclo-oxygenase enzyme. Therefore, cyclo-oxygenase inhibitors have been studied for their immunomodulating effects, and recent data have indicated that these inhibitors reverse the immunosuppressive effects of prostaglandins at a molecular level (52). Further research is necessary to determine if these effects can be translated into clinical measures of immunity.

Hormonal agents that appear to have an impact on immunity include sex hormones, growth hormone, and megestrol acetate (53–55). Estrogens have been found to have complex effects on immunity. This is evident as women tend to have more autoimmune disorders and diminished skin test responses (54). Growth hormone (GH) is another hormone that is used extensively in older adults, despite the fact that the clinical utility of GH has yet to be determined. GH levels diminish with age, and supplementation has been shown to have numerous beneficial effects on the immune system including a reversal of the involution of the thymus seen in older adults. In addition, GH enhances the activation of the immune system including a 50% increase in T-cell proliferative response and increased IL-2 receptor quantity on T cells (55). While these results are promising, much more research needs to be conducted to delineate the efficacy of GH supplementation in the healthy elderly.

8. CONCLUSION

Reduced immune functions contribute to increased risk of infections in older adults. Recent findings show that reduced immune functions in older adults caused by changes intrinsic to immune cells (i.e., primarily genetic changes) are nominal, compared to changes extrinsic to immune cells (i.e., environmental changes) (17). The significance of these findings is that successful intervention is more likely with environmental than genetic changes. This is supported by the relative ease in enhancing immune response of older adults through nutritional intervention, in contrast to intervention with stem cells.

The challenge we are now faced with is threefold: (a) to identify a simple clinical predictor of immunosenescence, (b) to identify immune cell(s) that are most vulnerable to environmental changes, and (c) to develop intervention models with high specificity in managing older adults with significant comorbidities. As to identifying a clinical predictor of immunosensescence, cytokine IL-6 and IL-10 are likely candidates based on recent epidemiological and experimental studies. With regard to identifying immune cells that are highly sensitive to changes in the environment, dendritic cells, which play a pivotal role in both innate and adaptive immune responses, are likely candidates. Finally, to develop intervention models with high specificity, much work will be needed, for there has been no systematic study on the immunologic consequence of modulating individual comorbidity. It would appear, therefore, that future studies on the impact of age and chronic illness-related immune dysfunction on risk of infections will require, unlike past studies, a team approach involving geriatricians/gerontologists, immunologists, infectious disease specialists, and epidemiologists.

ACKNOWLEDGMENTS

The U.S. Department of Veterans Affairs, through the Geriatric Research, Education and Clinical Center program, provides ongoing research support.

REFERENCES

1. Stevenson KB. Regional data set of infection rates for long-term care facilities: description of a valuable benchmarking tool. Am J Infect Control 1999; 27:20–26.
2. Castle SC, Uyemura K, Makinodan T. The SENIEUR Protocol after 16 years: a need for a paradigm shift? Mech Ageing Dev 2001; 122:127–140.
3. Pawelec G. Immunosenescence: impact in the young as well as the old? Mech Ageing Dev 1999; 108:1–7.
4. Ligthart GJ, Corberand JX, Fournier C, Galanaud P, Hijmans W, Kennes B. Admission criteria for immunogerontological studies in man: The SENIEUR Protocol. Mech Ageing Dev 1984; 28:47–55.
5. Wick G, Grubeck-Loebenstein B. The aging immune system: primary and secondary alterations of immune reactivity in the elderly. Exp Gerontol 1997; 32:401–413.
6. Mysliwska J, Bryl E, Foerster J, Mysliwski A. The upregulation of TNFα production is not a generalized phenomenon in the elderly between their sixth and seventh decades of life. Mech Ageing Dev 1999; 107:1–14.
7. Centers for Disease Control and Prevention. Influenza vaccination coverage among adults aged >50 years and pneumococcal vaccination coverage among adults aged >65 years United States, 2002. MMWR 2003; 52:987–992.
8. Centers for Disease Control and Prevention. Prevention and control of influenza: recommendations of the Advisory Committee on Immunization Practices (ACIP). MMWR 1999; 48:1–23.
9. Carson P, Nichol K, O'Brien J, Hilo P, Janoff E. Immune function and vaccine responses in healthy advanced elderly patients. Arch Intern Med 2000; 160:2017–2024.
10. Gravenstein S, Drinka PJ, Duthie EH, Miller BA, Brown CS, Hensley M, Circo R, Langer E, Ershler WB. Efficacy of an influenza hemagglutinin-diphtheria toxoid conjugate vaccine in elderly nursing home subjects during an influenza outbreak. J Am Geriatr Soc 1994; 42:245–251.
11. Bernstein E, Kaye D, Abrutyn E, Gross P, Dorfman M, Murasko DM. Immune response to influenza vaccination in a large elderly population. Vaccine 1999; 17:82–94.
12. Burns EA, Goodwin JS. Immunodeficiency of aging. Drugs Aging 1997; 11:374–397.
13. Fulop T, Wagner JR, Khalil A, Weber J, Trottier L, Payette H. Relationship between response to influenza vaccination and the nutritional status in institutionalized elderly subjects. J Gerontol A Biol Sci Med Sci 1999; 54A:M59–M64.
14. Potter JM, O'Donnel B, Carman WF, Roberts MA, Scott DJ. Serological response to influenza vaccination and nutritional and functional status of patients in geriatric medical long term care. Age Ageing 1999; 28:141–145.
15. Kout ML, Cooper MM, Knickolaus MS, Russell DR, Cunnick JE. Exercise and psychosocial factors modulate immunity to influenza vaccine in elderly individuals. J Gerontol A Biol Sci Med Sci 2002; 57A:M557–M562.
16. Menec V, MacWilliam L, Aoki FY. Hospitalizations and deaths due to respiratory illnesses during influenza seasons: a comparison of community residents, senior housing residents, and nursing home residents. J Gerontol A Biol Sci Med Sci 2002; 57A: M629–M635.
17. Hedlund JU, Kalin ME, Ortqvist A, Henrichsen J. Antibody response to pneumococcal vaccine in middle-aged and elderly patients recently treated for pneumonia. Arch Intern Med 1994; 154:1961–1965.

18. Hedlund J, Ortqvist A, Kndradsen HB, Kalin M. Recurrence of pneumonia in relation to antibody response after pneumococcal vaccination in middle-aged and elderly adults. Scand J Infect Dis 2000; 32:281–286.

19. Nuorti JP, Butler JC, Crutcher JM, Guevara R, Welch D, Holder P, Elliott JA. An outbreak of multidrug-resistant pneumococcal pneumonia and bacteremia among unvaccinated nursing home residents. N Engl J Med 1998; 338:1861–1868.

20. Orme I. Mechanisms underlying the increased susceptibility of aged mice to tuberculosis. Nutr Rev 1995; 53(S4):S35–S40.

21. Schmader K. Postherpetic neuralgia in immunocompotent elderly people. Vaccine 1998; 16:1768–1770.

22. Levine MJ, Ellison MC, Zerbe GO, Barber D, Chan C, Stinson D, Jones M, Hayward AR. Comparison of a live attenuated and an inactivated varicella vaccine to boost the varicella-specific immune response in seropositive people over 55 years of age and older. Vaccine 2000; 18:2915–2920.

23. Kaufman CA, Hedderwick SA, Bradley SF. Antibiotic resistance: issues in long-term care. Infect Med 1999; 16:122–128.

24. Banchereau J, Steinman RM. Dendritic cells and the control of immunity. Nature 1998; 392:245–252.

25. Ohwada A, Sekiya M, Hanaki H, Kuwahara A, Nagaoka I, Hori S, Tominaga S, Hiramatsu K, Fukuchi Y. DNA vaccination by *mecA* sequence evokes an antibacterial immune response against methicillin-resistant *Staphylococcus aureus*. J Antimicrob Chemother 1999; 44:767–774.

26. Son NH, Murray S, Yanovski J, Hodes RJ, Weng N. Lineage-specific telomere shortening and unaltered capacity for telomerase expression in human T and B lymphocytes with age. J Immunol 2000; 165:1191–1196.

27. Hodes RJ, Fauci AS, eds. Report of Task Force on Immunology and Aging. National Institutes of Aging and Allergy and Infectious Disease. U.S. Department of Health and Human Services, March 1996.

28. Miller RA. Cellular and biochemical changes in the aging mouse immune system. Nutr Rev 1995; 53:S8–S17.

29. Castle S, Uyemura K, Crawford W, Wong W, Klaustermeyer WB, Makinodan T. Age-related impaired proliferation of peripheral blood mononuclear cells is associated with an increase in both IL-10 and IL-12. Exp Gerontol 1999; 34:243–252.

30. Steger MM, Maczek C, Grubeck-Loebenstein B. Peripheral blood dendritic cells reinduce proliferation in in vitro aged T cell populations. Mech Ageing Dev 1997; 93:125–130.

31. Murasko DM, Bernstein ED, Gardner EM, Gross P, Munk G, Dran S, Abrutyn E. Role of humoral and cell-mediated immunity in protection from influenza disease after immunization of healthy elderly. Exp Gerontol 2002; 37:427–439.

32. Fraser GM, Ochana N, Fenyves D, Neumann L, Chazan R, Niv Y, Chaimovitch S. Increasing serum creatinine and age reduce the response to hepatitis B vaccine in renal failure patients. J Hepatol 1994; 21:450–454.

33. Ershler WB, Keller ET. Age-associated increased interleukin-6 gene expression, late-life diseases, frailty. Annu Rev Med 2000; 51:245–270.

34. Bermudez LE, Wu M, Petrofsky M, Young LS. Interleukin-6 antagonizes tumor necrosis factor-mediated mycobacteriostatic and mycobactericidal activities in macrophages. Infect Immun 1992; 60:4245–4252.

35. Reuben DB, Judd-Hamilton L, Harris TB, Seeman TE. The associations between physical activity and inflammatory markers in high-functioning older persons: MacArthur studies of successful aging. J Am Geriatr Soc 2003; 51:1125–1130.

36. Cesari M, Penninx B, Newman AB, Kritchevsky SB, Nicklas BJ, Sutton-Tyrell K, Rubin SM, Ding J, Simonsick EM, Harris TB, Pahor M. Inflammatory markers and onset of cardiovascular events: results from Health ABC study. Circulation 2003; 108:2317–2322.

37. Pedersen M, Bruunsgaard H, Weis N, Hendel HW, Andreassen BU, Eldrup E, Dela F, Pedersen BK. Circulating levels of TNF-alpha and IL-6-relation to truncal fat mass and

muscle mass in healthy elderly individual and in patients with type-2 diabetes. Mech Age Dev 2003; 124:495–502.

38. Roubenoff R. Catabolism of aging: is it an inflammatory process? Curr Opin Clin Nutr Metab Care 2003; 6:295–299.

39. Cappola AR, Xue QL, Ferrrucci L, Guralnik JM, Volpato S, Fried LP. Insulin-like growth factor I and interleukin-6 contribute synergistically to disability and mortality in older women. J Clin Endocrinol Metab 2003; 88:2019–2025.

40. Sala G, Galimberti G, Canevari C, Raggi ME, Isella V, Facheris M, Appollonio I, Ferrarese C. Peripheral cytokine release in Alzheimer patients: correlations with disease severity. Neurobiol Aging 2003; 24:909–914.

41. Bachen EA, Manuck SB, Cohen S, Muldoon MF, Raible R, Herbert TB, Rabin BS. Adrenergic blockade ameliorates cellular immune responses to mental stress in humans. Psychosom Med 1995; 57:366–372.

42. Rafi AW, Castle SC, Uyemura K, Makinodan T. Immune dysfunction in the elderly and its reversal by antihistamines. Biomed Pharmacother 2003; 57:246–250.

43. Elenkov IJ, Webster E, Papanicolaou DA, Fleisher TA, Chrousos GP, Wilder RL. Histamine potently suppresses human IL-12 and stimulates IL-10 production via H2 receptors. J Immunol 1998; 161:2586–2593.

44. Moharana AK, Bhattacharya SK, Mediratta PK, Sharma KK. Possible role of histamine receptors in the central regulation of immune responses. Indian J Physiol Pharmacol 2000; 44(2):153–160.

45. Komlos L, Notmann J, Arieli J, Hart J, Levinsky H, Halbrecht I, Sendovsky U. In vitro cell-mediated reaction in herpes zoster patients treated with cimetidine. Asian Pac J Allergy Immunol 1994; 12:51–58.

46. Harizi H, Juzan M, Pitard V, Moreau JF, Gualde N. Cyclooxygenase-2-issued prostaglandin E2 enhances the production of endogenous IL-10, which down regulates dendritic cell functions. J Immunol 2002; 168:2255–2263.

47. Phipps RP, Stein SH, Roper RL. A new view of prostaglandin E regulation of the immune response. Immunol Today 1991; 2:349–352.

48. Roper RL, Phipps RP. Prostaglandin E3 regulation of the immune response. Adv Prostaglandin Thromboxane Leukotrience Res 1994; 22:101–111.

49. Snijdewint FG, Kalinski MP, Wierenga EA, Bos JD, Kapsenberg ML. Prostaglandin E2 differentially modulates cytokine secretion profiles of human Th lymphocytes. J Immunol 1993; 150:S321.

50. Iniguez MA, Punzon C, Fresno M. Induction of cyclooxygenase-2 on activated T lymphocytes: regulation of T cell activation by cyclooxygenase-2 inhibitors. J Immunol 1999; 163:111–119.

51. Mantonvani F, Maccio A, Lai P, Massa E, Ghiani M, Santona MC. Cytokine involvement in cancer anorexia/cachexia: role of megestrol acetate and medroxy-progesterone acetate on cytokine down regulation and improvement in clinical symptoms. Crit Rev Oncogenes 1998; 9:99–106.

52. Rook GAW, Hernandez-Pando R, Lightman SL. Hormones, peripherally activated prohormones, and regulation of the Th1/Th2 balance. Immunol Today 1994; 15:301–303.

53. Khorram O, Yeung M, Vu L, Yen SSC. Effects of growth hormone-releasing hormone (GHRH) (1-29)-NH2 administration on the immune system of aging men and women. J Clin Endocrinol Metab 1997; 82:3590–3596.

SUGGESTED READING

Castle SC, Uyemura K, Makinodan T. The SENIEUR Protocol after 16 years: a need for a paradigm shift? Mech Ageing Dev 2001; 122:127–140.

Hodes RJ, Fauci AS, eds. Report of Task Force on Immunology and Aging.

National Institutes of Aging and Allergy and Infectious Disease. U.S. Department of Health and Human Services, March 1996.

Murasko DM, Bernstein ED, Gardner EM, Gross P, Munk G, Dran S, Abrutyn E. Role of humoral and cell-mediated immunity in protection from influenza diseases after immunization of healthy elderly. Exp Gerontol 2002; 37:427–439.

Rafi AW, Castle SC, Uyemura K, Makinodan T. Immune dysfunction in the elderly and its reversal by antihistamines. Biomed Pharmacother 2003; 57:246–250.

Roubenoff R. Catabolism of aging: is it an inflammatory process? Curr Opin Clin Nutr Metab Care 2003; 6:295–299.

4

Functional Assessment

Ronan Factora and Robert M. Palmer
Section of Geriatric Medicine, Department of General Internal Medicine, Cleveland Clinic Foundation, Cleveland, Ohio, U.S.A.

Key Points:

- Functional status affects both patient response to treatment of infection and clinical outcomes.
- Functional assessment involves evaluation of physical status, cognitive function, and social support resources available for the patient. Nurses, social workers, physical and occupational therapists, and other health professionals often assist physicians in this evaluation.
- Lower-extremity weakness and deconditioning are the common causes of impaired gait and mobility that can compromise an elderly patient's performance of activities of daily living, but are amenable to targeted interventions.
- Differentiation between acute delirium, depression, and dementia can be made based on history obtained from the patient and the caregiver, and is prompted by the utilization of valid and reliable tools that can direct appropriate therapies.
- Functionally impaired patients require extra resources to meet their families' care-giving needs; social workers and local health care agencies can provide invaluable community services.

1. INTRODUCTION

1.1. Homeostatic Reserve and Medical Illness

The process of aging depletes an individual's homeostatic reserve, the capacity of organ systems to adapt to physiologic stressors. Redundancy in physiological systems, abundant in youth, declines steadily over time. Consequently, the impact of a single acute illness or event affects the aging individual to a greater degree by both its effect on multiple organ systems and its duration. The loss of homeostatic reserve also diminishes the older individual's ability to recover from such an acute illness.

Acute illnesses, such as infection of the lungs or kidneys, can adversely affect the functional status of elderly patients, especially in those patients with multiple comorbid conditions and high severity of illness. A decline in physical functioning, or self-care capacity, predisposes the patient to further decline and complications

37

resulting from the illness itself or from its intended therapy. Even common symptoms of infectious diseases can affect daily activities. For example, fever, anorexia, malaise, diarrhea, and headache impair the ability to feed one's self, ambulate, perform daily chores, and drive; the resulting dehydration, malnutrition, immobilization, and social isolation reduce the patient's quality of life. The cascade of decline predisposes the patient to falls, delirium, incontinence, iatrogenic illness, and loss of independent living. However, this cascade can potentially be interrupted, and adverse effects of infections or their treatments can be avoided. An assessment of the older patient linked to therapies targeted to those at risk of functional decline can help to maintain or restore the patient's ability to function independently, thereby improving the clinical outcomes of a treated infection.

1.2. Demographics of Aging

The population of the elderly in the United States continues its steady growth. Currently, there are an estimated 35 million people aged 65 years or older. By the year 2020, and with the aging of the "baby boomers," estimates project that >53 million, or 16.5% of the U.S. population, will be of age 65 and older. Octogenarians are the fastest-growing group of the American elderly. For a community-residing woman of 65 years of age life expectancy is 19 years, and it is nearly 7 years for an 85-year-old person (1). Life expectancy is somewhat less for elderly men. Infections are common in elderly patients and are associated with substantial morbidity and mortality. Influenza and pneumonia are the fifth leading causes of death overall. Septicemia often arises from urinary tract infection (UTI), abdominal, skin, and wound infections, and is also a common cause of mortality in the older population.

1.3. Case Presentation

The following case study illustrates the relationship between functional status and infection. A 75-year-old independent male with a history of coronary artery disease, essential hypertension, diabetes mellitus, and benign prostatic hypertrophy presents to a local emergency room with confusion and anorexia. The history is negative for fever, cough, shortness of breath, abdominal pain, or change in bowel habits. His wife recently noted the odor of urine on his clothes. His physical examination is remarkable for the presence of orthostatic hypotension, lethargy, slow response to questioning, disorientation, and diminished ability to answer directed questions. An extensive evaluation reveals only the presence of a UTI, and he is admitted for treatment of dehydration. In hospital he develops pulmonary edema after vigorous intravenous hydration. Confusion persists and he becomes agitated, prompting the use of sedatives and antipsychotic medications, and physical restraints to prevent him from getting out of bed. He remains bed-bound throughout his hospitalization and becomes unable to stand or walk without assistance. Because of concerns regarding his personal safety he is sent to a skilled nursing facility for rehabilitation prior to a return home. However, the persistent confusion and weakness interfere with his ability to participate in physical therapy. He is subsequently transferred to a long-term care facility because he is unable to be cared for at home by his wife. Although the patient's infection was cured, he had lost the ability to function independently due to the cascade of functional decline. Improved medical care, better nutrition, improved mobility, avoidance of psychotropic medications in favor of behavioral methods for controlling agitation, and earlier introduction of physical therapy might have prevented this unfortunate outcome (2).

The case highlights many of the nonspecific manifestations of infections in elderly patients that result from the loss of homeostatic reserve, the severity of illness, and the presence of comorbidities. Common nonspecific symptoms include confusion, malaise, anorexia, and generalized weakness. Also, symptoms and signs of infectious diseases may be quite different in older compared with younger adult patients (3) with presenting symptoms being altered, blunted, or absent. Fever and leukocytosis, identifiable hallmarks of acute infection, may be absent in an elderly individual. Pneumonia and UTI commonly present as delirium in the elderly. Endocarditis can present very insidiously as otherwise unexplained weight loss. Many of these "atypical" symptoms go unnoticed or are attributed to normal aging, delaying diagnosis, and exacerbating the infection's impact on the patient's health and functional status (see also Chapter 2: Clinical Manifestations of Infections).

The high prevalence of chronic medical conditions further complicates the treatment of elderly patients with infections. Chronic diseases can exacerbate the loss of homeostatic reserve leading to greater functional decline. Specific diseases such as chronic obstructive pulmonary disease (COPD), congestive heart failure, and dementia affect both the respective organ system and the presentation of and response to the treatment of an acute infection. In the case presentation, the development of pulmonary edema was likely the result of diminished cardiovascular reserve or occult cardiovascular disease (e.g., diastolic dysfunction). Hypoxemia, resulting from COPD and pneumonia, exacerbated the delirium and likely precipitated myocardial ischemia. Dementia diminishes cognitive reserve increasing the risk of delirium from even the modest physiological insult of an infection; in turn, delirium increases the risk of aspiration, anorexia, and undernutrition (including subsequent dehydration and hypotension). In many instances, chronic illness itself is exacerbated by an acute infection. COPD exacerbations are common in pneumonia and bronchitis. Diabetic control commonly worsens in the face of new infections.

Even the appropriate management of acute infection by antibiotic therapy, hospitalization, or surgery has the potential to further complicate a patient's course of illness and recovery. Medication interactions are common and are especially troublesome in those individuals receiving medical therapy for multiple chronic illnesses. Addition of antibiotics to a patient's regimen has the potential to increase adverse drug events, side effects, and drug–drug interactions; these concerns are further augmented by renal insufficiency or liver dysfunction. For example, hospitalization of elderly patients with digoxin toxicity is associated with concomitant administration of the antibiotic clarithromycin, presumably due to inhibition of P-glycoprotein, which normally promotes clearance of digoxin (4). Hospitalization presents the possibility of iatrogenic complications, whose rates increase with the age of the patient. Peripheral and central venous catheters carry an inherent risk of infection. The common act of inserting a Foley catheter can lead to undesirable events such as development of simple and complicated UTI, delirium, and complications of enforced immobility, a result of the catheter acting as a tether that restrains the patient's movement.

Delirium occurs commonly within the context of acute infections and hospitalizations, often causing agitation, insomnia, and combative behavior; physical restraints and psychopharmacological agents, notably antipsychotics, diphenhydramine, and benzodiazepines, are often employed for control of these symptoms. However, these medications have the potential to cause serious adverse effects in elderly patients. For example, benzodiazepines can lead to paradoxical confusion and agitation and increase the risk of falling. Antipsychotic drugs (e.g., haloperidol) can cause movement disorders or postural hypotension. Diphenhydramine, an antihistamine with prominent anticholinergic effects, increases the risk of delirium. Though these medications may have a role in controlling symptoms of agitation, anxiety, and drug withdrawal (e.g., from alcohol and benzodiazepines), use of non-pharmacological interventions and close monitoring can more safely address undesirable behaviors. Medications to generally avoid in hospitalized elderly patients, and their alternatives, are summarized in Table 1.

The interactions of acute infection, chronic diseases, physiologic impairments, and elements of hospitalization often result in elderly patients being discharged from the hospital more dysfunctional than when they were admitted (5). Our patient entered the hospital from home, previously independent in the performance of daily activities, but was discharged with a nursing facility because of the cascade of decline that occurred during the hospital course for an uncomplicated UTI. His decline was likely multifactorial resulting from the initial infection and its impact on multiple organ systems, the unintended adverse effects of therapeutic interventions (such as intravenous fluids), and the elements of hospitalization (including the use of catheters and restraints). In order to prevent the cascade of decline, early detection of patients at risk begins with an assessment of physical functioning.

2. PHYSICAL FUNCTIONING

2.1. Impact on Prognosis and Therapy

Physical effects of infections can disturb the patient's level of independent physical functioning. For example, pathogens in pneumonia diminish respiratory function and bacterial infections of the heart can diminish cardiac output resulting in the patient's loss of ability to walk due to breathlessness or to conduct daily activities due to generalized weakness. Infections can also produce broader effects. Influenza, beyond its typical respiratory involvement, has been shown to be directly damaging to muscle tissue (6). In one observational study, development of and recovery from gram-negative sepsis led to self-perceived and measurable declines in the ability to work and perform activities of daily living (ADLs) (7). Beyond specific organ symptoms due to infection, general symptoms such as malaise, weakness, anorexia, and undernutrition arise and further increase the impact of illness on the individual. Consequently, increased and diminished nutritional status perpetuates physical weakness and functional decline resulting in loss of self-care ability. In one study, diminished functional capacity was linked to higher mortality in patients with lower respiratory tract infections (8).

2.2. Assessment of Physical Functioning

A systematic approach of an older adult, i.e., geriatric assessment, evaluates patients at risk for functional decline due to an acute infection, strives to reduce risk factors for functional decline, and intervenes quickly when functional problems arise, leading to improvements in clinical outcomes of hospitalization (2). Patients at risk of adverse outcomes of hospitalization (e.g., delirium and malnutrition) can be identified and interventions targeted to prevent the adverse event (2,9). Deficits in vision, hearing, strength, and gait contribute to risk of functional decline.

Table 1 Medications to Avoid in the Elderly: Side Effects and Alternatives

Medications of risk	Recommendations	Alternatives
• *Antihistamines*: Confusion, oversedation, orthostatic hypotension, falls, constipation, and urinary retention due to anticholinergic effects		
Diphenhydramine	Avoid use as hypnotic	*Hypnotics*
Hydroxyzine	Avoid use as opioid adjunct Use lowest effective dose for allergic reactions	Temazepam 7.5 mg hs
	Use a nonsedating antihistamine for seasonal allergy	Zolpidem 5 mg hs
		Trazodone 50 mg hs *Nonsedating antihistamines* Loratadine 10 mg daily Fexofenadine 60 mg daily or bid
• *Narcotic analgesics*: Meperidine—confusion, oversedation, orthostatic hypotension, falls, constipation, and urinary retention due to anticholinergic effects; metabolite may produce agitation and seizures; short duration of analgesia; Propoxyphene—poor analgesic effect with usual opioid anticholinergic effects		
Meperidine	Use alternative pain	Acetaminophen
Propoxyphene	medication	Provides analgesia equivalent to Propoxyphene and add codeine or oxycodone 2.5 mg q4–6h if pain relif is inadequate Morphine Initially low doses (e.g., 2–4 mg q3–4h) suffice
• *Benzodiazepines*: Confusion, sedation, and falls		
Diazepam	Use a shorter acting agent for	*Anxiety or withdrawal*
Chlordiazepoxide	anxiety, and for alcohol or benzodiazepine withdrawal Use a low-dose antipsychotic to treat agitation and psychosis	Lorazepam 0.5–1 mg q6h prn Oxazepam 10 mg q6h prn Agitation/psychosis Haloperidol 0.5–2 mg bid or tid Risperidone 0.5 mg bid
• *Tricyclic antidepressants (TCA)*: confusion, oversedation, orthostatic hypotension, falls, constipation, and urinary retenion due to anticholinergic effects		
Amitriptyline	Use less anticholinergic TCA	*Neuropathic pain*
Imipramine	for neuropathic pain; use	Desipramine 10–20 mg daily
Doxepin	alternative agents (e.g., SSRI) for depression	Nortriptyline 10–25 mg daily
• *Antiemetics*: Confusion, oversedation, orthostatic hypotension, falls, constipation, and urinary retention due to anticholinergic effects; Trimethobenzamide—low-potency antiemetic, highly anticholinergic		
Promethazine	Use lowest effective dose	Promethazine 12.5 mg q6h prn
Prochlorperazine	Avoid use as opioid adjunct	Prochlorperazine 5 mg q6h prn
Trimethobenzamide		
• *Histamine*: two-receptor blocker: confusion, depression, and headache due to decreased renal elimination		
Famotidine	Reduce usual dose by 50%	Famotidine 10–20 mg daily or 20 mg every other day

Abbreviations: qhs = at bed time; bid = twice a day; tid = three times a day; prn = as needed; SSRI = selective serotonin reuptake inhibitor.

Comprehensive geriatric assessment is the process of identifying medical, environmental, and psychosocial factors that impact on an elderly individual's functional capacity (10). Traditionally, comprehensive geriatric assessment is an extensive and lengthy process, usually performed by a multidisciplinary team that can include a physician, nurse, social worker, and any combination of physical therapists, occupational therapists, speech therapists, pharmacists, or nutritionists. Interdisciplinary geriatric evaluation has been studied extensively. Its effectiveness in identifying risk factors for functional loss, reducing the rate of functional decline in inpatient and outpatient settings, and improving the quality of life has been demonstrated in Refs. 10–12.

Assessment of physical functioning begins with cataloging the patient's chronic illnesses and other risk factors for decline in the ability to perform the ADL. The greater the number of chronic diseases identified in an individual, the greater the risk of functional decline. Standardized and validated measures of physical functioning can be applied to the evaluation of a patient with an infectious disease. Both self-report (or proxy report) and performance-based measures are available and can be completed efficiently, often by members of an interdisciplinary team. The instruments vary in their sensitivity and specificity for clinical conditions, but are still useful to detect at-risk patients or those with functional impairments.

Baseline information regarding a patient's ability to perform ADL is done readily through direct questioning of the patient or an accompanying caregiver (Table 2) (13). ADLs are commonly used as a surrogate marker for physical functional capacity. Capacity can be measured by determining how many of these activities the patient is capable of doing independently (that is, without another person's assistance); the physician can also determine how much assistance is required by the patient to complete these tasks. Loss of ability to perform any of these functions during the course of the illness is a marker of physical functional decline and can serve as a prompt for intervention to restore independent functioning.

Table 2 Activities of Daily Living

Assessment tool	Independent	Assistance needed
Basic activities (self care)		
Bathing	☐	☐
Dressing	☐	☐
Transferring from bed to chair	☐	☐
Toileting	☐	☐
Grooming	☐	☐
Feeding oneself	☐	☐
Instrumental activities		
Telephone use	☐	☐
Meal preparation	☐	☐
Doing laundry	☐	☐
Doing housework	☐	☐
Shopping	☐	☐
Managing transportation	☐	☐
Taking medications	☐	☐
Managing household finances	☐	☐

Source: From Ref. 12.

The patient's baseline level of ADL performance is a benchmark level of functioning that serves as a goal to be achieved during the course of recovery from the infection.

2.2.1. Vision

Vision is often impaired with aging due to disease processes such as age-related macular degeneration, glaucoma, diabetic retinopathy, and cataracts. The insidious progression of these diseases over the years coupled with infrequent medical evaluation obscures diagnosis of these entities until much vision is already lost. Corrective lenses' prescriptions are often not adjusted frequently enough to maximize their effectiveness. Vision impairment can reduce the patient's self-care ability, increase reliance on others for assistance, and increase caregiver burden. It is also a risk factor for incident delirium in hospitalized elderly patients (14). Simply asking the question "Do you have difficulty driving or watching television or reading or doing any of your activities because of your eyesight?" will identify at-risk patients. Follow-up evaluation with the Snellen chart for each eye can help to quantify the level of impairment (15).

2.2.2. Hearing

Hearing impairment is also a risk factor for delirium (14). Its presence can often be mistaken for cognitive impairment or dementia, as patients fail to "remember" what they did not hear. Hearing loss reduces the ability of the patient to follow physician instructions and can lead to poor compliance with treatment regimens. The history of hearing loss is usually obtained from the patient or family members, who might describe the patient's difficulty in hearing during simple conversations. Hearing impairment can be detected with instruments and a brief clinical examination (10,15).

2.2.3. Strength

Physical strength is an integral part of the performance of most basic ADLs. Reduction in the use of large muscle groups leads to weakness, loss of coordination, and atrophy; these are losses that take time to reverse. Prolonged bed rest, poor nutrition, and dehydration are all potential complications of acute infection, and can cause generalized weakness, especially of the lower extremities of the patient. Diminished ability to stand or ambulate reduces the ability to perform ADLs and increases the risk of falling (16). Assessment of strength during the physical examination can identify changes that may occur during illness. Particular attention is paid to lower-extremity strength (specifically the quadriceps and hip muscles) especially as it affects gait. In patients unable to get out of bed or ambulate without assistance, a bedside assessment of strength is useful. The identification of new weakness or limited range of motion may be the sign of the effects of deconditioning, a potentially reversible process.

2.2.4. Gait

Gait is the physical ability that contributes most to personal independence and is critical to the performance of most ADLs. For those patients who are able to ambulate, assessment of gait is easily performed. The brief timed up and go test (Table 3) provides qualitative information about level of independence in sit-to-stand transfers, identifies instability in change of positions (e.g., postural instability due to lightheadedness or dizziness), and instability with turns (e.g., due to ataxia or

Table 3 Timed Up and Go (TUG) Test

Ask patient to:
 rise from chair without assistance of arms
 walk 10 ft (3 m)
 turn around and return to chair
 sit back down in chair
Significance of time to execute sequence
 10–19 sec: fairly mobile
 20–29 sec: variable mobility
 $\geq$30 sec: dependent in balance and mobility
 Inability to rise from chair without the assistance of arms suggests lower extremity or
  quadriceps weakness, which is predictive of future disability; further evaluation is
  suggested when the TUG is $\geq$20 sec

Source: From Ref. 16.

lower-extremity weakness) (17). Patients unable to perform this task or requiring more than 20 sec to do so require further evaluation in order to improve gait and lower-extremity functioning and to reduce the risk of falling.

3. COGNITIVE FUNCTION

3.1. Delirium, Depression, and Dementia

Common causes of cognitive dysfunction in elderly patients are delirium, dementia, and depression. Delirium, an acute disorder of attention and global cognitive function, is a common and potentially preventable complication of infection in hospitalized patients (9). Clinical features of delirium include disturbance of consciousness (i.e., reduced awareness of the environment) with reduced ability to focus, sustain, or shift attention; change in cognition (e.g., memory deficit, disorientation, and language disturbance) or perceptual disturbance that is not better accounted for by a preexisting, established, or evolving dementia; increased or reduced psychomotor activity; disorganized sleep–wake cycle; acute onset of disturbance (usually from hours to days) with fluctuation over the course of the day (frequently vacillating between a hyperactive and a hypoactive state); and evidence from the history, physical examination, or laboratory findings that the disturbance is caused by an etiologically related general medical condition.

 Delirium is associated with prolonged hospitalization, increased risk of nursing home placement, persistent functional decline, and debilitating complications (e.g., falls, injury, and immobility). It is an independent marker for increased mortality among older medical inpatients during the 12 months after hospital admission, functional decline, and nursing home placement. Delirium is a particularly important prognostic marker among patients without dementia (18).

 A number of factors increase the risk of development of delirium in the elderly. These include age, hearing and vision impairment, presence of baseline cognitive dysfunction, number of medications being taken, and physical frailty. Although acute infection is among the most common etiologies of delirium, all potential contributing factors (e.g., hypoxemia, dehydration, and adverse drug effects) should be sought and treated.

Recognition of delirium can lead to interventions to reduce its impact and duration. Delirium is commonly recognized by the presence of agitation, aggression, hallucinations—hallmarks consistent with hyperactive delirium. Because these behaviors usually attract the attention of the caregivers and family members, hyperactive delirium is an easily recognized entity. Alternatively, delirium can present as lethargy, malaise, and somnolence—consistent with hypoactive delirium. This presentation is often mistaken for depression and is less often recognized as delirium, thus delaying identification, assessment, and treatment of the underlying problem.

3.2. Diagnosis of Cognitive Dysfunction

Delirium, dementia, and depression frequently coexist in the elderly population. Depression can be confused with dementia or delirium. As interventions for each of these differ, recognizing the difference between them aids in identifying their proper treatment. A three-item recall tool can detect the presence of a memory impairment characteristic of delirium, dementia, or depression (15). The clinician provides the patient with three items to remember (such as apple, table, and penny) and then asks the patient to recall those items after 1 min. A deficit in recall should prompt more extensive testing using instruments utilized for assessment of depression [15-item Geriatric Depression Scale (GDS), Table 4] (19), cognitive function [Mini-Mental State Examination (MMSE), Table 5] (20), and detection of delirium [Confusion Assessment Method (CAM) Table 6] (21).

Posing the question "Do you often feel sad or depressed" can detect depression with a fairly high sensitivity and specificity (15). Symptoms can be quantified with the brief GDS (19). Patients scoring six or more depressive symptoms on this scale are likely to be depressed. Patients with depression are alert and attentive compared with delirious patients. Simple tests of attention, such as a digit span (Table 7) or spelling the word "world" backward can help identify inattentive patients (unable to perform task) who have delirium rather than depression (10).

Dementia is the development of multiple cognitive deficits that include memory impairment and at least one of the following cognitive disturbances: aphasia, apraxia, agnosia, or a disturbance in executive functioning. The cognitive deficits must be sufficiently severe to cause impairment in occupational or social functioning. Patients with dementia are at very high risk for the development of delirium and commonly develop it within the context of acute infection.

Distinction between delirium and dementia can usually be made based on the acuity and chronicity of the cognitive decline. Undiagnosed patients with dementia are alert and attentive; they often have a history of memory loss and slow functional decline over several years, or an acute onset coincident with a remote stroke. Family members and caregivers should be interviewed in order to diagnose dementia, especially when the patient is unable to provide an adequate history or cooperate with the mental status examination. The interview can aid in determining the patient's baseline mental status and recent changes in the patient's behavior that may indicate development of delirium rather than dementia.

The MMSE provides a relatively easy and familiar method of quantifying cognitive functioning (20). Patients who score 26 or greater on this test usually have normal cognition. The MMSE cannot distinguish delirium from dementia, but dementia is likely when the score is low on the MMSE ($\leq$24) and the patient has a documented history of cognitive and functional impairment for six or more months.

Table 4 Geriatric Depression Scale (Short Form)

Are you basically satisfied with your life?	YES	**NO**
Have you dropped many of your activities or interests?	**YES**	NO
Do you feel your life is empty?	**YES**	NO
Do you often get bored?	**YES**	NO
Are you in good spirits most of the time?	YES	**NO**
Are you afraid that something bad is going to happen to you?	**YES**	NO
Do you feel happy most of the time?	YES	**NO**
Do you often feel helpless?	**YES**	NO
Do you prefer to stay at home, rather than go out and doing new things?	**YES**	NO
Do you feel you have more problems with memory than most?	**YES**	NO
Do you think it is wonderful to be alive now?	YES	**NO**
Do you feel pretty worthless the way you are now?	**YES**	NO
Do you feel full of energy?	YES	**NO**
Do you feel that your situation is hopeless?	**YES**	NO
Do you think that most people are better off than you are?	**YES**	NO

Note: Score bolded answers. One point for each of these answers. Cutoffs: normal is 0–5; above 5 suggests depression.
Source: From Ref. 18.

Table 5 MMSE Sample Items

Orientation to time: "What is the date?"
Registration: "Listen carefully. I am going to say three words. You say them back after I stop. Ready? Here they are . . .
HOUSE (pause), CAR (pause), LAKE (pause). Now repeat those words back to me."
(Repeat up to five times, but score only the first trial.)
Naming: "What is this?" (Point to a pencil or pen.)
Reading: "Please read this and do what it says."
(Show examinee the words on the stimulus form.)
CLOSE YOUR EYES

Source: Reproduced by special permission of the Publisher, Psychological Assessment Resources, Inc. (PAR, Inc.), 16204 North Florida Avenue, Lutz, FL 33549, from the MMSE, by Marshal Folstein and Susan Folstein, Copyright 1975, 1998, 2001 by Mini Mental LLC, Inc. Published 2001 by PAR, Inc.

Table 6 Confusion Assessment Method (CAM)

Acute onset and fluctuating course
Is there an acute change in mental status from the patient's baseline?
Did this fluctuate during the course of the interview?
Inattention
Was the patient easily distracted from, have difficulty focusing attention to, or have difficulty in keeping track of what was said in a conversation?
Disorganized thinking
Was the patient's thinking disorganized, incoherent, unclear, illogical, or did the patient switch from subject to subject?
Altered level of consciousness
Was the patient alert (normal), vigilant (hyperalert, very sensitive to stimuli, and startled very easily), lethargic (drowsy, easily aroused), stuporous (difficult to arouse), or comatose (unarousable)?

Note: Diagnosis of delirium by CAM requires the presence of 1, 2, and either 3 or 4.
Source: From Ref. 20.

The CAM instrument can be used to diagnose and monitor acute delirium. Characteristics of delirium as detected by the CAM distinguish it from dementia and depression. The CAM has demonstrated high interobserver reliability as well as high sensitivity and specificity for detecting delirium (21).

4. CAREGIVERS

4.1. Role of the Caregiver

The role of the caregiver in the context of acute illness can be easily overlooked. In many instances, previously robust individuals become debilitated and unable to function independently as a result of infections, as illustrated in the case presentation. Our patient who was previously independent left the hospital less able to perform his daily activities at discharge compared with his status prior to hospitalization. Relatively healthy, elderly are already at risk of functional decline because of the loss of homeostatic reserve associated with normal aging. For those frailer elderly, already with some level of disability and even less reserve, even a minor acute health insult predisposes them to greater functional loss and greater difficulty in regaining functioning, leading to more dependence on those who care for them.

The primary caregiver should be consulted regarding the home situation of the ill patient. In many instances, the caregiver of the acutely ill individual will be able to adjust to the increase in the patient's functional impairment or disability and will still

Table 7 Digit Span Test

Gain the patient's attention, eliminate extraneous noise.
Instruct the patient, "I am going to ask you to repeat some numbers after me. First I will say them, then you say them" (e.g., "If I say 3, 8 you would say—?").
Once the patient appears to understand the instructions, begin by asking him/her to repeat three random single numbers, spoken in a monotone at 1 sec intervals (e.g., 3, 8, 2).
Repeat the task by increasing the repetition from three to four, then five random numbers.

Note: Patients with delirium are usually unable to repeat five random numbers correctly.

provide adequate care. However, an already taxed caregiver, stretched to the limit of ability, might be unable to meet the increased needs of the patient with an infection, at least until the patient fully recovers. The caregiver could become ill and no longer be able to adequately support the needs of the patients who depend on them for help with basic ADLs. Other family members residing nearby should be identified as those who could assist with the patient's care. For the patient with a high risk of falls and inability to perform activities such as transferring, preparing and eating meals, or toileting, the family caregivers would need to provide a 24 hr supervision.

Provisions might be made to support the family (informal) caregivers at home with formal (paid) caregivers (for example, home-care services). Decision making concerning this issue revolves around the determination of the patient's current functional capacity, the resources currently available to meet any functional disabilities, and the expected level of the patient's recovery. Often this determination is performed in collaboration with nurses and social workers. The quality of care giving by family caregivers should also be assessed. Specific attention should be given in cases where gaps exist between the needs of the elderly patient and the level of care provided by the caregivers. Elder mistreatment or self-neglect can be suspected when the patient is noncompliant with therapies, has unexplained weight loss, numerous bruises, or multiple injuries at home.

4.2. Social Supports

Recovery from infections can be a lengthy process, depending on the patient's illness severity, baseline physical and functional capacity, and severity of cognitive and physical functional loss that may have occurred during the illness. Social support services in the community should be sought to aid the caregivers as the patient recovers (22). A listing of the available community support services can be obtained from the local area agency on aging (www.aoa.dhhs.gov). Useful resources for the patient include services such as visiting nurses, home care liaisons, or meals on wheels (www.mowaa.org); educational materials and information regarding support groups can also be made available for the family caregivers from local organizations (for example, Alzheimer's Association, www.alz.org). Available services can also be sought out through local religious and charitable organizations providing volunteer services for homebound individuals. Veterans may also have services available to them through a local veterans affairs hospital.

If the gap between needed and available supports for the patient is too large, then the decision for an alternative place of residence may be appropriate, even if it is only temporary. This may mean a short stay in a skilled nursing facility for rehabilitation during convalescence or permanent long-term care facility placement. A social worker helps families to identify and access resources to benefit the patient during and after hospitalization. A social worker or case manager in the hospital can perform an in-depth evaluation of these needs and determine available resources for the patient and the patient's caregiver.

5. PREVENTING FUNCTIONAL DECLINE

The severity of functional decline and the speed of recovery are both influenced by how quickly the infection is recognized and treated. A patient with an acute infection can be assessed quickly, provided with appropriate treatment for the infection, and

Table 8 Functional Assessment Measure

Physical functioning		
Activities of daily living (see Table 2)		
Change from baseline?	YES ___	NO ___
Dependent in ADL?	YES ___	NO ___
Basic	_____	
Instrumental	_____	
Vision		
Ask: "Do you have difficulty driving or watching television or reading or doing any of your activities because of your eyesight?"	YES ___	NO ___
*Positive: YES (perform Snellen Eye Chart)		
Snellen Eye Chart Score	RIGHT ___	LEFT ___
*Positive is best correction of worse than 20/40		
Hearing		
Self-report hearing loss	YES ___	NO ___
Or audioscope (40 dB)	RIGHT	LEFT
1000 Hz	_____	_____
2000 Hz	_____	_____
*Positive: inability to hear 1000 or 2000 Hz in one or both ears		

Strength and gait

	RIGHT	LEFT
Lower–extremity strength		
Hip flexion	_____	_____
Hip extension	_____	_____
Knee flexion	_____	_____
Knee extension	_____	_____

Timed Up and Go —   TIME: ___
*Positive: >20 sec
Cognitive functioning
Three-item recall
  Ask: "Remember these three items: apple, table, penny."
  *Positive: Unable to recall after 1 minute (perform MMSE, CAM)
Mood
  Ask: "Do you ever feel sad or depressed?"
  *Positive: YES (perform GDS)
Attention
  Ask: "Spell the word WORLD backward."
  Digit span (see Table 7)
  *Positive: Unable to spell WORLD backward or repeat digit span is <5

	SCORE
Geriatric Depression Scale (GDS)	_____
Mini-Mental State Examination (MMSE)	_____
Confusion Assessment Method (CAM)	_____

Caregiver assessment		
Family support available	YES ___	NO ___
If YES, who is primary caregiver?	_____	
Is family support adequate?	YES ___	NO ___
Does patient utilize community resources (e.g., visiting nurse, meals on wheels, home health aid, etc.)?	YES ___	NO ___

(Continued)

Table 8 Functional Assessment Measure (*Continued*)

If YES, which resources?	_____
Patient requires supervision for safety issues/concerns	YES ___ NO ___
Considering placement of patient into rehabilitation, assisted living, long-term care facility, or location other than current place of residence?	YES ___ NO ___
*Positive: Any BOLD answer—consider social worker consultation	

monitored closely for changes in cognitive or physical functioning. The identification of patient factors associated with functional decline can help to determine what measures can be placed for prevention.

Patients at risk of physical functional decline who have been identified by the interdisciplinary team (aided by the evaluation tools) may benefit from the services of physical therapy and occupational therapy for the purposes of prevention of deconditioning. Patient participation in supervised walks or physical therapy reduces the impact of immobility and promotes the maintenance of physical strength, balance, and coordination. In circumstances where therapists are already involved in the care of the patient, declines in function may be identified sooner and intervened upon more aggressively. Physical activity during treatment may help to prevent the need for rehabilitation and accelerate a return to baseline level of functioning, the goal of physical therapy (2).

Nonpharmacological interventions aid in the prevention of acute delirium (8). Reduction in immobility and promotion of ambulation during acute illness eliminate a primary factor responsible not only for deconditioning and physical decline, but also for delirium and cognitive decline. For patients with cognitive impairment, frequent and regular reorientation and participation in cognitively stimulating activities (such as discussing current events and word games) may serve to prevent delirium and agitation. For patients with hearing or vision impairment, glasses and hearing aids increase sensory input and the ability to accommodate to surroundings. Medications that may adversely affect an elderly patient's level of consciousness are avoided whenever possible (Table 1). Adequate hydration and nutrition can prevent delirium. Avoidance of instrumentation, restraints, catheters (urinary and vascular), and procedures that do not necessarily provide therapeutic or diagnostic value to the patient's care reduces the chances of iatrogenic illness.

The Hospital Elder Life Program, a model of hospital care incorporating these preventative measures, significantly lowers the incidence of delirium. In a controlled trial, patients assigned this multicomponent intervention had a 40% lower incidence of delirium in hospital and a significant reduction in total number of days and episodes of delirium compared to those assigned to usual care (9).

6. SUMMARY

A functional assessment linked to preventative and restorative therapies is an essential component of medical care in elderly patients with infectious diseases. Evaluation of functional capacity in the elderly patient with an acute infection has advantages to the clinician as well as the patient. Targeted interventions based on functional assessment can improve the patient's health and quality of life, and potentially reduce associated morbidity and mortality from an infection. The identification of patients at risk for adverse functional outcomes of therapy is easily achieved with the use of assessment tools, as summarized in Table 8.

REFERENCES

1. National Vital Stats Report. 2002; 51:2.
2. Landefeld CS, Palmer RM, Kresevic D, Fortinsky RH, Kowal J. A randomized trial of care in a hospital medical unit especially designed to improve the functional outcomes of acutely ill older patients. N Engl J Med 1995; 332:1338–1344.
3. Janssens JP, Krause KH. Pneumonia in the very old. Lancet Infect Dis 2004; 4:112–124.
4. Juurlink DN, Mamdani M, Kopp A, Laupacis A, Redelmeier DA. Drug–drug interactions among elderly patients hospitalized for drug toxicity. J Am Med Assoc 2003; 289:1652–1658.
5. Palmer RM, Counsell S, Landefeld CS. Clinical intervention trials: the ACE unit. In: Palmer RM, ed. Acute Hospital Care. Clin Geriatr Med 1998; 14:831–849.
6. Barker WH, Borisute H, Cox C. A study of the impact of influenza on the functional status of frail older people. Arch Intern Med 1998; 158:645–650.
7. Perl TM, Dvorak L, Hwang T, Wenzel W. Long-term survival and function after suspected gram-negative sepsis. J Am Med Assoc 1995; 274:338–345.
8. Mehr DR, Foxman B, Colombo P. Risk factors for mortality from lower respiratory infections in nursing home patients. J Fam Pract 1992; 34:585–591.
9. Inouye SK, Bogardus ST, Charpentier PA, Leo-Summers L, Acampora D, Holford TR, Cooney LM. A multicomponent intervention to prevent delirium in hospitalized older patients. N Engl J Med 1999; 340:669–676.
10. Palmer RM. Geriatric assessment. In: Lang RS, Isaacson JH, eds. Screening. Med Clin North Am 1999; 83:1503–1523.
11. Boult C, Boult LB, Morishita L, Doud B, Kane RL, Urdangarin CF. A randomized clinical trial of outpatient geriatric evaluation and management. J Am Geriatr Soc 2001; 49:351–359.
12. Cohen HJ, Feussner JR, Weinberger M, Carnes M, Hamdy RC, Hseih F, Phibbs C, Lavori P. A controlled trial of inpatient and outpatient geriatric evaluation and management. N Engl J Med 2002; 346:905–912.
13. Lawton MP, Brody EM. Assessment of older people: self-maintaining and instrumental activities of daily living. Gerontologist 1969; 9:179–186.
14. Inouye SK, Viscoli CM, Horwitz RI, Hurst LD, Tinetti ME. A predictive model for delirium in hospitalized elderly medical patients based on admission characteristics. Ann Intern Med 1993:474–481.
15. Moore AA, Siu AL. Screening for common problems in ambulatory elderly: clinical confirmation of a screening instrument. Am J Med 1996; 100:438–443.
16. Bean JF, Kiely DK, Herman S, Leveille SG, Mizer K, Frontera WR, Fielding RA. The relationship between leg power and physical performance in mobility-limited older people. J Am Geriatr Soc 2002; 50:461–467.
17. Podsiadlo D, Richardson S. The timed "Up & Go": a test of functional mobility for frail elderly persons. J Am Geriatr Soc 1991; 39:142–148.
18. McCusker J, Cole M, Abrahamowicz M, Primeau F, Belzile E. Delirium predicts 12-month mortality. Arch Intern Med 2002; 162:457–463.
19. Sheikh JL, Yesavage JA. Geriatric Depression Scale (GDS): recent evidence and development of a shorter version. Clin Gerontol 1986; 5:165.
20. Folstein MF, Folstein S, McHugh PR. "Mini-mental state." A practical method for grading the cognitive state of patients for the clinician. J Psychiatr Res 1975; 12:189–198.

21. Inouye SK, van Dyck CH, Alessi CA, Balkin S, Siegal AP, Horwitz RI. Clarifying confusion: the confusion assessment method. Ann Intern Med 1990; 113:941–948.
22. Anetzberger GJ. Community resources to promote successful aging. In: Palmer RM, ed. Successful Aging: Preventive Gerontology. Clin Geriatr Med 2002; 18:611–625.

SUGGESTED READING

Inouye SK. Prevention of delirium in hospitalized older patients: risk factors and targeted intervention strategies. Ann Med 2000; 32:257–263.
Moore AA, Siu AL. Screening for common problems in ambulatory elderly: clinical confirmation of a screening instrument. Am J Med 1996; 100:438–443.

5

Assessment of Nutritional Status and Interventions to Reduce Infection Risk in the Elderly

Kevin P. High
*Sections of Infectious Diseases and Hematology/Oncology, Wake Forest University
School of Medicine, Winston-Salem, North Carolina, U.S.A.*

Key Points:

- Older adults are at high risk of nutritional deficiencies; particularly, those who reside in long-term care facilities, have dental or medical problems, or suffer from depression.
- Data in older adults suggest that there is potential benefit of the following nutritional supplements:
    Multivitamin supplement daily
    Additional vitamin E up to a dose of 60–200 mg/day
    Trace minerals of zinc (20 mg/day of elemental zinc or its equivalent) and selenium (100 μg/day)
    Specific micronutrients in documented deficiency (e.g., vitamin B_{12})
- Supplementation of vitamin A or β-carotene in excess of the daily recommended amount is potentially harmful: decreasing bone density and increasing fracture risk in the elderly, and perhaps enhancing pneumonia and lung cancer risk in older smokers.
- Commercial high-protein/calorie supplements may reduce overall mortality risk in the acute care setting and perhaps long-term care, but they do not clearly reduce the risk of infection.
- Specific nutritional supplements may reduce the risk of some infections in older adults [e.g., cranberry juice to reduce the risk of urinary tract infection (UTI), and acute treatment with some nutritional interventions (e.g., vitamin C or commercial formulas as therapy in seniors with pneumonia)], but more data are needed to prove the clinical benefits of these dietary interventions.

Infectious diseases commonly afflict older adults, and the elderly are 2–10-fold more likely to die from specific infectious syndromes than young adults. This risk is influenced by a number of factors including senescent immunity, comorbidity, social and economic issues, and nutritional status. Malnutrition is extremely common in older adults and nutritional interventions among the best-studied preventive strategies for reducing infection risk. This chapter will examine the epidemiology of malnutrition in older adults, nutritional assessment in seniors, and critique the evidence behind specific nutritional interventions for preventing or treating infection in the elderly.

1. THE EPIDEMIOLOGY OF MALNUTRITION IN OLDER ADULTS AND ITS CLINICAL RELEVANCE

When compared with many areas of the world, malnutrition is rare in the United States and other developed countries. However, seniors represent a high-risk population (Table 1) (1,2). A variety of prevalent medical conditions, social, and economic circumstances form the root causes of malnutrition in this group (Table 2), but those living in long-term care facility (LTCF) or hospitalized are at the greatest risk. Up to 65% of older adults admitted in the hospital are undernourished (2), and malnutrition in hospitalized seniors is strongly associated with morbidity and mortality. In the community, depression, medications, poor oral health, cognitive impairment, and comorbid illness (e.g., cancer and poorly controlled diabetes mellitus) are the most common reversible causes of malnutrition (3).

Specific micronutrient (vitamins and trace minerals) deficiencies are also common in older adults (Table 1). Poor oral intake or absorption, increased metabolic demands, and comorbidities that may lead to specific deficiencies (e.g., atrophic gastritis and vitamin B_{12} deficiency) all increase the risk of micronutrient deficiency. Perhaps most subtle, dietary habits and changes in food preferences may lead to specific deficiency. For example, zinc intake declines throughout adult life, eventually falling below the U.S. recommended dietary allowance of 0.2 mg/kg (12–15 mg/

Table 1 Nutritional Deficiencies Prevalent in Older Adults

Nutrient	Estimated prevalence (%)[a] LTCF/hosp.	Community	Suspect the diagnosis if the following findings are present
Protein/ calorie	17–85	10–25	Weight loss, anorexia, depression, muscle wasting, low BMI, dermatitis, peripheral edema, low-serum albumin, and lymphopenia
Vitamin A	2–20	2–8	Dry skin, corneal changes, and night blindness
Vitamin B_{12}		7–15	Dementia, depression, neuropathy, and megaloblastic anemia
Vitamin D	20–40	2–10	Infrequent sun exposure, dairy intolerant, weakness, and osteoporosis/osteomalacia
Vitamin E	5–15		Cerebellar ataxia and decreased reflexes myopathy
Zinc		15–25	Loss of taste and poor wound healing

[a]Prevalence is dependent on the measure employed (dietary intake, serum levels, tissue levels, and change in physiologic measures).
Abbreviations: LTCF, long-term care facility; hosp, hospital; BMI, body mass index.

Table 2 Risk Factors for Malnutrition in Older Adults

Physical conditions
  Inability to feed oneself
  Medication-induced anorexia
  Poor dentition
  Swallowing dysfunction
  Gastro Intestinal (GE reflux, constipation)
  Restrictive diets
  Cachexia/anorexia of underlying disease (e.g., cancer, infection)
  Increased metabolic demand (e.g., wound healing/pressure ulcer)
  Metabolic disorders (diabetes, thyroid disease)
Cultural/psychosocial
  Food preferences
  Social isolation (e.g., living alone)
  Depression/bereavement
System barriers to oral intake
  Inadequate staffing in LTCFs
  Lack of food between meals (inability to "graze")
  Restrictive meal times

Abbreviations: GE, gastroesophageal; LTCF, long-term care facilities.

day) in the majority of older adults. This reduction may not always be reflected in serum zinc levels, but cellular levels are often reduced.

1.1. Nutritional Assessment in the Elderly

A high index of suspicion is the most important diagnostic tool for primary care physicians to detect malnutrition in older adults. Important clues include weight loss/low body weight, muscle wasting, sparse/thinning hair, dermatitis, cheilosis/angular stomatitis, poor wound healing, and peripheral edema (Table 1). A number of relatively easy-to-use office assessments of nutritional status have been validated in seniors, which provide a systematic approach to diagnosis (4,5). One helpful screen is simply to assess weight and recent weight changes, and calculate body mass index (BMI) in weight in kilograms/(height in meters)^2. Barrocas and colleagues (5) suggest that older adults who experience $\geq$5% loss of body weight in 1 month have a body weight 20% or more below ideal body weight, or a BMI >27 or <22, undergo a thorough assessment of nutritional status. One caution regarding BMI in this population: height is sometimes difficult to measure accurately in older adults due to kyphosis, osteoporosis, or inability to stand. The measure of "knee-height," which can be accomplished in the supine position with calculation of overall height using a specific validated formula can solve this problem and provide accurate height measures to calculate BMI.

A number of indicators that are readily available from common data acquired for all LTCF residents also correlate with more sophisticated measures of nutritional status. The weight and BMI measures available in the Minimum Data Set closely correlate with more complicated measures of nutritional status. Further, several studies have documented that a recent loss of >5% of body weight, a weight <90% ideal body weight for age/gender, and complaints of anorexia by LTCF residents correlate with poor nutritional status.

If one wishes to use a more formal, standardized approach several time-sensitive short-form assessments are available. One instrument validated for use in older adults both in the community and in the LTCF is the Mini-Nutritional Assessment (MNA) (6). This instrument is widely used in geriatric research. There is a relatively good correlation with BMI, but the MNA adds easy-to-answer questions regarding functional measures, dietary intake, and self-assessment of health data for a more complete picture of nutritional health. The MNA can be administered by healthcare professionals in <15 min. Electronic versions of the MNA and several other nutritional assessment tools can be accessed on-line via The Medical Algorithms Project (http://www.medal.org).

The MNA and other nutritional instruments include important physical examination measures that, in and of themselves, are good predictors of nutritional risk. These include BMI, midarm circumference (MAC), and calf circumference. A recent study in elderly LTCF residents suggested that MAC may the most important of these measures for predicting mortality (7). In that study, after controlling for demography, length of stay, functional status, and comorbidities, an MAC <26 cm was associated with a 4.24-fold increase in mortality risk, and an MAC of 26–29 cm was associated with a 2.93-fold increased risk vs. those with an MAC ≥29 cm. The MAC was more predictive than BMI, triceps skin-fold measures, or even lean body mass measured by bioelectric impedance (7). MAC can be obtained in a few seconds using a simple tape measure to assess circumference at the midpoint between the acromion and the olecranon processes.

Laboratory data are also widely used to assess nutritional fitness in older adults, and several laboratory parameters correlate with important clinical outcomes (4). Serum albumin, absolute lymphocyte count, and serum cholesterol are the most readily available measures and are strong predictors of mortality. For each 1 g/dL drop in serum albumin, mortality of hospitalized elderly subjects increases from 10% to 22%. Mortality increases fourfold when the absolute lymphocyte count is <1500/mm^3, and 10-fold when serum cholesterol is <120 mg/dL (4).

In summary, there are a variety of quick, easy, and accurate tools to assess nutritional risk in older adults. Simple measures such as assessing weight/weight loss, BMI, MAC, serum albumin, and serum cholesterol can be easily incorporated into outpatient and inpatient assessments and will detect the majority of nutritional problems. More complete measures, such as the MNA, are appropriate for research environments and high-risk populations such as LTCF residents, debilitated seniors that live in the community, or others suspected of malnutrition.

1.2. Nutritional Supplementation to Enhance Immune Responses and Prevent Infection

Despite the evidence that malnutrition in the elderly is associated with adverse outcomes, there are few studies that have shown that nutritional support can reduce the risk of infection (8). These studies are very difficult to perform, require large numbers of subjects for adequate power, and are rarely done in the most "at-risk" groups, hospitalized patients, or LTCF residents with extensive comorbidity. Most studies use surrogate markers of immune response [e.g., antibody titers, delayed-type hypersensitivity (DTH) responses] to assess efficacy.

1.2.1. Multivitamin Supplements

The high prevalence of multinutrient deficiencies in the older population and the recent understanding that older adults may have different daily requirements than young adults for many nutrients have resulted in trials examining the effect of multivitamin supplements on immune function. Most studies have only focused on surrogate markers of immune competence (e.g., DTH responses and cytokine production), but a few interventional studies have sufficient sample size to assess clinical events and have shown benefits in elderly outpatients or LTCF residents. One study of community-dwelling seniors used a specific formulation of multivitamins and minerals with retinol, β-carotene, thiamine, riboflavin, niacin, pyridoxine, folate, vitamins B_{12}, C, D, E, iron, zinc, copper, selenium, iodine, calcium, and magnesium. The 12-month, double-blind, and randomized placebo-controlled trial enrolled all subjects regardless of baseline nutritional status. Over the 12 months of the study, there was less overall vitamin deficiency and an increase in several parameters including CD4+ T-cell percentage, natural killer (NK) cell activity, mitogen-activated responses, and interleukin-2/interleukin-2 receptor expression in the supplemented group. "Illness days" were lowered from an average of 48 in the placebo group to 23 in the supplemented group ($p = 0.002$), and antibiotic use was reduced from an average of 32 days in the placebo group to 18 days in the supplemented group ($p = 0.004$) (9).

Other studies of multivitamin compounds in older adults have not replicated these results and show no benefit in a variety of settings (8,10–12). The different outcomes of such studies have been ascribed to population differences, study design/adequate sample size issues, and use of formulations that differed from the specific nutrients used in the noncommercial product. It has been reported in a review article (11) that a study of LTCF residents using the identical product that showed benefit in community-dwelling older adults (9) again resulted in reduced infection rates, but the primary data have not yet been published. While multivitamin supplement trials have inconsistently shown efficacy, all have demonstrated safety of these supplements.

1.2.2. Trace Mineral Supplementation

Several studies of the institutionalized elderly suggest that trace minerals, rather than vitamins, may be the key nutritional factors for preventing infection in older adults (13). Zinc (20 mg of elemental Zn^{2+}) + selenium (100 μg) daily have been examined vs. placebo and demonstrated decreased infection rates (13) in one small study, and barely missed significance in a similarly designed larger trial ($p = 0.06$) (14). Both studies used a factorial design (vitamins, trace minerals, both or neither) and exclusively enrolled LTCF residents. When compared with placebo recipients, the mean number of infections (respiratory and urinary tract) was reduced in groups taking trace elements alone or trace elements + vitamins, but not in the vitamin alone group.

The most likely mechanism underlying the benefits of trace element supplementation is a boosting of host immunity, perhaps, particularly in those who are deficient at baseline. Several studies of zinc supplementation in older adults suggest that DTH responses, lymphocyte counts, and the function of NK cells are all enhanced by zinc. However, there is little effect on humoral immune responses (e.g., antibody) (Table 3) (8,11–14).

No. of subjects	Duration/design	Nutrient(s)	Conclusions
103	3 months/R, P	Zn^{2+} acetate	No change in DTH/lymphocyte prolifer
63	1 year	Zn^{2+} acetate	⇑ DTH responses and NK cell activity
84	1 month/R, P	Zn^{2+} sulfate	No change in response to influenza vacc
30	1 month/Obs	Zn^{2+} sulfate	⇑ T lymphocytes/DTH responses
81	2 years/R, P, F	Zn^{2+} + selenium or vitamins A, C, E; both or neither	⇑ serum selenium levels in Zn^{2+}, + selenium group and both groups ⇓ infectious episodes in the Zn^{2+}, + s but not in group receiving vitamins al
118	3 months/R, P, F	Vitamin A, Zn^{2+}; both or neither	⇓ $CD3^+$ and $CD4^+$ in vitamin A group, $CD4^+$, $CD16^+$, and $CD56^+$, lymphoc Zn^{2+} group
384	2 months/R	Zn^{2+} or Zn^{2+} + arginine	No difference in response to influenza v
725	2 years/R, P, F	Zn^{2+} + selenium or vitamins A, C, E; both or neither	⇑ Serum micronutrient levels, no effect responses; improved Zn^{2+} influenza v Zn^{2+} + selenium groups, marginal re respiratory infection in Zn^{++} + seleni ($p = 0.06$), no effect of vitamins alone

ndomized; P, placebo controlled; F, factorial; Obs, observational; DTH, delayed-type hypersensitivity; ⇑, increased; ⇓, decreased; Zn^{2+}, zinc

8,11,12.

Recent data suggest that trace mineral malnutrition may not only impair immune response, but also directly enhance the virulence of pathogenic viruses. In selenium-deficient mice infected with either coxsackie (15) or influenza virus (16) viral replication leads to more severe pathology than in the nutrient-replete mice. Moreover, in the selenium-deficient host, this environment induces mutations in the virus that increase its virulence. These malnutrition-induced changes in virulence are long lasting and subsequent infection of either selenium-deficient or well-nourished mice with the mutated virus causes severe disease (Fig. 1). This suggests that nutritionally deficient hosts may promote mutations in the viral genome during replication resulting in spread of a virus to others that has enhanced virulence (16). This important host/organism interaction has only been demonstrated in murine models, and is not yet confirmed to occur in humans. If confirmed in human disease, outbreaks in the nursing home setting, or similar facilities such as senior day care centers, are the most likely sites for wild-type viruses to find malnourished hosts and a susceptible population. This hypothesis deserves further study.

1.2.3. Vitamin A/β-carotene

Vitamin A supplementation in children throughout the developing world has been a major public health success story reducing ocular and infectious complications.

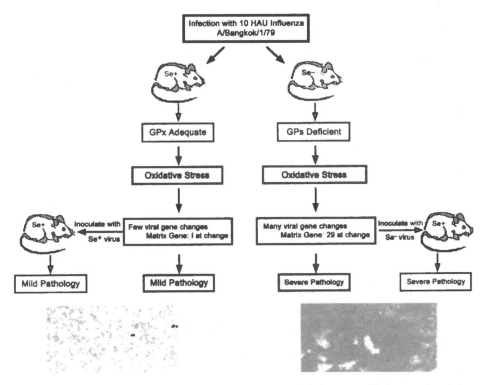

Figure 1 Influence of selenium deficiency on mutation and virulence of influenza virus infection. Passage of the virus through selenium deficient mice leads to mutations in a variety of viral genes, which results in a more virulent virus. Pathologic changes are more severe when this mutated virus is used to infect either selenium deficient or replete hosts. *Source*: From Ref. 16.

Older adults are frequently vitamin A deficient (Table 1), and several investigators have examined retinol (vitamin A) or β-carotene (a retinol precursor) supplements in aged adults in an effort to reduce infection risk. However, studies using different designs in both the community and the LTCFs have shown no benefit. In fact, some data suggest that older adults may experience adverse effects such as osteoporosis and fracture risk (17). Further, two large studies of retinol/β-carotene supplementation in smokers were prematurely halted due to increased risk of lung cancer. Thus, it is the opinion of the author that retinol/β-carotene supplementation above the recommended daily doses should be avoided in the elderly until further data are available from clinical trials.

1.2.4. Vitamin E

Vitamin E, an antioxidant vitamin that has been extensively investigated as a preventive measure for chronic illnesses including heart disease and cancer with disappointing results. However, vitamin E has also been examined as a means to boost immune responses and reduce infection in the elderly with greater success (Table 4). It is not clear how vitamin E augments immune responses, but the compound may alter cytokine generation from T-cells or macrophages (18). Vitamin E consistently improved DTH responses in elderly subjects in several studies using doses as low as 60 mg/day, and augmented antibody responses to T-cell-dependent antigens at higher doses (≥ 200 mg/day) (19). The vaccine effect occurred only after primary vaccination (there was no benefit with regard to booster responses to diphtheria or tetanus). There was also no benefit for humoral responses vs. a T-cell-independent antigen (pneumococcal polysaccharide).

None of the studies using vitamin E have demonstrated a significant reduction in disease incidence or severity. In fact, there is disagreement among published studies as to the effect of vitamin E on illness in elderly populations. In one large study, self-reported infections were 30% lower in vitamin E treated subjects vs. the placebo group ($p = 0.10$) (19). In contrast, another study specifically examined respiratory tract infections (RTIs) in older adults and showed no difference in RTI incidence but an increase in the severity of symptoms when RTIs occurred (20) (Table 4), although the number of subjects requiring medication for relief of symptoms was not different (31% vs. 31.7%, $p = 0.84$). Though it is purely a speculation at this juncture, one might hypothesize that enhanced immunity could underlie the increase in upper respiratory infection (URI) symptoms, since symptoms occur largely as a result of the immune response rather than due to pathogenic effects of the virus itself.

1.2.5. Commercial Nutritional Formulas

Commercial nutritional supplements are widely advertised to the public and touted to have immune benefits. Further, there is a "common sense" notion that nutritional supplements are likely to have benefit in malnourished elderly for promoting wound healing and overall health. However, there are few, well-controlled studies specifically in the elderly that demonstrate benefit. Two recent publications, one a carefully done meta-analysis of the overall benefits of nutritional supplements (21) and the other a well-designed, randomized controlled trial of a specific formulation in an older population (22), suggest that this common sense perception has merit.

Milne and colleagues (21) examined 31 randomized controlled trials of protein/energy supplements in hospitalized or community-dwelling seniors. The n E Supplementation Trials in Older Adults

No. of subjects	Duration/design	Vitamin E dose(s)	Conclusions
161	6 months/R, P	50 or 100 mg/day	Slight ⇑ DTH, IL-2 and IL-4, ⇑ I
88	8 months/R, P	60, 200, or 800 mg/day	⇑ DTH and primary Ab response T-cell-dependent antigens); no e T-cell-independent antigen or b responses; borderline reduction reported illness ($p = 0.10$); 200 mg/day = 800 mg/day; bot effective than 60 mg/day
52	3 months/R, P	100 mg/day	No effect on T-cell proliferation production
80	1–4.5 months/R, P	60, 200, and 800 mg/day	⇑ DTH responses at all doses
30	1 month/R, P	50 mg/day (with 100 mg/day vitamin C and, 8000 IU vitamin A)	⇑ CD4$^+$ cells, CD4/CD8 ratio, a lymphocyte proliferation
32	1 month/R, P	800 mg/day	⇑ DTH and IL-2 responses
652	15 months/R, P	200 mg/day	No change in RTI incidence, ⇑ ill severity when RTI did occur: m duration (19 vs. 14 days, $p = 0.02$), number of symptom (6 vs. 4, $p = 0.03$), presence of (36.7 vs. 25.2%, $p = 0.009$), anc activity (52.3 vs. 41.1%, $p = 0.02$)

ndomized; p, placebo controlled; DTH, delayed-type hypersensitivity; IL, interleukin; IFNγ, interferon gamma; Ab, antibody; IgG, immunc
eased; RTI, respiratory tract infection.
8,11,12.

main outcomes examined were mortality, morbidity (which included urinary and respiratory infections), and functional status. There was no clear effect on functional status, and morbidity was insignificantly reduced (though infections were not determined independently); however, overall mortality was 9.7% in the supplement recipients vs. 13.7% in the routine care group (relative risk reduction was 33% and the number needed to treat was 25).

Infectious symptoms of URI and response to influenza vaccines were specific outcomes measured in a recent randomized controlled trial of a commercial formula in assisted- and independent-living residents aged 65 years and older (22). This study was unique in that both control and experimental subjects received nutritional supplements; one group was administered a standard, commercial protein/calorie supplement, while the other group received an experimental formulation based on identical protein sources. The experimental formula also included a variety of vitamins, zinc, and selenium; specific carbohydrates were altered to include fructo-oligosaccharides, touted to maintain gastrointestinal (GI) integrity, and the lipid component included long- and medium-chain fatty acids that can be specifically utilized by leukocytes. There were minor and inconsistent benefits with regard to immunization response, but days of URI symptoms were reduced in the experimental supplement group vs. standard supplement recipients (median number of days 0 vs. 3, respectively; $p = 0.049$) over a 6-month follow-up period that spanned the winter months including influenza season. Another way to look at the data showed that 63% of the experimental formula recipients had 0 days of URI symptoms vs. 28% in the standard formula group ($p = 0.08$). Much larger studies are needed to provide evidence that such formulas reduce the risk of more serious illnesses such as pneumonia, and outcomes from this group of elderly with mild functional impairment (independent- or assisted-living) are difficult to extrapolate to more debilitated hosts.

There were a large number of dropouts in that study; 66 subjects were enrolled and only 34 completed the 6-month trial. There was not a difference in dropout rates or reasons for dropout between groups, but this highlights the difficulties in completing such studies in older adults. Many intervening events and changing patient preference are common in studies of the elderly. Frequent causes of withdrawal in the study described earlier included "unspecified" ($n = 14$), relocation to another facility after unrelated medical event ($n = 3$), suspected food–drug interaction ($n = 3$), and GI complaints or weight gain ($n = 10$).

1.2.6. Appetite Stimulants

Appetite stimulants have been studied in older adults but only for weight gain and other surrogate markers of nutritional status. No study has sufficient sample size to adequately assess infection as an end point. The Council for Nutritional Clinical Strategies in Long-Term Care recently reviewed this topic in the elderly and concluded that, of the appetite stimulants studied, the evidence supporting the use of megestrol acetate (MA) is strongest. In a recent randomized, double-blind trial in LTCF residents with weight loss or low body weight (23), they were given 800 mg/day of MA or placebo for 12 weeks to residents. Study participants were followed for an additional 13 weeks for specific outcomes, and the MA recipients were more likely to have gained weight than the placebo recipients.

Other appetite stimulants and anabolic agents have been sparingly studied in older adults. Dronabinol can be used for many patients with anorexia but should be given in a low dose (2.5 mg) in the evening, and increased as tolerated in 2–4 weeks until the desired effect is achieved. If depression is also present mirtazapine is an antidepressant with appetite-stimulating properties that may be of benefit. Anabolic agents such as oxandrolone may also lead to weight gain, but some authorities feel anabolic steroids should be used only in profound cachexia. An excellent review of the relative risks and benefits of these agents has recently been published (24); the reader is referred to this reference for greater detail.

2. NUTRITIONAL PREVENTION OF SPECIFIC INFECTIOUS SYNDROMES IN OLDER ADULTS

2.1. Pressure Ulcers

Common sense suggests that nutritional supplements may reduce the risk of developing wound infection and speed wound healing, but when this notion is tested in a scientific fashion, it is less clear that nutritional interventions are justified. Pressure ulcers are common wounds in older adults, particularly those in LTCFs. A recent multicenter trial demonstrated a slightly reduced risk of pressure ulcers in LTCF residents utilizing protein/calorie supplements, but other data demonstrate little if any benefit. More widely accepted, but just as lacking in well-controlled data, is the use of zinc supplements. Most data suggest that benefit to zinc supplements for preventing pressure ulcers is confined to those who are zinc deficient. Current recommendations are to provide adequate protein/calories and zinc sulfate at a dose of ≥ 220 mg/day to promote healing of pressure ulcers in patients with active wounds, but not provide nutritional supplements in an effort to prevent pressure ulcers.

2.2. Urinary Tract Infections

Nutritional intervention for the prevention of urinary tract infections (UTI) in elderly subjects may be useful and inexpensive. Cranberry juice has been touted as a preventive measure for UTI (25). This is supported by a study in young adult outpatients in which cranberry juice reduced the incidence of bacteriuria with pyuria (15% in the cranberry juice recipients vs. 28% in the placebo group; $p = 0.01$), but there was no change in symptomatic UTI. Asymptomatic bacteriuria is very common in older adults and should not be treated, so symptomatic UTI is the proper outcome to measure. One study of 500 + LTCF residents did examine cranberry juice for preventing UTI and found a benefit with reduced symptomatic UTI in the cranberry recipients. However, the trial has only been reported as an abstract, and never published in full form that would allow the primary data to be scrutinized. Cranberry juice has the potential to be of value in the elderly even if it does not reduce UTI. Cranberry juice may result in a reduction in malodorous urine, a common trigger for urinalysis and urine culture for the institutionalized elderly. This results in a substantial amount of inappropriate antibiotic use in LTCF residents where up to 75% of the antibiotics used are inappropriate. The randomized trial of cranberry juice in young adults showed a trend toward reduced antibiotic use in the treatment group (1.7 vs. 3.2 antibiotics per 100 patient-months) which, if true in the elderly LTCF population, would be of great value in, and of, itself to reduce antibiotic use in LTCF residents.

2.3. Respiratory Tract/Pneumonia

Many of the studies described earlier utilized URI and URI symptoms as an outcome measure, but two recent studies have examined culture-documented upper tract respiratory disease due to important viral etiologies [influenza and/or respiratory syncytial virus (RSV)], or lower respiratory tract disease (pneumonia).

During two different influenza seasons (2000 and 2001), nursing home patients were enrolled in a randomized, controlled study of ginseng extract (CVT-E002) for the prevention of laboratory-confirmed influenza or RSV (26). When compared with CVT-E002 recipients, placebo recipients had a higher risk of confirmed influenza (odds ratio = 7.73 and $p = 0.033$) and the combined end point of confirmed influenza or RSV (odds ratio = 10.5 and $p = 0.009$). The CVT-E002 was administered as a 200 mg dose twice daily for 12 weeks during the influenza season.

A different study evaluated whether vitamin E or β-carotene could reduce the risk of pneumonia requiring in-hospital treatment in older male smokers as part of a larger trial examining the effects of these compounds on lung cancer (27). Nearly 900 cases of pneumonia occurred in the 29,133 male smokers of age 50–69 years followed in this study for a median of 6 years. Overall, there was no effect on pneumonia risk. However, in a subanalysis of study subjects grouped by age at smoking onset, vitamin E was associated with a reduced risk in those who started smoking at or after 21 years of age (relative risk = 0.65), whereas β-carotene was associated with an increased risk in this group (relative risk = 1.42). This trial was stopped early due to an increased risk of lung cancer in the β-carotene recipients suggesting that β-carotene supplementation should be avoided in smokers for several reasons.

Nutritional interventions have also been examined as a treatment rather than prevention strategy for lower RTI in a small study in older adults. Vitamin C at 200 mg/day over 4 weeks showed a trend toward lower mortality and severity of symptoms, and a subanalysis of those with the most severe presenting complaints demonstrated statistical significance for symptom reduction. However, the small size of this trial and the statistical limitations of subanalysis suggest that these findings require validation. Other studies have assessed the utility of commercially available liquid supplements in elderly patients hospitalized with pneumonia, and demonstrated improved cognitive and physical function at 2 and 3 months postdischarge. Further research assessing the impact of interventions on debility and functional status is particularly important in older adults in whom survival, the most commonly targeted primary end point, is not always the most important outcome. Quality of the added life-years is sometimes even more important.

3. CONCLUSIONS AND RECOMMENDATIONS

The elderly are a population at special risk for malnutrition that may lead to an increased risk of infection. Reversible causes of malnutrition such as depression, dental disorders, and medication-induced anorexia are common in the elderly, underrecognized, and undertreated. Data suggest that a daily multivitamin/trace-mineral supplement may be beneficial for the prevention of infection and some data even suggest that antibiotic use may be reduced in elderly adults by this practice. While there are conflicting data regarding benefit, there is no study that indicates harm due to multivitamin/mineral supplements. The supplement provided should include zinc (20 mg/day of elemental zinc or its equivalent) and selenium (100 μg/day), with additional vitamin E to achieve a daily dose of 200 mg/day. Specific micronutrient replacement therapy makes sense and should be provided for those individuals with documented deficiencies, but data regarding protective efficacy of infection are lacking. Vitamin A and β-carotene supplements above the age-adjusted recommended daily intake should be avoided due to possible harm, particularly in seniors who smoke. Recent data support the use of commercial nutritional supplements to augment calories and protein in older adults in the hospital or LTCF and at-risk elderly living in the community, but there are no data favoring one formulation over another. Further, cost–benefit analysis to determine quality-adjusted life years gained using these supplements have not been performed, but one study suggests that nutritional supplements may improve functional status following hospitalization for pneumonia in the elderly. Other infectious diseases may be addressed by specific nutritional strategies (such as cranberry juice consumption to reduce UTI), potentially reducing unnecessary cultures and antibiotic use in older adults, particularly in LTCFs. Future clinical studies should be powered to adequately evaluate important clinical end points, not just surrogate markers of immune function.

Note added in proof: After this chapter was submitted, several important papers regarding vitamin E supplementation were published. A randomized trial of 200 IU/day of vitamin E vs. placebo in long-term care residents age ≥ 65 years demonstrated no difference in survival or incidence of lower respiratory tract infection, but a lower risk of upper respiratory tract infection (RR 0.88, $p = 0.048$) in vitamin E recipients (Meydani, et al. JAMA 2004;292: 828–836). Also, a meta-analysis of 19 clinical trials involving more than 135,000 subjects (of all ages) demonstrated an *increased* mortality risk in those receiving high dose vitamin E supplementation (≥ 400 IU/day) (Miller et al. Ann Intern Med 2005;142:37–46). While the methodology of this review is challenged in subsequent letters (Ann Intern Med 2005;143:150–157), a recommendation to avoid very high dose vitamin E supplementation (≥ 400 IU/day) would seem prudent until additional data are available.

REFERENCES

1. Marwick C. NHANES III health data relevant for aging nation. J Am Med Assoc 1997; 277:100–102.
2. Abbasi AA, Rudman D. Undernutrition in the nursing home: prevalence, consequences, causes, and prevention. Nutr Rev 1994; 52:113–122.
3. Wilson MG, Caswani S, Liu D, Morley JE, Miller DK. Prevalence and causes of undernutrition in medical outpatients. Am J Med 1998; 104:56–63.
4. Omran ML, Morley JE. Assessment of protein energy malnutrition in older persons, part I: history, examination, body composition, and screening tools. Nutrition 2000; 16:50–63.
5. Barrocas A, Belcher D, Champagne C, Jastram C. Nutrition assessment practical approaches. Clin Geriatr Med 1995; 11:675–713.
6. Guigoz Y, Vellas B, Garry PJ. Assessing the nutritional status of the elderly: the mini nutritional assessment as part of the geriatric evaluation. Nutr Rev 1996; 54:S59–S65.
7. Allard JP, Ashdassi E, McArthur M, McGeer A, Simor A, Abdolell M, Stephens D, Liu B. Nutrition risk factors for survival in the elderly living in Canadian long-term care facilities. J Am Geriatr Soc 2004; 52:59–65.
8. High KP. Nutrition and infection. In: Yoshikawa TT, Norman DC, eds. Infectious Disease in the Aging. Totowa, NJ: Humana Press, 2001:299–312.
9. Chandra RK. Effect of vitamin and trace-element supplementation on immune responses and infection in elderly subjects. Lancet 1992; 340:1124–1127.
10. Barringer TA, Kirk JK, Santaniello AC, Foley KL, Michielutte R. Effect of a multivitamin and mineral supplement on infection and quality of life, a randomized, double-blind, placebo-controlled trial. Ann Intern Med 2003; 138:365–371.
11. Chandra RK. Impact of nutritional status and nutrient supplements on immune responses and incidence of infection in older individuals. Ageing Res Rev 2004; 3:91–104.
12. Mitchell BL, Ulrich CM, McTiernan A. Supplementation with vitamins or minerals and immune function: can the elderly benefit? Nutr Res 2003; 23:1111–1139.

13. Girodon F, Lombard M, Galan P, Brunet-Lecomte P, Monget A-L, Arnaud J, Preziosi P, Hercberg S. Effect of micronutrient supplementation on infection in institutionalized elderly subjects: a controlled trial. Ann Nutr Metab 1997; 41:98–107.

14. Girodon F, Galan P, Monget AL, Boutron-Ruault MC, Brunet-Lecomte P, Preziosi P, Arnaud J, Manuguerra JC, Herchberg S. Impact of trace elements and vitamin supplementation on immunity and infections in institutionalized elderly patients: a randomized controlled trial. MIN. VIT. AOX. geriatric network. Arch Intern Med 1999; 159: 748–754.

15. Beck MA. Nutritionally induced oxidative stress: effect on viral disease. Am J Clin Nutr 2001; 71:1676S–1679S.

16. Nelson HK, Shi Q, Van Dael P, Schiffrin EJ, Blum S, Barclay D, Levander OA, Beck MA. Host nutritional selenium status as a driving force for influenza virus mutations. FASEB J 2001; 15:1846–1848.

17. Melhus H, Michaelsson K, Kindmark A, Bergstrom R, Holmberg L, Mallmin H, Wolk A, Ljunghall S. Excessive dietary intake of vitamin A is associated with reduced bone mineral density and increased risk for hip fracture. Ann Intern Med 1998; 129:770–778.

18. Wu D, Hayek MG, Meydani SN. Vitamin E and macrophage cyclooxygenase regulation in the aged. J Nutr 2001; 131:382S–388S.

19. Meydani SN, Meydani M, Blumberg JB, Leka LS, Siber G, Loszewski R, Thompson C, Pedrosa MC, Diamond RD, Stollar BD. Vitamin E supplementation and in vivo immune response in healthy elderly subjects. A randomized controlled trial. J Am Med Assoc 1997; 277:1380–1386.

20. Graat J, Schouten EG, Kok FJ. Effect of daily vitamin E and multivitamin-mineral supplementation on acute respiratory tract infections in elderly persons. A randomized controlled trial. J Am Med Assoc 2002; 288:715–721.

21. Milne AC, Potter J, Avenell A. Protein and energy supplementation in elderly people at risk from malnutrition. Cochrane Database Syst Rev 2002; 28(3):CD003288.

22. Langkamp-Henken B, Bender BS, Gardner EM, Herrlinger-Garcia KA, Kelley MJ, Murasko DM, Schaller JP, Steelmiller JK, Thomas DJ, Wood DM. Nutritional formula enhanced immune function and reduced days of symptoms of upper respiratory tract infection in seniors. J Am Geriatr Soc 2004; 52:3–12.

23. Yeh SS, Wu SY, Lee TP, Olson JS, Stevens MR, Dixon T, Porcelli RJ, Schuster MW. Improvement in quality-of-life measures and stimulation of weight gain after treatment with megestrol acetate oral suspension in geriatric cachexia: results of a double-blind, placebo-controlled study. J Am Geriatr Soc 2000; 48:485–492.

24. Morley JE. Orexigenic and anabolic agents. Clin Geriatr Med 2002; 18:853–866.

25. Raz R, Chazan B, Dan M. Cranberry juice and urinary tract infection. Clin Infect Dis 2004; 38:1413–1419.

26. McElhaney JE, Gravenstein S, Cole SK, Davidson E, O'neill D, Petitjean S, Rumble B, Shan JJ. A placebo-controlled trial of a proprietary extract of North American ginseng (CVT-E002) to prevent acute respiratory illness in institutionalized older adults. J Am Geriatr Soc 2004; 52:13–19.

27. Hemila H, Virtamo J, Albanes D, Kaprio J. Vitamin E and beta-carotene supplementation and hosptial-treated pneumonia incidence in male smokers. Chest 2004; 125:557–565.

SUGGESTED READING

Chandra RK. Impact of nutritional status and nutrient supplements on immune responses and incidence of infection in older individuals. Ageing Res Rev 2004; 3:91–104.

High KP. Nutrition and infection. In: Yoshikawa TT, Norman DC, eds. Infectious Disease in the Aging. Totowa, NJ: Humana Press, 2001:299–312.

Omran ML, Morley JE. Assessment of protein energy malnutrition in older persons, part I: history, examination, body composition, and screening tools. Nutrition 2000; 16:50–63.

6
Pharmacology

Jay P. Rho
Kaiser Foundation Hospital, Los Angeles, California, U.S.A.

Jiwon Kim
University of Southern California, Los Angeles, California, U.S.A.

Key Points:

- Age-related physiologic changes often require medication and or dosage adjustment.
- Most antimicrobial agents exert a pharmacological action through one of four distinct mechanisms: (1) inhibition of cell wall synthesis, (2) alteration in the permeability of cell membrane or active transport across cell membrane, (3) inhibition of protein synthesis, and (4) inhibition of nucleic acid synthesis.
- Diminished clearance of antimicrobials in the geriatric patient is primarily associated with the decline in renal excretion.
- Combination of two or more antimicrobial agents may be useful in certain clinical situations: (1) to broaden the antimicrobial spectrum, (2) to delay or prevent the emergence of resistant microbial strains, (3) to enhance the antimicrobial effect of another drug against a specific organism, and (4) to reduce the dose of an agent to avoid toxicity.
- Increased medication use by the geriatric patient is the highest risk factor for an adverse drug event.

1. INTRODUCTION

Pharmacology can be defined as the study of substances that interact with living systems through chemical processes, especially by binding to regulatory molecules and activating or inhibiting normal body processes (1). Drugs are defined as any substance that brings about change in biologic function through its chemical actions (1). For purposes of describing the manner in which a drug interacts with normal body processes, pharmacology is often subclassified into two functional areas: pharmacokinetics and pharmacodynamics. The term pharmacokinetics was introduced in 1953 to describe the movement of a drug through the body (2). Biologic rate processes control the onset, intensity, and duration of action of any drug by determining the concentration of the drug, its active metabolities, or both at the receptor site. Age-related changes in pharmacokinetics principally affect drug absorption, distribution, metabolism, and elimination. Pharmacodynamics governs the effect of a drug at the site of action or target organs. There is some evidence that changes in tissue sensitivity to drugs are altered with aging through changes in receptor activity, as well as a decline in cellular viability and the homeostatic mechanism (3).

Antimicrobial agents are widely used in the treatment of infection in the geriatric patient. Most antimicrobial agents exert a pharmacological action through one of four distinct mechanisms:

1. Inhibition of cell wall synthesis
2. Alteration in the permeability of cell membrane or active transport across cell membrane
3. Inhibition of protein synthesis (i.e., inhibition of translation and transcription of genetic material)
4. Inhibition of nucleic acid synthesis

Penicillins, cephalosporins, and vancomycin exert their antibacterial effects by inhibiting the synthesis of bacterial cell walls (4).

Microbial organisms must continually synthesize specific proteins to carry out cellular functions, including enzymatic reactions and membrane transport. Drugs that inhibit bacterial protein synthesis enter the bacterial cell and bind to specific ribosomal subunits (5). Agents that exert their antimicrobial effects by inhibiting or impairing the synthesis of these proteins include the aminoglycosides, macrolides, tetracyclines, and linezolids.

The pharmacological activity of antimicrobial inhibition is often described as bacteriostatic or bactericidal. The term "bacteriostatic" describes a drug that temporarily inhibits the growth of a microorganism. The therapeutic success of an antimicrobial agent often depends on the participation of host defense mechanisms. When the drug is removed, the organism will resume growth, and infection or disease may recur. The term "bactericidal" is applied to drugs that cause the death of the microorganism. However, the terms are relative, not absolute. Sometimes prolonged treatment with bacteriostatic drugs can kill certain microbial populations. In a host with adequate defenses a bacteriostatic effect may be sufficient to result in eradication of the infection.

Although there are reports that both the pharmacokinetics and the pharmacodynamics of antimicrobial agents are affected by age, the basic principles of therapy are no different from those applicable in younger patients. Consideration of the pharmacokinetic and pharmacokinetic changes in the geriatric patient described in this chapter can help guide decisions about dosing and monitoring of antimicrobial agents detailed in subsequent chapters.

2. PHARMACOKINETICS

2.1. Absorption

Drug absorption is a complex process that involves not only the physical and chemical properties of the drug but also its interaction with various parts of the gastrointestinal tract. The rate and extent of drug absorption can differ between individuals due to variability in gastric motility, gastric emptying time, and stomach acidity, which influence dissolution and absorption of drugs. Change in intestinal blood flow, a primary route of drug removal from the gut into the circulation, can also influence drug absorption.

There are several age-associated physiologic changes that may affect the absorption of drugs. Decrease in acid production and increase in gastric pH that can modify the ionization and solubility of some drugs can result from alterations in parietal and gastric cells in older individuals (6,7). Although absorption of drugs such as cefuroxime axetil is impaired at higher pH levels in the stomach (8), a recent study found no significant change in gastric acidity in the elderly (9). Other factors that may alter the absorption of drugs from the gastrointestinal tract are the blood flow of splanchnic vessels and the quantity of mucosal cells involved in absorption of drugs, both of which decrease with age (10,11). Atrophy of gastric mucosa and decreased gastrointestinal motility in the elderly (12) may not have an impact on drug absorption since this process is a simple passive diffusion in most cases that depends on concentration gradient or lipid–water partition coefficient. A few studies failed to show any evidence of reduced intestinal drug absorption in the elderly (13) and therefore the drug absorption is usually unchanged in the elderly despite the physiologic changes that may affect the absorption process.

2.2. Distribution

Distribution involves partitioning of drugs into fat and cellular and extracellular fluids. Several factors that may affect the distribution of drugs include body composition, plasma protein concentration, and distribution of blood flow to various organs and tissues. Reduced total body weight and a notable age-associated change in body composition result in alteration of drug distribution in older individuals. In addition to decline in total body water with age, continuous loss of lean body mass with aging also contributes to significant change in body composition (14). Age-related decrease in muscle and lean body mass is compensated by increase in total fat. The percentage of body fat may increase up to 45% in females and 36% in elderly males (15). Due to this increase in percentage of body fat, higher serum concentration of hydrophilic drugs is distributed primarily to lean body mass or body water. Conversely, the apparent volume of distribution of lipid-soluble drugs in turn increases with age. If the dose is unchanged in this population, increased volume of distribution can result in drug accumulation and prolonged effect (16). Decrease in cardiac output by about 1% per year during adult life (17) combined with decline in preferential regional blood flow in the elderly may influence drug distribution (18). Other factors suggested to alter the drug distribution in the geriatric patient include reduced physical activity (19) and variation in tissue permeability (20).

The decline in total body water, which occurs 10–15% over the adult life span, leads to a smaller volume of distribution for water-soluble drugs. Volume of distribution of a drug represents an extent of drug distribution to tissues relative to the plasma volume and also the relationship between plasma drug concentration and the total amount of drug in the body. For drugs that distribute extensively into total body water (i.e., hydrophilic drugs), reduced volume of distribution has been reported in the elderly (21). Without dosage adjustment of these drugs in the geriatric patient, the reduced volume of distribution can lead to a higher drug concentration per unit volume of drugs and subsequent drug toxicity. The alterations in the area under the plasma concentration time curve and plasma half-life due to the increase in volume of distribution in the aging population are expected to influence the time above minimum inhibitory concentrations for antimicrobial agents.

The decrease in plasma albumin is also well known to alter both the volume of distribution and the free fraction of highly protein-bound drugs in the elderly. The reduction in serum albumin levels due to lower dietary intake of protein and reduced synthesis in the liver is reported to be up to 25% in older population (22). The increased drug response often seen in the elderly may result from the higher free fraction of highly protein-bound drugs and greater concentration of pharmacologically active drugs. In the presence of lower serum albumin concentration, drug interactions affecting the displacement of drugs from albumin have been reported to increase in the elderly due to multiple-drug therapy (23).

2.3. Hepatic Metabolism

Hepatic metabolism is a process that facilitates the renal elimination of certain drugs by conversion to more water-soluble drugs. Although most drug metabolites are pharmacologically inactive, prolonged or toxic effects of certain drugs are due to the formation of active metabolites. Aside from factors associated with age-related changes in hepatic metabolism of drugs, considerable interindividual variation is seen in drug-metabolism capacity due to genetics, gender, and other environment factors. A selected list of antimicrobial agents with hepatic metabolism as a primary route of excretion is given in Table 1.

Factors that influence the rate of hepatic clearance of drugs include overall hepatic function, enzymatic activities in the liver, and hepatic blood flow. Age-associated decline in hepatic blood flow and structural and functional changes of the liver decrease the clearance of many drugs (24). Significant reduction in liver mass or volume occurs with the aging process, which was found to correlate with decline in clearance of certain drugs, and regional blood flow to the liver has been shown to be reduced by up to 45% between the age of 25 and 65 years (25). This reduction in blood flow and decreased liver size affects the phase I reactions (oxidation, reduction, and hydroxylation) of the hepatic microsomal enzymatic system and can change the biotransformation of drugs in the elderly. Several drugs, including commonly used cardiovascular and psychiatric drugs, have been identified to undergo phase I hydroxylation or demethylation with decreased metabolic capacity in older individuals (16). The decreased enzymatic activity in the liver reduces the transformation of lipid-soluble drugs to water-soluble metabolites and for those drugs that are extensively metabolized by phase I reaction, half-life may be prolonged and plasma clearance may be reduced, resulting in elevated serum drug levels and potential drug toxicity in the elderly (11). However, phase II reactions (conjugation, acetylation, and methylation) do not appear to be affected by age (26).

2.4. Renal Excretion

Renal excretion is an important process by which drugs and their metabolites are cleared from the body. The two most important physiologic processes involved in renal excretion are the glomerular filtration and active tubular secretion at the level of proximal tubules. Renal reabsorption, a passive process by which drugs enter back into the body through the peritubular capillary network, also determines the renal clearance of drugs. Antimicrobial agents that are primarily eliminated by renal excretion are listed in Table 1.

The decline in renal excretion of drugs in the aging population is primarily due to decreases in glomerular filtration rate (GFR) and renal blood flow, which can be reduced up to 50% in the elderly (27). This reduction is due to changes in several structural and functional aspects of the kidney in the elderly. Age-associated decline

Table 1 Routes of Antimicrobial Elimination

Drug	Primary route of elimination
Penicillins	
Ampicillin	Tubular secretion
Ampicillin/sulbactam	Tubular secretion
Methicillin	Tubular secretion
Nafcillin	Hepatic/biliary excretion/renal
Oxacillin	Hepatic/biliary excretion/renal
Penicillin G	Tubular secretion
Piperacillin	Tubular secretion/hepatic
Ticarcillin	Tubular secretion
Cephalosporins	
Cefazolin	Tubular secretion
Cephapirin	Tubular secretion
Cefotetan	Tubular secretion
Cefoxitin	Tubular secretion
Cefuroxime	Tubular secretion
Cefoperazone	Bilary excretion
Cefotaxime	Hepatic/tubular secretion
Ceftazidime	Tubular secretion
Ceftizoxime	Tubular secretion
Ceftriaxone	Renal/hepatic
Carbapenems	
Ertapenem	Tubular excretion
Imipenem/cilastatin	Tubular excretion
Meropenem	Tubular excretion
Monobactams	
Aztreonam	Glomerular filtration and tubular secretion
Quinolones	
Ciprofloxacin	Hepatic/tubular secretion
Ofloxacin	Tubular secretion
Lomefloxacin	Tubular secretion
Levofloxacin	Hepatic/tubular secretion
Moxifloxacin	Hepatic
Gatifloxacin	Hepatic/tubular secretion
Tetracyclines	
Doxycycline	Hepatic
Minocycline	Hepatic
Tetracycline	Glomerular filtration
Macrolides	
Azithromycin	Hepatic
Clarithromycin	Hepatic/renal
Erythromycin	Hepatic
Vancomycin	Glomerular filtration
Aminoglycosides	Glomerular filtration

in kidney volume and weight correlates well with the loss of the total number of glomeruli. Decrease in renal blood flow due to age-related intrarenal vascular changes and loss of tubular excretory and reabsorptive capacity in the aging population occur simultaneously with the decline in GFR. Apart from the usual decline of renal function with age, the geriatric patients are at risk for further decline in renal function due to pathologic processes commonly seen in this population (e.g., dehydration, congestive heart failure, hypertension). The antimicrobial agents that are cleared primarily through renal excretion and are subject to profound effects with age-related decline in renal function include most β-lactams and aminoglycosides.

The determination of the renal function in an older individual often utilizes serum creatinine levels, which provide unreliable measurement of the GFR due to reduced muscle mass and creatinine production. Although GFR is reduced in the elderly and a higher serum creatinine is expected, serum creatinine levels are similar in the young and old. Measurement of endogenous creatinine clearance utilized to determine GFR yields overestimation due to tubular secretion of creatinine. Although creatinine clearance estimated by a mathematical equation that accounts for the age and weight of the patient can be a convenient and useful way of estimating GFR, the resulting calculated value is an approximation of the actual GFR at best (28).

3. PHARMACODYNAMICS

Pharmacodynamics describes the pharmacologic effects of the drugs on receptors, tissues, and organ systems. The interaction of a drug on its receptor organ may produce either a desired beneficial therapeutic effect or a negative toxic effect. The elderly appear to be more sensitive to medications compared with younger individuals due to age-related changes in receptor selectivity and changes in homeostatic control mechanisms (29,30). Among the changes that may occur include impaired sympathetic and parasympathetic response, thermoregulation, and postural stability; glucose intolerance; and reduced immune response and cognitive function (31). Although age-related changes in response to drugs are observed for several drug classes (32), responsiveness to drugs in general declines with age partly due to diminished receptor density and reduced high affinity binding sites (33).

Factors that might explain the changes in drug response at the end organ in the aged population include age-related changes in homeostatic mechanisms, disease state-induced changes in organ systems, and drug–drug or drug–nutrient interactions. Postural hypotension commonly seen in the elderly taking antihypertensive agents is due to less active baroreceptor reflexes and a failure of cerebral blood flow autoregulation (34). The elderly with impaired cardiac output and those taking concurrent diuretic agents are especially at risk for inefficient homeostatic adjustments. The central nervous system in the elderly is especially susceptible to alterations in drug response. The aging brain not only loses a significant number of active cells during later life but also experiences reduction in cerebral blood flow and oxygen consumption (35). Decrease in cholinergic neurons in the neocortex and hippocoampal areas of the brain may explain the exaggerated adverse effects of anticholinergic agents in the elderly. The decline in the central nervous system dopamine synthesis is associated with increased sensitivity to dopamine blocking agents (36).

4. ANTIMICROBIAL COMBINATIONS

4.1. Advantages

The combination of two or more antimicrobial agents may be useful in certain clinical situations: (1) to broaden the antimicrobial spectrum to cover all potential or known pathogens; (2) to delay or prevent the emergence of resistant microbial strains; (3) to enhance the antimicrobial effect of another drug against a specific organism (i.e., synergism); or (4) to reduce the dose of an agent to avoid toxicity.

Broadening the antimicrobial spectrum to cover all potential or known pathogens is particularly important in treating mixed infections. For example, in a diabetic wound infection, an agent active against aerobic gram-negative bacilli, such as an aminoglycoside, can be combined with an agent active against aerobic gram-positive bacteria and anaerobic bacteria, such as clindamycin.

The use of combinations of antimicrobial agents to prevent the emergence of resistant organism is best illustrated in the treatment of tuberculosis and human immunodeficiency virus infection. In both infections, the prevalence of resistance to a first-line agent can be suppressed by the addition of two or more other active agents.

Synergism has been described as when the action of two drugs results in an effect (A + B) far greater than the maximum effects of either A alone or B alone. For example, combinations of aminoglycosides and β-lactam agents have been traditionally prescribed for the treatment of enterococcal endocarditis. When penicillin is used alone in an enterococcal endocarditis infection the effect is usually bacteriostatic. By adding an aminoglycoside to the penicillin regimen a rapid bactericidal effect is observed.

The use of a second agent to avoid higher doses of a potentially toxic antimicrobial agent has been attempted with limited success. Attempts to ameliorate the nephrotoxic effects of high-dose amphotericin B in the treatment of crytococcocal meningitis by adding flucytosine to a lower amphotericin B regimen have been shown to be occasionally successful.

4.2. Disadvantages

At times, the combination of antimicrobial agents can result in a negative effect (i.e., antagonism) where (A + B) results in an effect far less than the maximum effects of either A alone or B alone. Antagonism has been demonstrated when one drug interferes with the mechanism of action of a second drug. A bacteriostatic drug, such as tetracycline, acts as an inhibitor of bacterial growth and may inhibit the effect of a bactericidal drug, such as penicillin, that requires bacterial growth (cell wall synthesis) for killing. For example, the combination of chlortetracycline with penicillin cured fewer patients with pneumococcal meningitis than did the same dose of penicillin alone (37).

4.3. Adverse Drug Events and Reactions

Antimicrobial agents are among the most frequently prescribed drugs today, second only as a class to cardiovascular drugs. Unnecessary prescribing of antimicrobial agents is both expensive and potentially dangerous, especially, in geriatric patients. Antimicrobial agents may alter the geriatric patient's indigenous flora and favor either the emergence of resistant strains or the acquisition of new strains with multiple antimicrobial resistance. Antimicrobial agents also cause adverse drug reactions (ADRs) such as anaphylaxis with β-lactams, aplastic anemia with chloramphenicol, severe diarrhea from clindamycin, nephrotoxicity from aminoglycosides, and palpitations from fluoroquinolones.

It has been well documented that geriatric patients are at a greater risk of an ADR than their younger counterparts (38). One study found that nearly half of all ADRs reported to the Food and Drug Administration (FDA), with age information provided, occurred in patients over the age of 50, and 17.0% of reports were in patients aged 70 years or older (39).

An ADR is regarded as "any response to a drug which is noxious and unintended and which occurs at doses normally used in man for prophylaxis, diagnosis, or therapy of disease for the modification of physiological function." For reporting purposes, the U.S. FDA categorizes a serious adverse reaction (events relating to drugs or devices) as one in which "the patient outcome is death, life threatening (real risk of dying), hospitalization (initial or prolonged), disability (significant, persistent, or permanent), congenital anomaly, or required intervention to prevent permanent impairment or damage. Risk factors for ADRs associated with the geriatric population include increased medication use, the type of medications prescribed, altered pharmacological response, the number of illnesses, the severity of illness, the length of hospitalization, and lower compliance.

Increased use of medication by the geriatric patient is the highest risk factor for an ADR. As the number of medications taken increases, the risk of developing an adverse reaction increases exponentially. This effect may be due in part to the exponential number of possible drug interaction combinations created when additional drugs are added. Other risk factors include the type and dose of the drug taken. Certain physiological conditions, such as impaired renal function, may also increase the risk of an ADR. Although it may be difficult to prevent an ADR altogether, certain interventions or actions may help to minimize a potential occurrence.

Greater attention to the monitoring of drugs with predictable toxicity and avoidance of drugs that are considered problem prone can result in fewer ADRs and considerable cost reductions. Increased efforts should be made toward a better understanding of drug pharmacokinetics and dynamics of drugs with narrow therapeutic indices. Programs should also be implemented that improve medication use practices among healthcare providers.

REFERENCES

1. Katzung BG. Basic and Clinical Pharmacology. 8th ed. New York: McGraw-Hill Companies Inc., 2001.
2. Azarnoff DL. Use of pharmacokinetic principles in therapy. N Engl J Med 1973; 289:635–636.
3. Tumer N, Scarpace PJ, Lowenthal DT. Geriatric pharmacology: basic and clinical considerations. Annu Rev Pharmacol Toxicol 1992; 32:271–302.
4. Reynolds PE. Inhibitors of bacterial cell wall synthesis. Symp Soc Gen Microbiol 1985; 38:13.
5. Siegenthaler WE, Bonetti A, Luthy R. Aminoglycoside antibiotics in infectious diseases: an overview. Am J Med 1986; 80(suppl 6B):2.
6. Baron JH. Studies of basal and peak acid output with an augmented histamine test. Gut 1963; 4:136–144.
7. Swift CG. Clinical pharmacology in the older patients. Scott Med J 1979; 24:221–223.
8. Kekki M, Samloff IM, Ihamaki T, Varis K, Siurala M. Age and sex-related behavior of gastric acid secretion at the population level. Scand J Gastroenterol 1982; 17:737–743.
9. Hurwitz A, Brady DA, Schaal SE, Samloff IM, Dedon J, Ruhl CE. Gastric acidity in older adults. J Am Med Assoc 1997; 278:659–662.
10. Bender AD. The effect of increasing age on distribution of peripheral blood flow in man. J Am Geriatr Soc 1965; 13:192–198.
11. Warren PM, Pepperman MA, Montgomery RD. Age changes in small-intestinal mucosa. Lancet 1978; 2:849–850.

12. Evans MA, Triggs EJ, Cheung M, Broe GA, Creasey H. Gastric emptying rate in the elderly: implications for drug therapy. J Am Geriatr Soc 1981; 21:201–205.
13. Greenblatt DJ, Sellers EM, Shader RI. Drug disposition in old age. N Engl J Med 1982; 306:1081–1088.
14. Forbes GB, Reina JC. Adult lean body mass declines with age; some longitudinal observations. Metabolism 1970; 19:653–663.
15. Cusack B, Vestal RE. Clinical pharmacology. In: Beers MH, Merkow R, eds. Merck Manual of Geriatrics. New York: Merck & Co., Inc., 2000:54–74.
16. Greenblatt DJ, Allen MD, Shader RI. Toxicity of high-dose flurazepam in the elderly. Clin Pharmacol Ther 1977; 21:355–361.
17. Bender AD. The effect of increasing age on the distribution of peripheral blood flow in man. J Am Geriatr Soc 1965; 13:192–198.
18. Ho PC, Triggs EJ. Drug therapy in the elderly. Aust NZ J Med 1984; 14:179–190.
19. Levy G. Effect of bed rest on distribution and elimination of drugs. J Pharm Sci 1967; 56:928–929.
20. Crooks J, O'Malley K, Stevenson IH. Pharmacokinetics in the elderly. Clin Pharmacokinet 1976; 1:280–296.
21. Chapron DJ. Drug disposition and response in the elderly. In: Delafuente JC, Stewart RB, eds. Therapeutics in the Elderly. 2nd ed. Harvey Whitney Books, 1995:190–211.
22. Greenblatt DJ. Reduced serum albumin concentration in the elderly: a report from the Boston Collaborative Drug Surveillance Program. J Am Geriatr Soc 1979; 27:20–22.
23. Wallace S, Whiting B, Runcie J. Factors affecting drug binding in plasma of elderly patients. Br J Clin Pharm 1976; 3:327–330.
24. James OFW. Gastrointestinal and liver function in old age. Clin Gastroenterol 1983; 12:671–691.
25. Bach B, Molholm HJ, Kampmann JP, Rasmussen SN, Skovsted L. Disposition of antipyrine and phenytoin correlated with age and liver volume in man. Clin Pharmacokinet 1981; 6:389–396.
26. Sotaniemi EA, Arranto AJ, Pelkonen O, Pasanen M. Age and cytochrome P450-linked drug metabolism in humans: an analysis of 226 subjects with equal histopathologic conditions. Clin Pharmacol Ther 1996; 61:331–339.
27. Chutka DS, Evans JM, Fleming KC, Mikkelson KG. Drug prescribing for elderly patients. Mayo Clin Proc 1995; 70:685–693.
28. Smythe MA, Hoffman JC, Kizy K, Dmuchowski C. Estimating creatinine clearance in elderly patients with low serum creatinine concentrations. Am J Hosp Pharm 1994; 51:198–204.
29. Collins KJ, Dore C, Exton-Smith AN, Fox RH, MacDonald IC, Woodward PM. Accidental hypothermia and impaired temperature homeostasis in the elderly. Br Med J 1977; 1:353–356.
30. Feldman RD, Limbird LE, Nadeau J, Robertson D, Wood AJ. Alterations in leukocyte beta-receptor affinity with aging. A potential explanation for altered beta-adrenergic sensitivity in the elderly. N Engl J Med 1984; 310:815–819.
31. Feely J, Coakley D. Altered pharmacodynamics in the elderly. Clin Geriatr Med 1990; 6:269–282.
32. Hale WE, Stewart RB, Marks RG. Central nervous system symptoms of elderly subjects using antihypertensive drug. J Am Geriatr Soc 1984; 32:5–10.
33. Hammerlein A, Derendorf H, Lowenthal DT. Pharmacokinetic and pharmacodynamic changes in the elderly. Clin Pharmacokinet 1998; 35:49–64.
34. Lipsitz LA. Orthostatic hypotension in the older patients. N Engl J Med 1989; 321:952–957.
35. Smith BH, Sethi PK. Aging and the nervous system. Geriatrics 1975; 30:109–112.
36. Samorajski T. Age-related changes in brain biogenic amines. In: Schneider EL, ed. Aging. Clinical, Morphologic and Neurochemical Aspects in the Aging Central Nervous System. Vol. I. New York: Raven Press, 1975:199.

37. Lepper MH, Dowling HF. Treatment of pneumococcal meningitis with penicillin compared with penicillin plus aureomycin. Arch Intern Med 1951; 88:489–494.

38. Tanner LA, Baum C. Spontaneous adverse reaction reporting in the elderly. Lancet 1998; 2:580.

39. Faich GA. National adverse drug reaction reporting. Arch Intern Med 1991; 151: 1645–1647.

SUGGESTED READING

Cusack B, Vestal RE. Clinical pharmacology. In: Beers MH, Merkow R, eds. New York: Merck Manual of Geriatrics. New York: Merck & Co., Inc., 2000:54–74.

Hammerlein A, Derendorf H, Lowenthal DT. Pharmacokinetic and pharmacodynamic changes in the elderly. Clin Pharmacokinet 1998; 35:49–64.

7

Penicillins

Sanjeet Dadwal
City of Hope Medical Center, Duarte, California, U.S.A.

Key Points:

- Penicillins remain an important and effective group of antibiotics for treatment of select infections in the elderly.
- A variety of gram-positive (streptococci, staphylococci, clostridia, listeria), gram-negative [meningococci, Enterobacteriacea, *Pseudomonas aeruginosa*, anaerobes/streptococci, *Actinomyces*, *Fusobacterium*, and spirochetes (*Treponema*, *Leptospira*, *Borrelia*)] are effectively treated with different groups of penicillins.
- Penicillins enter most tissues and body cavities at therapeutic concentrations for susceptible pathogens. However, it penetrates the cerebrospinal fluid poorly except in the presence of inflammation.
- Serum drug levels are not necessary for monitoring penicillins; however, declining renal function can increase serum levels and risk dose-related toxicities.
- Adverse effects of penicillin may be immune and nonimmune mediated with type I, IgE-mediated reactions being the most serious and life-threatening event.

1. INTRODUCTION

Penicillins are a group of antibiotics sharing a common β-lactam ring with varying antimicrobial spectrum based on the acyl side chain substitutions. Penicillin, since its discovery more than six decades ago by Alexander Fleming, continues to be an important antibiotic in the management of both mild and serious infections. It constitutes one of the largest and most important groups of antibiotics. It has been successfully used for various infections in the geriatric population. The elderly now account for approximately 13% of the entire U.S. population, and the numbers are expected to grow considerably, with the 65 and older age group constituting about 21% of population in the next 30 years. Infectious diseases are the fourth leading cause of death in this group, which results in increased utilization of antibiotics. Elderly patients have a higher risk of morbidity and mortality from infections, and these infections include pneumonia, skin and soft tissue infections, urinary tract infection (UTI), meningitis, infective endocarditis, septic arthritis, and intra-abdominal infections (1,2). Many of these infections can be effectively treated with penicillins alone or in combination with another antibiotic. When prescribing in

77

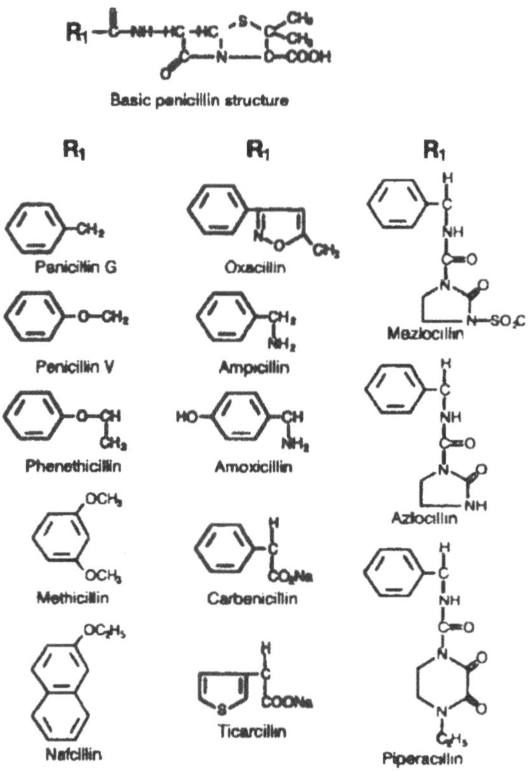

Figure 1 Chemical structure of penicillins. *Source*: From Ref. 3.

elderly patients one has to keep in mind the safety profile and the influence of age-related physiological changes on pharmacokinetics and pharmacodynamics of the antibiotic used. Penicillin use in the elderly is safe due to its wide therapeutic window; however, close attention should be given to the renal function.

The penicillins are classified into the following groups (Fig. 1):

1. Natural penicillins—penicillin G (oral and parenteral forms) and penicillin Vee K
2. Penicillinase-resistant penicillins—oxacillin, nafcillin, cloxacillin, and dicloxacillin
3. Aminopenicillins—ampicillin, amoxicillin, and bacampicillin
4. Carboxypenicillins—ticarcillin and carbenicillin
5. Ureidopenicillins—piperacillin, azlocillin, and mezlocillin

2. CHEMISTRY AND MECHANISM OF ACTION

The rudimentary structure of the penicillins is the β-lactam ring (thiazolidine and acyl side chain), which is formed by the condensation of alanine and β-dimethylcysteine (Fig. 2). The thiazolidine nucleus confers the bactericidal activity, whereas acyl side chain substitutions determine the antibacterial spectrum, pharmacological properties, and β-lactamase susceptibility.

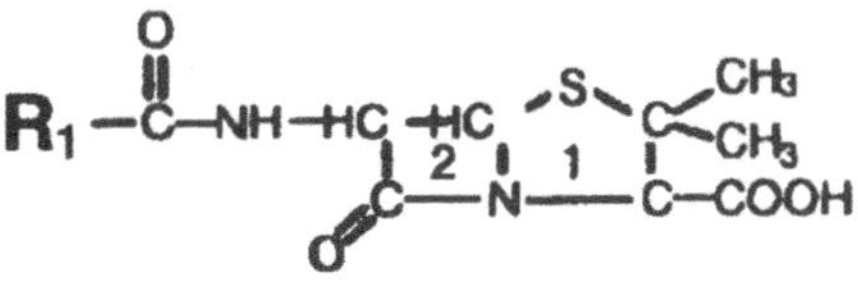

1-thiazolidine ring

2-β-lactam ring

R₁-acyl side chain

Figure 2 Basic structure of penicillin. *Source*: From Ref. 10.

Penicillins inhibit bacterial cell wall synthesis, which leads to activation of the endogenous autolytic enzymes. Penicillins bind to the penicillin-binding protein (PBPs) (enzymes involved in the synthesis of bacterial cell wall) and prevent cross-linkage of the peptide chains, i.e., transpeptidation (final step in the synthesis of peptidoglycan) process, thereby resulting in disruption of the synthesis of peptidoglycan.

β-Lactam antibiotics bind to the serine residue on the active site of PBPs by covalent acylation and thereby inhibiting both low and high molecular weight PBPs. The lethal effect is probably due to inactivation of multiple PBPs. The bactericidal effect is cell-cycle dependent, with most activity occurring while bacterial cells are dividing. Effectiveness of β-lactam drugs is also dependent on the permeability/penetrability across the cell wall and the degree of affinity for and concentration of PBPs. Penicillins by inhibiting cell-wall synthesis lead to activation of the endogenous autolysins through a two-component system, which initiates a cell death program (3). PBPs are membrane bound except for the β-lactamase, which is either secreted or membrane bound (4).

Peptidoglycan is the backbone of the bacterial cell wall and each chain comprises *N*-acetylglucosamine and *N*-acetylmuramic moieties, which alternate in a linear form. These individual chains are cross-linked by short peptides joined in amide linkage to the penultimate D-alanyl group of the *N*-acetylmuramic acid. In gram-negative species the 6-amino group of diaminopimelic acid is linked to the carboxyalanine terminus of another chain. PBPs mediate the transpeptidation and carboxypeptidation processes.

3. ANTIMICROBIAL SPECTRUM

Penicillins continue to be effective for a wide array of infections and retain their effectiveness as the first choice of treatment for several infections. They are generally safe, cost-effective treatment in geriatric patients for common skin soft tissue infections, urinary tract infections, and upper respiratory tract infections.

3.1. Gram-Positive Organisms

Streptococcus pyogenes, *Streptococcus bovis*, peptostreptococci, and anaerobic streptococci remain highly susceptible to penicillin G. Viridans streptococci also largely remain highly susceptible to penicillin G. Susceptible *Staphylococcus aureus*, *Staphylococcus epidermidis*, and *Streptococcus pneumoniae* may also be effectively killed with penicillin. In case of penicillinase-producing strains of *S. aureus* and *S. epidermidis*, oxacillin and nafcillin may be effective although methicillin-resistant *S. aureus* (MRSA) is increasing in frequency. Susceptible strains of enterococci may be treated with ampicillin, and an aminoglycoside may be added if synergy is documented on susceptibility testing.

3.2. Gram-Positive Bacilli

Clostridium perfringens, C. tetani, Erysipelothrix rhusiopathiae, Listeria monocytogenes, and non-β-lactamase-producing *Bacillus anthracis* are generally susceptible to penicillin G.

3.3. Gram-Negative Cocci

Neisseria meningitidis that do not produce lactamase can be effectively treated with penicillin G or ampicillin. Penicillin is no longer effective against *N. gonorrhoeae* due to the high incidence of resistance.

3.4. Gram-Negative Bacilli

Depending on the penicillin type, the spectrum includes *Proteus mirabilis* and other Enterobacteriacea, *Pseudomonas aeruginosa, Eikenella corrodens, Fusobacterium* sp., *Spirillum minus, Streptobacillus moniliformis,* and *Pasteurella multocida.* Extended-spectrum penicillins, such as carboxy and ureidopenicillins, are the agents of choice for *P. aeruginosa* and Entereobacteriacea bacteria. This is due to a high incidence of resistance to penicillin G and aminopenicillins. Piperacillin in combination with a β-lactamase inhibiting agent (tazobactam) continues to provide excellent antibacterial activity against most strains of *P. aeruginosa.*

3.5. Miscellaneous

Penicillin G remains the drug of choice for spirochetal diseases caused by *Treponema pallidum, Leptospira,* and *Borrelia. Actinomyces israelii* is also generally susceptible to penicillin.

4. CLINICAL PHARMACOLOGY

Tables 1 and 2 summarize the pharmacokinetic information for most penicillins. The use of penicillin antibiotics in the elderly merits consideration regarding certain factors:

1. Declining renal function with age, in terms of glomerular filtration and tubular secretion, can lead to prolongation of half-life of the administered penicillin.
2. In individuals aged 65 years and older, renal function declines progressively, and this necessitates adjustment in dose based on the creatinine clearance (6).
3. In the use of antistaphylococcal penicillins hepatic function should be monitored.
4. Reduced serum albumin levels and uremia may lead to higher serum levels of penicillin due to decreased protein binding (7).

cokinetic Profile of Natural, Amino, and Isoxazyl Penicillins

Oral absorption (%)	Protein binding (%)	Half-life (hr)	Route of excretion	Removal by dialysis	Dose change for renal failure	Route of administration	Cost ($ do
—	45–68	0.5	Renal	Yes	Yes	i.m., i.v.	5.30/20
60–73	75–89	0.5	Renal	Yes	Minimal	Oral	0.96/0 n
30–55	15–25	0.7–1.4	Renal	Yes	Yes	Oral, i.m., i.v.	0.82/5016.29/12
—	15–25	0.7–1.4	Renal	Yes	Yes	i.m., i.v.	55.88/12
75–90	17–20	0.7–1.4	Renal	Yes	Minimal	Oral	0.89/50
75–90	17–20	0.7–1.4	Renal	Yes	Minimal	Oral	12.95/50
37–60	90–96	0.3–0.9	Renal, partially hepatic	Minimal	No	Oral	1.11/50
35–76	95–97	0.3–0.9	Renal, partially hepatic	Minimal	No	Oral	1.68/50
Poor, erratic	70–90	0.5–1.5	Hepatic	Minimal	No	i.m., i.v.	47.42/12
30–35	89–94	0.3–0.9	Hepatic	Minimal	No	Oral, i.m., i.v.	68.10/12
Minimal, acid labile	30–50	0.3–0.9	Renal	Minimal	Yes	i.m., i.v.	—[b]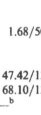

costs to pharmacy ("Red Book"), 1998.
e United States.
ntramuscular; i.v., intravenous; q.i.d., four times a day.

Pharmacokinetic Profile of Carboxy and Ureidopenicillins

Sodium content (mEq/g)	Protein binding (%)	Half-life (hr)	Distribution volume (L)	Accumulation of drug with renal dysfunction	Urinary excretion in 24 hr (%)	Biliary excretion (%)	Route of administration
4.7	50–60	1.1	12–16	Yes	90–95	0.2	p.o., i.m., i.v.
5.2	50–60	1.2	14–16	Yes	80–90	3–5	i.m., i.v.
5.2	50–60	1.2	14–16	Yes	80–90	3–5	i.v.
1.85	20–40	1.0	18–19	Minimal	50–70	20–30	i.m., i.v.
1.85	15–20	1.0	16–19	Minimal	60–80	20–30	i.m., i.v.
1.85	15–20	1.0	16–19	Minimal	60–80	20–30	i.v.
2.17	20–40	1.0	18–19	Minimal	50–70	20–30	i.m., i.v.

costs to pharmacy ("Red Book"), 1998.
he United States.

g.
every 6 hr.
intramuscular; i.v., intravenous; p.o., perorally.
10.

4.1. Natural Penicillins

This penicillin group is available in both oral and parenteral formulations. As a group, oral absorption is not very good due to their inactivation at acidic pH of the stomach. Penicillin G is absorbed poorly; however, penicillin V can achieve good levels, which can be twice the levels of benzyl penicillin. Coadministration with food leads to reduced serum levels and delayed absorption of these penicillins. Intravenous formulation is available as aqueous penicillin G, which can be administered intermittently or as a continuous infusion. Continuous infusion results in higher sustained levels and is associated with a short duration of postantibiotic effect with staphylococci and streptococci ($\approx$1.5–1.9 hr) (8). However, continuous infusion is not recommended in the elderly group due to concerns of drug accumulation. Intramuscular formulations are available as procaine penicillin and benzathine penicillin. These depot formulations provide extended absorption with steady serum and tissue levels up to 12 hr for procaine penicillin and 15–30 days with benzathine penicillin in a young host; in the elderly the levels will be longer than those of young adults. Penicillin is primarily excreted unchanged by the kidneys. Higher serum levels have been observed in the elderly compared with young patients when penicillin is given orally or parenterally. This has been attributed to reduced renal clearance (9).

4.2. Penicillinase-Resistant Penicillins

This group includes nafcillin and the isoxazyl penicillins (oxacillin, cloxacillin, and dicloxacillin). Emergence of resistant *S. aureus* (β-lactamase producing) led to development of this group of penicillins. Methicillin was the first member, which is infrequently prescribed now because of high rates of interstitial nephritis. Nafcillin is mainly used parenterally for staphylococcal infections. However, with the increasing prevalence of MRSA (which are resistant to all penicillins, and most cepahlosporins, and carbapenems), the role of these penicillins in treating staphylococcal infections is decreasing. Nafcillin excretion is primarily via the liver; therefore, the dose may not require adjustment in patients with mild to moderate renal dysfunction. Serum levels and half-life can be increased by coadministration of probenicid. Nafcillin is highly protein bound (90%).

The isoxazyl penicillins include oxacillin, cloxacillin, and dicloxacillin. The last two are available in oral formulation while oxacillin is available in both oral and parenteral formulations. Oral absorption in decreasing order is dicloxacillin > cloxacillin > oxacillin. Intravenous route is preferred for administration of oxacillin. All are highly protein bound (oxacillin 94%). Excretion is primarily via the liver. No reduction in dose is required for renal dysfunction (10). These agents are also ineffective against MRSA.

4.3. Aminopenicillins

This group of penicillins includes ampicillin and amoxicillin. They have extended the antimicrobial spectrum against gram-negative and gram-positive organisms compared with penicillin G and penicillin V. They are not stable to β-lactamases.

Ampicillin is stable in gastric acid and absorption is unaffected by food. With oral formulation peak levels are delayed in patients with diabetes mellitus, neurological disease, and heart failure (4). The parenteral form should be used for serious infections. The drug is only 15–24% protein bound and is rapidly excreted by the kidneys. The dose needs to be adjusted for renal dysfunction. Ampicillin is also manufactured in combination with sulbactam (See Chapter on "β-lactam/β-lactamase Inhibitors").

Amoxicillin is quite similar to ampicillin in antibacterial activity and chemical structure. It is available only in oral formulation. It has more complete absorption than ampicillin and achieves twice the serum levels. Due to its complete absorption from the gastrointestinal tract the occurrence of diarrhea with amoxicillin is less compared with ampicillin. It is also marketed in combination with clavulanic acid (See Chapter on "β-lactam/β-lactamase Inhibitors").

4.4. Antipseudomonal Penicillins

These are extended-spectrum penicillins (consisting of carboxypenicillins and ureido-penicillins), which were developed because of increasing resistance in gram-negative bacilli. The carboxypenicillins consists of carbenicillin and ticarcillin. Carbenicillin is synthesized by substitution of a carboxyl group for an amino group on ampicillin and, in turn, ticarcillin is derived by substitutions on carbenicillin. This group has increased activity against *P. aeruginosa* (ticarcillin is two to four times as active as carbenicillin) (10). However, this additional spectrum is not true for *Klebsiella* and *Serratia*, and these agents' binding to PBP of enterococci is poor, resulting in decreased activity against these organisms. The parenteral formulation is available for both carbenicillin and ticarcillin, while the oral form is only for carbenicillin. The oral form is used to treat chronic bacterial prostatitis in the elderly (9). Before selecting a carboxypenicillin an assessment of patient's risk (underlying cardiac or renal disease) for fluid overload should be made because these drugs have a high sodium content. Excretion is primarily via the renal tubular system and dosing should be based on creatinine clearance in the elderly to reduce the risks of complications. It is recommended not to mix carboxypenicillins and aminoglycosides, since it can lead to inactivation of aminoglycosides.

Mezlocillin, azlocillin, and piperacillin belong to the ureidopenicillin group of antipseudomonal penicllins. Their antipseudomonal activity is superior to that of carboxypenicillins. The most important drug of this group is piperacillin. It is commonly used in combination with the β-lactamase inhibitor tazobactam (see also the chapter "β Lactam/β-lactamase Inhibitors"). Ureidopenicillins are dispensed as monosodium salts with lower sodium concentrations than carboxypenicillins; however, caution still needs to be exercised when treating elderly patients with cardiac or renal disease. These agents are minimally metabolized (< 10%) and mainly eliminated in active form by glomerular filtration and tubular secretion. They have considerable biliary excretion, which results in high levels in the biliary system. An important pharmacokinetic consideration is that increasing doses of these antibiotics result in nonlinear increased antibiotic levels and decreased clearance. Due to their structure, penetration of bacterial cell wall is enhanced and their affinity for PBP is also increased. An additional feature possessed by ueidopenicillins is inhibitory activity on the septum of the dividing bacteria (10).

All penicillins achieve good levels in body fluids (synovial fluid, peritoneal fluid, pleural fluid, and pericardial fluid). The penetration of penicillins across intact blood–brain barrier is poor; however, in the presence of inflammation (such as meningitis) therapeutic levels are achieved.

5. CLINICAL INDICATIONS

5.1. Natural Penicillins

Penicillin G (aqueous) is administered intravenously for serious infections such as infective endocarditis, meningitis, septic arthritis, and pneumonia caused by *S. pyogenes*, viridans streptococci and penicillin-sensitive *S. pneumoniae* as well as susceptible staphylococci species. The drug is also the agent of choice for all forms of tertiary syphilis/neurosyphilis, fusospirochetal gingivostomatitis, and leptospirosis. Penicillin G is effective in treating serious skin and soft tissue infections such as necrotizing fasciitis due to group A streptococci, streptococcal impetigo, erysipelas, perianal streptococcal dermatitis, and cellulitis secondary to animal bites, and human bites; however, amoxicillin-clavulanate or ampicillin-sulbactam is preferable in most animal bites. Brain abscess, several odontogenic infections, and lung abscesses caused by susceptible anaerobic bacteria may be treated with penicillin G intravenously. All forms of actinomycosis can be effectively managed with high-dose penicillin G or ampicillin. Oral penicillin G or V still remains the drug of choice for most cases of streptococcal pharyngitis.

Penicillin G may also be considered in the therapy of erythema migrans with Lyme's disease, actinomycosis, and possibly in treatment of pemphigus, dermatitis herpetiformis, lupus vulgaris, psoriasis vulgaris, and lichen planus (5). A recent study evaluated the effect of various antibiotics on risk for stroke in the elderly. Results showed that penicillin was the only individual antibiotic class that showed a protective association across different time windows. This is a very interesting finding, which merits further study (11).

5.2. Aminopenicillins

5.2.1. Amoxicillin

Amoxicillin is indicated for uncomplicated upper and lower respiratory tract bacterial infections (otitis media, sinusitis, and bronchitis), and urinary tract infections caused by susceptible gram-negative organisms and enterococci. The drug is also active against agent of Lyme's disease and *Helicobacter pylori*. The American Heart Association recommends its use for oral prevention (chemoprophylaxis) of infective endocarditis in patients at risk undergoing certain dental, oral, respiratory tract, or esophageal procedures.

5.2.2. Ampicillin

Ampicillin's indications are similar to those for amoxicillin but it is used when parenteral therapy is required. Its use in the elderly extends to treatment of *Listeria monocytogenes* meningitis/brain abscess, infections by β-lactamase-negative *Haemophilus influenzae*, and infections by susceptible Enterobacteriaceae, with exception of *Klebsiella, Serratia, Enterobacter*, and *Pseudomonas*.

5.3. Antistaphylococcal Penicillins

These agents have activity against both streptococcal and β-lactamase-producing staphylococcal infections. They are primarily indicated for treatment of staphylococcal infections caused by penicillinase-producing strains. However, all antistaphylococcal penicillins are ineffective against MRSA. Dicloxacillin and cloxacillin are used as oral formulations for mild to moderate infections of skin and soft tissue.

Nafcillin and oxacillin are used primarily as intravenous formulation for treating more serious staphylococcal infections (e.g., infective endocarditis).

5.4. Antipseudomonal Penicillins

The most frequently used antipseudomonal penicillins are piperacillin and ticarcillin and they are usually prescribed in combination with a β-lactamase inhibitor, i.e., tazobactam with piperacillin and clavulanate with ticarcillin. Azlocillin, mezlocillin, and carbenicillin are used less frequently. Their main indication is treatment of *P. aeruginosa* and other resistant gram-negative pathogens, primarily Enterobacteriaceae. Piperacillin with tazobactam has been recommended for treatment of patients with febrile neutropenia. These antibiotics are not active against β-lactamase-producing strains of *S. aureus* and MRSA.

6. ADMINISTRATION OF DRUG

Oral or parenteral routes are used depending on the clinical indication and the type of penicillin used. Oral penicillin and its cogeners are used for mild to moderate infections of the upper and lower respiratory tract infections, uncomplicated skin and soft tissue infections, and various other conditions as mentioned before. Table 3 shows commonly prescribed oral penicillins and their dosage. Table 4 summarizes the commonly prescribed parenterally administered penicillins and their dosages.

7. DRUG MONITORING AND ADVERSE EFFECTS

Elderly patients are predisposed to a higher risk of adverse reactions from medications and drug interactions. This has been attributed to changes related to aging such as declining renal function and low serum albumin concentration, which may lead to higher serum levels of penicillin, as well as polypharmacy.

Drug monitoring for penicillin is achieved by assessing the patient periodically for side effects and signs of toxicity. This includes anaphylaxis after the first dose of penicillin, electrolyte imbalances (sodium/potassium), and neuromuscular hypersensitivity. The latter are more prone to develop in the elderly due to the aforementioned age-related changes and coexistent multiple morbid conditions (renal failure /heart failure). With prolonged use and high dose, monitoring hematological indices, renal function, and liver functions are recommended (Table 5).

Table 3 Oral Formulations of Penicillins

Oral formulation	Dosage
Penicillin VK	125–500 mg Q 6–8 hr
Amoxicillin	250–500 mg Q 6–8 hr
Ampicillin	250–500 mg QID
Dicloxacillin	125–500 mg QID
Cloxacillin	250–500 mg QID

Abbreviation: QID, four times a day.

Table 4 Parenteral Formulations

Parenteral formulation	Dosage
Penicillin G (IM, IV)	2–24 µ/day divided Q 4–6 hr
Ampicillin (IM, IV)	0.5–1.5 g Q 4–6 hr for IM, and 0.5–3 g Q 4–6 hr for IV
Nafcillin (IM, IV)	0.5 g q 4–6 hr for IM, and 0.5–2 g IV
Oxacillin (IM, IV)	2 g q 4–6 hr
Ticarcillin (IM, IV)	3 g q 4–6 hr
Piperacillin (IV)	3–4 g q 4–6 hr

Abbreviations: IV, intravenous; IM, intramuscular; µ, million units.

7.1. Adverse Effects

Penicillins have been used safely in the elderly patient; however, they are predisposed to certain side effects more so than the younger group of patients based on pharmacokinetic and pharmacodynamic changes seen with aging.

Adverse reactions can be broadly categorized as immune and nonimmune mediated. Immune-mediated reactions can be classified based on the mechanism (Gell and Coombs classification) or by the time to onset after the patient is started on penicillin (Levine's classification) (12,13). Immune-mediated reactions of the utmost importance are IgE-mediated type I reactions, which manifest with diffuse erythema, urticaria, pruritis, laryngeal edema, angiodema, bronchospasm, and hypotension. Concurrent use of β-adrenergic blockers may increase the risk of death (14). These anaphylactic reactions occur in ≈0.004–0.015% of patients receiving penicillin (15). It has been thought that these reactions may occur less commonly in the elderly; however, no objective data are available (16). Type II reactions result in hemolytic anemia, leucopenia, and thrombocytopenia; type III reaction leads to a serum sickness syndrome (vasculitis, fever); and type IV reaction manifests as contact dermatitis, when penicillin is used topically. Increased risk of hypersensitivity is associated with high doses of penicillin, previous untoward reactions, and mode of administration (16).

Cutaneous reactions vary from a relatively innocuous morbilliform rash to life-threatening skin eruptions such as Stevens–Johnson syndrome and exfoliative dermatitis. When the latter occurs it is prudent to discontinue penicillin and avoid reintroduction in the future. Patients should also not be subjected to skin testing with penicillin antigens.

Table 5 Drug Monitoring

Watch for anaphylaxis
Rash
Electrolytes (sodium, potassium)
Hematological indices (WBC, HgB, platelets), bleeding time
Signs of neurotoxicity
LFT and RFT with prolonged use

Abbreviations: WBC, white blood cell; Hgb, hemoglobin; LFT, liver function test; RFT, renal function test.

Rash has been associated at a higher rate with amoxicillin and ampicillin, especially in patients with infectious mononucleosis, cytomegalovirus infections, chronic lymphocytic leukemia, acute lymphocytic leukemia, hyperuricemia, and those receiving allopurinol (17).

Acute interstitial nephritis manifesting as oliguric vs. nonoliguric renal failure, nephrotic syndrome, and glomerulonephritis can occur with penicillin (17). Diarrhea, *Clostridium difficile* colitis, elevated aminotransferases with isoxazyl penicillins and carbenicillin, neutropenia, platelet dysfunction, and bleeding are potentially adverse events with penicillins. Neurological adverse effects of seizures occur more often in those with epilepsy, renal insufficiency, low serum albumin levels, meningitis, and intraventricular antibiotic therapy as well as patients undergoing cardiopulmonary bypass (18). Seizures are most commonly of the myoclonic type, but they can evolve into generalized seizures. Other neurological events include dysphagia, hyperreflexia, hallucinations, paraplegia, hemiplegia, and radiculitis (8). To avoid these adverse effects, penicillin dose should be calculated on the basis of creatinine clearance (Clcr). Based on the linear relationship between total plasma clearance of penicillin G and endogenous Clcr, upper dosage limits have been established by using the following equation:

$$\text{Dose (millions of units/day)} = 3.2 + (\text{endogenous Clcr}/7)$$

Caution should be exercised when using penicillins concurrently with methotrexate, warfarin, and tetracycline. Increased levels of methotrexate and warfarin can result, while tetracycline interferes with the bactericidal action of penicillins. Cyclosporine levels can be decreased by concomitant use of nafcillin. Prolonged neuromuscular blockade can result when neuromuscular blockers are used concurrently with ticarcillin or piperacillin. Anticoagulant effect of heparin can be potentiated with penicillins.

REFERENCES

1. Yoshikawa TT. Epidemiology of aging and infectious diseases. In: Yoshikawa TT, Norman DC, eds. Infectious Disease in the Aging. Totowa, NJ: Humana Press, 2001:3–6.
2. Yoshikawa TT. Antimicrobial resistance and aging: beginning of the end of the antibiotic era? J Am Geriatr Soc 2002; 50(suppl 7):S226–S229.
3. Novak R, Charpentier E, Braun JS, Tuomanen E. Signal transduction by a death signal peptide: uncovering the mechanism of bacterial killing by penicillin. Mol Cell 2000; 5:49–57.
4. Chambers HF. Penicillins. In: Mandell GL, Bennett JE, Dolin R, eds. Principles and Practice of Infectious Diseases. Philadelphia, PA: Churchill Livingstone, 2000:261–274.
5. Kadurina M, Bocheva G, Tonev S. Penicillin and semisynthetic penicillins in dermatology. Clin Dermatol 2003; 21:12–23.
6. Bressler R, Bahl JJ. Principles of drug therapy for the elderly patient. Mayo Clin Proc 2003; 73:1564–1577.
7. Barrons RW, Murray KM, Richey RM. Populations at risk for penicillin-induced seizures. Ann Pharmacother 1992; 26:26–29.
8. MacGowan AP, Bowker KE. Continuous infusion of b-lactam antibiotics. Clin Pharmacokinet 1998; 35(5):391–402.
9. Yoshikawa TT. Antimicrobial therapy for the elderly patients. J Am Geriatr Soc 1990; 38(12):1353–1372.
10. Wright AJ. The penicillins. Mayo Clin Proc 1999; 74:209–307.

11. Brassard P, Bourgault C, Brophy J, Kezouh A, Suissa S. Antibiotics in primary prevention of stroke in the elderly. Stroke 2003; 34(9):163–166.
12. Gell PGH, Coombs RRA. Classification of allergic reactions responsible for clinical hypersensitivity and disease. In: Gell PGH, Coombs RRA, Hachmann PJ, eds. Clinical Aspects of Immunology. Oxford: Blackwell Scientific Publications, 1975:761–781.
13. Levine BB. Immunological mechanisms of penicillin allergy. A haptenic model system for study of allergic diseases of man. N Engl J Med 1966; 275:1115–1125.
14. Salkind AR, Cuddy PG, Foxworth JW. Is this patient allergic to penicillin? An evidence-based analysis of the likelihood of penicillin allergy. J Am Med Assoc 2001; 285(19): 2498–2500.
15. Idsøe O, Guthe T, Willcox RR, De Weck A. Nature and extent of penicillin side-reactions, with particular reference to fatalities from anaphylactic shock. Bull WHO 1968; 38:159–188.
16. Weiss ME, Adkinson FN Jr. Beta-lactam allergy. In: Mandell GL, Bennett JE, Dolin R, eds. Principles and Principles of Infectious Diseases. Philadelphia, PA: Churchill Livingstone, 2000:299–304.
17. Erffmeyer JE. Adverse reactions to penicillins—part II. Ann Allergy 1981; 47:294–300.
18. Bryan CS, Stone WJ. Comparably massive penicillin G therapy in renal failure. Ann Intern Med 1975; 82:189–195.

SUGGESTED READING

Chambers HF. Penicillins. In: Mandell GL, Bennett JE, Dolin Dolin, eds. Principles and Practice of Infectious Diseases. Philadelphia, PA: Churchill Livingstone, 2000:261–274.
Wright AJ. The penicillins. Mayo Clin Proc 1999; 74:290–307.
Yoshikawa TT. Antimicrobial therapy for the elderly patient. J Am Geriatr Soc 1990; 38(12):1353–1372.

8

Cephalosporins

Jack D. McCue
*University of Maryland School of Medicine, Franklin Square Hospital Center,
Baltimore, Maryland, U.S.A.*

Key Points:

- Oral cephalosporins have different pharmacokinetics and spectra of activity; they should not be used as follow-up therapy to parenteral regimens without careful thought to alternatives.
- Cross-sensitivity between penicillins and cephalosporins is characteristic only of first-generation cephalosporins; it is rarely encountered with higher-generation cephalosporins.
- The inadequate coverage of enterococci and methicillin-resistant *Staphylococcus aureus* (and in some cases methicillin-sensitive strains) in all cephalosporins and *Bacteroides* spp. in noncephamycins should be taken into account when using cephalosporins in empirical regimens in the elderly.
- Dose-related toxicity is rare, and dosing of cephalosporins is generally the same in elderly and younger patients.
- The "generation" categorization of cephalosporins is often misleading; it is better to become familiar with a few drugs that are used frequently than to assume similarity among drugs within a generation.

There are a greater number of biochemically and/or clinically distinctive antimicrobials within the cephalosporins than any other group of antibacterial agents, and as a group they are one of the most widely used throughout the world. All are derived from the cephem nucleus, which is the core of the β-lactam compound cephalosporin C (Fig. 1). Cephalosporin C is a natural antimicrobial fermentation product isolated from the fungus *Cephalosporium acremonium* (now *Acremonium chrysogenum*), which was grown from the sewage in Sardinia in the first half of the last century. The cephem nucleus, a six-membered dihydrothiazine ring, has proved to be a remarkably versatile clay from which the more than 25 different cephalosporin antibiotics currently in clinical use have been crafted.

The safety of the cephalosporins has made them especially useful for the elderly; as a group they are renally excreted, but rarely cause toxicity when accidentally overdosed in patients with renal insufficiency, are not a cause of delirium, and are rarely of concern for drug interactions. They are available in both parenteral and

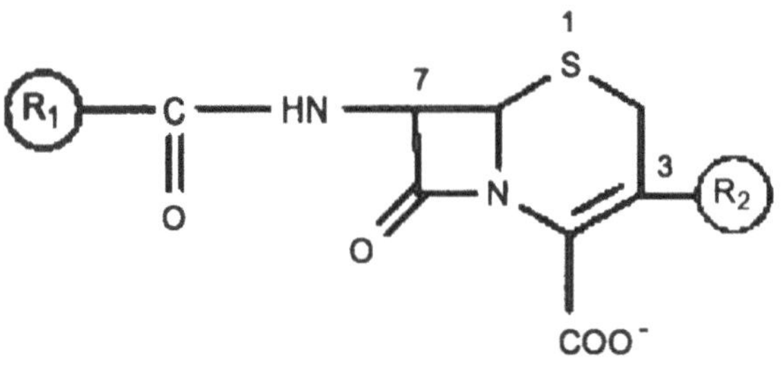

Figure 1 The cephem nucleus. All cephalosporins, except the three cephamycins, are directly derived from substitutions at the R_1 or R_2 positions of the cephem molecule.

oral formulations, although the latter is useful only for minor, nongenitourinary tract infections, or selectively for follow-up of parenteral therapy after defervescence. Most important, however, the breadth of their spectrum of activity makes them useful for empirical treatment of the presumed bacterial infections in the elderly that frequently defy attempts to define an etiology.

No new cephalosporins have been introduced in clinical testing for more than a decade—the late 1970s and the 1980s were the years of intense clinical investigation and a proliferation of new drugs. In 1997, cefepime—the last cephalosporin introduced for clinical use—was marketed, but its utility in comparison to older drugs is still not well defined. It may be that the versatility of the cephem nucleus has been exhausted and the clinical applicability of new cephalosporins has been vitiated by the emergence of resistant *Staphylococcus* spp., as well as the near-universal resistance of *Enterococcus* spp., to the cephalosporins as a class. Nevertheless, within the framework of use for community-acquired infections in which resistant organisms do not pose a significant threat or use for infections in which the pathogens and antimicrobial susceptibilities have been defined, they remain a safe, effective, and potentially cost-effective choice.

1. CHEMISTRY AND MECHANISM OF ACTION

The chemistry of the cephalosporins is at once simple and complex. All but three drugs are directly derived from substitutions at the R_1 or R_2 positions of the cephem molecule (Fig. 1); these substitutions can alter most relevant clinical properties of the drugs, including activity, pharmacokinetics, and, to a minor degree, adverse effects. The cephamycins cefoxitin, cefotetan, and cefmetazole derive from a different fungus, *Streptomyces lactamdurans*, and have a substitution of a methoxy group at the 7th position. This substitution creates 7-aminocephalosporanic acid as the drug nucleus and gives these three drugs enhanced anaerobic activity which is not characteristic of the cephalosporins as a group. Because they otherwise behave as cephalosporins, for clinical considerations the cephamycins are traditionally included in the cephalosporin category.

Despite decades of research, the precise mechanism of the antibacterial effects of cephalosporins remains incompletely understood (1). Characteristic of the β-lactam antibiotics, cephalosporins interfere with the synthesis of the peptidoglycan component of the bacterial cell wall. The peptidoglycan layer is external to the bacterial cell membrane; it is relatively thick in Gram-positive bacteria and thin in Gram-negative bacteria. The peptidoglycan component attacked by β-lactam antibiotics is a long polysaccharide chain composed of alternating *N*-acetylglucosamine and *N*-acetylmuramic acid residues that is transported to the outer surface of the cell membrane after synthesis in the cytoplasm. It is then inserted by transpeptidases, endopeptidases, and carboxypeptidases into the existing acid residues that are cross-linked by oligopeptide bridges, forming a lattice structure. It is these peptidases that are involved in creating the peptidoglycan component of the cell wall that is the target of the action of the β-lactam antibiotics. These peptidases are termed penicillin-binding proteins (PBPs) because of their affinity for the amide component of the β-lactam antibiotics, which is structurally similar to the D-alanyl–D-alanine bond of peptidoglycan pentapeptides—the usual substrate. When the peptidases bind to the β-lactam antibiotic with a long-lived covalent bond, instead of the usual D-alanyl–D-alanine substrate, they are rendered inactive (2). The number and makeup of PBPs vary among different bacteria, and the affinity of the PBPs for various β-lactam antibiotics varies, as does the binding with a cephalosporin affect cell wall synthesis. For example, cephalosporins are bactericidal against organisms that produce autolytic enzymes, e.g., *Streptococcus pneumoniae*, and bacteriostatic against organisms, e.g., *Pseudomonas aeruginosa*, that do not have such enzymes (3).

Resistance to cephalosporins occurs by three mechanisms: alterations in target PBPs, production of β-lactamases that inactivate the cephalosporin, or prevention of the cephalosporin from reaching its target PBPs. Multiple mechanisms may be relevant in the interaction between a specific antibiotic and a species of bacteria (4). Resistance may be present intrinsically in the bacterium, or it may result from selection of subclones or mutants during exposure of the bacterium to a cephalosporin.

First, alterations in target PBPs yielding decreased affinity for the cephalosporin is the mechanism by which methicillin-resistant *S. aureus* (MRSA) and penicillin-resistant *S. pneumoniae* have become resistant to cephalosporins (5,6). The PBP 2a, which is produced by MRSA, has very low affinity for cephalosporins and confers resistance MRSA of to all β-lactam antibiotics. Second, the production of β-lactamases, bacterial enzymes that are widely distributed in Gram-negative bacteria, is responsible for most clinically relevant resistance encountered in Gram-negative infections. The β-lactamases hydrolyze the critical amide bond of the β-lactam ring, reducing or eliminating the affinity of the PBP for the cephalosporin. The ability of a β-lactamase to protect the bacterium depends on a complex interaction among the antibiotic concentration, the affinity of the cephalosporin for the β-lactamase, and the concentration of the β-lactamase in the environment of the bacterial cell (7). This results in a great variation in the susceptibility of bacterial species and strains to individual cephalosporins. Genetic information that codes for β-lactamases can be carried chromosomally or on transposons on plasmids; production of the β-lactamase can be induced by exposure to a cephalosporin or can be constitutive (8). Third, Gram-negative, but not Gram-positive, bacteria have a complex outer membrane composed of lipids, polysaccharides, and proteins that is a significant barrier to cephalosporins (9). While not conferring resistance per se, the reduced rate of penetration of a β-lactam antibiotic through the outer membrane is strongly related to cephalosporin resistance (10).

2. ANTIMICROBIAL SPECTRUM AND CLASSIFICATION

The cephalosporins have been grouped into so-called generations since the introduction of cefotaxime, the first clinically available third-generation cephalosporin. What was probably a marketing concept has nevertheless become entrenched as a way of organizing cephalosporins for clinicians. It is important to keep in mind that the separation into generations is potentially arbitrary and confusing; not only are dissimilar drugs grouped together (e.g., placing the cephamycins in the second generation because they have activity against ampicillin-resistant community-acquired respiratory pathogens), but distinguishing features of a generation may also have disappeared over time (e.g., antipseudomonas activity of cefotaxime), and many clinically important distinctions (e.g., antistreptococcal and antistaphylococcal activity of some third-generation cephalosporins) are not considered.

3. CLINICAL PHARMACOLOGY

3.1. Parenteral Cephalosporins

Table 1 lists the selected parenteral cephalosporins in each of the four generations of cephalosporins that a physician who cares for elderly patients might consider selecting for empirical, and in some cases, definitive therapy. Usual doses, dose intervals, and half-lives are listed. Cephalosporins, except for cefoperazone (not included), are renally excreted largely as active drug. However, ceftriaxone has about 40% hepatic excretion, which accounts for the use of daily dosing even with moderate renal failure. Dosing is usually more determined by the severity of infection than renal function. For a typical geriatric patient, e.g., a 60 kg 75-year-old woman with a serum creatinine of 1.2 mg/dL (calculated creatinine clearance of about 40–50 mL /min, depending on the method employed), dosing does not differ from that prescribed for younger adults.

Table 1 Selected Parenteral Cephalosporins and Cephamycins with Representative Trade Names and Usual Dose Range, and Usual Geriatric Doses for Severe Infection

Parenteral cephalosporin	Trade names and generic availability	Half-life (hr)	Usual dose and dose interval range for mild to severe infections
Cefazolin	Ancef, Kefzol, generic	1.9	1–2 g every 8 hr, up to 12 g
Cefuroxime	Zinacef, Kefurox, generic	1.2	0.75–1.5 g every 8 hr, up to 9 g
Cefoxitin	Mefoxin, generic	0.8	1–2 g every 6–8 hr, up to 12 g
Cefotetan	Cefotan	3.5	1–2 g every 12 hr, up to 6 g
Ceftriaxone	Rocephin	6.4	1–2 g every 12–24 hr, up to 4 g
Ceftazidime	Fortaz, Tazidime, Ceptaz, Tazicef, generic	2.0	1–2 g every 8 hr, up to 6 g
Cefepime	Maxipime	2.1	1–2 g every 12 hr, up to 6 g

Note: All may be administered intravenously or intramuscularly with the same dose, resulting in similar pharmacokinetics.
Source: Adapted from Ref. (3).

However, when the creatinine clearance is 10–30 mL/min, the dose interval is usually lengthened, except for ceftriaxone (11).

All the parenteral cephalosporins have excellent tissue penetration, except for central nervous system and the cerebrospinal fluid (CSF). Cefuroxime and the third-generation cephalosporins have clinically useful CSF concentrations (12). All parenteral cephalosporins may be given intramuscularly. Although they are believed to cause pain with intramuscular injection, except for cephalothin they are actually well tolerated and yield pharmacokinetics comparable to intravenous administration.

3.2. Oral Cephalosporins

The orally absorbed cephalosporins, which are widely used in pediatrics, have limited usefulness for geriatric patients. The parenteral cephalosporins are not orally absorbed, with the exception of cefuroxime axetil, which is an esterified prodrug that is cleaved to its active form by gastrointestinal (GI) esterases. It is clinically important to recognize that the oral cephalosporins cannot be administered in doses comparable to those used for the parenteral cephalosporins because of GI intolerance at higher doses. Similarly, it is important to recognize that the oral cephalosporins are, with the exception of cefuroxime, different drugs with different pharmacokinetics and antibacterial activity from the parenteral cephalosporins usually listed in the same generation. If they are to be used for follow-up therapy, these differences must be taken into account. Cephalexin (first generation) or cefaclor (second generation), for example, are used for follow-up therapy for the commonly used parenteral first-generation cefazolin. They are, however, administered to patients in much lower doses than cefazolin, achieve <20% of the peak serum concentration, have shorter half-lives, and do not have comparable antimicrobial activity against Gram-negative bacilli. In general, the oral cephalosporins are well absorbed; cefuroxime axetil and cefpodoxime proxetil are exceptions, having only about 50% bioavailability. Absorption may be affected by food. Absorption of cefuroxime axetil and cefpodoxime proxetil is improved by administration with food—although the effect of food is not uniform, the remainder are best taken on an empty stomach. Table 2 lists four selected oral cephalosporins that might be considered for mild infections or follow-up therapy following a course of parenteral antibiotic therapy for more severe infections.

Table 2 Selected Oral Cephalosporins with Representative Trade Names and Usual Dose Range

Oral cephalosporin	Trade names and generic availability	Half-life (hr)	Usual dose and dose interval range
Cephalexin	Keflex, generic	0.9	0.25–0.5 g every 6 hr
Cefaclor	Ceclor, generic	0.6	0.25–0.5 g every 8 hr
Cefuroxime axetil	Ceftin	1.3	0.125–0.5 g every 12 hr[a]
Cefpodoxime proxetil	Vantin	2.2	0.2–0.4 g every 12 hr[a]

[a]Absorption is increased with food.

4. ANTIMICROBIAL SPECTRUM

The generations are used as a short-hand for grouping cephalosporins according to antimicrobial activity. However, one must be careful of such generalizations because there are important exceptions. Except for the fourth-generation cefepime, antistaphylococcal activity declines as one goes from the first- to the third-generation cephalosporins, and the third generation should not be used for serious staphylococcal infections. Gram-negative antimicrobial activity increases as one progresses through the generations of cephalosporins. Antistreptococcal activity stays the same, except for the cephamycins, which are less active against Gram-positive cocci. The cephalosporins have activity against the penicillin-susceptible anaerobic organisms that are encountered in the oropharynx, but only the cephamycins cefoxitin and cefotetan, have reliable activity against *Bacteroides fragilis*.

4.1. First-Generation Cephalosporins

The parenteral first-generation cephalosporin cefazolin has activity typical of its generation, but has superior pharmacokinetics and is the only parenteral agent in its generation that is commonly used today. It is very active against Gram-positive cocci and has moderate activity against the community-acquired Gram-negative bacteria *Moraxella catarrhalis*, *Escherichia coli*, indole-negative *Proteus mirabilis*, and *Klebsiella pneumoniae*. First-generation cephalosporins cannot be assumed to be active against hospital-acquired Gram-negative bacilli and other Enterobacteriaceae, and are not active against *B. fragilis*, *Haemophilus influenzae*, enterococci, penicillin-resistant *S. pneumoniae*, or MRSA (10). Cefazolin is used for methicillin-sensitive *S. aureus* (MSSA) infections and for empirical therapy of community-acquired cellulitis. It is the prophylactic antibiotic of choice for most elective surgery with the exception of those in which enterococci or *B. fragilis* is a potential pathogen.

The oral cephalosporin cephalexin is nearly totally absorbed from the GI tract, although its serum concentrations are <20% of those of cefazolin in usual doses and it is rapidly excreted in the urine. It is moderately active against streptococci and MSSA, but it has no useful Gram-negative activity. It is used for streptococcal pharyngitis and community-acquired skin and soft infections. In general, it should not be used for moderate to severe infections and despite its urinary excretion it should not be used for urinary tract infections (UTIs).

4.2. Second-Generation Cephalosporins

The true cephalosporins, such as cefuroxime or cefamandole, and the cephamycins (cefoxitin and cefotetan) are quite different drugs, but are both included in this category.

Cefuroxime has an iminomethoxy group that lends enhanced stability against the β-lactamases produced by *H. influenzae*, *Neisseria gonorrhoeae*, *Neisseria meningitidis*, *M. catarrhalis*, and Enterobacteriaceae, such as *E. coli*, *P. mirabilis*, *K. pneumoniae*, *Citrobacter* spp., and *Morganella* spp.(13). It has enhanced activity against streptococci but reduced activity against MSSA. It does not have reliable activity against *Serratia* spp., *Providencia* spp., and *Proteus vulgaris*. It is used for upper and lower respiratory infections, such as community-acquired pneumonia, sinusitis, and skin and soft tissue infections (SSTI). It has been used for bacterial meningitis, but was shown to be inferior to ceftriaxone in a study in children (14).

Cefoxitin has Gram-negative activity that is similar to cefuroxime. However, compared with other first- and second-generation cephalosporins, its activity against streptococci and MSSA is significantly reduced (15). It is the most active cephalosporin against *B. fragilis*, although its activity against the other *Bacteroides* spp., such as *B. thetaiotaomicron* or *B. ovatus*, is less. It is highly active against *N. gonorrhoeae*, and is used in empirical therapy for pelvic inflammatory disease. Cefotetan is similar to cefoxitin except for a long half-life that permits twice-daily dosing, and less activity against the non-*fragilis Bacteroides* spp.(16). Unlike cefoxitin, it has an *N*-methylthiotetrazole (NMTT) group, which has been associated with hypoprothrombinemia and bleeding. Most hospital pharmacies consider cefoxitin and cefotetan interchangeable, and may have only one on their formulary. The cephamycins are effective in the treatment of mixed aerobic–anaerobic infections, such as pelvic, abdominal, or diabetic foot infections. However, metronidazole and clindamycin have superior activity against *Bacteroides* spp. The cephamycins should not be used as monotherapy for nosocomial infections and serious nursing-home infections, or when reliable coverage against MSSA is needed. They are used for antimicrobial prophylaxis of colorectal surgery or for appendectomy, which would have clinical relevance to the elderly.

There is, in general, limited use for the second-generation oral cephalosporins in the elderly. Cefuroxime axetil can be used for mild to moderate community-acquired respiratory or SSTI; it should not be used for UTIs in the elderly unless there is no alternative. Cefaclor is similar to cephalexin in its pharmacokinetics but has somewhat improved activity against *H. influenzae*, *M. catarrhalis*, *P. mirabilis*, and *E. coli* and is available in generic form. Its indications are similar to cefuroxime axetil, although overall it is an inferior drug in antimicrobial activity and pharmacokinetics. However, in all cases, more effective and less expensive alternatives are available to either of these oral cephalosporins.

4.3. Third-Generation Cephalosporins

The third-generation cephalosporins were the first true broad-spectrum antibiotics with activity against a wide range of community-acquired and nosocomial pathogens, including highly resistant Gram-negative bacilli, such as *P. aeruginosa*, indole-positive *Proteus* spp., *Providencia* spp., and *Serratia* spp.—organisms that had generally required use of the relatively toxic and difficult-to-use aminoglycoside antibiotics (17). They all have excellent activity against streptococci, including most strains of penicillin-resistant *S. pneumoniae*, and while variable, all have less activity than first-generation cephalosporins against MSSA, and all are inactive against MRSA and enterococci. Unfortunately, inducible and plasmid-mediated β-lactamases are threatening the utility of these antibiotics against Gram-negative bacteria (10). They are generally divided according to their activity against *P. aeruginosa*: Ceftazidime and cefoperazone have antipseudomonal activity and the others, such as ceftriaxone, do not.

Ceftriaxone differs from all other parenteral cephalosporins in its long half-life, which permits once-daily dosing. It is the most potent cephalosporin against *N. meningitidis*, *N. gonorrhoeae*, and *H. influenzae*. It has good penetration into the cerebrospinal fluid and, as such, is a first-choice antibiotic for empirical treatment of bacterial meningitis; notably, however, it lacks activity against an important pathogen in meningitis in the elderly, *Listeria monocytogenes*. Because it has nearly equal biliary and renal excretion, it can be used without dose modification in most patients with chronic diseases and, except for meningitis, it is dosed once-daily.

Ceftazidime has Gram-negative activity similar to ceftriaxone except for its excellent activity against *P. aeruginosa*. It has the weakest activity against MSSA among the cephalosporins and is relatively weaker against *B. fragilis* than most cephalosporins. It has the advantage of being a weak inducer of β-lactamases as well as having a weak affinity for many of the inducible β-lactamases (18). Because it penetrates into the cerebrospinal fluid reasonably well, it is an antibiotic of choice (usually in combination with an aminoglycoside) for pseudomonas meningitis (12).

The oral cephalosporin cefpodoxime proxetil is an esterified prodrug like cefuroxime axetil; it is classified as a third-generation cephalosporin because of its broad range of activity that includes *S. aureus*, *S. pneumoniae*, *M. catarrhalis*, *Neisseria* spp., and many Enterobacteriaceae. It is only 50% absorbed and has a limited spectrum of activity compared with parenteral third-generation cephalosporins, and should not be considered as oral follow-up therapy without serious thought to reliably achievable serum concentrations and sensitivity of the pathogens being treated. Fluoroquinolone antibiotics, for example, have far superior pharmacokinetics and antimicrobial activity, and are significantly less expensive. Cefpodoxime proxetil may be used for follow-up therapy of community-acquired pneumonia in which atypical pathogens are unlikely or for acute exacerbation of chronic obstructive pulmonary disease (COPD).

4.4. Fourth-Generation Cephalosporins

Cefepime has both positive and negative charges on its molecule, which gives it zwitterionic properties; their zwitterionic nature permits rapid movement across the outer membrane of Gram-negative bacilli and the achievement of higher concentrations in the periplasmic space. Additionally, it is relatively resistant to a broader range of β-lactamases and has a high affinity for the PBPs of Gram-positive and Gram-negative bacteria (19). Hence, it is active against MSSA, *S. pneumoniae*, the Enterobacteriaceae, and about 50% of strains of *P. aeruginosa*. Its anaerobic activity is similar to other cephalosporins, as is its lack of activity against *L. monocytogenes*. Despite its broader range of activity, there is as yet no clearly defined clinical role for cefepime. It is most often used in intensive care units, although its antipseudomonas activity is inferior to that of ceftazidime. In clinical trials it has been comparable to, but not superior to, other cephalosporin and noncephalosporin regimens (19).

5. CLINICAL INDICATIONS

Clinical uses of cephalosporins as empirical therapy have diminished considerably over the past decade as a result of the emergence of resistance in common pathogens (e.g., MRSA and penicillin-resistant *S. pneumoniae*), the introduction of antibiotics with superior pharmacokinetics and spectrum of activity (e.g., the fluoroquinolones), and new clinical trials showing advantages of other regimens (e.g., as in coverage of atypical pathogens in community-acquired pneumonia in the elderly) (20).

5.1. Urinary Tract Infection

Parenteral cephalosporins are indicated as empirical therapy for febrile older patients with UTI or pyelonephritis. A third-generation cephalosporin is usually chosen, although the spectrum of activity of second-generation cephalosporins is sufficient for elderly persons with truly community-acquired, noncatheter-associated UTI. However, nursing-home-acquired UTI or UTI in older patients with a urinary catheter should receive an antibiotic with antipseudomonas activity. In general, an oral or parenteral fluoroquinolone such as levofloxacin or ciprofloxacin is a better choice, especially in older men for whom penetration of antibiotic into the prostate is important. Oral cephalosporins should be used for UTI only when there is no better option, such as a fluoroquinolone or trimethoprim–sulfamethoxazole.

5.2. Lower Respiratory Tract Infections

Once the cornerstone of monotherapy for elderly patients with community- or nursing-home-acquired lower respiratory tract infections (LRTI), parenteral cephalosporins, such as ceftriaxone, should be prescribed in an empirical regimen that includes a fluoroquinolone or macrolide (21). In most circumstances, it is doubtful that ceftriaxone gives a significant advantage over a fluoroquinolone alone, or a macrolide alone for older adults with uncomplicated community-acquired pneumonia. Ceftriaxone is active against most penicillin-tolerant or many penicillin-resistant strains of *S. pneumoniae*, but treatment failures occur. Ceftazidime or cefepime, in combination with a fluoroquinolone, is commonly used for severe LRTI in which infection with *P. aeruginosa* or Enterobacteriaceae may be present in the elderly. Oral cephalosporins have a limited role in community-acquired pneumonia, but cefpodoxime may be chosen for follow-up therapy, or for acute exacerbations of COPD. However, fluoroquinolones are less expensive, probably a more effective choice.

5.3. Upper Respiratory Infections

Second-generation oral cephalosporins have a long history of use in pediatric patients with otitis media. While sinusitis, otitis, or soft-tissue infections are more complicated in the elderly, cefpodoxime may still be a reasonable choice. However, amoxicillin-clavulanate or a fluoroquinolone is at least as effective and costs less.

5.4. Skin and Soft Tissue Infections

The emergence of MRSA in community-acquired SSTI has shaken the traditional role of cefazolin for empirical therapy. However, in uncomplicated infections it is still a safe, reasonable choice. Complicated infections (e.g., elderly with infected pressure ulcers or cellulitis complicated by diabetes mellitus or peripheral vascular disease) call for broader coverage (bearing in mind the possibility of MRSA, which would require specific coverage); a second-, third-, or fourth-generation parenteral cephalosporin is an appropriate choice. Specific coverage for *B. fragilis* and other anaerobes, as is offered by the second-generation cephamycins, for elderly patients with diabetes mellitus or severe peripheral vascular disease with SSTI, is assumed and recommended, but there are limited data to support this assumption; debridement, along with antibiotic therapy for anaerobic organisms, is required.

Oral first- or second-generation cephalosporins are good choices for initial or follow-through therapy of minor SSTs, or for follow-up therapy, cefpodoxime may be chosen for follow-through therapy of a complicated SSTI that has clearly responded to parenteral therapy.

5.5. Abdominal Infections

Elderly patients with febrile intra-abdominal infections such as acute cholecystitis or diverticulitis require therapy that is active against *B. fragilis*. A second-generation cephamycin or a third-generation cephalosporin with metronidazole is a good choice, depending on how likely infection with a resistant hospital- or nursing-home-acquired Gram-negative pathogen is. Oral cephalosporins have no role in the treatment of intra-abdominal infections.

5.6. Meningitis

Only third- and fourth-generation cephalosporins achieve therapeutic levels in cerebrospinal fluid. Since *S. pneumoniae* is the most common pathogen in elderly patients, the possibility of a resistant strain must be borne in mind. Ceftriaxone, ceftazidime, and cefepime are chosen for central nervous system infections for which cephalosporins are indicated. Cephalosporins are not active against *L. monocytogenes*, which may cause meningitis in the elderly, so a parenteral penicillin should be added, pending culture results.

5.7 Bone and Joint Infections

Keeping in mind the possibility of MSSA causing bone and joint infections (BJI), cefazolin may be a good choice, but would not be effective for MRSA. The relatively inferior antistaphylococcal activity of parenteral second- and third-generation cephalosporins limits their utility in empirical therapy for which culture data are not available. The relatively superior antistaphylococcal activity of cefepime makes it a reasonable choice for complicated BJI infections, although there are many options that are at least as effective. Oral first- or second-generation cephalosporins may be chosen for long-term follow-up therapy, of BJI that have responded to cefazolin, although the difficulty of treating these often recalcitrant infections has led most clinicians to favor outpatient parenteral antibiotic therapy.

5.8. Sepsis of Unclear Cause

A parenteral third- or fourth-generation cephalosporin is a good choice for sepsis in an elderly patient in whom the etiology is unclear, as is often the case. The lack of activity of ceftriaxone against *P. aeruginosa*, the unreliable activity of ceftazidime against MSSA and lack of activity against *B. fragilis*, and the lack of activity of cephalosporins against MRSA must be borne in mind when considering cephalosporin therapy for sepsis in the elderly. Ceftazidime or cefepime is used as monotherapy or combined with an aminoglycoside for presumed severe infection in patients with febrile neutropenia.

5.9. Bacterial Endocarditis

Cephalosporins that are highly active against the infecting bacterium may be used in the treatment of bacterial endocarditis. Ceftriaxone's long half-life and intramuscular administration should be considered for *Streptococcus bovis* and viridans streptococcal bacterial endocarditis.

5.10. Penicillin Allergy

Cephalosporins have historically been prescribed as an alternative regimen in patients with penicillin allergy manifested by rash or drug fever. Cross-reactivity between penicillins and cephalosporins is almost always a first-generation drug phenomenon; cross-reactivity between penicillins and second- and third-generation cephalosporins, which have side chains, is not generally a concern. However, in the case of type I allergic reactions to penicillins, such as urticaria or anaphylaxis, cephalosporins are not recommended. There is almost always an alternative regimen that can be prescribed instead of a cephalosporin.

6. ADMINISTRATION OF DRUG

Since cephalosporins are associated with minimal dose-related toxicities, recommendations for reduction in dosage are generally limited to patients with significant renal insufficiency or in the undernourished frail elderly of advanced age.

The efficacy of β-lactam antibiotics appears to be related to the amount of time that serum or tissue concentrations exceed the minimum inhibitory concentration (MIC) of the pathogens—so-called time-dependent killing, as opposed to concentration-dependent killing such as is seen with the fluoroquinolones. The best method of administration of cephalosporins is one that would maintain concentrations above the MIC for as much of the dose interval as possible. Because of the minimal toxicity of cephalosporins, negligible age-related differences in GI absorption, and often reduced drug clearance in elderly persons, increasing the dosing intervals may be preferred to lowering the dose. This approach yields higher concentrations than would be obtained by dose reduction, and offers theoretical advantages of reducing the emergence of resistant organisms and may increase concentrations in tissues that do not ordinarily have high drug concentrations. By reducing the number of doses, there may be significant cost savings (22): Standard preprepared doses can be used, and the time and supplies associated with administration costs are less with fewer doses. Less frequent dosing may permit nursing-home or home-antibiotic administration allowing earlier hospital discharge—always to be preferred in elderly patients.

Dosing guidelines are listed in Tables 1 and 2. If in doubt, it is safest to administer the higher dose initially and titrate down as the infection responds or the clinical situation is clarified.

7. ADVERSE EFFECTS

The elderly are well known to suffer greater consequences from drugs that have serious toxicities, such as hepatic, renal, hematologic, or neurologic adverse events.

Cephalosporins have a wide margin of safety—the only toxicity encountered with any frequency is drug allergy, and that is relatively uncommon as well. In addition, dose-related toxicity is quite uncommon, allowing greater latitude in empirical dosing. Table 3 lists reported adverse events with cephalosporins.

7.1. Hypersensitivity Reactions

Maculopapular rashes occurring after several days of therapy are the most frequently reported hypersensitivity reaction with cephalosporins, occurring in a few percentage of patients. Serious reactions, such as IgE-mediated bronchospasm, urticaria, and anaphylaxis, are very uncommon. Patients who are allergic to penicillins develop cross-hypersensitivity with first-generation cephalosporins at a frequency of <5–10%, and very rarely to never with higher-generation drugs. The likelihood of cross-reactivity appears to be related to the presence or absence of side chains. If it is absolutely necessary to use a cephalosporin in an older patient with a past history of a severe type 1 hypersensitivity reaction to penicillins, desensitization is prudent (23). Drug fever is a clinically perplexing complication that occurs with longer courses of therapy.

Table 3 Adverse Events with Cephalosporins

Hypersensitivity
  Maculopapular rash
  Pruritis
  Drug fever
  Serum sickness and toxic epidermal necrolysis
  Urticaria, anaphylaxis, and angioedema
Hematologic and hemostasis
  Impaired platelet aggregation
  Interference with vitamin-K dependent clotting factors
  Thrombocytopenia
  Eosinophilia
  Neutropenia (reversible)
  Hemolytic anemia
Nephrotoxicity
  Interstitial nephritis
GI/hepatobiliary
  Nausea and vomiting
  Cholelithiasis (ceftriaxone)
  Diarrhea and pseudomembranous colitis
  Transient increase in hepatic transaminases
Neurotoxicity
  Seizures
  Aseptic meningitis
Drug interactions
  Disulfiram reaction with alcohol (cephalosporins with NMTT side chain)
Local
  Pain injection (intramuscular or intravenous)

Abbreviation: NMTT, *N*-methylthiotetrazole.
Source: From Marshall W, Blair J. Mayo Clin Proc 1999; 74:187–195.

7.2. Bleeding and Coagulopathies

Many of the cephalosporins that have been most associated with bleeding and coagulopathies, such as moxalactam, cefoperazone, and cefamandole, are rarely used. All contain an NMTT side chain. The cephalosporins in common usage that contain an NMTT side chain include cefotetan, ceftriaxone, and cefepime. However, confusing the issue is the observation that other cephalosporins that do not have an NMTT side chain have also been associated with bleeding disorders. Possible mechanisms of coagulopathies are many: interference with intestinal synthesis of vitamin K_2, inhibition of hepatic carboxylation of vitamin K, irreversible inhibition of platelet function (moxalactam), thrombocytopenia, inhibition of fibrin polymerization, potentiation of warfarin effects, and eradication of vitamin K-producing bacterial flora in the gut (24).

It is clear that the elderly patient is at greater risk for the occurrence of coagulopathies—malnourished patients and those receiving vitamin K-deficient enteral/parenteral/oral feedings, which is typical of many older patients, appear to be at increased risk of bleeding disorders. Although rarely considered by physicians, such at-risk patients should receive vitamin supplementation when treated with cephalosporins. Patients receiving warfarin should have cephalosporins administered with caution, if at all.

7.3. Hematologic Reactions

Direct and/or indirect Coombs tests are occasionally positive for patients receiving cefamandole, cefoxitin, cephalexin, cephaloridine, cephalothin, and moxalactam. However, actual clinically significant hemolytic anemia is uncommon. Immune-mediated reversible thrombocytopenia has been rarely reported with cephalosporins, such as ceftriaxone and cefotaxime. Similarly, reversible neutropenia has occasionally been reported with high doses of cephalosporins or when prolonged courses are employed.

7.4. Nephrotoxicity

Cephalosporins are rarely associated with nephrotoxicity, except with cephaloridine—a cephalosporin no longer available in the United States. Modest reductions in renal function have been reported in patients with preexisting renal impairment, but in general it is not a concern with cephalosporin use in the elderly. Reversible interstitial nephritis very rarely occurs.

7.5. GI Effects

Symptoms with oral cephalosporins include nausea, vomiting, anorexia, and diarrhea—especially with doses in the higher range. Cefuroxime axetil and cefpodoxime proxetil, because they are prodrugs with variable absorption, cause more GI side effects than other oral cephalosporins. Diarrhea is more common with parenteral drugs that have hepatic/biliary excretion—cefoperazone and ceftriaxone. All cephalosporins, not surprisingly, have been associated with diarrhea and colitis due to *Clostridium difficile*, which is particularly hazardous in frail elderly patients.

7.6. Hepatobiliary

Clinically apparent hepatobiliary toxicity is rare. Ceftriaxone has been reported to produce pseudolithiasis, biliary sludge, and gallstones, but primarily in children. Whether aging is a risk factor for these biliary complications is unknown. Transient elevation of the hepatic transaminases and reversible hepatotoxicity may occur.

7.7. Neurological Effects

Patients of all ages with severe renal impairment who receive high doses of cephalosporins may have seizures. Other neurological side effects such as headache or paresthesias have been reported (24).

7.8. Thrombophlebitis and Pain with Intramuscular Injection

Intravenously administered cephalosporins may cause thrombophlebitis in a small percentage of patients or pain at the site of the intravenous catheter. Pain may occur with intramuscular injection, but in general appears to have been exaggerated as a complication. Most elderly patients tolerate intramuscular injections of cephalosporins without complaint; if it does occur, it may be lessened if lidocaine is combined in the syringe with the cephalosporin (25).

REFERENCES

1. Dunn G. Ceftizoxime and other third-generation cephalosporins: structure-activity relationships. Antimicrob Chemother 1982; 10(suppl C):1–10.
2. Yocum R, Rasmussin J, Strominger S. The mechanism of action of penicillin: penicillin aculates the active site of *Bacillus stearothermophilus* D-alanine carboxypeptidase. J Biol Chem 1980; 255:3977–3986.
3. Marshall W, Blair J. The cephalosporins. Mayo Clin Proc 1999; 74:187–195.
4. Pitout J, Sanders C, Sanders WJ. Antimicrobial resistance with focus on beta-lactam resistance in Gram-negative bacilli. Am J Med 1997; 103:51–59.
5. Utsui YT. Role of an altered penicillin-binding protein in methicillin- and cephem-resistant Staphylococcus aureus. Antimicrob Agents Chemother 1985; 28:397–403.
6. Hartman B, Tomasz A. Low affinity penicillin binding proteins associated with β-lactam resistance in *Staphylococcus aureus*. J Bacteriol 1984; 158:513–516.
7. Sanders C. Beta-lactamases of Gram-negative bacteria: new challenges for new drugs. Clin Infect Dis 1992; 14:1089–1099.
8. Sanders WJ, Sanders C. Inducible beta-lactamases: clinical and epidemiologic implications for use of newer cephalosporins. Rev Infect Dis 1988; 10:830–838.
9. Nikaido H, Nakae T. The outer membrane of Gram-negative bacteria. Adv Microb Physiol 1979; 20:163–250.
10. Karchmer A. Cephalosporins. In: Mandell G, Bennett J, Dolin R, eds. Practice and Principles of Infectious Disease. Philadelphia, Philadelphia: Churchill Livingstone, 2000: 274–291.
11. Patel I, Kaplan S. Pharmacokinetic profile of ceftriaxone in man. Am J Med 1984; 77(suppl 4C):17–25.
12. Cherubin C, Eng R, Norrby R, Modai J, Humbert G, Overturf G. Penetration of newer cephalosporins into cerebrospinal fluid. Rev Infect Dis 1989; 11:526–548.

13. Neu H, Fu K. Cefuroxime, a beta-lactamase-resistant cephalosporin with a broad spectrum of Gram-positive and -negative activity. Antimicrob Agents Chemother 1978; 13:657–664.
14. Schaad U, Suter S, Gianella-Borradori A, Pfenninger J, Auckenthaler R, Bernath O, Cheseaux JJ, Wedgwood J. A comparison of ceftriaxone and cefuroxime for the treatment of bacterial meningitis in children. N Engl J Med 1990; 322:141–147.
15. Birnbaum J, Stapley E, Miller A, Wallick H, Hendlin D, Woodruff H. Cefoxitin, a semisynthetic cephamycin: a microbiological overview. J Antimicrob Chemother 1978; 4(B):15–32.
16. Ward A, Richards D. Cefotetan. A review of its antibacterial activity, pharmacokinetic properties, and therapeutic use. Drugs 1985; 30:382–426.
17. Thornsberry C. Review of in vitro activity of third-generation cephalosporins and other newer beta-lactam antibiotics against clinically important bacteria. Am J Med 1985; 79(2A):14–20.
18. Neu H. Beta-Lactam antibiotics: structural relationships affecting in vitro activity and pharmacologic properties. Rev Infect Dis 1986; 8(suppl 3):S237–S259.
19. Garau J, Wilison W, Wood M, Carlet J. Fourth generation cephalosporins: a review of in vitro activity, pharmacokinetics, pharmcodynamics, and clinical utility. Clin Microbiol Infect 1997; 3(suppl 1):S87–S101.
20. McCue J, Tessler E. Cephalosporins. In: Yoshikawa T, Norman D, eds. Antimicrobial Therapy in the Elderly Patient. New York: Marcel Dekker, 1994:99–123.
21. Mandell L, Bartlett J, Dowell S, et al. Update of practice guidelines for the management of community-acquired pneumonia in immunocompetent adults. Clin Infect Dis 2003; 37:1405–1433.
22. McCue J. The Cost-Conscious Antibiotic Formulary: An Ideabook for Hospitals and Physicians. New York: Raven Health Care Communications, 1987.
23. Sanford J. Penicillin desensitization. J Crit Illn 1992; 7:791–795.
24. Fekety F. Safety of parenteral third generation cephalosporins. Am J Med 1990; 88(suppl 4A):38–44.
25. Schichor A, Bernstein B, Weinerman H, Fitzgerald J, Yordan E, Schechter N. Lidocaine as a diluent for ceftriaxone in the treatment of gonorrhea: does it reduce the pain of the injection? Arch Pediatr Adolesc Med 1994; 148:72–75.

SUGGESTED READING

Garau J, Wilison W, Wood M, Carlet J. Fourth generation cephalosporins: a review of in vitro activity, pharmacokinetics, pharmcodynamics, and clinical utility. Clin Microbiol Infect 1997; 3(suppl 1):S87–S101.
Karchmer A. Cephalosporins. In: Marchall G, Bennett J, Dolin R, eds. Practice and Principles of Infectious Disease. Philadelphia, Philadelphia: Churchill Livingstone, 2000:274–291.
Marshall W, Blair J. The cephalosporins. Mayo Clin Proc 1999; 74:187–195.

9

The Carbapenems

David R. P. Guay
*Department of Experimental and Clinical Pharmacology and Institute for the
Study of Geriatric Pharmacotherapy, University of Minnesota, College of Pharmacy and
Division of Geriatrics, HealthPartners Inc., Minneapolis, Minnesota, U.S.A.*

Key Points:

- Imipenem/cilastatin, meropenem, and ertapenem are not interchangeable agents (imipenem/cilastatin and meropenem compared with ertapenem have different in vitro activities against Gram-negative aerobes).
- Caution should be employed when contemplating the use of carbapenems in patients with preexisting seizures or other risk factors for seizures.
- The seizurogenic potential of imipenem/cilastatin is higher than those of meropenem and ertapenem.
- Imipenem/cilastatin and meropenem should be considered the carbapenems of choice for the empirical therapy of nosocomial infections and ertapenem for community-acquired infections.
- Carbapenems and penicillins/cephalosporins cross-react in allergic individuals (extent is unknown but may be up to one-third) and carbapenems should be avoided in individuals with anaphylactic/anaphylactoid or other immediate allergic reactions to other β-lactams.

1. INTRODUCTION

Imipenem, the first marketed carbapenem, is a synthetic derivative of the naturally occurring carbapenem thienamycin. Thienamycin was discovered in the 1970s during a large screening process as a product of *Streptomyces cattleyea*. The stable derivative of thienamycin, known as *N*-formimidoyl thienamycin or imipenem, possessed the necessary chemical stability without sacrificing the antibacterial activity of the parent compound. Unfortunately, imipenem proved to be chemically unstable during clinical trials. The drug proved to have an unexpectedly low and variable urinary recovery, due to the activity of a zinc-containing dipeptidase found in the brush border of the renal tubule, dehydropeptidase I (DHP-I). This phenomenon complicated the clinical development of the drug [especially for treatment of urinary tract infections (UTIs)], leading to a search for an inhibitor of DHP-I. The search ended successfully with the discovery of cilastatin, a very specific DHP-I inhibitor which has no relevant effects on physiologic peptides and does not interact with

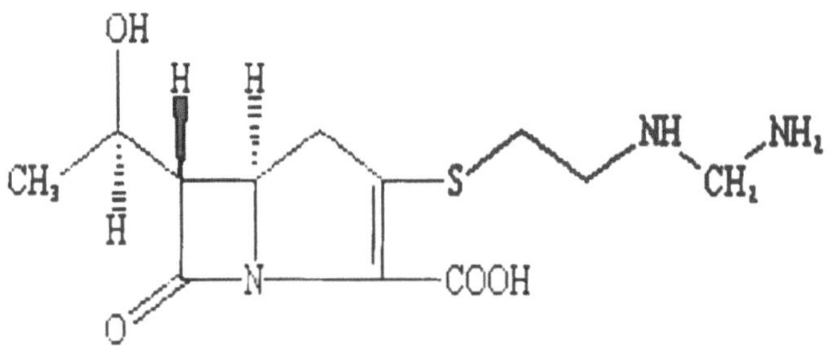

Figure 1 Chemical structure of imipenem.

imipenem. Development then continued with the imipenem/cilastatin combination (administered in equal amounts by weight). This culminated in the Food and Drug Administration approval of the drug in 1985 (1). This was followed by the discovery of other carbapenems, resulting in the approval of meropenem in 1996 and ertapenem in 2001. In contrast to imipenem/cilastatin, these newer agents are more stable to hydrolysis by DHP-I and do not require coadministration with a DHP-I inhibitor. This stability is the product of 1-β-methyl substitution.

Figure 1 illustrates the chemical structure of imipenem.

2. CHEMISTRY AND MECHANISM OF ACTION

The carbapenems are a unique class of antimicrobial agents that are structurally related to the penicillins and cephalosporins. They differ from the penicillins by the substitution of a carbon atom by a sulfur atom at the C-1 position and the addition of a C=C double bond in the five-membered ring. The marketed agents are small molecules, with molecular weights of 317.37 (imipenem), 437.52 (meropenem), and 497.50 (ertapenem).

Similar to other β-lactam antimicrobials, the carbapenems inhibit cell wall synthesis by binding to peptidases known as penicillin-binding proteins (PBPs), proteins involved in bacterial cell wall cross-linking and elongation. This usually results in cell lysis and death. These agents bind to several PBPs, which occurs more easily in gram-positive than Gram-negative organisms due to the differences in PBP location. Antimicrobials relatively easily traverse the peptidoglycan cell wall to access the cell surface PBPs of gram-positive organisms. In contrast, the periplasmic space location of PBPs in Gram-negative organisms is more difficult to access, although the molecular size and charge of the carbapenems allows them to use porin channels to do so (2–4).

3. ANTIMICROBIAL SPECTRUM

The carbapenems exhibit an unusually broad in vitro spectrum of activity (Tables 1 and 2) (2–7). These agents are active against most Gram-positive pathogens, including methicillin-susceptible staphylococci, *Streptococcus pyogenes*, *Streptococcus agalactiae*, and *Streptococcus pneumoniae* (although susceptibility to carbapenems falls as the degree of penicillin resistance increases for the latter). Most Enterobacteriaceae are susceptible to the carbapenems although minimum inhibitory concentrations (MICs) are higher in isolates producing extended-spectrum β-lactamases or AmpC β-lactamase. The common Gram-negative respiratory

Table 1 In Vitro Activity of Marketed Carbapenems

Organism	MIC_{90} values (mg/L)		
	Ertapenem	Imipenem	Meropenem
Gram-positive aerobes			
Methicillin sensitive			
Staphylococcus aureus	0.25–0.5	0.03–0.12	0.25
Methicillin sensitive			
S. epidermidis	0.5	0.06	0.5
Gram-negative aerobes			
Escherichia coli	0.016–0.03	0.25–0.5	<0.06
Klebsiella pneumoniae	0.016–0.06	0.5–1	0.06
Klebsiella oxytoca	0.016–0.03	0.5	0.06
Citrobacter species	0.016–0.25	1–2	≤0.06
Enterobacter aerogenes	0.25–1	1	0.13
Enterobacter cloacae	0.125–1	2	0.25
Acinetobacter baumannii	≥16	2–16	2
Morganella morganii	0.06	8	0.25
Proteus mirabilis	≤0.016–0.06	4–8	0.25
Proteus vulgaris	0.03–0.25	8	0.25
Serratia marcescens	0.12	2	0.25
Pseudomonas aeruginosa	≥16	8–16	4

Note: For pneumococci and anaerobes (Table 2). Data from studies evaluating at least 300 clinical isolates/study.
Abbreviations: MIC_{90}, minimum medium concentration inhibiting the growth of 90% of organisms.

pathogens (*Haemophilus influenzae* and *Moraxella catarrhalis*) are very susceptible as well. Gram-positive and -negative anaerobes, with a few exceptions, are readily inhibited by the carbapenems. Based on MIC_{90} values, imipenem is slightly more potent than meropenem and ertapenem against gram-positive pathogens while the converse is true for the Gram-negatives. These generalizations are made on the basis of pooling all in vitro activity studies although technically they should be made only on the basis of data from in vitro studies evaluating all three agents against the same isolate pools. The latter has only occurred in six published studies, evaluating activity against either pneumococci or anaerobes (Table 2).

Carbapenems are rapidly bactericidal in time-killing assays. The best surrogate marker for in vivo efficacy, as with the other β-lactams, is the proportion of the dosing interval over which the plasma/serum concentration exceeds the MIC. For carbapenems, therapeutic efficacy is generally achieved when this value exceeds 30% of the dosing interval (in contrast to the 50% reported for most β-lactams).

Relatively few microorganisms are intrinsically resistant to the carbapenems. These agents are not reliably active against methicillin-resistant *Staphylococcus aureus*. Enterococci, corynebacteria, *Stenotrophomonas maltophilia*, *Burkholderia cepacia*, and *Flavobacterium*, *Mycobacterium*, *Mycoplasma*, *Chlamydia*, and *Legionella* species are carbapenem resistant. In addition, ertapenem is inactive against *Pseudomonas aeruginosa*, *Acinetobacter* species, and highly penicillin-resistant pneumococci (in contrast to the other two agents) (2–7). Resistance can also develop during the therapy with these agents. Mechanisms include alterations in PBP, bacterial production of carbapenemases (a type of β-lactamase), impermeability which

Table 2 In Vitro Activity of Marketed Carbapenems from Published Studies in Which All Agents were Evaluated Against the Same Isolates

	MIC_{90} values (mg/L)		
Organism (No.)	Ertapenem	Imipenem	Meropenem
Aerobes			
Streptococcus pneumoniae			
Pen-sensitive (125)[1]	0.03	$\leq$0.008	0.016
Pen-intermediate (74)[1]	0.5	0.25	0.5
Pen-resistant (86)[1]	1	0.25	1
Pooled (102)[a,2]	2	0.5	1
Anaerobes			
Bacteroides fragilis group (442)[3,4]	2	1–2	0.5–1
B. fragilis (286)[3–5]	1–2	0.5–1	0.5–2
Bacteroides thetaiotaomicron (69)[3,4]	1–2	0.5–4	0.5–1
Porphyromonas spp. (10)[5]	0.062	0.062	0.062
Prevotella spp. (50)[5]	0.25	0.062	0.12
Prevotella bivia (30)[4]	0.5	0.06	0.125
Campylobacter gracilis (24)[5,6]	0.06–0.12	0.125–0.5	0.03–0.25
Fusobacterium nucleatum (24)[4,5]	0.062–2	0.06–0.12	0.062–1
Clostridium difficile (41)[4–6]	8	4–8	2–4
Clostridium perfringens (37)[4,5]	0.062–0.125	0.125	0.03–0.062
Peptostreptococci (93)[4–6]	0.12–1	0.06–0.5	0.062–0.5
Propionibacteria (21)[4]	0.5	0.03	0.5
Veillonella spp. (15)[6]	1	0.5	0.125

Note: Where studies had $\geq$10 isolates of the organism of interest, used a National Committee for Clinical Laboratory Standards-approved methodology, and used an inoculum of 10^4–10^6 organisms. For entries with multiple studies, data are the range.
[a]Twenty-six isolates were penicillin (pen)-sensitive, 33 isolates were pen-intermediate, and 43 isolates were pen-resistant.
Abbreviations: MIC_{90}, minimum medium concentration inhibiting the growth of 90% of organisms; Pen, penicillin.
Sources: 1. Antimicrob Agents Chemother 2002; 46:42–46. 2. Int J Antimicrob Agents 2002; 20:136–140. 3. Antimicrob Agents Chemother 2001; 45:2372–2374. 4. Antimicrob Agents Chemother 2002; 46: 220–224. 5. Antimicrob Agents Chemother 2000; 44:2222–2224. 6. Antimicrob Agents Chemother 2002; 46:1136–1140.

limits target site access, and efflux pumps which actively remove drug from the cell. However, the general resistance patterns of these agents have remained quite stable despite an excess of 15 years' use, with the exception of increasing resistance among nonfermentative Gram-negative bacilli. This resistance is generally mediated by acquired metallo-β-lactamases.

4. CLINICAL PHARMACOLOGY

4.1. Imipenem–Cilastatin

Parenteral administration is necessary as neither component is absorbed via the oral route. Imipenem bioavailability after intramuscular injection is approximately a mean of 60% compared with intravenous (IV) injection data. The time to peak plasma imipenem concentrations after intramuscular administration is ≈2 hr (2,5).

The degree of plasma protein binding of imipenem is the subject of controversy, with one study finding a value up to 20% and two studies finding values <10%. Imipenem penetrates reasonably well into colonic, lung, sinus, pancreatic, peritoneal, prostatic, and gynecologic tissues; bile; synovial, ascitic, and skin window fluids; and renal medullary and cortical tissues. Lower concentrations are found in tonsillar tissues, sputum, prostatic fluid, and cerebrospinal fluid (with inflamed meninges). Mean imipenem volumes of distribution range from 0.23 to 0.31 L/kg (2,5).

Imipenem is nearly completely eliminated by the renal route in the presence of cilastatin, a mean of 70% as the parent compound and 20% as an inactive metabolite. Renal handling involves both glomerular filtration and tubular secretion. Biliary excretion of parent compound is minimal, constituting less than a mean of 0.3% of the administered dose. Less than 1% of the dose is recovered as parent compound in the feces. The mean terminal disposition half-life of imipenem in the presence of normal renal function is $\approx$1 hr while mean renal and total body clearances are 0.15 and 0.20 L/hr/kg, respectively. Imipenem/cilastatin does not accumulate to a clinically significant degree upon repeated dosing. In addition, imipenem exhibits dose-independent pharmacokinetics (2,5).

The presence of renal impairment significantly reduces imipenem/cilastatin elimination, necessitating dose adjustment for reduced renal function. Although little change occurs in the volume of distribution as creatinine clearance falls, terminal disposition half-life and area under the serum concentration vs. time curve (and hence, total body clearance) of imipenem are significantly inversely correlated with creatinine clearance (e.g., mean terminal disposition half-life rises from 55 min in healthy volunteers to 173 min in hemodialysis patients on an off-dialysis day while area under the curve rises from 1073 to 4477 mg/L/min in corresponding populations). The inverse correlations of creatinine clearance with both imipenem renal and total body clearances are significant ($r = 0.88$ and 0.91, respectively). Hemodialysis readily clears both imipenem (80–90%) and cilastatin (40–60%), necessitating supplemental dosing. Extensive use in the critically ill has led to a large literature regarding the effects of slow hemodialysis, continuous arteriovenous hemofiltration, continuous arteriovenous hemodiafiltration, and intermittent hemofiltration on imipenem/cilastatin pharmacokinetics (2,5).

Several studies have evaluated the pharmacokinetics of imipenem/cilastatin in the elderly. In one study, six healthy elderly males (66–75 years old) received single and multiple (four times daily) 0.5 g IV doses. Pharmacokinetic parameters were similar to those noted in younger volunteers with mild renal insufficiency (day 1 mean $\pm$ standard deviation imipenem terminal disposition half-life 0.97 ± 0.18 hr, volume of distribution 0.24 ± 0.04 L/kg, total body clearance 175 ± 40 mL/hr/kg, renal clearance 94.8 ± 32.8 mL/hr/kg, and fraction renally eliminated unchanged 0.56 ± 0.13). Both total body and renal clearances of imipenem significantly correlated with creatinine clearance ($r = 0.80$ and 0.73, respectively) (8). Pharmacokinetic parameters were similar to those noted in younger volunteers with moderate renal impairment in a pharmacokinetic evaluation performed in six elderly patients treated for lower respiratory tract infection (creatinine clearances 31–80 mL/min, mean 51). Age did not correlate with any parameter, unlike the significant correlation of renal function with imipenem total body clearance and elimination rate constant (9).

Steady-state imipenem/cilastatin pharmacokinetics were evaluated after 0.5 g twice-daily intramuscular doses for 5–14 days in 13 elderly patients with various degrees of renal impairment. After stratifying by creatinine clearance (group I = 51–84 mL/min, group II = 20–50 mL/min, group III = <20 mL/min), peak and trough serum imipenem concentrations and area under the serum concentration vs. time curve were significantly higher in group III patients than those in groups I and II. Total body clearance in group III patients was significantly lower than that in group I patients (10). In a study of imipenem/cilastatin pharmacokinetics during high-dose therapy for serious infections involving 40 adults aged 21–83 years (32 received 4 g/day), imipenem total body clearance was significantly inversely correlated with age (11).

Other studies have evaluated the effect of disease states on the pharmacokinetics of imipenem/cilastatin (colonic surgery, complete obstruction of the common bile duct, lower respiratory tract infection, skin and skin-structure infection) (2,5).

4.2. Meropenem

Meropenem is not bioavailable by the oral route and must be administered parenterally. After intramuscular dosing, the time to peak plasma/serum concentration ranges from 0.2–2 hr after dosing. Compared with IV dosing, the mean intramuscular bioavailability is $94 \pm 8\%$. The peak plasma concentration after intramuscular administration is about 20% of that seen after IV bolus administration and 50% of that seen after IV infusion administration (3,6,7).

Steady-state volume of distribution ranges from 12.5 to 20.7 L and 15 to 20 L. Plasma protein binding is minimal (2%). Meropenem penetrates well into noninflammatory and inflammatory blister fluid (surrogates for interstitial fluid), with mean values compared to serum of 87% and 111%, respectively. Meropenem penetrates into a range of body tissue and fluid compartments. Penetration is adequate but not outstanding into lung, pleural, bronchial mucosa, intra-abdominal, skin, prostatic, and atrial tissues; peritoneal fluid; and sputum, with tissue or fluid to plasma concentration ratios generally ≤ 1.0 (3,6,7).

Metabolism constitutes a minor pathway of drug elimination, about 19–27% of total body clearance, with the main product being a ring-cleaved lactam generated by chemical hydrolysis in the plasma, kidney, and nonrenal organs. Renal excretion of parent compound ranges from 60% to 80% of the dose in healthy volunteers. Renal elimination involves both glomerular filtration and tubular secretion (as evidenced by studies with probenecid and renal clearance values exceeding that of creatinine clearance) (3,6,7).

Meropenem pharmacokinetics are slightly dose-nonproportional over the dose range of 250 to 1000 mg but this is clinically insignificant. The drug also does not accumulate to a clinically significant degree upon multiple dosing.

The presence of renal impairment significantly reduces meropenem elimination, necessitating dose adjustment for creatinine clearance values <50 mL/min. Although there is little change in peak plasma concentration or steady-state volume of distribution over the entire creatinine clearance range, terminal disposition half-life and area under the plasma concentration vs. time curve (and hence, total body clearance) are significantly inversely correlated with creatinine clearance (e.g., area under the plasma concentration vs. time curve rises from 28 mg/L/hr in healthy volunteers to 416 mg/ L/hr in anuric patients and terminal disposition half-life from 1.2 to >10 hr and 0.9 to 6.8 hr in corresponding populations). Nonrenal clearance as a percentage of total body clearance rises as renal clearance falls. Meropenem is readily cleared by hemodialysis (terminal disposition half-life is reduced from mean 7.0 to 2.9 hr). Thus, the regular dose should be administered after dialysis or a supplemental dose be given at that time. Due to the extensive use of meropenem in the critically ill patient population, a large volume of literature exists regarding the effect of veno-venous hemofiltration and hemodiafiltration on meropenem pharmacokinetics (3,6,7).

Hepatic disease has no significant effect on meropenem pharmacokinetics. The effect of aging on meropenem pharmacokinetics has been the focus of one study. This study compared meropenem pharmacokinetics in eight healthy elders (67–80 years old) and eight healthy young volunteers (20–34 years old). Terminal disposition half-life was significantly higher in the elders compared with the young (harmonic means of 1.27 and 0.81 hr, respectively) as was mean residence time (1.85 ± 0.29 hr and 1.22 ± 0.12 hr, respectively). Total body, renal, and nonrenal clearances were significantly lower in the elders compared with the young (139 ± 20 mL/min/1.73 m^2 vs. 203 ± 28 mL/min/1.73 m^2, respectively; 99 ± 13 mL/min/1.73 m^2 vs. 137 ± 25 mL/min/1.73 m^2, respectively; 39 ± 15 mL/min/1.73 m^2 vs. 66 ± 18 mL/min/1.73 m^2, respectively). Total body and renal clearances significantly correlated with creatinine clearance ($r = 0.94$ and 0.87, respectively). Most of these changes can be accounted for by the reduction in renal function with age (12).

Other studies have evaluated the effect of disease states on meropenem pharmacokinetics (ventilator-associated pneumonia, sepsis, respiratory tract infection, moderate-severe infections in surgical patients) (3,6,7).

4.3. Ertapenem

Ertapenem is not bioavailable by the oral route and must be administered parenterally. After intramuscular administration, the mean time to peak plasma concentration is ≈2.3 hr. Mean bioavailability by the intramuscular route is ≈90% compared with that after IV dosing (4).

Mean steady-state volume of distribution is ≈8.2 L. The plasma protein binding of ertapenem is extensive and concentration dependent. Binding falls from ≈95% (concentrations <100 mg/L) to 85% (concentrations of 300 mg/L). This results in the drug exhibiting nonlinear pharmacokinetics (vida infra). Few data are available regarding the tissue and body fluid penetration of ertapenem. Penetration into suction-induced blister fluid (a surrogate for noninflammatory interstitial fluid) approximates mean 61% (4).

Ertapenem is metabolized to a minor degree to an inactive ring-opened metabolite formed by hydrolysis of the β-lactam ring. Following IV administration in healthy volunteers, a mean of ≈80% of the dose is recovered in the urine and 10% in the feces. Of the 80% in the urine, 38% is parent compound and 37% is metabolite. The mean terminal disposition half-life and total body clearance are 4 hr and 1.8 L/hr, respectively, in healthy volunteers (4).

Area under the plasma concentration vs. time curve of ertapenem increases less than dose proportionally based on total drug concentrations over the dose range of 0.5–2 g while the converse occurs based on unbound concentrations. The concentration dependence of plasma protein binding probably accounts for this (4).

The effects of renal impairment on the pharmacokinetics of ertapenem have been studied in 26 adults, 31–80 years of age, encompassing a wide range of renal functional capacity. Following single 1 g IV doses, the mean unbound areas under the plasma concentration vs. time curve rose 1.5-, 2.3-, 4.4-, and 7.6-fold in patients with creatinine clearances (in mL/min) of 60–90, 31–59, 5–30, and <10 (on hemodialysis), respectively, compared with that in healthy volunteers (≥91 mL/min). The total area under the curve results had a similar pattern but were of a smaller magnitude. A 4 hr hemodialysis session cleared approximately mean 30% of the dose (4).

The effects of hepatic disease on ertapenem pharmacokinetics have not been evaluated but would not be expected to be substantial based on the mass balance data cited previously. Gender exerts no significant effect on drug pharmacokinetics (4).

One study has evaluated the pharmacokinetics of total and unbound ertapenem in healthy elderly volunteers, comparing the results with historic results obtained in healthy young volunteers under the same study conditions. Single and multiple 1 g IV doses (the latter being administered once daily for 7 days) were administered to eight males and six females at least 65 years old (mean age, 73 ± 5). Ertapenem pharmacokinetics were statistically indistinguishable by gender, allowing pooling of the data. Compared with historic data, total and unbound areas under the plasma concentration vs. time curve were 39% and 71% higher in the elders ($p < 0.0001$). Mean terminal disposition half-life was 5.1 hr in the elders and 3.8 hr in the historical younger subjects. Renal clearance was reduced by 30% (based on total drug) and 45% (based on unbound drug) in the elders, mirrored by the lower fractional excretion of parent compound in urine over 24 hr in elders (37%) compared with the historical younger subjects (44%). Of interest, nonrenal clearance was lower in the elderly, whether based on total drug (17%) or unbound drug (34%). As a result, total body clearance was lower in elders (26% based on total drug and 40% based on unbound drug). Ertapenem did not accumulate over time. The unbound fraction of drug was consistently higher in the elders (5–11%) compared with the historical young (5–8%). For example, at the end of drug infusion, the unbound fraction was significantly higher in the elders (11% vs. 8%, $p < 0.0001$) while the intergroup differences fell at the lower plasma concentrations observed at later time points. The results can be explained by the concentration dependence of plasma protein binding and the decline in renal function with advancing age (13).

5. CLINICAL INDICATIONS

Table 3 illustrates the microorganisms for which the carbapenems are either drugs-of-choice or among the alternatives (14). For few organisms are the carbapenems considered the drugs-of-choice.

Although there are clinical data supporting the efficacy of the carbapenems in community-acquired bacterial pneumonia, there are many other alternative agents available and guidelines do not support their general use. One potential exception is the use of intramuscular ertapenem in the initial treatment of nursing home-acquired bacterial pneumonia in patients who are not ill enough to require hospitalization but require parenteral therapy initially or patients with "Do Not Hospitalize" orders who would otherwise require hospitalization. Even in this case, there is much greater clinical experience with intramuscular ceftriaxone.

However, hospital-acquired bacterial pneumonia is frequently caused by Gram-negative bacilli that may be multiply antimicrobial resistant. Among numerous alternatives, a combination of aminoglycoside with either imipenem/cilastatin or meropenem as empirical therapy is reasonable. Due to the negligible activity of ertapenem against *Acinetobacter* species and *P. aeruginosa*, ertapenem should not be used empirically in treating hospital-acquired bacterial pneumonia.

Meningitis in the elderly is frequently caused by enteric Gram-negative bacilli. Meropenem monotherapy is a reasonable alternative for empirical therapy. Imipenem/cilastatin therapy should be avoided due to the elevated risk of seizures in these patients and the lack of *P. aeruginosa* and *Acinetobacter* species coverage makes empirical use of ertapenem difficult to justify.

Table 3 Indications for Carbapenems by Organism

Organism (infection)	Drug-of-choice	Alternative
Methicillin sensitive		
Staphylococcus aureus		X
Streptococcus pneumoniae		
(penicillin susceptible)		X
(penicillin high-level resistant)		Imipenem–cilastatin and meropenem
Bacillus cereus, subtilis		X
Clostridium perfringens		X
Bacteroides species		X
Campylobacter fetus	X	
Citrobacter freundii	X	
Enterobacter species	X	
Escherichia coli		X
Klebsiella pneumoniae		X
Proteus mirabilis		X
Indole-positive *Proteus*		X
Providencia stuartii		X
Serratia species	X	
Acinetobacter species	Imipenem/cilastatin and meropenem	
Aeromonas species		Imipenem/cilastatin and ertapenem
Burkholderia cepacia		Imipenem/cilastatin
Burkholderia mallei		Imipenem/cilastatin
Burkholderia pseudomallei	Imipenem/cilastatin	
Capnocytophaga canimorsus		X
Haemophilus influenzae (meningitis, arthritis, other serious infections; not upper respiratory infections or bronchitis)		Meropenem and ertapenem only (if meningitis) (otherwise X)
Pseudomonas aeruginosa		Imipenem/cilastatin and meropenem
Nocardia species		X
Rhodococcus equi	X	

Note: X, any carbapenem can be used.

In life-threatening sepsis, carbapenem therapy either alone or in combination with an aminoglycoside is one of the several alternatives for empirical therapy, especially if anaerobes are potentially involved (e.g., pelvic, intra-abdominal, or complicated skin and skin-structure infections). If microorganism acquisition in the hospital environment is suspected, ertapenem may be a poor choice of carbapenem due to its lack of activity against *P. aeruginosa* and *Acinetobacter* species.

Carbapenem monotherapy of community-acquired complicated skin and skin-structure infections (e.g., infected pressure ulcers, diabetic limb ulcers), intra-abdominal infections, and acute pelvic infections is one of several reasonable alternatives, based on their excellent activity against the most common pathogens of these infections.

Empirical carbapenem therapy of complicated UTIs requiring hospitalization is one of the many alternatives. Their use is more easily justified in the context of empirical therapy of serious nosocomial UTI, especially if associated with sepsis. Again, the caveat with ertapenem applies.

Table 4 illustrates the clinical studies of the carbapenems as conducted in predominantly or exclusively elderly (≥60 years old) patients. These studies made up fully one-quarter of the 101 efficacy/tolerability papers reviewed. Reviews of these data do not reveal any reason for concern regarding the use of these drugs in the elderly, from either an efficacy or a tolerability perspective.

6. DOSING AND ADMINISTRATION

Imipenem–cilistatin is available in 250 and 500 mg vials for preparation of doses for IV administration and 500 and 750 mg vials for preparation of doses for intramuscular administration (calculated on imipenem content). Two percent lidocaine should be used in reconstituting the vials for intramuscular dosing to reduce the pain of injection. For IV administration in mild, moderate, and severe infections, the usual dosage regimens are 250–500 mg four times daily, 500 mg three or four times daily to 1 g three times daily, and 500 mg four times daily to 1 g three or four times daily, respectively. For uncomplicated and complicated UTI, the usual IV dosage regimens are 250 mg four times daily and 500 mg four times daily, respectively. For intramuscular administration (in mild or moderate infections only), the usual dosage regimen is 500–750 mg twice daily. For intramuscular use in intra-abdominal infections, the usual dose is 750 mg twice daily. Dose adjustment is recommended when creatinine clearance is ≤70 mL/min (15).

Meropenem is available in 0.5 and 1 g vials for preparation of doses for IV administration. The usual dosage is 1 g thrice daily and dose adjustment is recommended when creatinine clearance is 50 mL/min or less (15).

Ertapenem is available in 1 g vials for preparation of IV and intramuscular doses. Doses for intramuscular administration should be reconstituted with 1% lidocaine to reduce the pain of injection. The usual dosage is 1 g once daily. Dosage adjustment is recommended when creatinine clearance is 30 mL/min or less. If ertapenem is administered within 6 hr of a hemodialysis session, a supplemental 150 mg dose should be administered at the end of dialysis (15).

7. ADVERSE EVENTS

The most common adverse effects seen with the carbapenems include reactions at the administration site (phlebitis, pain, erythema), rash, diarrhea, nausea/vomiting, headache, vaginitis, and elevated serum transaminase concentrations (2–7).

The tolerability of meropenem in the elderly and chronic renal failure subpopulations was evaluated using a pooled analysis of 843 elders (65 years and older) and 436 chronic renal failure (creatinine clearance <51 mL/min) patients participating in 26 phase 3 clinical trials (16). These trials compared meropenem 0.5–1 g thrice daily (or dose adjusted for renal function) to other antimicrobials in hospitalized patients (trials in pediatrics, meningitis, cystic fibrosis, and fever of unknown origin were excluded). The overall pattern and frequency of adverse events were similar in the elderly and nonelderly and chronic renal failure and nonchronic renal failure cohorts and to the comparators imipenem–cilastatin and injectable third-generation cephalosporins. Adverse event patterns/frequencies were similar in the <75- and

(text continued on p. 126)

Study design	Type of infection	N	Treatment regimens	Clinical results	Adverse ev
R	CAP	71	Mero 0.5 g tid × mean 10 days (range, 4–20)	At the end of treatment, clinical cure or improvement occurred in 89% of mero ($N = 64$) and 91% of imi–cil ($N = 66$) recipients. At the 2–4 weeks follow-up, a satisfactory response was seen in 100% of patients in both groups (mero $N = 36$, imi–cil $N = 32$); at the end of therapy, bacteriological eradication occurred in 100% of mero ($N = 8$) and 93% of imi–cil ($N = 14$) patients; at the 2–4 week follow-up, bacteriological eradication occurred in 100% of mero ($N = 6$) and imi–cil ($N = 5$) patients	Treatment-emerg events occurred mero and 11% patients (rash i cil patient, the were abnormal
		73	Imi–cil 1g bid × mean 9.7 days (range, 4–16)		
R	CAP	52	Mero 0.5 g tid × mean 8.7 days (range, 7–13)	At the end of treatment, clinical cure or improvement occurred in 87% (mero), 86% (imi–cil), 69% (clari + ceftriax) and 86% (clari + amik); at the end of treatment, bacteriological eradication occurred in 77% (mero $N = 26$), 71% (imi–cil $N = 24$), 61% (clari + ceftriax $N = 23$), and 77% (clari + amik $N = 26$); at 2–3 weeks posttherapy, clinical cure or improvement rates were 96, 100, 92, and 96%, respectively	Adverse events o three mero pati diarrhea, glossi each), three imi (dizziness in tw one), four clari patients (↑ AST three, ↓ leukoc three clari + am (↑ serum creati
		51	Imi–cil 0.5 g tid × mean 9.1 days (range, 8–14)		
		49	Clari 0.5 g bid + ceftriax 1 g bid × mean 12.8 days (range, 9–16)		
		49	Clari 0.5 g bid + amik 250 mg bid × mean 8.9 days (range, 7–14)		

Study design	Type of infection	N	Treatment regimens	Clinical results	Adverse
O	AECB	9	Mero 3 g qd IV × 7–10 days (outpatient)	Eight of nine clinically improved; bacteriological eradication occurred by day 6 of treatment in five of six in whom a pathogen was cultured	No mention wa: adverse events
R	Serious infections (82 CAP, 69 nosocomial P, 29 sepsis, 40 complicated UTI, 1 uncomplicated UTI, 8 SSSI)	116	Mero 1 g tid × mean 8.8 days	Clinical cure or improvement occurred in 93% CAP, 81% nosocomial P, 83% sepsis, 87% complicated UTI, 100% uncomplicated UTI, 100% SSSI with mero; corresponding values for clinical cure or improvement with ceftaz + amik were 79, 72, 94, 100,—, 60% (none of these intergroup differences were significant); bacteriological eradication occurred in 100% CAP, 71% nosocomial P, 100% sepsis, 56% complicated UTI, and 100% SSSI for mero; corresponding values for bacteriological eradication with ceftaz + amik were 87, 76, 100, 100, and 25%; the intergroup differences in bacteriological eradication rates were significant for CAP ($p = 0.038$) and complicated UTI ($p = 0.01$)	Adverse events 42% of mero ceftaz + amik (similar types, in the 2 group: emergent adve occurred in 2(and 11% of c(patients (mos↑ transaminas groups)
		121	Ceftaz 2 g tid + amik 15 mg/kg/d × mean 8.3 days		
R	Sepsis	61	Mero 0.5–1 g tid × mean 9.8 days	At the end of therapy, clinical cure/improvement occurred in 84%/8% mero and 87%/7% ceftaz ± amik patients; at the 2–4 week posttherapy follow-up, corresponding values were 97%/0% and 100%/0%;	Treatment-emer, events occurre mero and 15% ceftaz ± amik (similar types/ in the 2 group:

		70	Ceftaz 0.25–1 g tid or Ceftaz 2 g tid ± amik 15 mg/kg/day (× mean 9.6 days)	bacteriological eradication occurred in 100% of patients in both groups; one superinfection occurred in the mero group and one relapse in the ceftaz ± amik group.	
R	Serious (pneumonia in 41, intra-abdominal in 10, UTI in 11, sepsis in 7, other in 1; 18 bacteremic)	37 / 33	Mero 1 g tid × mean 7.5 days (range, 3–21) / Cefurox 1.5 g tid + gent 4 mg/kg/day × mean 7.4 days (range, 3–17) (could add metro 0.5 g qid if intra-abdominal)	Clinical cure or improvement at the end of treatment occurred in 70% (mero) and 73% (cefurox + gent) of patients (NS); deleting the UTI data, the corresponding rates were 74% and 75% (NS); at follow-up, the corresponding rates (all infections) were 78% and 64% (NS); bacteriological eradication occurred in 68% (mero) and 63% (cefurox + gent) of patients (NS); deleting the UTI data, the corresponding rates were 79% and 71% (NS)	Adverse events o◖ 49% of mero a◗ cefurox + gent ▮ (NS). Renal fai◗ occurred in 5% and 13% of cef◗ patients during therapy (NS)
R	VAP	69 / 71	Mero 1 g tid × mean ± SD, 9.3 ± 4.2 days / Ceftaz 2 g tid + amik 7.5 mg/kg bid × mean ± SD, 8.3 ± 4 days	By intent-to-treat analysis, clinical cure or improvement rates at the end of treatment were 68% (mero) and 55% (ceftaz + amik); by evaluable patient-only analysis, corresponding rates were 83% and 66% ($p = 0.044$); in this analysis, the corresponding rates at 2 weeks posttherapy follow-up were 90% and 84% (NS); bacteriological eradication rates were 75% (mero $N = 51$) and 53% (ceftaz + amik $N = 45$) ($p = 0.03$); superinfection occurred in 9% of mero and 5% of ceftaz + amik patients	Treatment-emerg◖ event rates wer◗ (mero) and 17% (ceftaz + amik)

Study design	Type of infection	N	Treatment regimens	Clinical results	Adverse
R	Serious (mostly sepsis and/or intra-abdominal)	68	Mero 1 g tid × mean ± SD, 6.6 ± 2.2 d	Clinical cure or improvement rates at the end of treatment were 93% (mero) and 92% (cefotax + metro) and at long-term follow-up of up to 8 weeks. later, 91% (mero) and 93% (cefotax + metro) (both NS); bacteriological eradication rates at the end of treatment were 86% (mero) and 88% (cefotax + metro) (NS)	Adverse event r (mero) and 2. (cefotax + me
		63	Cefotax 1 g tid + Metro 0.5 g tid × mean ± SD, 6.0 ± 2.0 days		
O	Serious infections (11 UTI, 3 LRTI, 6 SSSI, 3 IA, 3 misc.)	25	Imi–Cil 0.5 g qid × mean 11.1 days (range, 5–28)	Clinical cure or improvement occurred in 96% of 26 infection sites (in 24 patients); for individual infection types, rates were as follows: LRTI 100%, UTI 91%, SSSI 83%, IA 100%, misc. 67%	Adverse events 67% of patier 13; thromboc infusion phle N ± V and eo three each; ve and positive candidosis, a tachycardia/ one each)
O	Serious infections (primarily intra-abdominal)	19	Imi–cil up to 4 g/day (qid) × ≥5 days	Clinical cure or improvement occurred in 79% of patients; superinfection occurred in one patient	Nausea and dia occurred in t patient, respe
O	Mod. severe to severe infections (8 UTI, 6 LRTI, 6 sepsis, 1 peritonitis)	21	Imi–cil 0.25–3g/ day × median 6 days (range, 5–16)	Clinical cure was noted in 86% of patients and bacteriological eradication in 88% of pathogens; resistance and persistence occurred with two *Pseudomonas* species (*aeruginosa* and *fluorescens*)	Infusion phlebi four patients.

O	Pneumonia	21	Imi–cil 0.5–1 g qid × mean 9.2 days (range, 4–35)	Clinical cure in 95% and bacteriological eradication in 84% of patients	Pseudomembranou hypotension, inc seizure frequency in one patient ea
O	COPD with RTI	40	Imi–cil 0.5 g qid × mean ± SD, 6.3 ± 1.6 days (range, 5–11)	Ninety five percent improved clinically; the two nonresponders had *P. aeruginosa* as the pathogen (one isolate was sensitive and one was resistant to imi–cil after the end of therapy); bacteriological eradication occurred in 94% of patients; relapse occurred in two patients (*P. aeruginosa*, *H. influenzae*) and superinfection in one patient (*S. maltophilia*)	IV site phlebitis oc 50% of patients; adverse events in sleep disturbance patients, diarrhe thrush in two pa each, and pedal paresthesias and one patient each
O	Variety of infections (37 RTI, 18 UTI, 14 SSSI, 11 sepsis, 2 IA, 1 misc.)	83 (87 episodes)	Imi–cil 0.5–1 g tid–qid (duration not stated)	Clinical cure or improvement occurred in 88% of patients; bacteriological eradication occurred in 71% of pathogens; reinfection, colonization, and superinfection occurred in seven, eight, and two patients, respectively	Minor clinical adv possibly or prob related occurred patients; these in phlebitis at the i site, diarrhea, na dizziness, headac moniliasis most severe adverse ev occurred in two (cerebral ischemi seizure and strok patient each)

(

Study design	Type of infection	N	Treatment regimens	Clinical results	Adverse e
O	Variety of infections (44 sites: 17 SSSI, 11 UTI, 8 RTI, 5 B+J, 3 misc.)	39	Imi–cil 1–2 g/day (qid) (duration not stated)	Clinical cure occurred in 85% and improvement in 10% while bacteriological eradication occurred in 82% of patients; superinfection occurred in 5% and colonization in 15% during therapy; 8/11 (73%) colonizing pathogens were resistant to imi–cil	There was one c. diarrhea, IV si rash, and seizu
O	Serious infections in high-risk immunosuppressed patients	30	Imi–cil 1–3 g/day (bid–tid)× mean ± SD, 8.6 ± 3.1 days	Clinical cure and improvement occurred in 80% and 10% of patients, respectively; bacteriological eradication occurred in 83% of pathogens	No "important" events per auth
O	Severe infections in cancer patients	30	Imi–cil 2–4 g/day (bid–tid)× mean ± SD, 9.6 ± 2.1 days	Clinical cure occurred in 77% of patients and bacteriological eradication in 80% of pathogens	"No important a events" occurr authors; rash a occurred in on patients, respe
O	Variety of infections after failing other therapy (18 RTI, 9 IA, 8 UTI, 4 sepsis)	39	Imi–cil 0.5–1 g bid (duration not stated)	"Excellent" or "good" clinical outcomes occurred in 77% of patients (for 18 RTI, 56%; for 9 intra-abdominal infections, 89%; for 8 UTI, 100%; for 4 sepsis, 100%; $p < 0.01$); bacteriological eradication occurred in 44% of patients	"None noted" p

R	Acute bacterial peritonitis	19	Imi–cil 0.5 g qid × ≥5 days	Clinical cure or improvement occurred in 84% of imi–cil and 92% of amp + metro + gent patients (NS)	Adverse events o one patient in (infusion site r imi–cil and ras amp + metro +
		24	Amp 0.5 g qid + metro 0.5 g tid + gent 80 mg tid × ≥5 days		
R	Intra-abdominal infections	38	Imi–cil 0.5 g qid × mean 5 days (range, 5–8)	Treatment was successful in 71% of imi–cil and 64% of clinda + aztreo patients	Phlebitis due to antimicrobials 26% of imi–cil clinda + aztreo (NS); diarrhea vasculitis occu imi–cil patient transiently ↑ tr in three; transi creatinine occu clinda + aztreo
		42	Clinda 0.6 g tid + Aztreo 1 g tid × mean 5 d (range, 5–8)		
R, DB	Pneumonia	24	Cipro 400 mg tid × mean 11 days	Bacteriological eradication occurred in 71% of cipro and 67% of imi–cil patients (NS); at the end of therapy, clinical cure or improvement occurred in 71% of cipro and 67% of imi–cil patients while the corresponding values at 2 weeks after the end of therapy were 71% and 57%; most failures occurred due to the emergence of resistance in *P. aeruginosa* (resistance occurred in 42% of baseline isolates while on cipro and 78% of baseline isolates while on imi–cil)	No "significant" events were see either therapy
		21	Imi-Cil 1 g tid × mean 10 days		

Study design	Type of infection	N	Treatment regimens	Clinical results	Adverse
R, DB	Pneumonia	200	Imi–cil 1 g tid (duration not stated)	At 3–7 days after the end of treatment, clinical resolution occurred in 64% of cipro and 56% of imi–cil patients (NS); bacteriological eradication occurred in 66% of cipro and 57% of imi–cil patients (NS); bacteriological eradication occurred in 73% of pathogens with cipro and 66% with imi–cil; premature drug discontinuation due to failure occurred in 12% of cipro and 20% of imi–cil patients ($p = 0.032$)	Adverse events 65% of cipro imi–cil patien seizures occur cipro and 6% patients ($p = $
		202	Cipro 400 mg tid (duration not stated)		
R	Severe nosocomial pneumonia	41	Cipro 800–1200 mg/ d × mean ± SD, 9.3 ± 3.8 days	Clinical cure or improvement occurred in 71% (cipro) and 79% (imi–cil) of patients (NS); when *P. aeruginosa* was the causative agent, the corresponding rates were 71% (cipro $N = 14$) and 67% (imi–cil $N = 12$) (NS); bacteriological eradication occurred in 49% (cipro) and 50% (imi–cil) of patients (NS); resistant organisms developed in 7% of cipro and 33% of imi–cil patients (NS)	Possibly drug-re events occurr cipro and 12% patients (NS)
		34	Imi–cil 2–4 g/ day × mean ± SD, 10.1 ± 3.2 days		

| R, DB | CAP | 148 | Erta 1 g qd → PO agent × mean 12 days (range, 3–21) | At the end of parenteral therapy, clinical cure rates were 96% (erta) and 93% (ceftriax) (NS) and, 7 14 days after the end of therapy, 94% (erta) and 90% (ceftriax) (NS); similar results were found when the analysis was confined to subjects ≥75 years old; bacteriological eradication rates were 93% in both groups | Treatment-emerge adverse events in 16% of erta 22% of ceftriax treatment-emerg adverse events in 10% of erta 13% of ceftriax infusion site rea occurred in 6% 8% of ceftriax |
| | | 125 | Ceftriax 1 g qd → PO agent × mean 13 days (range, 1–21) | | |

dy populations were predominantly or exclusively over 60 years old (≥50%) or mean age was ≥60 years (overall or in all groups). Unless oth
tered by the IV route.

ndomized; CAP, community-acquired pneumonia; mero, meropenem; tid, thrice daily; imi–cil, imipenem–cilastatin; bid, twice daily; SD, stand
te exacerbation of chronic bronchitis; qd, once daily; cefotax, cefotaxime; metro, metronidazole; clari, clarithromycin; ceftriax, ceftriaxone; am
sminase; VAP, ventilator-associated pneumonia; ALT, alanine transaminase; ceftaz, ceftazidime; cipro, ciprofloxacin; ↓, decreased; NS, nc
nary tract infection; cefurox, cefuroxime; gent, gentamicin; qid, four times daily; DB, double-blind; erta, ertapenem; PO, oral; SSSI, skin and s
iratory tract infection; B + J, bone + joint; clind, clindamycin; aztreo, aztreonam; COPD, chronic obstructive pulmonary disease; LFTs, liver f
, intra-abdominal; N ± V, nausea with/without vomiting; IV, intravenous.

xp Clin Res 1999; 25:243–252. 2. J Chemother 2002; 14:609–617. 3. J Antimicrob Chemother 2000; 45:247–250. 4. J Antimicrob Chemother 1
timicrob Chemother 1995; 36(suppl A):179–189. 6. Antimicrob Agents Chemother 1998; 42:1233–1238. 7. J Chemother 2001; 13:70–81. 8.
:631–638. 9. Rev Infect Dis 1985; 7(suppl 3):S506–S512. 10. NZ Med J 1991; 104(904):22–23. 11. J Antimicrob Chemother 1986; 18(supp
Chemother 1995; 15:233–238. 13. J Antimicrob Chemother 1988; 21:107–112. 14. J Antimicrob Chemother 1988; 21:481–487. 15. Am
, Drugs Expt Clin Res 1989; 15:17–20. 17. Drugs Expt Clin Res 1990; 16:293–297. 18. Clin Ther 1991; 13:448–456. 19. Scand J Infect Di
nicrob Chemother 1993; 32:491–500. 21. Drugs 1995; 49(suppl 2):436–438. 22. Drugs 1995; 49(suppl 2):439–441. 23. Thorax 2000; 55:1033–
oc 2003; 51:1526–1532.

≥75-year-old cohorts and in the 0.5 and 1 g dose cohorts in elders without chronic renal failure. Even when patients with chronic renal failure were not dose-adjusted for renal function, there was no change in the pattern or frequency of events (unfortunately, this happened in 86% of cases). No evidence of nephrotoxicity or hepatotoxicity was noted. Only four seizures (0.1%) were felt to be related to meropenem to some degree (all four occurred in elders, two also having chronic renal failure), a pattern similar to those of the comparators mentioned previously.

An important issue in the potential use of intramuscular carbapenems in the treatment of infections in the long-term care setting is local tolerability. One of the reasons for the extensive use of intramuscular ceftriaxone in this setting (in lieu of hospitalization) is the good tolerability of this agent if reconstituted with lidocaine to reduce the pain of injection. A study was performed to compare the local tolerabilites of intramuscular ertapenem and intramuscular ceftriaxone, both reconstituted with lidocaine. Although not primarily an efficacy study, it was a double-blind, randomized study of ertapenem 1 g intramuscular daily vs. ceftriaxone 1 g intramuscular daily in the treatment of lower respiratory tract, skin and skin structure, and UTIs in adults. After 2 days, patients could be switched to oral therapy. The total study population was 117 patients (27% were ≥65 years old) (87 ertapenem, 30 ceftriaxone who received intramuscular therapy for mean 4.1 and 3.8 days, respectively). During treatment, local site reactions occurred in 36% of ertapenem and 43% of ceftriaxone recipients (most commonly, tenderness followed by pain) (not significant). Local symptoms were moderate to severe in 1% of ertapenem and 10% of ceftriaxone recipients (not significant). Mean serum creatine kinase concentrations at the end of intramuscular therapy were 205 ± 235 U/L in ertapenem and 383 ± 721 U/L in ceftriaxone recipients (17).

A major tolerability issue involving the use of imipenem–cilastatin but less so with the other two carbapenems is seizurogenic potential. Numerous case reports have described generalized tonic–clonic seizures occurring in imipenem–cilastatin recipients, frequently in elderly individuals receiving full doses (2–4 g/day) of drug. Other neurological reactions include flapping tremor and myoclonus. Population-based studies suggest that the seizure risk is about 1–2% in the general population. Known risk factors include preexisting central nervous system disease, preexisting seizure disorder, and abnormal renal function. Assiduous monitoring of recipients for the presence of risk factors and dose adjustments for renal impairment can reduce the seizure risk down to 0.2% (i.e., by 5- to 10-fold).

Cross-allergenicity exists between β-lactams and carbapenems. One case report documented two cases of cross-reactivity to cefotaxime and meropenem, leading to toxic epidermal necrolysis and death (18). In a case series of febrile bone marrow transplant patients with a history of penicillin allergy, the cross-reactivity rate was about 10% overall (7% in self-reported penicillin allergy, 33% in skin test or RAST-verified penicillin allergy) (19).

REFERENCES

1. Birnbaum J, Kahan FM, Kropp H, McDonald JS. Carbapenems, a new class of β-lactam antibiotics. Discovery and development of imipenem/cilastatin. Am J Med 1985; 78(suppl 6A):3–21.
2. Clissold SP, Todd PA, Campoli-Richards DM. Imipenem/cilastatin. A review of its antibacterial activity, pharmacokinetic properties and therapeutic efficacy. Drugs 1987; 33:183–241.

3. Wiseman LR, Wagstaff AJ, Brogden RN, Bryson HM. Meropenem: a review of its antibacterial activity, pharmacokinetic properties and clinical efficacy. Drugs 1995; 50:73–101.
4. Curran MP, Simpson D, Perry CM. Ertapenem. A review of its use in the management of bacterial infections. Drugs 2003; 63:1855–1878.
5. Balfour JA, Bryson HM, Brogden RN. Imipenem/cilastatin. An update of its antibacterial activity, pharmacokinetics, and therapeutic efficacy in the treatment of serious infections. Drugs 1996; 51:99–136.
6. Lowe MN, Lamb HM. Meropenem. An updated review of its use in the management of intra-abdominal infections. Drugs 2000; 60:619–646.
7. Hurst M, Lamb HM. Meropenem: a review of its use in patients in intensive care. Drugs 2000; 59:653–680.
8. Toon S, Hopkins KJ, Garstang FM, Aarons L, Rowland M. Pharmacokinetics of imipenem and cilastatin after their simultaneous administration to the elderly. Br J Clin Pharmacol 1987; 23:143–149.
9. Finch RG, Craddock C, Kelly J, Deaney NB. Pharmacokinetic studies of imipenem/cilastatin in elderly patients. J Antimicrob Chemother 1986; 18(suppl E):103–107.
10. Pietroski NA, Graziani AL, Lawson LA, Bland JA, Rogers JD, MacGregor RR. Steady-state pharmacokinetics of intramuscular imipenem-cilastatin in elderly patients with various degrees of renal function. Antimicrob Agents Chemother 1991; 35:972–975.
11. MacGregor RR, Gibson GA, Bland JA. Imipenem pharmacokinetics and body fluid concentrations in patients receiving high-dose treatment for serious infections. Antimicrob Agents Chemother 1986; 29:188–192.
12. Ljungberg B, Nilsson-Ehle I. Pharmacokinetics of meropenem and its metabolite in young and elderly healthy men. Antimicrob Agents Chemother 1992; 36:1437–1440.
13. Musson DG, Majumdar A, Holland S, Birk K, Xi L, Mistry G, Sciberras D, Muckow J, Deutsch P, Rogers JD. Pharmacokinetics of total and unbound ertapenem in healthy elderly subjects. Antimicrob Agents Chemother 2004; 48:521–524.
14. Anonymous. The choice of antibacterial drugs. Med Lett Drugs Ther 2001; 43:69–78.
15. Anonymous. Drug Facts and Comparisons. St. Louis, Facts and Comparisons (Wolters Kluwer).
16. Cunha BA. Meropenem in elderly and renally impaired patients. Int J Antimicrob Agents 1999; 11:167–177.
17. Legua P, Lema J, Moll J, Jiang Q, Woods G, Friedland I. Safety and local tolerability of intramuscularly administered ertapenem diluted in lidocaine: a prospective, randomized, double-blind study versus intramuscular ceftriaxone. Clin Ther 2002; 24:434–444.
18. Paquet P, Jacob E, Damas P, Pierard GE. Recurrent fatal drug-induced toxic epidermal necrolysis (Lyell's syndrome) after putative beta-lactam cross reactivity: case report and scrutiny of antibiotic imputability. Crit Care Med 2002; 30:2580–2583.
19. McConnell SA, Penzak SR, Warmack TS, Anaissie EJ, Gubbins PO. Incidence of imipenem hypersensitivity reactions in febrile neutropenic bone marrow transplant patients with a history of penicillin allergy. Clin Infect Dis 2000; 31:1512–1514.

SUGGESTED READING

Balfour JA, Bryson HM, Brogden RN. Imipenem/cilastatin. An update of its antibacterial activity, pharmacokinetics, and therapeutic efficacy in the treatment of serious infections. Drugs 1996; 51:99–136.
Curran MP, Simpson D, Perry CM. Ertapenem. A review of its use in the management of bacterial infections. Drugs 2003; 63:1855–1878.
Hurst M, Lamb HM. Meropenem: a review of its use in patients in intensive care. Drugs 2000; 59:653–680.
Lowe MN, Lamb HM. Meropenem. An updated review of its use in the management of intra-abdominal infections. Drugs 2000; 60:619–646.

10
Monobactams

Jay P. Rho
Kaiser Foundation Hospital, Los Angeles, California, U.S.A.

Key Points:

- Aztreonam is a monobactam antibiotic with considerable β-lactamase stability.
- Aztreonam has a narrow spectrum of activity, limited primarily to Gram-negative bacilli.
- Aztreonam should be used in combination with other agents when polymicrobial infection is suspected.
- Aztreonam is well tolerated without major renal toxicity or ototoxicity.
- Aztreonam is weakly immunogenic and can be used with caution in patients with β-lactam hypersensitivity.

1. INTRODUCTION

The monobactams are unique monocyclic β-lactam antibiotic compounds that have been discovered in various soil bacteria. Naturally occurring monobactams have been isolated from *Chromobacterium violaceum* but show generally weak antibacterial activity due to enzymatic inactivation. Synthetic monobactams, such as aztreonam, contain a 3-aminomonobactamic acid (3-AMA) nucleus that provides protection against hydrolytic activation, resulting in enhanced spectra of activity and antimicrobial potency. Although additional monobactams [i.e., carumonam (1), tigemonam (2)] are under investigation, the only commercially marketed monobactam is aztreonam. Similar to the aminoglycosides, aztreonam has a purely Gram-negative aerobic spectrum. However, aztreonam is better tolerated than aminoglycosides, demonstrating no major renal toxicity or ototoxic potential. Because of this feature, aztreonam is often prescribed in geriatric patients in lieu of aminoglycosides. Another benefit associated with aztreonam is its weak immunogenicity, allowing its use in patients with penicillin hypersensitivity reactions.

Approved indications for aztreonam include infections of the urinary tract, lower respiratory tract, skin and skin structure, and intra-abdominal and gynecological logical organs, as well as septicemia caused by susceptible microorganisms. In polymicrobial infections or when used for empirical therapy, aztreonam must be given in combination with other antimicrobial agents that are active against Gram-positive and anaerobic species.

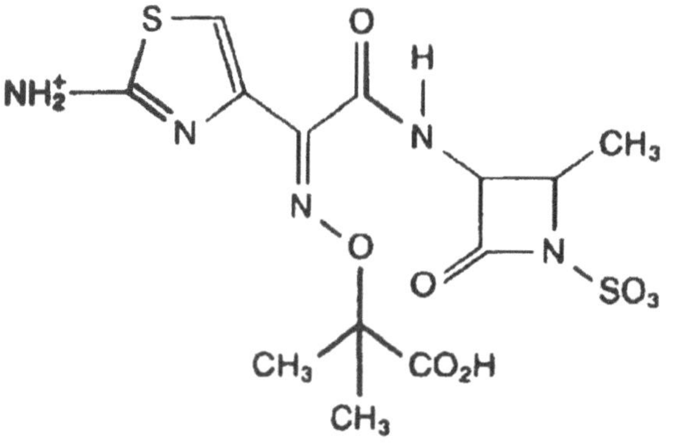

Figure 1 Chemical structure of aztreonam.

2. CHEMISTRY

Aztreonam is a synthetic monocyclic β-lactam antibiotic (Fig. 1) that contains a 3-AMA nucleus. The addition of various substituents on the 3-AMA nucleus results in monobactam derivatives that differ in spectra of activity, antimicrobial potency, and stability against hydrolysis by β-lactamases. Aztreonam contains a sulfonic acid group on the nitrogen at the 1-position of the 3-AMA nucleus, which activates the β-lactam moiety, an aminothiazolyl oxime side chain in the 3 position and a methyl group in the 4-position that confers the specific antibacterial spectrum and β-lactamase stability.

Aztreonam is generally stable against hydrolysis by β-lactamases classified as Richmond–Sykes types I, III (TEM-1, TEM-2, SHV-1), and V (PSE and OXA types). However, aztreonam can be hydrolyzed by a chromosomally mediated Richmond–Sykes type IV enzyme K1 produced by some *Klebsiella* species and Richmond–Sykes type V enzyme PSE-2 produced by some species of *Pseudomonas aeruginosa*. The drug does not induce production of β-lactamases in *Pseudomonas*, *Citrobacter*, *Enterobacter*, or *Serratia* species (3) and generally is a weak inducer of chromosomally mediated β-lactamases (4).

3. MECHANISM OF ACTION

The mode of action of aztreonam resembles that of cephalosporins and penicillins by inhibiting mucopeptide synthesis in the bacterial cell wall. Aztreonam has a high affinity for and preferentially binds to penicillin-binding protein (PBP) 3, with complete binding at 0.1 μg/mL of susceptible Gram-negative bacteria (5). The drug also has moderate affinity for PBP 1a of these bacteria, but little or no affinity for PBPs 1b, 2, 4, 5, or 6, with complete binding at ≥ 100 μg/mL. Because PBP 3 is involved in septation, aztreonam causes the formation of abnormally elongated or filamentous forms in susceptible Gram-negative bacteria. As a consequence, cell division is inhibited and breakage of the cell wall occurs, resulting in lysis and death. Aztreonam has poor binding affinity to the PBP of gram-positive bacteria and anaerobic bacteria (5).

4. ANTIMICROBIAL SPECTRUM

The in vitro spectrum of activity of aztreonam includes most Gram-negative bacilli. The drug has been shown to be active in vitro against most strains of *Citrobacter* species, including *Citrobacter freundii*, *Enterobacter* species, including *Enterobacter cloacae*, *Escherichia coli*, *Haemophilus influenzae*, *Klebsiella oxytoca*, *Klebsiella pneumoniae*, *Proteus mirabilis*, *Proteus aeruginosa*, *Serratia* species, including *Serratia marcescens*.

Most strains of Enterobacteriaceae are inhibited at concentrations of $<1\mu g/mL$ (6); however, *C. freundii*, *Enterobacter aerogenes*, and *E. cloacae* are sometimes resistant to aztreonam, as they are to cefotaxime and ceftazidime (7,8). Enterobacteriaceae are killed at concentrations of two to four times the minimum inhibitory concentration (MIC). Aztreonam reportedly kills *P. aeruginosa* at 4–16 times the MIC with MICs ranging from $4–50\mu g/mL$ (6). All *Neisseria meningitidis* and *Neisseria gonorrhoea* organisms are inhibited at $0.03–0.06\mu g/mL$, including penicillinase-producing gonorrhea (9). β-lactamase- and β-lactamase-producing strains of *H. influenzae* are inhibited by $0.03–0.25\mu g/mL$ of aztreonam (6).

Aztreonam exhibits in vitro MICs of $8\mu g/mL$ or less against most strains of *Aeromonas hydrophilia*, *Morganella morganii*, *N. gonorrhoeae*, *Pasteurella multocida*, *Proteus vulgaris*, *Providencia stuartii*, *Providencia rettgeri*, and *Yersinia enterocolitica* (6).

Limited activity has been noted against strains of *Acinetobacter*, *Alcaligenes*, *Flavobacterium*, *Pseudomonas fluorescens*, and *Stenotrophomonas maltophilia* (6). Synergy may be demonstrated with aminoglycosides in vitro in 30–60% of Gram-negative organisms tested; however, the drug has not been shown to produce synergy with other β-lactam agents (10–13). Antagonism between aztreonam and other β-lactam drugs has also been demonstrated. For example, cefoxitin antagonizes the activity of aztreonam against *Enterobacter* species; this antagonism probably relates to the cefoxitin-induced production of β-lactamase (10,11).

Aztreonam has little or no activity against gram-positive aerobic bacteria or against anaerobic bacteria. Aztreonam is inactive against *Chlamydia*, *Mycoplasma*, fungi, and viruses (6).

5. CLINICAL PHARMACOLOGY

Aztreonam may be administered intramuscularly or intravenously. Aztreonam exhibits linear, dose-independent pharmacokinetics. After a 30 min intravenous (IV) infusion of 500 mg, 1 g, and 2 g doses in healthy subjects, mean peak serum concentrations of 54, 90, and $204\mu g/mL$, respectively, have been recorded. Eight-hour concentrations average 1, 3, and $6\mu g/mL$, respectively (14,15). Aztreonam is widely distributed into body tissues and fluids including skeletal muscle, adipose tissue, skin, bone, gallbladder, liver, lungs, kidneys, atrial appendage, intestines, prostatic tissue, myometrium, endometrium, fallopian tubes, ovaries, and cervical and vaginal tissue. Aztreonam is also distributed into saliva, sputum, bronchial secretions, aqueous humor, bile, pericardial, pleural, peritoneal, synovial, and blister fluids (15). Aztreonam is distributed into cerebrospinal fluid (CSF) following IV administration. CSF concentrations are generally higher in patients with inflamed meninges. In patients with uninflamed meninges, a 2 g dose of aztreonam produces concentrations of 0.5 and $1\mu g/mL$ in the CSF at 1 and 4 hr, respectively, compared with mean CSF levels of 2 and $3.2\mu g/mL$, respectively, when administered to patients with inflamed meninges (16,17). Protein binding has been measured at 56–71% (18). In biliary T-tube studies, Martinez and associates (19) found less than 1% of the total dose in the bile.

Aztreonam is partially metabolized to several microbiologically inactive metabolites. The elimination half-life in patients with normal renal function and hepatic function is 1.5–2.1 hr (18). The elimination half-life is slightly longer in geriatric adults than in younger adults and ranges from 1.7 to 4.3 hr in adults 64–82 years of age. Urinary excretion of unchanged drug via glomerular filtration and tubular secretion is the primary route of elimination. In adults with normal renal function, urinary concentrations reached 250–330 μg/mL and 710–720 μg/mL, 4–6 hr after IV administration of single 0.5 and 1 g doses, respectively. The elimination half-life of aztreonam in anephric patients is 6–8 hr (20). The elimination half-life during hemodialysis may decrease to 2.7 hr; approximately, 38% of an administered dose may be cleared during an average hemodialysis. Aztreonam is removed by hemodialysis; therefore, administration of a small supplementary dose of aztreonam after dialysis is recommended. The drug is cleared much more slowly by peritoneal dialysis (21).

In seriously ill patients, especially those with *P. aeruginosa* infection, a dosage of 2 g every 6–8 hr has been suggested. Otherwise, the recommended dosage is 1 g every 8 hr for patients with normal renal function. Urinary infections caused by Gram-negative bacteria may be treated by intramuscular administration of 500 mg once or twice daily. Organisms with an MIC of 8 μg/mL or less are considered susceptible, whereas those with an MIC of 32 μg/mL or more are resistant.

6. CLINICAL INDICATIONS

The narrow Gram-negative aerobic spectrum of aztreonam limits its use as a single agent for empirical therapy for potential polymicrobial infections. Aztreonam has Food and Drug Administration (FDA) approved indications for the treatment of urinary tract infections (UTIs), lower respiratory tract infections (LRTIs), septicemia, skin and skin-structure infections, intra-abdominal infections, and gynecologic infections caused by susceptible Gram-negative microorganisims. Although not FDA-approved, aztreonam has also been shown to be effective in the treatment of infections in bone and joints (22), cystic fibrosis (23), digestive tract decontamination (24), and febrile neutropenia (25), as well as therapy for gonorrhea (26), meningitis (27), peritonitis (28), surgical prophylaxis (29), and traveler's diarrhea (30).

6.1. Urinary Tract Infections

Aztreonam can be used as a single agent for treatment of complicated UTIs, including pyelonephritis and initial and recurrent cystitis, caused by Enterobacteriaceae, *P. aeruginosa*, and *Providencia* (31,32). In controlled studies in men and women with UTIs, aztreonam was shown to be at least as effective as aminoglycosides or a parenteral cephalosporin over a 5–14-day course.

Swabb et al. (33) reported the summary results of worldwide clinical trials of aztreonam in patients with UTIs. Aztreonam was administered to a total of 681 patients with UTIs due to susceptible Gram-negative bacteria; 56 patients received a single 1 g intramuscular dose for acute uncomplicated cystitis, and 625 patients received multiple parenteral doses (usually a 5-day course of 1 g two or three times daily) for a variety of UTIs, including pyelonephritis, cystitis, prostatitis, and epididymitis. Microbiologic cure was achieved in 84% of patients in the single-dose study and in 85% of patients in the multiple-dose studies. In the latter studies the microbiologic cure rates for infections with *E. coli*, the *Klebsiella–Enterobacter–Serratia* group, and *P. aeruginosa* were 87%, 90%, and 76%, respectively.

Childs et al. (31) assessed the possible advantages of the monobactam antibiotic aztreonam in the treatment of hospital-acquired UTI in a study comparing aztreonam (0.5–1 g twice daily or three times daily) to cefamandole (1 g three times daily) in 159 patients. Initial pathogens were eradicated in 91.7% of the patients of the aztreonam group who were treated three times daily, in 82.7% of the group treated twice daily, and in 78.3% of the patients receiving cefamandole. Enterococci was most commonly responsible for reinfection and superinfection in the aztreonam groups, whereas *P. aeruginosa* was most commonly responsible in the cefamandole group. In a subset study, 35 patients infected with multidrug-resistant organisms were treated with aztreonam 1–6 g per day for 8 days. The overall cure rates were 93% for *Pseudomonas* infections, 87.5% for *E. coli* infections, and 100% for other pathogens.

Cox et al. (32) administered aztreonam to 145 consecutive patients with complicated UTIs caused by multidrug-resistant, aztreonam-sensitive bacteria. Multidrug resistance was defined by disk diffusion testing as resistance to aminopenicillins and to first- and second-generation cephalosporins, with or without resistance to aminoglycosides. The first 40 assessable patients received 1 g of aztreonam intravenously three times daily for a median period of 8 days; the remaining 95 assessable patients received 0.5 g twice daily for a median period of 9 days. Fifty-five patients were infected with *P. aeruginosa*, 24 with *E. coli*, 18 with *S. marcescens*, 13 with *M. morganii*, 12 with *P. rettgeri*, and 10 with *Enterobacter* species. Bacteriologic cure rates were 98% for the group given 3 g daily and 96% for that given 1 g daily. Minimal and transient adverse reactions occurred with both dosages.

6.2. Lower Respiratory Tract Infections

Aztreonam is used for the treatment of LRTIs, including pneumonia, bronchitis, or lung abscess, caused by susceptible Gram-negative microorganisms such as *E. coli*, *K. pneumoniae*, *H. influenzae*, *P. mirabilis*, *Enterobacter* species, and *S. marcescens*. Because LRTIs are commonly caused by mixed flora, including gram-positive and anaerobic bacteria, the American Thoracic Society has suggested aztreonam be combined with other antimicrobial agents (e.g., clindamycin) as initial empirical treatment until the causative organism (or organisms) has been determined in patients who are seriously ill or at risk for Gram-positive or anaerobic infections. Gram-negative pneumonia has been shown to respond to the combination of aztreonam and clindamycin as effectively as the combination of tobramycin and clindamycin. Rodriguez et al. reported the safe and effective use of an aztreonam–clindamycin combination for the treatment of LRTIs caused by aerobic Gram-negative bacilli when the organisms are susceptible (34). A total of 80 patients were randomized to receive either aztreonam–clindamycin or tobramycin–clindamycin for the treatment of LRTIs caused by Gram-negative bacilli. The most common pathogens isolated from the patients were *K. pneumoniae*, *E. coli*, and *P. aeruginosa*. All of the isolated organisms were susceptible to both tested antibiotics, except for a strain of *Pseudomonas cepacia* resistant to both tested antimicrobial agents and a strain of *E. aerogenes* and one of *P. aeruginosa* that were resistant to aztreonam. A total of 53 patients were randomized to receive aztreonam–clindamycin; of these, 46 were clinically evaluable and 39 were bacteriologically evaluable. Of the 46 clinically evaluable patients, 41 were considered cured, 3 failed to be cured, and 2 died during the study period of unrelated causes. Of the 39 bacteriologically evaluable patients, 36 were considered cured and 3 failed to be cured. A total of 26 clinically evaluable patients were randomized to receive tobramycin–clindamycin, of which 22 patients were considered cured, 3 failed to be cured, and 1 died of unrelated causes during the study period. There were 18 bacteriologically evaluable patients in the tobramycin–clindamycin group; 17 were cured and 1 failed to be cured. Transient abnormal renal function tests were noted in 7.7% of the patients randomized to receive tobramycin–clindamycin while none were observed in the patients randomized to receive aztreonam–clindamycin.

Rivera-Vazquez et al. (35) reported on 110 patients randomized to receive one of the following antibiotic combinations: aztreonam + clindamycin, tobramycin + clindamycin, or amikacin + mezlocillin for the treatment of LRTIs caused by Gram-negative bacilli, most commonly *K. pneumoniae*, *E. coli*, and *P. aeruginosa*. Of the 68 patients who received aztreonam + clindamycin, 60 were clinically evaluable and 50 were bacteriologically evaluable. Of the 60 clinically evaluable patients, 54 were cured and 5 were treatment failures or died during the study period. Of the 50 bacteriologically evaluable patients, 46 were cured and 3 failed to respond to therapy. Of the 26 clinically evaluable patients in the tobramycin + clindamycin group, 22 were cured and 4 either failed to respond or died during the study period. Of the 18 bacteriologically evaluable patients in this group, 16 were cured and 2 failed to respond. In the amikacin + mezlocillin group, 14 of the 15 clinically and bacteriologically evaluable patients were cured, and 1 failed to respond. The very few adverse drug reactions that were seen were transient and comparable in all three groups except for renal function parameters, which deteriorated in 6–8% of patients receiving the aminoglycoside combination. All three antibiotic combinations were similar in effectiveness and safety.

6.3. Septicemia

Scully and Henry (36) reported the efficacy of aztreonam in the treatment of Gram-negative bacteremia in 101 patients. Each patient was treated with aztreonam 1–8 g daily for 5–34 days (mean, 12 days). Thirty-four patients also received a second antibiotic for suspected or documented gram-positive or anaerobic infection. The sources of bacteremia were the urinary tract (50 patients), an intra-abdominal site (17), the respiratory tract (8), an intravascular site (9), and an unknown site (17). The clinical response was 92% (91 of 99 evaluable patients). The bacteriologic response rate was 97% (98 of 101 patients), including six of seven patients with *P. aeruginosa* bacteremia. Superinfection with gram-positive cocci or *Candida* species occurred in 12 patients and 1 patient developed diarrhea associated with *Clostridium difficile*. No other serious adverse effects were noted.

McKellar (37) reported the use of aztreonam for the treatment of 26 serious infections due to Gram-negative bacteria in 23 patients: nine cases of bacteremia, one of infective endocarditis, one of pneumonia, one of septic arthritis, six of osteomyelitis, five of abscess or soft tissue infection, and three of meningitis. The majority of patients had serious underlying disease, and 18 were in critical or poor condition. The mean age of the patients was 62 years, and the mean duration of therapy was

19 days. The clinical condition of all 23 patients improved during therapy; 20 infections were cured according to clinical criteria. Three of the six instances of therapy failure were due to inadequate debridement. No superinfections, resistant pathogens, or significant adverse reactions were seen.

6.4. Skin and Skin-Structure Infections

Winner et al. (38) reported a case of an 81-year-old man admitted with severe cellulitis of the left arm and bacteremia due to *P. multocida* successfully treated with aztreonam. The patient demonstrated a complete resolution of the infection after 14 days of treatment.

6.5. Intra-abdominal Infections

Henry (39) summarized the overall results of a multiclinic study of 113 patients with intra-abdominal infections due to Gram-negative aerobic organisms. Appropriate therapy with an antibiotic (usually clindamycin) active against Gram-positive or anaerobic organisms was administered concomitantly with aztreonam for mixed-pathogen infections. A favorable clinical response and microbiologic cure occurred in 90% of the patients treated. All of the 13 patients with infections due to *P. aeruginosa* responded clinically, and 11 of the 13 patients experienced microbiologic cure. In a comparative study, 59 patients were treated with aztreonam and 56 were treated with tobramycin (3–5 mg/kg/day); 95% of the patients in the aztreonam group and 81% of those in the tobramycin group experienced microbiologic cure.

Birolini (40) reported the activity of aztreonam in hospitalized patients with severe intra-abdominal infections due to Gram-negative pathogens, either alone or in association with other bacteria. Of a total study population of 156 patients, 76 were assigned to treatment with aztreonam + clindamycin, and the remaining 80 were treated with tobramycin + clindamycin. Patients underwent a variety of surgical procedures involving the peritoneal cavity. The efficacy of two treatment groups was considered equal with satisfactory results reported in 86.8% for the patients in the aztreonam-treated group and 86.2% for the tobramycin-treated patients. Among the patients who had a poor therapeutic result, Gram-negative bacteria, either alone or associated with gram-positive pathogens, were considered responsible for 50% of the infections in the aztreonam group; the percentage increased to 82% among those treated with tobramycin.

6.6. Gynecologic Infections

Henry (41) summarized the effectiveness of aztreonam in 73 women with gynecologic infections (primarily endometritis and pelvic inflammatory disease). Each of the women were randomized to receive aztreonam + clindamycin or a control regimen. For 72 of the 73 women, a microbiologic cure and a satisfactory clinical response were achieved. Twenty-three of the 73 patients were treated with aztreonam in an open study; all experienced a microbiologic cure and a favorable clinical response. Fifty of the 73 patients treated with aztreonam + clindamycin were entered into a comparative study that included 38 patients who received gentamicin (3–5 mg/kg per day) plus clindamycin (600 mg three times a day). In 49 (98%) of the aztreonam-treated patients and in 36 (95%) of the gentamicin-treated patients, the causative organism was eradicated, and in 98% and 89% of the patients, respectively, a favorable clinical response was achieved.

7. ADMINISTRATION OF DRUG

Aztreonam may be administered intravenously or by intramuscular injection. The IV route is recommended for patients requiring single doses greater than 1 g or those with bacterial septicemia, localized parenchymal abscess, peritonitis, or other severe systemic or life-threatening infections. Specific dosage, route of administration, and duration of therapy in older patients should be determined by the severity of infection, general condition of the patient, and renal impairment. Dosage recommendations for the treatment of UTI are 500 mg or 1 g every 8 or 12 hr. The dosage recommendation for moderately severe systemic infections is 1 or 2 g every 8 or 12 hr. The dosage recommendation for severe systemic or life-threatening infections is 2 g every 8 or 12 hr.

Although a specific adjustment for age is not indicated, the renal status of the elderly patient needs to be considered. For elderly patients, the dosage should be halved in patients with an estimated creatinine clearance between 10 and 30 mL/min/1.73 m^2 after an initial loading dose of 1 or 2 g. In patients with a creatinine clearance below 10 mL/min/1.73 m^2 the maintenance dose should be one-fourth of the usual initial dose given at the usual fixed interval of 6, 8, or 12 hr, following a loading dose of 500 mg, 1 g, or 2 g. The same dosage recommendation should be followed in patients undergoing hemodialysis, with an additional one-eighth of the initial dose given after each hemodialysis session.

8. DRUG MONITORING AND ADVERSE EFFECTS

Aztreonam is devoid of major toxicities with the most common adverse effects of a minor nature. In one review, the overall rate of adverse reactions to aztreonam among 2700 patients was 6.8% (42). Local reactions at the site of injection were most common, followed by rash, diarrhea, nausea, and vomiting. Renal impairment was reported only rarely. Clinical bleeding did not occur, and platelet abnormalities were observed infrequently. Pseudomembranous colitis occurred in only 3 of 2388 patients who received the drug and had appropriate follow-up.

A number of minor laboratory test abnormalities reported during clinical trials included increased levels of aspartate aminotransferase, alanine aminotransferase, and alkaline phosphatase, but symptoms or signs of hepatobiliary dysfunction were evident in less than 1%. Increases in prothrombin time and partial thromboplastin time, eosinophilia, positive Coombs' test, and some instances of increased creatinine concentration were noted.

Saxon et al. (43) described 26 patients with positive results of skin tests for penicillin who safely received 1 g doses of aztreonam without a reaction, as measured by IgE antibody titers. Immunologic recognition of aztreonam, when it occurs, is due to antibodies specific for the side chain of aztreonam rather than the nucleus, as shown with penicillins and cephalosporins.

Immediate hypersensitivity in temporal relationship to administration of aztreonam, however, has been reported (44,45). The manufacturer indicates that the incidence of anaphylaxis with the use of aztreonam alone is less than 1% (15).

REFERENCES

1. Drabu YJ, Mehtar S, Blakemore PH. Clinical efficacy of carumonam. Drugs Exp Clin Res 1988; 14:665–667.
2. Nelet F, Gutmann L, Kitzis MD, Acar JF. Tigemonam activity against clinical isolates of Enterobacteriaceae and Enterobacteriaceae with known mechanisms of resistance to beta-lactam antibiotics. J Antimicrob Chemother 1989; 24:173–181.
3. Sykes RB, Bonner DP, Bush K, Georgopapadakou NH. Azthreonam (SQ 26,776), a synthetic monobactam specifically active against aerobic Gram-negative bacteria. Antimicrob Agents Chemother 1982; 21:85–92.
4. Bush K, Sykes RB. Interaction of new beta-lactams with beta-lactamases and beta-lactamase-producing Gram-negative rods. In: Neu H, ed. New Beta-Lactam Antibiotics: A Review from Chemistry to Clinical Efficacy of the New Cephalosporins. Philadelphia, PA: Francis Clark Wood Institute for the History of Medicine, College of Physicians of Philadelphia, 1982:47–64.
5. Georgopapadakou NH, Smith SA, Sykes RB. Mode of action of azthreonam. Antimicrob Agents Chemother 1982; 21(6):950–956.
6. Neu HC, Labthavikul P. In vitro activity and beta-lactamase stability of a monobactam, SQ 26,917, compared with those of aztreonam and other agents. Antimicrob Agents Chemother 1983; 24:227–232.
7. Barry AL, Thornsberry C, Jones RN, Gavan TL. Aztreonam: antibacterial activity, beta-lactamase stability, and interpretive standards and quality control guidelines for disk-diffusion susceptibility tests. Rev Infect Dis 1985; 7(suppl 4):S594–S604.
8. Livermore DM, Williams JD. In-vitro activity of the monobactam, SQ 26,776, against Gram-negative bacteria and its stability to their beta-lactamases. J Antimicrob Chemother 1981; 8(suppl E):29–37.
9. Strandberg DA, Jorgensen JH, Drutz DJ. Activity of aztreonam and new beta-lactam antibiotics against penicillinase-producing Neisseria gonorrhoeae. Curr Ther Res Clin Exp 1983; 34:955–959.
10. Stutman HR, Welch DF, Scribner RK, Marks MI. In vitro antimicrobial activity of aztreonam alone and in combination against bacterial isolates from pediatric patients. Antimicrob Agents Chemother 1984; 25:212–215.
11. Buesing MA, Jorgensen JH. In vitro activity of aztreonam in combination with newer beta-lactams and amikacin against multiply resistant Gram-negative bacilli. Antimicrob Agents Chemother 1984; 25:283–285.
12. Aronoff SC, Klinger JD. In vitro activities of aztreonam, piperacillin, and ticarcillin combined with amikacin against amikacin-resistant Pseudomonas aeruginosa and P. cepacia isolates from children with cystic fibrosis. Antimicrob Agents Chemother 1984; 25:279–280.
13. Van Laethem Y, Husson M, Klastersky J. Serum bactericidal activity of aztreonam, cefoperazone, and amikacin, alone or in combination, against Escherichia coli, Klebsiella pneumoniae, Serratia marcescens, and Pseudomonas aeruginosa. Antimicrob Agents Chemother 1984; 26:224–227.
14. Scully BE, Swabb EA, Neu HC. Pharmacology of aztreonam after intravenous infusion. Antimicrob Agents Chemother 1983; 24:18–22.
15. E. R. Squibb & Sons, Inc. Azactam (package insert). Princeton, NJ: E. R. Squibb & Sons, Inc., 1991.
16. Duma RJ, Berry AJ, Smith SM, Baggett JW, Swabb EA, Platt TB. Penetration of aztreonam into cerebrospinal fluid of patients with and without inflamed meninges. Antimicrob Agents Chemother 1984; 26:730–733.
17. Modai J, Vittecoq D, Decazes JM, Wolff M, Meulemans A. Penetration of aztreonam into cerebrospinal fluid of patients with bacterial meningitis. Antimicrob Agents Chemother 1986; 29:281–283.

18. Swabb EA, Singhvi SM, Leitz MA, Frantz M, Sugerman AA. Metabolism and pharmacokinetics of aztreonam in healthy subjects. Antimicrob Agents Chemother 1983; 24: 394–400.

19. Martinez OV, Levi JU, Devlin RG. Biliary excretion of aztreonam in patients with biliary tract disease. Antimicrob Agents Chemother 1984; 25:358–361.

20. Mihindu JCL, Scheld WM, Bolton ND, Spyker DA, Swabb EA, Bolton WK. Pharmacokinetics of aztreonam in patients with various degrees of renal dysfunction. Antimicrob Agents Chemother 1983; 24:252–261.

21. Gerig JS, Bolton ND, Swabb EA, Scheld WM, Bolton WK. Effect of hemodialysis and peritoneal dialysis on aztreonam pharmacokinetics. Kidney Int 1984; 26:308–318.

22. Conrad DA, Williams RR, Couchman TL. Efficacy of aztreonam in the treatment of skeletal infections due to *Pseudomonas aeruginosa*. Rev Infect Dis 1991; 13(suppl 7): S634–S639.

23. Jensen T, Pedersen SS, Hoiby N, Koch C. Safety of aztreonam in patients with cystic fibrosis and allergy to beta lactam antibiotics. Rev Infect Dis 1991; 13(suppl 7): S594–S597.

24. de Vries-Hospers HG, Sleijfer DT, Mulder NH, van der Waaij D, Neiweg HO, van Saene HK. Bacteriological aspects of selective decontamination of the digestive tract as a method of infection prevention in granulocytopenic patients. Antimicrob Agents Chemother 1981; 19:813–820.

25. Rolston KVI, Bodey GP, Elting L. Aztreonam in the prevention and treatment of infection in neutropenic cancer patients. Am J Med 1990; 88(suppl 3C):24S–42S.

26. Evans DTP, Crooks AJR, Jones C. Treatment of uncomplicated gonorrhoea with single dose aztreonam. Genitourin Med 1986; 62:318–320.

27. Daikos GK. Clinical experience with aztreonam in four Mediterranean countries. Rev Infect Dis 1985; 7(suppl 4):S831–S835.

28. Dratwa M, Glupezynski Y, Lameire N. Treatment of Gram-negative peritonitis with aztreonam in patients undergoing continuous ambulatory peritoneal dialysis. Rev Infect Dis 1991; 13(suppl 7):S645–S647.

29. Mozzillo N, Dionigi R, Ventriglia L. Multicenter study of aztreonam in the prophylaxis of colorectal, gynecologic and urologic surgery. Chemotherapy 1989; 35(suppl 1):58–71.

30. DuPont HL, Ericsson CD, Mathewson JJ, de la Cabada FJ, Conrad DA. Oral aztreonam, a poorly absorbed yet effective therapy for bacterial diarrhea in US travelers to Mexico. J Am Med Assoc 1992; 267:1932–1935.

31. Childs SJ. Aztreonam in the treatment of urinary tract infection. Am J Med 1985; 78(suppl 2A):44–46.

32. Cox CE. Aztreonam therapy for complicated urinary tract infections caused by multidrug-resistant bacteria. Rev Infect Dis 1985; 7(suppl 4):S767–S771.

33. Swabb EA, Jenkins SA, Muir JG. Summary of worldwide clinical trials of aztreonam in patients with urinary tract infections. Rev Infect Dis 1985; 7(suppl 4):S772–S777.

34. Rodriguez JR, Ramirez-Ronda CH, Nevarez M. Efficacy and safety of aztreonam-clindamycin versus tobramycin-clindamycin in the treatment of lower respiratory tract infections caused by aerobic Gram-negative bacilli. Antimicrob Agents Chemother 1985; 27:246–251.

35. Rivera-Vazquez CR, Ramirez-Ronda CH, Rodriguez JR, Saavedra S. A comparative analysis of aztreonam + clindamycin versus tobramycin + clindamycin or amikacin + mezlocillin in the treatment of Gram-negative lower respiratory tract infections. Chemotherapy 1989; 35(suppl 1):89–100.

36. Scully BE, Henry SA. Clinical experience with aztreonam in the treatment of Gram-negative bacteremia. Rev Infect Dis 1985; 7(suppl 4):S789–S793.

37. McKellar PP. Clinical evaluation of aztreonam therapy for serious infections due to Gram-negative bacteria. Rev Infect Dis 1985; 7(suppl 4):S803–S809.

38. Winner JS, Gentry CA, Machado LJ, Cornea P. Aztreonam treatment of *Pasteurella multocida* cellulitis and bacteremia. Ann Pharmacother 2003; 37:392–394.

39. Henry SA. Overall clinical experience with aztreonam in the treatment of intraabdominal infections. Rev Infect Dis 1985; 7(suppl 4):S729–S733.

40. Birolini D, Moraes MF, de Souza OS. Comparison of aztreonam plus clindamycin with tobramycin plus clindamycin in the treatment of intra-abdominal infections. Chemotherapy 1989; 35(suppl 1):49–57.

41. Henry SA. Overall clinical experience with aztreonam in the treatment of obstetric-gynecologic infections. Rev Infect Dis 1985; 7(suppl 4):S703–S708.

42. Newman TJ, Dreslinski GR, Tadros SS. Safety profile of aztreonam in clinical trials. Rev Infect Dis 1985; 7(suppl 4):S648–S655.

43. Saxon A, Beall GN, Rohr AS, Adelman DC. Immediate hypersensitivity reactions to beta-lactam antibiotics. Ann Intern Med 1987; 107:204–215.

44. Soto Alvarez J, Sacristan del Castillo JA, Sampedro Garcia I, Alsar Ortiz MJ. Immediate hypersensitivity to aztreonam. Lancet 1990; 335:1094.

45. Hantson P, de Coninck B, Horn JL, Mahieu P. Immediate hypersensitivity to aztreonam and imipenem. Br Med J 1991; 302:294–295.

SUGGESTED READING

Henry SA. Overall clinical experience with aztreonam in the treatment of intraabdominal infections. Rev Infect Dis 1985; 7(suppl 4):S729–S733.

Rivera-Vazquez CR, Ramirez-Ronda CH, Rodriguez JR, Saavedra S. A comparative analysis of aztreonam + clindamycin versus tobramycin + clindamycin or amikacin + mezlocillin in the treatment of Gram-negative lower respiratory tract infections. Chemotherapy 1989; 35(suppl 1):89–100.

11

β-Lactam/β-Lactamase Inhibitors

Robert A. Bonomo
Section of Infectious Diseases, Department of Medicine, Louis Stokes Veterans Affairs Medical Center, Cleveland, Ohio, U.S.A.

Key Points:

- Despite the introduction of highly potent β-lactam antibiotics, bacterial resistance enzymes called β-lactamases have emerged that compromise the clinical efficacy of β-lactam antibiotics.
- There are a growing number of bacterial β-lactamases. An extremely effective method to nullify the unwelcome consequences of these enzymes is to combine β-lactams with β-lactamase inhibitors.
- Increasing numbers of bacterial β-lactamase are being found that are resistant to β-lactamase inhibitors.
- As a rule, β-lactam β-lactamase inhibitor combinations are indicated for the empirical treatment of community-acquired, nosocomial, or aspiration pneumonia in the elderly; complicated refractory rhinosinusitis; oral and dental infections; diabetic foot infections; intra-abdominal infections; pelvic and complicated genitourinary infections; skin and soft tissue infections; and neutropenic fever.
- Despite the efficacy of β-lactamase inhibitors in use, there is an urgent need to develop novel β-lactamase inhibitors that will be effective against bacteria possessing multiple β-lactamases.

1. β-LACTAM ANTIBIOTICS, β-LACTAMASES, AND β-LACTAMASE INHIBITION

1.1. β-Lactamases Emerge in Response to β-Lactams

β-Lactam antibiotics (penicillins, cephalosporins, monobactams and carbapenems) are among our oldest, most successful, and safest class of antimicrobial agents. These antibiotics are effective at killing bacteria by interfering with the synthesis of the bacterial cell wall (1). In forming a covalent bond with the cell wall-synthesizing enzymes [herein referred to as penicillin-binding proteins (PBPs)], the β-lactam mimics closely the amino acid building blocks that are used to define the architectural integrity of the bacterial cell wall. As a result of β-lactam action, the cell wall-synthesizing enzymes are unable to further build new cell wall. Simultaneously, bacterial enzymes that are responsible for breaking down the cell wall are unabated (autolysins). Bacteria become highly permeable to water, cells rapidly increase in size, and lyse (burst). Hence, β-lactam antibiotics are the premier bactericidal agent.

In this context, it is readily appreciated why the clinical introduction of penicillin in the 1940s resulted in previously unimaginable success in treating serious infections caused by *Staphylococcus aureus* and *Streptococcus pyogenes* (2). β-Lactams were truly "the magic bullet" and were curative. Before long, however, *S. aureus* strains resistant to penicillin, by virtue of production of an enzyme able to degrade penicillin, a β-lactamase, were observed. The introduction of β-lactam antibiotics stable in the presence of the β-lactamase enzymes partially addressed this problem (e.g., oxacillin, nafcillin, and other semisynthetic penicillins referred to as isoxazolyl penicillins). But this bonus was short-lived. Initial control over gram-positive bacteria in the hospital setting also led to the emergence of gram-negative bacilli, primarily *Escherichia coli*, as an important community-acquired and nosocomial pathogen. Although ampicillin represented the first truly effective β-lactam against *E. coli*, many strains were found resistant to ampicillin through the production of an acquired plasmid encoded, β-lactamase, designated TEM-1, different from the β-lactamase found in *S. aureus* (PC 1). Other important gram-negative pathogens (*Haemophilus influenzae*, *Klebsiella pneumoniae*, *Enterobacter aerogenes*, and *Enterobacter cloacae*, *Serratia* spp., and *P. aeruginosa*) were also found to be resistant to ampicillin due to production of a plasmid or a chromosomally encoded β-lactamase. Paradoxically, each new β-lactam agent introduced into clinical use was soon greeted by the discovery of a clinical isolate able to resist the action of that β-lactam via an enzyme-mediated process. It has been remarked that the evolution and dissemination of β-lactamases have been fueled by each generation of β-lactam antibiotic introduced into the clinical arena (1).

At the present time, there are more than 470 different β-lactamases found in bacteria. β-lactamases are members of a bacterial protein superfamily of active site serine proteases (D,D-peptidases) that catalytically disrupt the β-lactam (amide) bond to form an acyl enzyme complex. A critically positioned water molecule completes hydrolysis to regenerate the free enzyme: water disrupts the covalent (ester) linkage and releases the penicilloyl and cephalosporyl moieties (Fig. 1). The large majority of these enzymes possess a conserved serine in the active site (Ser70 in class A and Ser67 in class C, Ser64 in class D) that acts as the reactive nucleophile for the catalysis of the amide bond. Other β-lactamases use a metal ion (zinc) as the catalytic residue for hydrolysis (3).

The nomenclature used in describing β-lactamases is often problematic. These enzymes are usually designated with three-letter abbreviations, but there are exceptions. Sometimes, the enzymes are named after the patient from whom they are isolated (e.g., "TEM" after the child with the infection resistant to penicillin); a biochemical property [e.g., sulfyhydryl variable (SHV) or hydrolyzing oxacillin— "OXA"]; or the hospital where the enzyme was found (e.g., MIR-1 for Miriam Hospital in Rhode Island). β-lactamases are classified into four groups (1–4) or classes (A–D) (Table 1). The Bush–Jacoby–Medeiros classification system arranges β-lactamases using functional characteristics (susceptibility to β-lactamase inhibitors or ethylenediaminetetracetic acid), and the Ambler classification system uses amino

$$\beta\text{-lactam} + \beta\text{-lactamase} \leftrightarrow \beta\text{-lactamase:}\beta\text{-lactam} \rightarrow \beta\text{-lactamase-}\beta\text{-lactam} \xrightarrow{H_2O} \beta\text{-lactam} + \text{hydrolyzed }\beta\text{-lactam}$$

Figure 1 The β-lactam and β-lactamase first form a Michaelis complex (β-lactam: β-lactamase) and then form an acyl enzyme (β-lactam-β-lactamase). The acyl enzyme is hydrolyzed in the presence of water.

ation Schemes for β-Lactamases

leiros functional group	Ambler molecular classification (classes A–D)	Comment
sporinases	Class C—cephalosporinase	Examples include AmpC of *E. coli* and P99 of *E* spp; these enzymes are usually clavulanic acid and are usually chromosomally encoded; there number of these cephalosporinases that are pl encoded (e.g., CMY-2, ACT-1)
inases (clavulanate taphylococcal penicillinase; HV-1 β-lactamases; ectrum β-lactamases; istant β-lactamases; hydrolyzing β-lactamases; nases inhibited by arbapenem hydrolyzing	Class A—penicillinases	Examples are penicillinases of *E. coli*, *K. pneume* *S. aureus*; these enzymes are usually clavulanic susceptible, with notable exceptions (IRTs an enzymes) of the 2br group; it is noteworthy th extended spectrum and carbapenemases found group are all clavulanic acid susceptible
	Class D—cloxacillin hydrolyzing enzymes (OXA)	These enzymes are less clavulanic acid susceptib 2b, or 2be; these represent a growing group o lactamases in which are found many carbapen
3c) (5)	Class B—metallo-β-lactamases (zinc)	Metal ion is necessary for hydrolysis; these enzy resistance to carbapenems and are not inhibit clavulanic acid; it is notable that some are inh aztreonam
	Unknown	Miscellaneous or unsequenced/uncharacterized that do not fit into any function or molecular

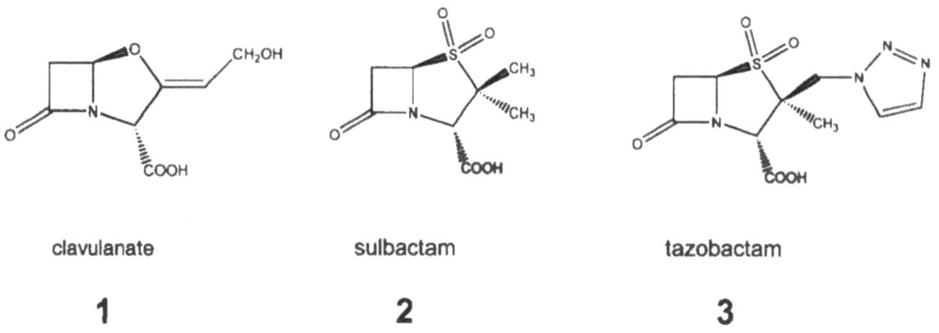

clavulanate   sulbactam   tazobactam

1   **2**   **3**

Figure 2 Chemical structures of β-lactamase inhibitors: clavulanate, sulbactam, and tazobactam.

acid sequence identity (4). For the sake of simplicity, we will use the Ambler classification system (classes A–D) in this chapter.

1.2. Combating β-Lactamases: The Discovery and Synthesis of β-Lactamase Inhibitors

To combat the growing problem of β-lactamase-mediated resistance, two strategies became evident: either design β-lactams resistant to the hydrolytic action of β-lactamases or find inhibitors of these enzymes. Clavulanate 1, sulbactam 2, and tazobactam 3 are the major β-lactamase inhibitors used in combination with β-lactams for the treatment of community and nosocomially acquired infections (Fig. 2). Clavulanate is produced naturally by the fungus *Streptomyces clavuligerus*. Sulbactam and tazobactam are synthetic penicillins that are the product of the pharmaceutical industry medicinal chemists. The contribution of this class of antibiotics (also termed "suicide" inhibitors) to our therapeutic armamentarium cannot be overstated. In this chapter, we will first address how β-lactamase inhibitors inactivate class A β-lactamases, describe briefly the problem of inhibitor-resistant β-lactamases, review important pharmacological and clinical issues related to their use, and discuss the most appropriate application in a clinical setting the geriatrician is likely to encounter.

2. CHEMISTRY AND MECHANISM OF ACTION

As these β-lactamase inhibitors were introduced into clinical practice, interest was (and still is) keen on determining the mechanism by which they inhibited β-lactamase activity. Among the most notable early studies performed here were those done by Knowles and colleagues at Harvard University (6–8). Based on a series of elegant investigations published more than two decades ago, a general mechanism of inactivation by clavulanic acid and sulbactam of the TEM-2 β-lactamase was proposed. The critical intermediates in the inactivation process and formation of stable end products formed the basis of our early understanding of how these inhibitors worked. The "state of the art" on how β-lactamase inhibitors inactivate β-lactamases can be summarized.

   As is evident by examination of their chemical structure, β-lactamase inhibitors are essentially β-lactam compounds. Hence, they are rapidly acylated by the class A β-lactamase to form the acyl enzyme. Once acylated, there is a secondary ring opening (either simultaneously or sequentially), and there is formation of two highly important and reactive intermediates (imine and enamie). Here, the water molecules in the active site of the enzyme modify the chemical structures attached to the enzyme and result in a series of smaller inhibitor fragments still covalently bonded to the β-lactamase. In the process of generating smaller and smaller fragments, there are a series of other intermediates formed that are able to modify the β-lactamase at more than one site on the enzyme. The precise details and importance of each of these steps is still being actively investigated (Fig. 3).

In a practical and clinical sense, once the β-lactamase is acylated and unable to hydrolyze the β-lactams that are targeting the PBPs, the task of the "suicide" inhibitor is accomplished. Consequently, the effective or potent β-lactamase inhibitor

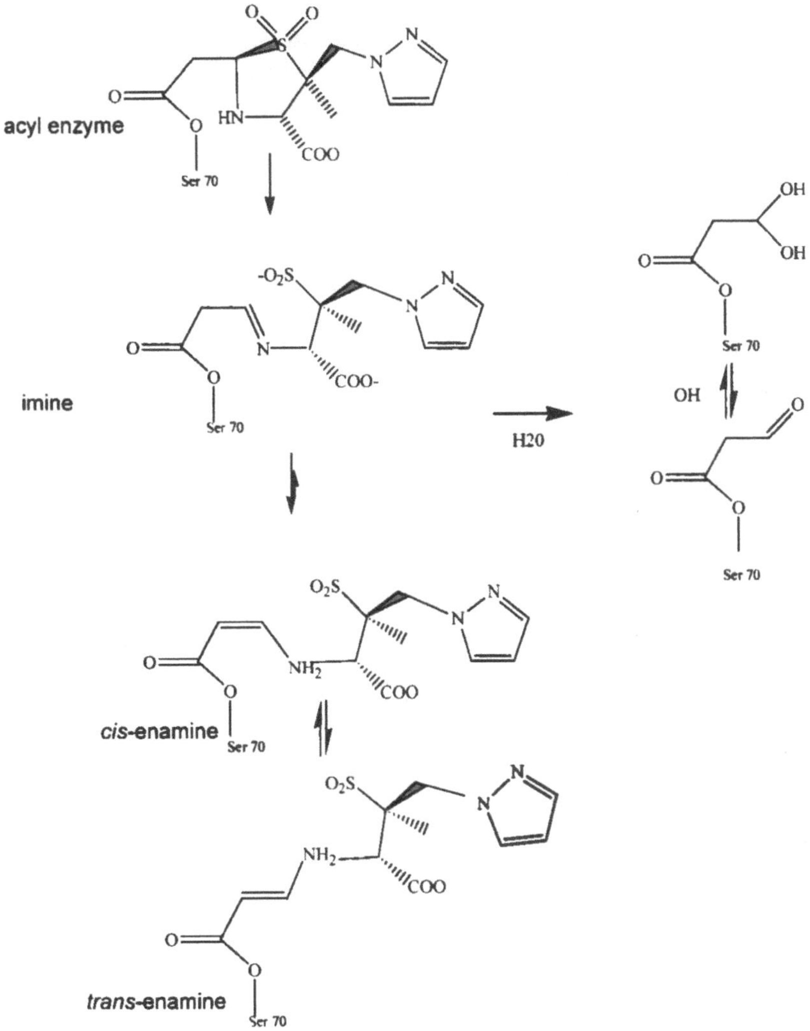

Figure 3 Proposed reaction mechanism of tazobactam, a β-lactamase inhibitor, with a class A β-lactamase. Note the opening of the two β-lactam rings and the fragmentation of the molecule while still attached to the β-lactamase.

requires sufficient affinity for the active site to be readily incorporated as another β-lactam (hence, the name "suicide"), be broken down slowly relative to the β-lactam, and form inactive stable end products that regenerate the free β-lactamase (9). An unappreciated notion is that the effective inhibitor stays in the active site of the β-lactamase for a prolonged period—longer than the normal substrate does. Ideally, this would be at least the half-life of the cell (20 min). This strategic considera-tion is essential in successful use of these agents and for the future design of novel compounds. It is interesting to ponder that the most potent β-lactam antibiotics we have (carbapenems, aztreonam, and cefepime) stay attached to the β-lactamase for a long time and have a low turnover number relative to the other β-lactams. This duality (part β-lactam and part β-lactamase inhibitor) may explain the superior per-formance of carbapenems, monobactams, and cefepime in the clinical setting (10–12).

In 1992 the first clinical report emerged describing an inhibitor-resistant strain of *E. coli* infecting a neonate (13). Prior to this time, rare *E. coli* isolates were found that were resistant to ampicillin/sulbactam (14). The mechanism responsible for this was believed to be overproduction of the TEM-1 beta-lactamase. Similarly, experi-mental work generating mutants of TEM-1 also revealed that TEM-1 β-lactamase could be resistant to inactivation by sulbactam and clavulanic acid (15–17). Unfortunately, the full implications of these finding were largely unappreciated by physicians and microbiologists at that time (i.e., mutations in the promoter region of the *bla*$_{TEM}$ gene and mutations affecting the affinity of clavulanate and sulbactam for the active site of TEM-1). Once the clinical isolate was discovered, sequencing of the *bla*$_{TEM}$ gene revealed a substitution that resulted in a single amino acid change from Arg244 to Ser (Ambler numbering system). This report stressed the importance of substitutions at certain amino acid positions that gave rise to the inhibitor-resistant phenotype in class A β-lactamases and confirmed the importance of heralding work performed in the laboratory (18). These β-lactamases are now referred to as inhibitor-resistant TEMs (IRTs). Intensive studies examining clinical isolates, using site-directed mutagenesis, kinetics, and crystal structure determinations of class A β-lactamase with and without inhibitors have followed (3,19). A full discussion of these exciting findings is beyond the scope of this chapter. The reader is referred to the website www.lahey.org for a comprehensive list of β-lactamases of the TEM and SHV variety possessing the amino acid mutations responsible for resistance to inhibitors.

There are currently 22 IRTs (e.g., TEM-30, TEM-31, etc.) and 3 SHV β-lactamases (SHV-10, SHV-26, and SHV-49) described that are resistant to inactivation. Three com-plex mutants of TEM (CMT-1 → CMT-3) also are known that are IRTs with amino acid mutations that also increase resistance to ceftazidime and other third-generation cepha-losporins. These unique β-lactamases possess amino acid mutations that define the extended-spectrum β-lactamase (ESBL) phenotype (mutations at Glu104Lys, Arg164-Ser, Gly239Ser, Glu240Lys) as well as resistance to inhibitors. All of the IRTs and inhibitor-resistant SHVs have the mutations located at amino acids Met69 (-Ile, -Leu, and -Val), Ser130 (-Gly), Arg244 (-Ser, -Cys, -Gly, -His, -Leu), Arg275 (-Leu), and Asn276 (-Asp).

3. MICROBIAL SPECTRUM

In the strictest sense, the current β-lactam β-lactamase inhibitor combinations are primarily agents effective against community-acquired pathogens such as *E. coli*, *K. pneumoniae*, *Neiserria gonorrhoeae*, *S. aureus*, *H. influenzae*, *Bacteroides fragilis*, other *Bacteroides* spp., *Moraxella catarrhalis*, *Proteus mirabilis*, *Proteus vulgaris* and other common oral, respiratory, abdominal, and genitourinary anaerobes (e.g., *Prevotella*, *Fusobacterium*, and *Veillonella*). The microbiological data presented to the clinician reveal that these pathogens will be resistant to ampicillin and susceptible to ampicillin/sulbactam or amoxicillin/clavulanate. In the main, these pathogens usually possess a single class A β-lactamase (20).

In combination with a β-lactam, β-lactamase inhibitors lower the minimum inhibitory concentrations (MICs) against class A β-lactamase-producing bacterial isolates. This clinical finding is central to understanding why organisms which process class A β-lactamases can be effectively treated. As stated above, β-lactam β-lactamase inhibitor combinations in conventional dosages are principally effective against pathogens expressing low or moderate expression levels of TEM-1 and SHV-1 β-lactamases. In addition, β-lactam β-lactamase inhibitor combinations are also effective against carbapenemases of the type A class. These are a unique group of β-lactamases that can hydrolyze carbapenems (Sme-1 → 3, KPC 1→ 3, etc.) (21–23). It should be kept in mind that β-lactam β-lactamase inhibitors must be present above the MIC for greater than 40–50% of the dosing interval to optimize bacterial killing and reduce emergence of resistant strains. Generally, streptococci and pneumococci are susceptible to the penicillin alone, so the need of a β-lactamase inhibitor is not required.

Although it is appreciated that β-lactamase inhibitors may inactivate class C and D β-lactamases in vitro, they are not recommended for treatment of bacteria possessing these β-lactamases (9,24). In contrast to class A enzymes like TEM, the amount of β-lactamase inhibitor required to inactivate the other classes of β-lactamases is significantly greater. Thus, the application of β-lactam β-lactamase inhibitor therapy is not generally advocated against bacteria-possessing classes C, D, or B β-lactamases (e.g., some *Enterobacter* spp., *Citrobacter freundii*, *Aeromonas* spp., *Serratia* spp., *Pseudomonas* spp., and *Stenotrophomonas maltophilia*). Hence, the decision to use β-lactam β-lactamase inhibitor therapy must be made on a careful and considered clinical judgment. The clinician then must decide on the basis of interpretation of susceptibility data whether β-lactam β-lactamase inhibitor therapy is appropriate for treatment of these pathogens. Herein, the choice of β-lactam β-lactamase inhibitor is also important. Piperacillin is the most active β-lactam against PBP-3, thus explaining the better activity against nonfermenting gram-negative bacteria. In contrast to ampicillin/sulbactam, the combination piperacillin/tazobactam is more active against nosocomial pathogens. As will be discussed below, although β-lactam β-lactam inhibitor combinations may prove to be an excellent choice for the treatment of ceftazidime-resistant *E. coli* and *K. pneumoniae* possessing ESBLs, their use cannot be advocated without more clinical data to support this practice (5,25,26). In contrast, clavulanate but not sulbactam or tazobactam, induces class C β-lactamases in vitro and this raises significant concern that during the treatment of *P. aeruginosa* infections with ticarcillin/clavulanate acid the effect of ticarcillin can be compromised (27,28). Most clinical experts feel in this context that drugs such as piperacillin or cefoperazone have less ability to induce class C β-lactamase production and when partnered with β-lactamase inhibitor combinations are effective.

3.1. Clinical Pharmacology

The pharmacodynamics and pharmacokinetics (PD and PK) of β-lactamase inhibitors are critical concerns in the use with their partner antibiotic. With an accompanying penicillin (or cephalosporin), β-lactam β-lactamase inhibitor combinations exhibit time-dependent bacterial killing (29–31). β-Lactamase inhibitor combinations also demonstrate a post-antibiotic effect (30). The target of penicillin action used with the β-lactamase inhibitor is PBP-1, -2, or -3. As a drug itself, only sulbactam processes intrinsic antimicrobal activity, usually demonstrated against PBP-2 of *Acinetobacter* spp. (32,33). Sulbactam also processes some intrinsic activity against *N. gonorrhoeae* PBP-3 (31).

Most β-lactamase inhibitors have half-lives that last between 30 and 60 min and the usual administration interval is 6–8 hr (31). As a rule, these compounds are often dosed up to four times a day (except for amoxicillin/clavulanate, an oral preparation). Usually, sulbactam when added to ampicillin is dosed on a 6–8 hr basis. Amoxicillin/clavulanate acid can be dosed on a 12 hr basis when given orally. Ticarcillin can be dosed up to every 4–6 hr depending on whether *P. aeruginosa* is being treated or not.

The amount of β-lactamase inhibitor varies with each formulation. In the formulations containing ampicillin/sulbactam, ampicillin is usually in a 2:1 ratio with sulbactam. The dose of 3 g of Unasyn® is 2 g of ampicillin and 1 g of sulbactam. Augmentin® is 250, 500, 750, or 1000 mg of amoxicillin and 125 mg of clavulanate. In contrast, piperacillin is delivered with tazobactam in an 8:1 ratio (4 g piperacillin, 0.5 mg tazobactam). The peak serum levels of the β-lactamase inhibitor parallel the β-lactam (31).

The kidneys usually excrete tazobactam and sulbactam, while clavulanate acid undergoes extensive metabolism into inactive metabolites by other mechanisms (31). In patients with renal failure the dose of the β-lactam β-lactamase inhibitor combinations must be adjusted. Usually, this is done by decreasing the dose and increasing the dosing interval. Excretion of cefoperazone in the bile often offers a theoretical advantage in treating biliary tract infections (cholecystitis or gall stone-induced obstruction). However, this agent is not widely used in the United States due to the ability of multiple β-lactamases able to hydrolyze cefoperazone.

Generally, β-lactamase inhibitors penetrate well into the middle ear, lung, biliary tract, peritoneum, and pelvic tissues, with sulbactam having the largest volume of distribution. They are not considered first-line therapy for treating serious central nervous system infections.

There are certain side effects that are notable with β-lactam β-lactamase inhibitor combinations. These side effects are generally predictable (as the inhibitors are very similar in structure to β-lactams). For example, diarrhea, abnormal liver function, or skin rashes have been reported with these compounds. It is suspected that antibiotic associated *Clostridium difficile* diarrhea occurs less frequently in patient treated with piperacillin/tazobactam than with cephalosporins, which is probably related with the activity against the anaerobes. In contrast, ampicillin/sulbactam and amoxicillin/clavulante acid are more controversial in this respect. Oral amoxicillin/clavulante acid has been associated with dose-dependent diarrhea (>250 mg clavulanate dose) in up to 10–18% of children given amoxicillin/clavulante acid. Occasionally, clavulanate will form dose-related nonfatal cholestatic hepatitis. In Europe cefoperazone when used with β-lactamase inhibitors has been associated with a reversible coagulopathy. This author has noted the same effect with ampicillin/sulbactam (unpublished findings).

3.2. Clinical Indications

The overall antibacterial spectrum and clinical use of β-lactam β-lactamase inhibitor combinations depend on the activity of the penicillin as well as the characteristic of the particular β-lactamases inhibitor (34). As a rule, β-lactam β-lactamase inhibitor combinations are used for the empiric treatment of community-acquired or aspiration pneumonia in the elderly, complicated sinus, dental infections, bites (human, dog, cat), epiglottitis, pharyngitis due to *Prevotella* spp., exacerbations of chronic obstructive pulmonary disease, hospital-acquired pneumonia, diabetic foot infections, intra-abdominal infection, pelvic and complicated genitourinary infections, skin and soft tissue infection, and neutropenic fever (www.idsociety.org) (35). When compared with more conventional regimens, β-lactam β-lactamase inhibitor combinations are relatively well tolerated and are at least as efficacious if not superior to comparator β-lactams. The therapy of mixed infections (aerobe and anaerobe, gram-positive and gram negative pathogens) leads logically to the use of these agents.

The available oral formulations such as amoxicillin/clavulante acid provide convenient outpatient step-down therapy against susceptible pathogens. Although not a first-line agent according to the Infectious Disease Society of America (IDSA), the use of amoxicillin/clavulante acid as an oral therapy in outpatient community-acquired pneumonia is permissible (36). Apparently, the PK and PD charactistics of amoxicillin/clavulante make it effective against penicillin-resistant *Streptococcus pneumoniae*. Amoxicillin/clavulanate is superior to oral cephalosporins, macrolides, or cotrimoxazole. This slightly lower MIC of amoxicillin in vitro compared with penicillin is a possible explanation. Despite the net reduction in failure rate noted in penicillin-resistant *S. pneumoniae* using amoxicillin/clavulanic acid, the best treatment for penicillin-resistant *S. pneumoniae* may require the use of a non-β-lactam antibiotic (36).

Up to 99% *H. influenzae* and *M. catarrhalis* are susceptible to amoxicillin/clavulanate acid and this combination is superior to most oral cephalosporins. For the treatment of seriously ill patients with community-acquired pneumonia in the medical intensive-care units, piperacillin/tazobactam is used intravenously as a drug of choice (36). Using piperacillin/tazobactam coadministered with a macrolide or fluoroquinolone can be an effective combination. Further prospective studies are warranted to demonstrate this. For nosocomial and ventilator-associated pneumonia, an aminoglycoside and piperacillin/tazobactam, ticarcillin/clavulanate, or cefoperazone/sulbactam provide empirical therapy especially against methicillin-sensitive *S. aureus*, *Enterobacteriaceae*, and *P. aeruginosa*. Up to 80% clinical success rate has been demonstrated for piperacillin/tazobactam, which is comparable to rates achieved with ceftazidime plus amikacin or monotherapy with imipenem/cilastatin (37).

In complicated urinary tract infections in our hospital due to *E. coli*, up to 60% of isolates will be eradicated with ampicillin/sulbactam. However, the emergence of *P. mirabilis* and other more resistant gram-negative bacteria limits the use of ampicillin/sulbactam in this setting. Piperacillin/tazobactam tends not to select for these pathogens and remains effective in complicated urinary tract infections that are acquired as a result of indwelling bladder catheters.

For intra-abdominal infections due to gram-negative bacilli and anaerobes such as *B. fragilis*, β-lactam β-lactamase inhibitor combinations containing sulbactam and tazobactam are particularly superior because activities against gram-negative bacilli are equal, if not superior to, clindamycin, cefoxitin, or metronidazole

(38). Standard regimens involving combinations consisting of cephalosporins and aminoglycosides are not as effective as piperacillin/tazobactam. Clinical response rates reach up to 90% effectiveness against these pathogens (38). Similar evidence suggests that ampicillin/sulbactam is useful for surgical chemoprophylaxis, especially in the course of elective colorectal surgery to prevent postoperative wound infections (31). However, the increasing extent of *B. fragilis* resistance to sulbactam (up to 7%) deserves attention. Notably, β-lactam β-lactamase inhibitor combinations containing ampicillin, amoxicillin, and piperacillin as initial treatment for enterococci are effective. In addition, the complication of pelvic inflammatory disease also merits β-lactam β-lactamase inhibitor combination therapy.

In the setting of neutropenia, fever is considered a medical emergency. In this context, piperacillin/tazobactam plus amikacin as well as piperacillin/tazobactam alone have been used effectively in the empirical treatment of neutropenic fever (37). Most clinicians favor the use of piperacilin/tazobactam combined with amilkacin for this purpose, although it is unclear if amikacin really adds anything to this regimen. The IDSA has specific guidelines for this (37).

In skin and soft tissue infection β-lactam β-lactamase inhibitor combinations provide the necessary broad-spectrum antimicrobial activity to overcome mixed infections (staphylococci, streptococci, gram negatives, etc.). In the setting of diabetic foot infections and complicated soft tissue infections in intravenous drug users and nursing home residents, these drugs serve an important role.

Against ESBL-producing *E. coli* and *K. pneumoniae*, carbapenems are the only reliable therapy that can be used in the presence of these β-lactamase-producing organisms. In many parts of the world, 5–25% of *E. coli*, *Klebsiella* spp., and *Pseudomonas* spp. now produce ESBLs. These TEM and SHV-derived β-lactamases generally appear more susceptible to tazobactam or clavulanate acid, but in clinical trials this has not been shown to be the case. Carbapenems constitute the only reliable treatment here (21–23).

The emergence of inhibitor-resistant β-lactamase has been a significant concern. The discovery of these enzymes has been an unwelcome consequence of the extensive use of many of the β-lactam β-lactamase inhibitor combinations. Fortunately, these β-lactamase enzymes that are resistant tend to be more susceptible to cephalosporins and hence, a therapeutic alternative for this type of infection by organisms possessing β-lactamase inhibitor resistant enzymes exists.

It should be noted that β-lactam β-lactamase inhibitor combinations are ineffective against methicillin-resistant *S. aureus* or *Mycoplasma*, *Chlamydia*, and *Legionella* spp.

4. NOVEL AGENTS

The finding of inhibitor-resistant variants of TEM and SHV and the challenge of inhibiting other classes of β-lactamases have stimulated interest in developing novel inhibitors (39,40). The reader is also referred to a comprehensive reviews, summarizing the "state of the art" in academia and industry (12, and assigned readings). Recent work in a number of laboratories has explored new classes of inhibitors and novel reaction chemistry. There are a series of novel inhibitors in development that are directed against class C, A, and B enzymes. So far, trials are limited and most of the work has been in vitro. The direction taken in these approaches capitalizes upon unique reaction chemistry. Specifically, they preferentially form the acyl enzyme, displace the position of a water molecule in the active site, and follow secondary ring closure. Peptide base inhibitors of class A enzymes like TEM and Sme as well as the anthracis β-lactamase are also in development. These exciting advances are setting the stage for a major breakthrough in the near future.

ACKNOWLEDGMENT

This work was supported by grants from the Department of Veterans Affairs Merit Review Program and the National Institutes of Health.

REFERENCES

1. Medeiros AA. Evolution and dissemination of β-lactamases accelerated by generations of β-lactam antibiotics. Clin Infect Dis 1997; 24:S19–S45.
2. Bradford PA. Extended-spectrum β-lactamases in the 21st century: characterization, epidemiology, and detection of this important resistance threat. Clin Microbiol Rev 2001; 14:933–951.
3. Helfand MS, Bonomo RA. β-Lactamases: a survey of protein diversity. Curr Drug Targets Infect Disord 2003; 3:9–23.
4. Ambler RP, Coulson AF, Frere JM, Ghuysen JM, Joris B, Forsman M, Levesque RC, Tiraby G, Waley SG. A standard numbering scheme for the class A β-lactamases. Biochem J 1991; 276:269–270.
5. Paterson DL, Ko WC, Von Gottberg A, Mohapatra S, Casellas JM, Goossens H, Mulazimoglu L, Trenholme G, Klugman KP, Bonomo RA, Rice LB, Wagener MM, McCormack JG, Yu VL. Antibiotic therapy for Klebsiella pneumoniae bacteremia: implications of production of extended-spectrum β-lactamases. Clin Infect Dis 2004; 39: 31–37.
6. Charnas RL, Fisher J, Knowles JR. Chemical studies on the inactivation of Escherichia coli RTEM β-lactamase by clavulanic acid. Biochemistry 1978; 17:2185–2189.
7. Charnas RL, Knowles JR. Inactivation of RTEM β-lactamase from Escherichia coli by clavulanic acid and 9-deoxyclavulanic acid. Biochemistry 1981; 20:3214–3219.
8. Fisher J, Charnas RL, Knowles JR. Kinetic studies on the inactivation of Escherichia coli RTEM β-lactamase by clavulanic acid. Biochemistry 1978; 17:2180–2184.
9. Bush K, Macalintal C, Rasmussen BA, Lee VJ, Yang Y. Kinetic interactions of tazobactam with β-lactamases from all major structural classes. Antimicrob Agents Chemother 1993; 37:851–858.
10. Maveyraud L, Mourey L, Kotra LP, Pedelacq J-D, Guillet V, Mobashery S, Samama J-P. Structural basis for clinical longevity of carbapenem antibiotics in the face of challenge by the common class A β-lactamases from the antibiotic-resistant bacteria. J Am Chem Soc 1998; 120:9748–9752.
11. Monks J, Waley SG. Imipenem as substrate and inhibitor of β-lactamases. Biochem J 1988; 253:323–328.
12. Page MG. β-Lactamase inhibitors. Drug Resist Updat 2000; 3:109–125.
13. Vedel G, Belaaouaj A, Gilly L, Labia R, Philippon A, Nevot P, Paul G. Clinical isolates of Escherichia coli producing TRI β-lactamases: novel TEM-enzymes conferring resistance to β-lactamase inhibitors. J Antimicrob Chemother 1992; 30:449–462.
14. Page JW, Farmer TH, Elson SW. Hyperproduction of TEM-1 β-lactamase by Escherichia coli strains. J Antimicrob Chemother 1989; 23:160–161.
15. Zafaralla G, Manavathu EK, Lerner SA, Mobashery S. Elucidation of the role of Arginine-244 in the turnover processes of class A β-lactamases. Biochemistry 1992; 31: 3847–3852.

16. Imtiaz U, Billings EM, Knox JR, Manavathu EK, Lerner SA, Mobashery S. Inactivation of class A β-lactamases by clavulanic acid: the role of Arginine-244 in a proposed non-concerted sequence of events. J Am Chem Soc 1993; 115:4435–4442.

17. Imtiaz U, Billings EM, Knox JR, Mobashery S. A structure-based analysis of the inhibition of class A β-lactamases by sulbactam. Biochemistry 1994; 33:5728–5738.

18. Vakulenko SB, Geryk B, Kotra LP, Mobashery S, Lerner SA. Selection and characterization of β-lactam-β-lactamase inactivator-resistant mutants following PCR mutagenesis of the TEM-1 β-lactamase gene. Antimicrob Agents Chemother 1998; 42: 1542–1548.

19. Knox JR. Extended spectrum and inhibitor resistant TEM type β-lactamases: mutations, specificity and three-dimensional structure. Antimicrob Agents Chemother 1995; 39: 2593–2601.

20. Livermore DM. Evolution of β-lactamase inhibitors. Intensive Care Med 1994; 20(suppl 3): S10–S13.

21. Queenan AM, Torres-Viera C, Gold HS, Carmeli Y, Eliopoulos GM, Moellering RCJ, Quinn JP, Hindler J, Medeiros AA, Bush K. SME-type carbapenem-hydrolyzing class A β-lactamases from geographically diverse *Serratia marcescens* strains. Antimicrob Agents Chemother 2000; 44:3035–3039.

22. Yigit H, Queenan AM, Anderson GJ, Domenech-Sanchez A, Biddle JW, Steward CD, Alberti S, Bush K, Tenover FC. Novel carbapenem-hydrolyzing β-lactamase, KPC-1, from a carbapenem-resistant strain of *Klebsiella pneumoniae*. Antimicrob Agents Chemother 2001; 45:1151–1161.

23. Yigit H, Queenan AM, Rasheed JK, Biddle JW, Domenech-Sanchez AA, Iberti S, Bush K, Tenover FC. Carbapenem-resistant strain of *Klebsiella oxytoca* harboring carbapenem-hydrolyzing β-lactamase KPC-2. Antimicrob Agents Chemother 2003; 47: 3881–3889.

24. Bonomo RA, Liu J, Chen Y, Ng L, Hujer AM, Anderson VE. Inactivation of CMY-2 β-lactamase by tazobactam: initial mass spectroscopic characterization. Biochim Biophys Acta 2001; 1547:196–205.

25. Paterson DL, Ko WC, Von Gottberg A, Mohapatra S, Casellas JM, Goossens H, Mulazimoglu L, Trenholme G, Klugman KP, Bonomo RA, Rice LB, Wagener MM, McCormack JG, Yu VL. International prospective study of *Klebsiella pneumoniae* bacteremia: implications of extended-spectrum β-lactamase production in nosocomial infections. Ann Intern Med 2004; 140:26–32.

26. Paterson DL, Ko WC, Von Gottberg A, Casellas JM, Mulazimoglu L, Klugman KP, Bonomo RA, Rice LB, McCormack JG, Yu VL. Outcome of cephalosporin treatment for serious infections due to apparently susceptible organisms producing extended-spectrum β-lactamases: implications for the clinical microbiology laboratory. J Clin Microbiol 2001; 39:2206–2212.

27. Akova M, Yang Y, Livermore DM. Interactions of tazobactam and clavulanate with inducibly- and constitutively-expressed Class I β-lactamases. J Antimicrob Chemother 1990; 25:199–208.

28. Livermore DM, Akova M, Wu PJ, Yang YJ. Clavulanate and β-lactamase induction. J Antimicrob Chemother 1989; 24(suppl B):23–33.

29. Li C, Nicolau DP, Lister PD, Quintiliani R, Nightingale CH. Pharmacodynamic study of β-lactams alone and in combination with β-lactamase inhibitors against *Pseudomonas aeruginosa* possessing an inducible β-lactamase. J Antimicrob Chemother 2004; 53: 297–304.

30. Lavigne JP, Bonnet R, Michaux-Charachon S, Jourdan J, Caillon J, Sotto A. Post-antibiotic and post-β-lactamase inhibitor effects of ceftazidime plus sulbactam on extended-spectrum β-lactamase-producing Gram-negative bacteria. J Antimicrob Chemother 2004; 53:616–619.

31. Lee N, Yuen KY, Kumana CR. Clinical role of β-lactam/β-lactamase inhibitor combinations. Drugs 2003; 63:1511–1524.

32. Rahal JJ, Urban C, Segal-Maurer S. Nosocomial antibiotic resistance in multiple gram-negative species: experience at one hospital with squeezing the resistance balloon at multiple sites. Clin Infect Dis 2002; 34:499–503.
33. Urban C, Segal-Maurer S, Rahal JJ. Considerations in control and treatment of nosocomial infections due to multidrug-resistant *Acinetobacter baumannii*. Clin Infect Dis 2003; 36:1268–1274.
34. Gorbach SL. Piperacillin/tazobactam in the treatment of polymicrobial infections. Intensive Care Med 1994; 20:S27–S34.
35. Lipsky BA, Berendt AR, Deery HG, Embil JM, Joseph WS, Karchmer AW, LeFrock JL, Lew DP, Mader JT, Norden C, Tan JS. Diagnosis and treatment of diabetic foot infections. Clin Infect Dis 2004; 39:885–910.
36. Mandell LA, Bartlett JG, Dowell SF, File TM Jr, Musher DM, Whitney C. Update of practice guidelines for the management of community-acquired pneumonia in immunocompetent adults. Clin Infect Dis 2003; 37:1405–1433.
37. Hughes WT, Armstrong D, Bodey GP, Bow EJ, Brown AE, Calandra T, Feld R, Pizzo PA, Rolston KV, Shenep JL, Young LS. 2002 guidelines for the use of antimicrobial agents in neutropenic patients with cancer. Clin Infect Dis 2002; 34:730–751.
38. Solomkin JS, Mazuski JE, Baron EJ, Sawyer RG, Nathens AB, DiPiro JT, Buchman T, Dellinger EP, Jernigan J, Gorbach S, Chow AW, Bartlett J. Guidelines for the selection of anti-infective agents for complicated intra-abdominal infections. Clin Infect Dis 2003; 37:997–1005.
39. Livermore DM. The need for new antibiotics. Clin Microbiol Infect 2004; 10(suppl 4): 1–9.
40. Georgopapadakou NH. β-Lactamase inhibitors: evolving compounds for evolving resistance targets. Expert Opin Investig Drugs 2004; 13:1307–1318.

SUGGESTED READING

Georgopapadakou NH. β-lactamase inhibitors: evolving compounds for evolving resistance targets. Expert Opin Investig Drugs 2004; 13:1307–1318.

12

Glycopeptides

Burke A. Cunha
Infectious Disease Division, Winthrop-University Hospital, Mineola and Department of Medicine, State University of New York School of Medicine, Stony Brook, New York, U.S.A.

Key Points:

- The two important glycopeptides are vancomycin and teichoplanin, the latter drug being unavailable in the United States.
- Vancomycin's spectrum is primarily Gram-positive bacteria including staphylococci and streptococci as well as *Clostridium difficile*.
- Vancomycin is available in oral (PO) and intravenous (IV) preparations. Except for treating *C. difficile* diarrhea with oral vancomycin, the vancomycin is administered by the IV route for systemic infections.
- The usual dose of vancomycin for elderly patients with relatively normal renal function and moderate to severe infection is 1 g (IV) every 12 hr.
- Vancomycin, contrary to common belief, is not nephrotoxic. In renal insufficiency, vancomycin dosing should be based on CrCl and not vancomycin serum levels.

1. INTRODUCTION

Glycopeptides are antibiotics with anti-Gram-positive activity. Vancomycin has been used worldwide for decades to treat serious staphylococcal infections. Teicoplanin has not been available in the United States, but has been used worldwide as an alternative to vancomycin. Intravenous (IV) vancomycin's main use has been against staphylococci, e.g., coagulase-negative *Staphylococcus epidermidis* (CoNS), methicillin-sensitive *Staphylococcus aureus* (MSSA), and methicillin-resistant *S. aureus* (MRSA). Oral vancomycin is the preferred drug against *Clostridium difficile* diarrhea. Vancomycin has been used extensively to treat penicillin-allergic infections due to susceptible organisms and Gram-positive shunt infections/bacteremias in dialysis patients. The use of vancomycin has been limited by the emergence of vancomycin-resistant enterococci (VRE) during/following vancomycin therapy. Another concern is decreasing susceptibility of *S. aureus* to vancomcyin, i.e., vancomycin-intermediate *S. aureus* (VISA). Fortunately, high-level resistance of *S. aureus* to vancomycin, i.e., vancomycin-resistant *S. aureus* (VRSA), remains rare (1–5).

Teicoplanin's structure and use is similar to vancomycin. An advantage of teicoplanin over vancomycin is that it may be given intramuscularly. Teicoplanin-resistant staphylococci were detected before vancomycin-resistant strains, and cross-reaction between vancomycin and teicoplanin is a concern (6–10).

2. CHEMISTRY AND MECHANISM OF ACTION

Glycopeptides are chemically complex antimicrobial compounds that contain a heptapeptide connected to a variety of sugar groups. Vancomycin was isolated from *Nocardia orientalis*. Teicoplanin is derived from the Actinomycete, *Actinoplanes teichomyceticus*. Both vancomycin and teichoplanin were discovered in the 1950s. Vancomycin was introduced into clinical use in 1956, and since that time, teicoplanin has been used extensively in Europe but not in the United States. Glycopeptides have a larger structure and molecular weight than do β-lactams and aminoglycosides. Both vancomycin and teicoplanin act on the peptidoglycan component of bacterial cell walls in Gram-Positive Organisms. Vancomycin has an effect on intracellular or RNA synthesis, but teichoplanin does not. Pharmacokinetically, vancomycin and teicoplanin exhibit concentration-dependent killing kinetics and are bactericidal at high concentrations and are bacterostatic at lower concentrations (4–7).

3. ANTIMICROBIAL SPECTRUM

Vancomycin is highly active against Gram-positive aerobic and anaerobic organisms. Vancomycin has a high degree of activity against *S. aureus* (both MSSA and MRSA strains), CoNS, *Streptococcus pneumoniae* (including highly penicillin-resistant strains), *Streptococcus bovis*, groups A, B, C, and G streptococci, viridans streptococci, and *Enterococcus faecalis* (non-VRE strains). Vancomycin is also active against Actinomyces, *Propionibacterium acnes*, *Bacillus anthracis*, *Listeria monocytogenes*, *Corynebacterium diphtheriae*, *Corynebacterium jaeikelium* (JK), *Rhodococcus equi*, *Clostridium perfringens*, *C. difficile*, and *Borellia burgdorferi* Vancomycin has little activity against most *Enterococcus faecium* (VRE), Gram-negative organisms, anaerobic organisms (excluding clostridia), rickettsiae, and atypical pathogens (e.g., Legionella, Mycoplasma, Chlamydia). Against even-sensitive strains of group D enterococci, e.g., *E. faecalis*, vancomycin is bacteriostatic rather than bactericidal. Bactericidal activity is achieved if a β-lactam, e.g., penicillin, or an aminoglycoside is given together with vancomycin. Vancomycin plus gentamicin is bactericidal against nearly all strains of *E. faecalis*. Vancomycin has little or no activity against *Leukonostoc*, *Lactobacillus*, and *Erysipelothrix rhusiopathiae*, *Flavobacterium meningosepticum*, and *Neisseria* species (11–17).

Teicoplanin has the same spectrum of activity as vancomycin. There are subtle differences in activity, particularly with respect to Gram-positive cocci. Teicoplanin has lower minimum inhibitory concentrations (MICs) than vancomycin with respect to *S. aureus*, *Streptococcus pyogenes*, *S. pneumoniae*, and *E. faecalis*. Vancomycin and teicoplanin are equally active against *C. difficile*. Teicoplanin is less active than vancomycin is against *Streptococcus hemolyticus*. Neither vancomycin nor teicoplanin is active against most *E. faecium* (VRE) strains. The oral administration of vancomycin results in a high intraluminal concentration of the drug because it is not significantly absorbed from the gastrointestinal (GI) tract. After a 500 mg oral dose of vancomycin, intraluminal levels in the colon are ≈3000–5000 μg/mL (17–23) (Tables 1 and 2).

Table 1 In Vitro Antibacterial Activity of Teicoplanin Compared with Vancomycin Against Selected Gram-Positive Organisms

	Reported range of MIC_{90} values (μg/mL)	
Organism	Teicoplanin ($\leq$8 μg/mL)	Vancomycin ($\leq$4 μg/mL)
Staphylococci		
S. aureus		
Methicillin sensitive (MSSA)	0.2–1.6	0.78–3.1
Methicillin resistant (MRSA)	0.195–3.12	0.5–3.12
S. epidermidis		
Methicillin sensitive (MSSE)	1.56–6.3	1.56–6.3
Methicillin resistant (MRSE)	3.1–12.5	3.1–4.0
S. haemolyticus	2.0 > 16	1
S. saprophyticus	0.78–3.1	1.56
Streptococci		
S. pneumoniae	0.1–0.2	0.25–0.8
S. pyogenes	0.1–0.5	0.78–1.0
S. agalactiae	0.2–0.4	0.78–1.0
Group C	0.1	
S. bovis	0.4–0.5	1
Group F	0.12–0.2	1
Group G	0.12–0.2	0.5
Viridans group	0.25–0.4	1
Enterococci	1–4	0.12–0.5
Listeria monocytogenes	0.2–3.1	1.56–4.0
Corynebacterium jeikeium (JK)	0.8	1.8
C. difficile	0.2–0.8	1.0–1.6

Note: All studies used standard broth or agar dilution techniques.
Abbreviation: MIC_{90}, minimum inhibitory concentration.
Source: Adapted from Ref. 9.

4. CLINICAL PHARMACOLOGY

Vancomycin, given as a 1 g IV dose achieves peak serum concentrations of $\approx$60 μg/mL. Ninety percent of vancomycin is excreted unchanged in the urine. The plasma-protein binding of vancomycin is 55%, and its volume of distribution (V_d) is 0.7 L/kg. The half-life of vancomycin with normal renal function is $\approx$6 hr and in anuria, 180 hr. Given as 1 g every 12 hr dose, therapeutic serum concentrations of vancomycin are 25–40 μg/mL (peak concentrations), and 5–12 μg/mL are the trough concentrations. Vancomycin penetrates well into most body sites except cerebrospinal fluid (CSF), peritoneal fluid, and synovial fluid. Penetration of vancomycin into noninflamed meninges is nil, and in the presence of meningitis, $\approx$25%. The intraperitoneal absorption of vancomycin is $\approx$40%, and the biliary excretion of vancomycin is $\approx$50% (1,5,24–27).

Like vancomycin, teicoplanin does not significantly absorb from the GI tract and for this reason it may be administered orally to treat *C. difficile* diarrhea, as with vancomycin (Section 3). IV teicoplanin given in a dose of 6 mg/kg results in peak serum concentrations of $\approx$112 μg/mL. Doses of 3 mg/kg of teicoplanin administered intravenously yield peak serum concentrations of $\approx$54 μg/mL. After a 6 mg/kg dose of teicoplanin, the serum concentrations at 24 hr are $\approx$4 μg/mL. Teicoplanin may be

Table 2 Effective Clinical Spectrum of Vancomycin and Teicoplanin

Susceptible organisms	Nonsusceptible organisms
S. aureus	VISA
MSSA	VRSA
MRSA	S. haemolyticus
S. epidermidis[a]	E. faecium (VRE)
Groups A, B, C, GG streptococci	Aerobic Gram-negative bacilli
Viridans streptococci	Anaerobic Gram-negative bacilli
Streptococcus pneumoniae	(Bacteroides fragilis)
S. bovis	Nocardia
Enterococcus faecalis (non-VRE)	Lactobacilli
Coryneacterium diphtheriae	Leuconostoc
Corynebacterium JK	
Propionibacterium acnes	
Bacillus anthracis	
Actinomyces	
Anaerobic streptococci	
Clostridia perfringens	
C. difficile	
Lactobacilli	

[a] Teicoplanin relative resistance may occur with strains of S. epidermides/S. haemolyticus. Teicoplanin resistant isolates reported which are cross-resistant to vancomycin. Teicoplanin has no activity against Neisseria.

Abbreviations: VISA, vancomycin-intermediate Staphylococcus aureus; VRSA, vancomycin-resistant Staphylococcus aureus; VRE, vancomycin resistant enterococci.

given by rapid IV injection in contrast to vancomycin, which should be administered slowly over a 60 min period. Teicoplanin may be given intramuscularly (bioavailability 90%), which achieves peak concentrations ≈2 hr after intramuscular (IM) injection. Teicoplanin is 90% protein bound, and has a large volume of distribution. The half-life of teicoplanin is 50–100 hr with normal renal function. The dose of teicoplanin should be decreased in renal failure; the dose of teicoplanin per day is decreased proportionately with decrease in creatinine clearance. Approximately 80% of teicoplanin should be eliminated via the urine, and it is not removed by hemodialysis or peritoneal dialysis. Teicoplanin penetrates most tissues well, as does vancomycin, but like vancomycin its penetration into synovial fluid, peritoneal fluid, and CSF is limited. Although teicoplanin is excreted via urine and feces, it is metabolized in the liver. Teicoplanin does not penetrate cardiac tissue well, and concentrates in phagocytic white cells (28–32) (Tables 3 and 4).

5. CLINICAL INDICATIONS

5.1. *C. difficile* Diarrhea

Vancomycin is clinically used in an oral formulation for the treatment of *C. difficile* diarrhea and in an IV preparation for the treatment of Gram-positive coccal infections. The use of vancomycin orally to treat *C. difficile* diarrhea is based on the fact that oral vancomycin is poorly absorbed and concentrates intraluminally in the colon, the site of *C. difficile* diarrhea. Oral doses of 125–250 mg given every 6 hr result in intraluminal

Table 3 Clinical Uses of Vancomycin and Teicoplanin

Prophylaxis	Therapy
Prosthetic valve endocarditis prophylaxis (procedures below the waist)	Bacterial endocarditis (Gram+)
Hemodialysis shunt infections (Gram+ bacteria)	Serious MSSA/MRSA infections (in penicillin allergic patients)
Open heart surgery (if infection incidence of TCV MRSA infection >20%)	Highly penicillin resistant strains of *Streptococcal pneumoniae* (excluding CNS infections)
	Streptococcal infections (excluding VRE)
	CAPD peritonitis (IP)
	Hemodialysis shunt infections (Gram+ bacteria)
	C. difficile diarrhea (PO)

Abbreviations: TCV, tricuspid valve; MRSA, methicillin-resistant *Staphylococcus aureus*; MSSA, methicillin-sensitive S. *aureus*; CNS, central nervous system; VRE, vancomycin-resistant enterococci; CAPD, chronic ambulatory peritoneal dialysis; IP, intraperitoneal; PO, oral.

concentrations of 3000–5000 μg/mL of vancomycin. Such concentrations are extremely effective for *C. difficile* diarrhea and do not lead to the emergence of VRE.

Elderly patients given many drugs, particularly antibiotics, often get *C. difficile* diarrhea. Oral metronidazole is often used to treat *C. difficile* diarrhea in adults as well as elderly patients. Oral metronidazole used to treat *C. difficile* diarrhea, in the author's experience, not infrequently fails, requiring retreatment with oral vancomycin. Oral vancomycin is uniformly effective in treating *C. difficile* diarrhea. In *C. difficile* colitis, oral vancomycin has no role. *C. difficile* colitis causes an ileus of the colon. Orally administered vancomycin does not reach the site of the infection and pools in the small bowel rendering it useless in *C. difficile* colitis. IV vancomycin also has no place in the treatment of *C. difficile* colitis. Vancomycin given intrave-

Table 4 Suboptimal use of Vancomycin and Teicoplanin

Avoid vancomycin for:	Avoid teicoplanin for:
Gram(−) aerobic bacillary infection	Gram(−) aerobic bacillary infection
VRE infection	*Enterococcus faecalis* infection
C. difficile colitis (IV/PO)	VRE infections
Nocardia infections	*C. difficile* colitis (IV/PO)
Erysipelothrix rhusiopathiae infections	Nocardia infections
Leuconostoc infections	*Erysipelothrix rhusiopathiae* infections
Lactobacillus infections	*Leuconostoc* infections
Empirical therapy of IV line infections (if incidence of IV MRSA line infections MRSA ≤20%)	*Lactobacillus*
	S. haemolyticus infection
Febrile neutropenia	
Treatment of CNS infections[a] (IV)	
Surgical prophylaxis (if incidence of surgical MRSA infection ≤20%)	

[a]Vancomycin penetration of CSF limited. If no alternative to vancomycin, use vancomycin IV plus IT.
Abbreviations: VRE, vancomycin-resistant enterococci; IV, intravenous; PO, oral; MRSA, methicillin-resistant *Staphylococcus aureus*; CNS, central nervous system.

nously does not result in effective intraluminal concentrations of vancomycin as does orally or intravenously administered metronidazole. Therefore, the cornerstone of treatment of *C. difficile* colitis remains metronidazole given intravenously/orally, and in conjunction with another drug active against the aerobic Gram-negative pathogens, which are permissive pathogens in this setting.

C. difficile diarrhea may initially be treated with metronidazole, and oral vancomycin used for metronidazole failures, or oral metronidazole may be used primarily to treat *C. difficile* diarrhea. Oral vancomycin does not appear to increase the prevalence of VRE in these patients (1–3).

5.2. Serious MSSA/MRSA

Vancomycin was originally used to treat Gram-positive coccal infections in penicillin-allergic patients. With the emergence of MRSA worldwide, vancomycin use has changed and it has been employed as primary therapy for serious MRSA infections. The extensive use of vancomycin for MRSA has led to its overuse and misuse, which is responsible for our current problems with VRE and vancomycin-resistant staphylococci.

Because of its long half-life in anuria, vancomycin is particularly useful in patients on hemodialysis, who have staphylococcal infections either due to MSSA or due to MRSA. Because vancomycin is not removed by dialysis, it may be given as a once-weekly dose, which is cost-effective and convenient for the patient. While VRE colonization or infection may follow vancomycin usage for dialysis, the clinical advantages override these concerns. In elderly patients with renal failure due to diabetes mellitus, hypertension, or glomerulonephritis, vancomycin is an ideal drug to treat staphylococcal infections in patients on hemodialysis (2–5).

5.3. Central Nervous System Infections

The kinetics of vancomycin permit the treatment of staphylococcal infections in most parts of the body, but its structural and physiochemical characteristics limit its usefulness in the Central Nervous System (CNS) infections, and in joint infections due to Gram-positive organisms. Penetration of vancomycin into the CSF is ≈40% of simultaneous serum levels. This may or may not be adequate to treat CNS infections due to susceptible organisms where ideally CSF concentrations should exceed the MIC of the infecting organism by a factor of 10. In other words, the vancomycin concentration should be 10 times higher than the MIC of the organism in the CSF for optimal effectiveness. If such concentrations cannot be achieved, then an alternate antibiotic with excellent CSF penetration characteristics should be used instead, e.g., linezolid, to treat staphylococcal infections of the CNS (1,2).

5.4. Septic Arthritis

Vancomycin is a suboptimal therapy in treating septic arthritis. The large size of the vancomycin molecule does not permit ready entry into infected synovial fluid. Treatment of MRSA or MSSA in patients with septic arthritis can be achieved with vancomycin, but are better treated with drugs that penetrate well into synovial fluid and have activity against staphylococci, e.g., daptomycin, quinupristin–dalfopristin, or linezolid (1,3,4).

5.5. Infective Endocarditis

The treatment of staphylococcal bacteremias or endocarditis with vancomycin has been problematic. In spite of adequate serum concentrations, some patients with staphylococcal bacteremias are not cleared with vancomycin therapy. Several explanations have been advanced to explain this therapeutic problem. Some believe that because vancomycin is a bacteriostatic drug, it clears bacteremias and treats endocarditis due to staphylococci less optimally than bactericidal drugs. Others have suggested that the reason for vancomycin's inability to clear these infections is due to vancomycin-tolerant or -resistant strains. Heterogenous vancomycin resistance (hVISA) has been put forth as a cause for the lack of therapeutic response in such patients. Some patients with staphylococcal bacteremias treated with vancomycin, not infrequently have bacteremias that fail to clear on the drug. Patients do not worsen, but the bacteremia does not clear and they do not improve clinically until switched to another agent with activity against MSSA/MRSA, e.g., linezolid, quinupristin–dalfopristin, or daptomycin (1–4).

5.6. Summary

IV vancomycin is the best used to treat MRSA/MSSA serious infections in hemo-dialysis patients because of its pharmacokinetics and nondialyzability. Vancomycin should be used with caution in treating certain MSSA/MRSA infections, i.e., parti-cularly septic arthritis, staphylococcal bacteremias, and staphylococcal endocarditis. Linezolid, quinupristin–dalfopristin, and daptomycin may be the preferable agents to use in this situation. For MSSA/MRSA infections involving the CSF, linezolid is pre-ferred to vancomycin because of superior CSF penetration of linezolid compared with vancomycin. Empirical vancomycin use for surgical prophylaxis and in treating staphylococcal infections in general should be minimized because of potential con-cerns regarding vancomycin resistance and the emergence of VRE. Vancomycin was initially used to treat staphylococcal infections in penicillin-allergic patients, but this justification is no longer applicable since there are other drugs available that can be used to treat staphylococcal infections that do not cross-react with β-lactam antibiotics. Vancomycin's usefulness is limited not by its toxicity but by its side effects and resistance potential.

6. ADMINISTRATION OF DRUG

Vancomycin is available for parenteral or oral administration. Oral vancomycin used to treat *C. difficile* diarrhea is administered as a 125 or 250 mg dose every 6 hr. IV vancomycin is usually administered as 1 g every 12 hr. Vancomycin should not be administered intramuscularly because it is painful when administered via the IM route. In patients with chronic ambulatory peritoneal dialysis, vancomycin may be administered intraperitoneally (IP); 2 g of vancomycin is given IP in the dialysis fluid. Alternatively, vancomycin may be given as a 30 mg/kg dose IP into the dialysis fluid. Because of shifts between the peritoneal compartment and the peripheral compartments, intraperitoneal vancomycin should always be given with IV vancomy-cin. After a loading dose of 30 mg/kg of vancomycin IP, a maintenance dose of 30 mg/L of vancomycin may be given IP per dialysis. Vancomycin to treat CNS infections due to susceptible organisms is administered intravenously supplemented by intrathecal doses of 10–20 mg/day. In hemodialysis patients, vancomycin is given

1g (IV) on a once-weekly basis. Vancomycin is not significantly removed by hemodialysis or peritoneal dialysis (1–5).

Teicoplanin dosing for severe infections is 400 mg (IV) every 12 hr for three doses, then 400 mg every 24 hr. For moderately severe infections, an initial 400 mg IV loading dose on day 1 is given for one dose, followed by 200 mg IV every 24 hr. Teicoplanin may be given intramuscularly and concentration time kinetics are similar with IV or IM administration. The bioavailability of teicoplanin after IM administration is ≈90%. Patients with anuria should be given teicoplanin in a daily dosage which is approximately one-third of the dose with normal renal function, i.e., 6 mg/kg (IV) every 72 hr. Alternatively, teicoplanin in anuria may be given as a 2 mg/kg (IV) dose every 24 hr. Patients with moderate renal insufficiency, with a creatinine clearance of ≈50 mL/min, should be given approximately half the daily dosage. Teicoplanin may be given either as 6 mg/kg (IV) every 24 hr dose or as 3 mg/kg (IV) dose every 24 hr, alternatively. Hemodialysis and peritoneal dialysis do not remove teicoplanin. Therefore, teicoplanin should be dosed for the degree of renal insufficiency and postdialysis dose is unnecessary. Teicoplanin may be used to treat CAPD peritonitis due to susceptible organisms; 50 mg is added to each 2 L of dialysate daily for 1 week. During the second week of treatment, 50 mg of teicoplanin is added to every other 2 L bag of dialysate fluid. Oral teicoplanin may be used to treat *C. difficile* diarrhea. The usual dose for teicoplanin to treat *C. difficile* diarrhea ranges from 200 mg oral (PO) every 12 hr to 500 mg (PO) every 6 hr (7–10).

7. DRUG MONITORING AND ADVERSE EFFECTS

7.1. Vancomycin and Teicoplanin Serum Levels

Serum concentrations of antibiotics are measured to determine if therapeutic levels are being achieved or to monitor for toxicity. Vancomycin serum levels have been employed for many years, primarily to monitor for potential vancomycin nephro- and ototoxicity, and rarely have been used to monitor efficacy. The notion that vancomycin serum levels were needed to monitor potential vancomycin toxicity was based on the toxicity of the early preparations of vancomycin. Vancomycin was introduced in the era then aminoglycosides were the mainstay of the therapeutic armamentarium. Obtaining vancomycin serum concentrations continued even after it was demonstrated that vancomycin was not a nephrotoxic antibiotic. To this day, no study has clearly shown a relationship between nephrotoxicity ozuromycin serum levels. In studies where vancomycin is implicated as a potential cause of nephrotoxicity, there are always one or more other drugs with a known nephrotoxic potential that are responsible for the nephrotoxicity in the combination. During the past decade, the clinical usefulness of vancomycin levels has been questioned by many authorities. To get peak and serum vancomycin concentrations to monitor toxicity makes sense only if the drug is nephrotoxic or ototoxic, which ozuromycin is not. In renal insufficiency, vancomycin dosing should be based on CrCl and not vancomycin serum levels (1–4).

Vancomycin serum concentrations are used primarily now to check the therapeutic efficacy and not toxicity. If vancomycin serum levels are desired to check for efficacy, peak serum concentrations should be checked in patients who are likely to have different pharmacokinetic profiles, e.g., burn patients, those with obesity, etc. Vancomycin serum concentrations should be obtained after the drug has reached a steady state, i.e., four to five half-lives ($t_{1/2}$). Trough concentrations should be obtained 30 min prior to the next dose and peak concentrations 30 min after the dose is given. Pharmacokinetically, it is not rational to obtain vancomycin levels after a single dose or on patients on hemodialysis. Therapeutic vancomycin serum concentrations are 20–40 µg/mL. In summary, vancomycin serum levels should be obtained only in special situations where pharmacokinetic considerations in certain host subsets require monitoring for adequacy of therapy (1,33–37).

7.2. Teicoplanin Serum Levels

Because teicoplanin is potentially ototoxic, serum levels are recommended in situations where teicoplanin accumulation is likely. Teicoplanin levels are also useful to verify the adequacy of therapy in treating serious infections, e.g., infective endocarditis, where serum concentrations should be maintained to ≥ 10 µg/mL. Teicoplanin serum trough concentrations should be maintained in the range of 20–60 µg/mL. Teicoplanin ototoxicity has been associated with peak serum concentrations ≥ 85 µg/mL, and trough concentrations > 40 µg/mL.

7.3. Vancomycin Adverse Effects

The most common vancomycin adverse effects are "red man or red neck syndrome" and hematologic side effects. The administration of vancomycin by rapid IV infusion may result in a reddening of the neck or body shortly after vancomycin infusion. This has been termed "red man or red neck syndrome" depending on the distribution of the rash. Red neck/red man syndrome is a histamine-mediated, short-lived response that is self limiting after minutes or hours. It requires no treatment and does not indicate an allergy to vancomycin.

Vancomycin has frequently been responsible for a variety of hematologic side effects including leukopenia or thrombocytopenia. Anemia is not a side effect of vancomycin use. Leukopenia and thrombocytopenia are the most common side effects seen in clinical practice associated with vancomycin use. Rarely, vancomycin use has also been associated with cardiac arrest. Because vancomycin is not a nephrotoxic antibiotic, increases in the blood urea nitrogen (BUN) or serum creatinine in patients receiving vancomycin should not be ascribed to vancomycin nephrotoxicity. In such patients, other causes of an increased BUN/increased creatinine should be sought as the explanation for these abnormalities rather than ascribing it to vancomycin.

An important consequence of vancomycin therapy is that its use predisposes to the emergence of VRE. Intravenous but not oral vancomycin often leads to an increase in the prevalence of VRE. Enterococci are intestinal organisms, 90% of which are *E. faecalis*, which is sensitive to vancomycin. The remaining $\leq 10\%$ of unaltered enterococcal gut flora is due to *E. faecium*. Virtually all strains of *E. faecium* are vancomycin resistant and hence *E. faecium* has become synonymous with VRE. The overuse and misuse of vancomycin over the years has not resulted in an increased *E. faecalis* resistance. Rather, it has increased the prevalence of the normally present, naturally vancomycin-resistant strains of *E. faecium* in the gut flora. Intravenous therapy with vancomycin alters the gut flora and decreases the number of *E. faecalis* sensitive to vancomycin and causes an increase in the normally resistant strains of *E. faecium* to become more prevalent. The increase in "enterococcal resistance" in the literature refers to an increase in the prevalence of *E. faecium* strains rather than an increase in resistance per se. It is not clear why vancomycin administered intravenously predisposes to VRE, while oral vancomycin administration does not. The association of IV vancomycin use and the

Table 5 Adverse Effects of Vancomycin and Teicoplanin

Vancomycin	Teicoplanin
Fever/chills	Mild pain on IM injection
Phlebitis	Potential ototoxicity
Pain on IM injection	Thrombocytopenia
"Red man" syndrome	Eosinophilia
Leukopenia	Skin rash
Thrombocytopenia	Mild ↑ serum transaminases
Sudden death syndrome	

subsequent emergence of VRE have been noted in patients with normal renal function and in those with renal failure on hemodialysis. The oral treatment of *C. difficile* with vancomycin does not predispose to VRE. Vancomycin use should be minimized and carefully considered because of its propensity to increase the prevalence of VRE in an institution.

Prolonged IV vancomycin use has also been associated with vancomycin resistance. Vancomycin with reduced susceptibility or so-called intermediate sensitivity, e.g., VISA strains, has been related to prolonged vancomycin usage. Staphylococci that have intermediate susceptibility to vancomycin have developed thick cell walls. It is thought that VISA strains represent a permeability barrier to the entrance of vancomycin into the cell. In summary, vancomycin usage should be minimized, not only because of its hematologic side effects, but also more importantly because of its propensity to foster the development of vancomycin-resistant strains of *S. aureus* and increase the prevalence of vancomycin-resistant enterococci (1,37–39).

7.4. Teicoplanin Side Effects

Teicoplanin side effects are uncommon. Eosinophilia is uncommon, and leukopenia is rare. Thrombocytopenia and uremia are not teicoplanin side effects. Teicoplanin is potentially ototoxic. Unlike vancomycin, teicoplanin has not been associated with red man syndrome. Skin rash has rarely been reported with teicoplanin (40–44) (Table 5).

REFERENCES

1. Cunha BA. Vancomycin. Med Clin North Am 1995; 79:817–831.
2. Alexander MR. A review of vancomycin after 15 years of use. Drug Intell Clin Pharm 1974; 8:520–524.
3. Cook FV, Farrar WE Jr. Vancomycin revisited. Ann Intern Med 1978; 88:813–818.
4. Cunha BA. Vancomycin Serum Levels: unnecessary, unhelpful, and costly. Antibiotics for Clinicians. 2004; 8:273–277.
5. Kucers A. Vancomycin. In: Kucers A, Crowe SM, Grayson ML, Hoy JF, eds. The Use of Antibiotics. Oxford: Butterworth Heinemann, 1997:763–790.
6. Reynolds PE. Structure, biochemistry, and mechanisms of action of glycopeptide antibiotics. Eur J Clin Microbiol Infect Dis 1989; 8:943–950.
7. Williams AH, Gruneber RN. Teicoplanin. J Antimicrob Chemother 1984; 14:441–445.

8. Trautman M, Wiedeck H, Ruhnke M, Oethinger M, Marre R. Teicoplanin: 10 years of clinical experience. Infection 1994; 22:430–436.

9. Shea KW, Cunha BA. Teicoplanin. Med Clin North Am 1995; 79:833–844.

10. Kucers A. Teicoplanin. In: Kucers A, Crowe SM, Grayson ML, Hoy JF, eds. The Use of Antibiotics. Oxford: Butterworth Heinemann, 1997:791–801.

11. Watanakunakorn C, Bakie C. The antibacterial action of vancomycin. Rev Infect Dis 1981; 3:S210–S215.

12. Hiramatsu K, Aritaka AN, Hanaki H, Kawasaki S, Hosoda Y, Hori S, Fukuchi Y, Kobayashi I. Dissemination in Japanese hospitals of strains of *Staphylococcus aureus* heterogeneously resistant to vancomycin. Lancet 1997; 350:1670–1673.

13. Hiramatsu K, Hanaki H, Ino T, Yabuta K, Oguri T, Tenover FC. Methicillin-resistant *Staphylococcus aureus* clinical strain with reduced vancomycin susceptibility. J Antimicrob Chemother 1997; 40:135–136.

14. Chang S, Sievert DM, Hageman J, Boulton M, Tenover FC, Downes FP, Shah S, Rudrik J, Pupp GR, Brown WJ, Cardo D, Fridkin SK. Infection with vancomycin-resistant *Staphylococcus aureus* containing the vanA resistance gene. N Engl J Med 2003; 348: 1342–1347.

15. Liu C, Chambers HF. *Staphylococcus aureus* with heterogeneous resistance to vancomycin: epidemiology clinical significance, critical assessment of diagnostic methods. Antimicrob Agents Chemother 2003; 47:3040–3045.

16. Howden BP, Ward PB, Charles PGP, Korman TM, Fuller A, du Cross P, Brabsch EA, Roberts SA, Robson J, Read K, Bak N, Hurley J, Johnson PDR, Morris AJ, Mayall BC, Grayson L. Treatment outcomes for serious infections caused by methicillin-resistant *Staphylococcus aureus* with reduced vancomycin susceptibility. Clin Infect Dis 2004; 38:521–528.

17. Tenover F, Biddle J, Lancaster AM. Increasing resistance to vancomycin and other glycopeptides in *Staphylococcus aureus*. Emerg Infect Dis 2001; 7:327–332.

18. Bannerman TL, Wadiak DL, Kloos WE. Susceptibility of penicillin-sensitive and -resistant strains of *Streptococcus pneumoniae* to new antimicrobial agents, including daptomycin, teicoplanin, cefpodoxime and quinolones. J Antimicrob Chemother 1991; 35:1919–1922.

19. Campoli-Richards DM, Brogden RN, Faulds D. Teicoplanin. A review of its antibacterial activity, pharmacokinetic properties, and therapeutic potential. Drugs 1990; 40: 449–486.

20. Mainardi J-L, Shlaes DM, Goering RV, Shlaes JH, Acar JF, Goldstein FW. Decreased teicoplanin susceptibility of methicillin-resistant strains of *Staphylococcus aureus*. J Infect Dis 1995; 171:1646–1650.

21. Shlaes DM, Shlaes JH. Teicoplanin selects for *Staphylococcus aureus* that is resistant to vancomycin. Clin Infect Dis 1995; 20:1071–1073.

22. Verbist L, Tjandramaga B, Hendrickx B, Van Hecken A, Van Melle P. In vitro activity and human pharmacokinetics of teicoplanin. Antimicrob Agents Chemother 1984; 26:881–886.

23. Watanakunakorn C. In-vitro selection of resistance of *Staphylococcus aureus* to teicoplanin and vancomycin. J Antimicrob Chemother 1990; 25:69–72.

24. Moellering RC Jr, Krogstad D, Greenblatt DJ. Pharmacokinetics of vancomycin in normal subjects and in patients with reduced renal function. Rev Infect Dis 1981; 3:S230–S235.

25. Moellering RC Jr, Krogstad DJ, Greenblatt DJ. Vancomycin therapy in patients with impaired renal function: a nomogram for dosage. Ann Intern Med 1981; 94: 343–346.

26. Daschner FD, Frank U, Kümmel A, Schmidt-Eisenlohr E, Schlosser V, Spillner H, Schuster B, Schindler M. Pharmacokinetics of vancomycin in serum and tissue of patients undergoing open-heart surgery. J Antimicrob Chemother 1987; 19:359–362.

27. Cunha BA, Quintiliani R, Deglin JM, Izard MW, Nightingale CH. Pharmaco-kinetics of vancomycin in anuria. Rev Infect Dis 1981; 3:S269–S272.

28. Carver PL, Nightingale CH, Quintiliani R, Sweeney K, Stevens RC, Maderazo E. Pharmacokinetics of single- and multiple-dose teicoplanin in healthy volunteers. Antimicrob Agents Chemother 1989; 33:82–86.

29. Falcoz C, Ferry N, Pozet N, Cuisinaud G, Zech PY, Sassard J. Pharmacokinetics of teicoplanin in renal failure. Antimicrob Agents Chemother 1983; 31:1255–1262.

30. Lam YWF, Kapusnik-Uner JE, Sachdeva M, Hackbarth C, Gambertoglio JG, Sande MA. The pharmacokinetics of teicoplanin in varying degrees of renal function. Clin Pharmacol Ther 1990; 47:655–661.

31. Guay DRP, Awni WM, Halstenson CE, Kenny MT, Keane WF, Matzke GR. Teicoplanin pharmacokinetics in patients undergoing continuous ambulatory peritoneal dialysis after intravenous and intraperitoneal dosing. Antimicrob Agents Chemother 1989; 33:2012–2015.

32. Wilson APR, Gruneberg RN, Neu H. Dosage recommendations for teicoplanin. J Antimicrob Chemother 1993; 32:792–796.

33. Beckers B, Broderson HP, Stolpmann RM, Jansen G, Larbig D. Efficacy and pharmacokinetics of teicoplanin in hemodialysis patients. Infection 1993; 21:71–74.

34. Levy JH, Marty AT. Vancomycin and adverse drug reactions. Crit Care Med 1993; 21:1107–1108.

35. Goetz MB, Sayers J. Nephrotoxicity of vancomycin and aminoglycoside therapy separately and in combination. J Antimicrob Chemother 1993; 32:325–334.

36. Bailie GR, Neal D. Vancomycin ototoxicity and nephrotoxicity. A review. Med Toxicol Adverse Drug Exp 1988; 3:376–386.

37. Pauly DJ, Musa DM, Lestico MR, Lindstrom MJ, Hetsko CM. Risk of nephrotoxicity with combination vancomycin-aminoglycoside antibiotic therapy. Pharmacotherapy 1990; 10:378–382.

38. Sorrell TC, Collignon PJ. A prospective study of adverse reactions associated with vancomycin therapy. J Antimicrob Chemother 1985; 16:235–241.

39. Terol MJ, Sierra J, Gatell JM, Rozman C. Thrombocytopenia due to use of teicoplanin. Clin Infect Dis 1993; 17:927.

40. Davey PG, Williams AH. A review of safety profile of teicoplanin. J Antimicrob Chemother 1991; 27(suppl B):69–73.

41. Davenport A. Allergic cross-reactivity to teicoplanin and vancomycin. Nephron 1993; 63:482.

42. McElrath MJ, Goldberg D, Neu HC. Allergic-cross reactivity of teicoplanin and vancomycin. 1986; 1(8471):47.

43. Schlemmer B, Falkman H, Boudjadja A, Jacob L, LeGall JR. Teicoplanin for patients allergic to vancomycin. New Engl J Med 1988; 318:1127–1128.

44. Smith SR, Cheesebrough JS, Makris M, Davies JM. Teicoplanin administration in patients experiencing reactions to vancomycin. J Antimicrob Chemother 1989; 23:810–812.

SUGGESTED READING

Cunha BA. Antibiotic Essentials. Michigan: Physicians Press, 2005.

Greenwood D. Glycopeptides. In: Finch RG, Greenwood D, Norrby SR, Whitley RJ, eds. Antibiotic Chemotherapy. London: Churchill Livingstone, 2003:300–304.

13
Quinolones

Thomas J. Marrie
Department of Medicine, University of Alberta, Edmonton, Alberta, Canada

Susan Fryters
Department of Regional Pharmacy Services, Capital Health, Edmonton, Alberta, Canada

Key Points:

- Quinolones are synthetic antibiotics with broad-spectrum antimicrobial activity against gram-positive, gram-negative. But, not all quinolones are active against and anaerobic bacteria, nor against *Chlamydia* spp., *Mycoplasma* spp., and *Legionella* spp.
- The newer quinolones, i.e., levofloxacin, gatifloxacin, moxifloxacin, and gemifloxacin are well absorbed orally. With the exception of gemifloxacin, the agents can also be administered intravenously.
- The pharmacokinetics of levofloxacin, gatifloxacin, moxifloxacin, and gemifloxacin are not altered substantially with age.
- The quinolones are indicated for a wide variety of infections caused by susceptible pathogens but are prescribed most often for urinary tract and respiratory tract infections, which are the two most common infections in the elderly.
- Drug interactions of quinolones with other compounds are common. Multivalent ions (e.g., iron, zinc, magnesium, aluminum) may interfere with absorption of quinolones from the gastrointestinal tract.

1. INTRODUCTION

Quinolones are synthetic antibiotics. In the early 1960s, a by-product of the commercial preparation of chloroquine, 7-chloro-1-ethyl, 1,4-dihydro-4-oxoquinolone-3-carboxylic acid, was found to have antibacterial activity and it was subsequently modified to produce nalidixic acid (the first quinolone), a 1, 8-naphthyridine (1). Just 2 years later nalidixic acid was marketed for the treatment of urinary tract infections (2).

The next major event was the development of the first fluoroquinolone, norfloxacin, by combining both the 7-piperazine and the 6-fluorine groups (2). Like nalidixic acid it was poorly absorbed, only available as an oral preparation and its only indication was treatment of urinary tract infections (2). Norfloxacin became available to clinicians in 1984.

Table 1 Currently Available Quinolone Antibiotics Classified According to Generation

Generation	Generic name	Trade name	Route	Comments[a]
First	Nalidixic acid	NegGram	PO	A
Second	Norfloxacin	Noroxin	PO	A
	Ciprofloxacin	Cipro	PO, IV	B
	Ofloxacin	Floxin	PO	C
	Enoxacin	Penetrex	PO	
Third	Levofloxacin	Levaquin	PO, IV	D
	Gatifloxacin	Tequin	PO, IV	E
Fourth	Moxifloxacin	Avelox	PO, IV	E
	Gemifloxacin	Factive	PO	E

[a]A—Poorly absorbed, useful for UTIs. Mainly active against Gram-negative organisms but no activity against *P. aeruginosa*. B—Well absorbed from the GI tract. Available as both oral and intravenous formulations. Excellent aerobic Gram-negative rod activity including *P. aeruginosa*; *Neisseria gonorrheae*, *Legionella* spp, *Mycoplasma, and Chlamydia* spp. C—Activity as for B except *Pseudomonas aeruginosa*. D—Better Gram-positive activity than A,B,C agents—especially *S. pneumoniae* and E—Gram-positive activity as for D agents. Active against anaerobic bacteria.
Abbreviations: PO, oral; IV, intravenous.

The modern era of quinolone antibiotics began in 1987 with the introduction of ciprofloxacin (2). This quinolone, which is available in both intravenous and oral formulations, was reasonably well absorbed and had a considerable spectrum of antibacterial activity. Most importantly, it was the first oral antimicrobial agent that was effective for the treatment of *Pseudomonas aeruginosa* at sites of infection other than the urinary tract.

Ofloxacin became available in 1990. It was extremely well absorbed from the gastrointestinal (GI) tract but had little activity against *P. aeruginosa*.

The next major event in the history of quinolone antibiotics was the development of levofloxacin, the L-isomer of ofloxacin. This and subsequent newer quinolones had much better Gram-positive activity than did the older quinolones. In particular, levofloxacin and its followers (moxifloxacin, gatifloxacin, gemifloxacin) were active against *Streptococcus pneumoniae*.

The increasing antimicrobial activity of the quinolones over the years has led to the concept of first, second, third, and fourth generations of these antibiotics (Table 1), with the implication that an increase in the generation means an increase in antimicrobial spectrum.

2. CHEMISTRY AND MECHANISM OF ACTION

In general, all quinolones consist of a bicyclic aromatic core composed of two fused six-membered rings (Fig. 1) Modifications at various positions on the molecule result in changes in spectrum and potency of antimicrobial activity and adverse effects.

The R1 moiety influences antibacterial activity and theophylline interaction (2). Cyclopropyl at R1, as in ciprofloxacin and some of the newer fluoroquinolones, results in a major increase in antimicrobial activity. Carboxylic acid at position 3 and a carbonyl group at position 4 are present in all fluoroquinolones and are important in cell entry and binding the DNA/DNA gyrase complex, and in interactions with magnesium, aluminum, and iron.

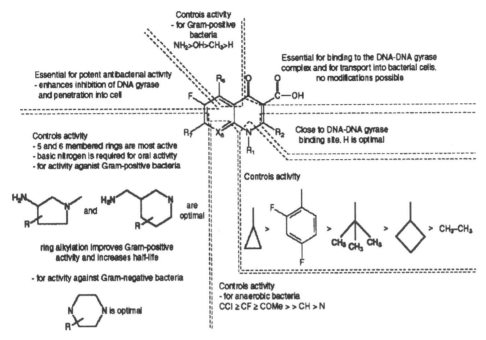

Figure 1 Quinolone molecule showing activity and adverse effects influenced by various chemical groups at different positions on the molecule. *Source*: From Ref. 3.

The R5 substituents are important for phototoxicity and genetic toxicity. All of the newer quinolones have a fluoro substituent at the C6 position, hence the name fluoroquinolone.

Modifications at R7 control gamma-amino-butyric acid (GABA) binding and it is this property that determines the extent of neurotoxicity, especially seizures, and the potential for drug interactions with theophylline and nonsteroidal anti-inflammatory drugs (NSAIDs) (3). In addition, changes at R7 also affect antibacterial activity and pharmacokinetics.

Changes at position 8 influence activity against anaerobic bacteria, and phototoxicity. The latter is pronounced for compounds with a halogen at this position, such as fluoro for sparfloxacin and chloro for clinafloxacin. A methoxy group confers antianaerobic activity, e.g., moxifloxacin and gatifloxacin. The fluoroquinolone/theophylline interaction is also affected by R8 substitution (3).

The mechanism of action of quinolones is inhibition of DNA synthesis by interfering with topoisomerase II (DNA gyrase) and topoisomerase IV. DNA gyrase maintains supercoiling in the bacterial chromosome and topoisomerase IV partitions the daughter chromosomes following DNA replication (4). DNA gyrase is composed of two subunits encoded by *gyr*A and *gyr*B genes while topoisomerase IV is encoded by *par*C and *par*E genes. Topoisomerase II in Gram-negative bacteria is more sensitive to quinolones while topoisomerase IV is more affected in Gram-positive bacteria (5). Inhibition of both enzymes is necessary for bactericidal activity and the relative affinity of a fluoroquinolone for both target enzymes dictates the in vitro activity (6). Resistance to fluoroquinolones arises through mutations in the genes that encode topoisomerases II and IV. *Gyr*A and *par*C are more frequently involved (4). Resistance due to these target site alterations tends to develop in a stepwise manner with the minimum inhibitory concentration (MIC) of the mutants increasing with each additional mutation in the topoisomerase (4).

Efflux can also be a mechanism whereby bacteria become resistant to fluoroquinolones. This is especially true for *P. aeruginosa*. Indeed, in Gram-negative microorganisms these efflux pumps have broad specificity often including aminoglycosides and beta-lactams as well as fluoroquinolones (4). Hydrophilic quinolones, such as ciprofloxacin, are more prone to efflux than hydrophobic quinolones, such as gatifloxacin, levofloxacin, and moxifloxacin (3).

3. ANTIMICROBIAL SPECTRUM

Fluoroquinolones are active against a wide spectrum of bacteria as well as *Chlamydia*, *Mycoplasma*, and *Legionella* species (Table 2). However, as seen in Table 2, fluoroquinolones are generally inactive against *Enterococcus* spp., methicillin-resistant *Staphylococcus aureus*, and *P. aeruginosa* (with the exception of ciprofloxacin—although in many centers 30–40% of *P. aeruginosa* isolates are now resistant to ciprofloxacin). Ciprofloxacin is the most active fluoroquinolone against Gram-negative organisms, including *P. aeruginosa* (10).

Table 2 Summary of the Antimicrobial Activity [MIC_{90} (mg/L)] of Selected Fluoroquinolones

Microorganism	Levo	Moxi	Gati	Cipro	Gemi
Gram-positive microorganisms					
PSSP	1	0.25	0.5	2	0.03–0.06
PRSP	1–2	0.25	0.5	2–4	0.06
Enterococcus faecalis	8– > 32	8–16	≥16	> 2– > 32	2
Streptococcus pyogenes	0.5–1	0.25	0.25	1	0.03
Streptococcus agalactiae (3)	1	0.25	0.4	2	0.06
MSSA	0.25–0.5	0.06–0.13	0.12–0.25	0.5– > 2	0.03
MRSA	4– > 32	2–4	4– > 32	> 2– > 32	8
Gram-negative microorganisms					
E. coli	≤0.12	≤0.5	≤0.1	≤0.25	0.015
P. aeruginosa	8–16	8–16	8	4	4–8
H. influenzae	≤0.03	≤0.03	≤0.03	≤0.016	0.008
M. catarrhalis	< 0.06	0.06	< 0.03	0.03	0.008
Haemophilus ducreyi				0.02	
Neisseria gonorrheae (9)	0.008	0.03	0.015	0.008	0.008
Miscellaneous microorganisms					
Chlamydia trachomatis	0.5	0.06	0.12	2	
Chlamydophila pneumoniae	1	1	0.25	2	0.25
Mycoplasma pneumoniae	0.5	0.12	0.12	2	0.12
Legionella pneumophila	0.015	0.015	0.015	0.03	0.03
Anaerobic microorganisms					
Anaerobic bacteria	NA	Act	Act	NA	Act
B. fragilis (3)	8	1	1	16	2

Abbreviations: PSSP, penicillin-susceptible *S. pneumoniae*; PRSP, penicillin-resistant *S. pneumoniae*; MSSA, methicillin-susceptible *Staphylococcus aureus*; MRSA, methicillin resistant *Staphylococcus aureus*; *Sources*: From Refs. 3,7,11.

Published susceptibility of the available systemic quinolones to relevant organisms is summarized in Table 3. *Haemophilus influenzae* and *Moraxella catarrhalis* were 99.9–100% susceptible to the quinolones tested—ciprofloxacin, levofloxacin, gatifloxacin, moxifloxacin, and gemifloxacin (12,22–24). *S. pneumoniae* resistance to fluoroquinolones (levofloxacin) increased from 0.6% in 1998–1999 to 0.9% in 2001–2002 in the United States (17). In Canada, fluoroquinolone resistance increased from 0.5% in 1997–1998 to 1.1% in 2001–2002 (14).

In some species of bacteria, such as *Neisseria gonorrheae,* resistance has been rapidly emerging. For example in the Philippines, high-level ciprofloxacin resistance (MIC > 4 mg/L) increased from 9% in 1994 to 49% by 1997 (25). In Ohio, USA, the incidence of gonococci with reduced susceptibility to ciprofloxacin rose from 2% in 1991 to 16% in 1994 (26). Another organism in which there has been a marked increase in resistance is *Campylobacter.* In Minnesota, the rate of quinolone resistance in *Campylobacter* spp. rose from 1.3% in 1992 to 10.2% in 1998 (27). In the same study, 14% of *Campylobacter jejuni* isolated from poultry were resistant to ciprofloxacin. There are 11 quinolones licensed for use in animals in various parts of the world and about 50 tons of proprietary quinolones and 70 tons of generic quinolones were consumed in 1 year in this industry (28). There are several lines of evidence that quinolone use in food animals leads to resistance among microorganisms in humans. First, the quinolones lead to resistance of the bacterial flora of animals. These resistant microorganisms are then transmitted to humans via direct contact with animals or through the consumption of contaminated food and water.

Moxifloxacin, gatifloxacin, and gemifloxacin are active against anaerobic bacteria (10,29,30). *Peptostreptococci* and most *Prevotella* and *Fusobacterium* spp. were inhibited by gatifloxacin at ≤1 mg/L in a U.S. study while higher values (≤25 mg/L) were noted in a Japanese study (29). This antibiotic is also active against *Bacteroides* spp. (27). Moxifloxacin inhibited 90% of 410 clinically important anaerobic bacterial strains at 2 mg/L (30). *Clostridium, Fusobacterium, Eubacterium, Prevotella* and *Peptostreptococcus* spp., *Propionibacterium acnes* and some *Bacteroides* spp. were susceptible (MIC$_{90}$ ≤ 2 mg/L) (30).

As with many other antibiotics there is a relationship between fluoroquinolone use and susceptibility of common pathogens. Zervos et al. found that from 1991 to 2000 in 10 teaching hospitals in the United States the overall susceptibility to fluoroquinolones decreased significantly and that the change in percentage of susceptibility was related to fluoroquinolone use (31). *P. aeruginosa, Proteus mirabilis,* and *Escherichia coli* showed decreases of 25.1%, 11.9%, and 6.8%, respectively.

4. PHARMACOLOGY

4.1. Pharmacokinetics

The newer fluoroquinolones, levofloxacin, gatifloxacin, and moxifloxacin, are extremely well absorbed from the GI tract. Gemifloxacin is 71% absorbed (34,35). All of the available fluoroquinolones achieve maximum concentration in the plasma within 1–2 hr after oral administration (3).

The volume of distribution ranges from 1.1 L/kg for levofloxacin to 1.8 L/kg for gatifloxacin, 3.3 L/kg for moxifloxacin, and 3.5 L/kg for both ciprofloxacin and gemifloxacin (3,32).

The new fluoroquinolones do not penetrate cerebrospinal fluid (CSF) very well but they do penetrate neutrophils, alveolar macrophages, bronchial mucosa,

Table 3 Susceptibility of Available Quinolones

Organism	Ref.	Program[a]	Year(s)	Geographic area	Source of isolates	Patients	Type of isolates	No. of isolates	% Susceptible			
									Cipro-floxacin	Levo-floxacin	Gati-floxacin	Moxi-floxacin
Gram-positive *S. pneumoniae*	12	SENTRY	2000	North America	5 Cdn and 25 U.S. medical centers	Inpatients with pneumonia	RT	246		98.8	99.2	
	13	CBSN	2000	Canada (10 provinces)	63 private, community, and university hospital labs	Inpatients and outpatients	Blood 40%, LRT 24%, conjunct 20%, ear swabs 10%, CSF 2%, other 2%	2,245	95.6	98.1	98.0	98.0
	14	CROSS	1997–2002	Canada (nine provinces)	25 medical centers	54% inpatients, 46% outpatients	RT	6,991		99.2	99.1	99.4
	15	ABC	2002	USA (nine states)	Labs of acute care hospitals	Inpatients	Invasive isolates	3,120		99.5		
	16	—	1999–2000	USA	33 medical centers	Inpatients and outpatients	RT 65.8%, blood, CSF, or other sterile body fluid 32.1%	1,531[b]	98.6	99.3	99.6	99.7

Gram-negative Enterobacteriaceae

Organism	Ref	Study	Year	Country	Labs	Patient population	Site	No.	%	%	%
Citrobacter spp.	17	TRUST	1998–2002	USA	Up to 240 labs	Inpatients and outpatients	Any site (61.3% from RT)	27,828			99.2
	18	TSN	2000	USA	257 labs	NR	NR	>3,800		90.5	91.8
	18	TRUST	2000	USA	26 hospital labs	Inpatients and outpatients	Any site	190	96.3	93.7	95.8
Enterobacter spp.	12	SENTRY	2000	North America	5 Cdn and 25 U.S. medical centers	Inpatients with pneumonia	RT	156	96.2		96.2
Enterobacter aerogenes	18	TSN	2000	USA	257 labs	NR	NR	>2,200		93.9	95.1
	18	TRUST	2000	USA	26 hospital labs	Inpatients and outpatients	Any site	161	96.9	96.3	97.5
Enterobacter cloacae	18	TSN	2000	USA	257 labs	NR	NR	>4,700		86.7	89.4
	18	TRUST	2000	USA	26 hospital labs	Inpatients and outpatients	Any site	297	96.0	91.3	95.6
E. coli	18	TSN	2000	USA	257 labs	NR	NR	>55,000		96.0	95.4
	18	TRUST	2000	USA	26 hospital labs	Inpatients and outpatients	Any site	655	94.7	94.5	94.7
	19	SENTRY	2000	North America	hospital labs	Inpatients	Urinary	635		95.0	

(Continued)

Table 3 Susceptibility of Available Quinolones (*Continued*)

Organism	Ref.	Program[a]	Year(s)	Geographic area	Source of isolates	Patients	Type of isolates	No. of isolates	% Susceptible			
									Cipro-floxacin	Levo-floxacin	Gati-floxacin	Moxi-floxacin
	12	SENTRY	2000	North America	5 Cdn and 25 U.S. medical centers	Inpatients with pneumonia	RT	105	93.3	94.3	93.3	
Klebsiella spp.	19	SENTRY	2000	North America	Hospital labs	Inpatients	Urinary	176	96.0			
	12	SENTRY	2000	North America	5 Cdn and 25 U.S. medical centers	Inpatients with pneumonia	RT	203	97.5	97.5	98.0	
Klebsiella pneumoniae	18	TSN	2000	USA	257 labs	NR	NR	>12,000	93.9	94.4		
	18	TRUST	2000	USA	26 hospital labs	Inpatients and outpatients	Any site	550	94.2	95.5	96.0	
Proteus mirabilis	18	TSN	2000	USA	257 labs	NR	NR	>7,400	87.4	90.9		
	18	TRUST	2000	USA	26 hospital labs	Inpatients and outpatients	Any site	430	87.7	94.0	87.7	
Serratia spp.	12	SENTRY	2000	North America	5 Cdn and 25 U.S. medical centers	Inpatients with pneumonia	RT	96	94.8		96.9	
S. marcescens	18	TSN	2000	USA	257 labs	NR	NR	>2,700	88.7	93.2		
	18	TRUST	2000	USA	26 hospital labs	Inpatients and outpatients	Any site	161	89.4	94.4	92.6	

Organism	Ref	Program	Year	Country	Source	Setting	Site	No. isolates	%	%	%
Providencia spp.	18	TSN	2000	USA	257 labs	NR	NR	>700	47.1	50.8	
	18	TRUST	2000	USA	26 hospital labs	Inpatients and outpatients	Any site	75	37.3	42.7	42.7
Other											
Acinetobacter baumanii	20	TSN	1998–2001	USA	65 hospital labs	ICU	Any site	Cipro 4,442, levo 2,691	49.2	55.1	
	18	TSN	2000	USA	257 labs	Non ICU	NR	>1,400	41.0	47.6	
						NR			47.8	54.3	
	18	TRUST	2000	USA	26 hospital labs	Inpatients and outpatients	Any site	82	47.6	50.0	56.1
P. aeruginosa	20	TSN	1998–2001	USA	65 hospital labs	ICU	Any site	Cipro 54,721, levo 33,361	75.7	72.5	
	18	TSN	2000	USA	257 labs	non-ICU	NR	>18,000	73.2	71.4	
						NR			66.4	66.3	
	18	TRUST	2000	USA	26 hospital labs	Inpatients and outpatients	Any site	404	73.5	73.0	71.0
	19	SENTRY	2000	North America	Hospital labs	Inpatients	Urinary	106	66.0		
	12	SENTRY	2000	North America	5 Cdn and 25 U.S. medical centers	Inpatients with pneumonia	RT	543	72.4	71.5	67.0

(Continued)

Table 3 Susceptibility of Available Quinolones (*Continued*)

Organism	Ref.	Program[a]	Year(s)	Geographic area	Source of isolates	Patients	Type of isolates	No. of isolates	% Susceptible Cipro-floxacin	Levo floxacin	Gati-floxacin	Moxi-floxacin
Neisseria gonorrheae	21	National Laboratory for STD	2001	Canada	Provincial labs	NR	Urethra, cervix, rectum; excl. pharynx	NR	97.9			

[a]Programs: ABC, Active Bacterial Core Surveillance; CBSN, Canadian Bacterial Surveillance Network; CROSS, Canadian Respiratory Organism Susceptibility Study; SENTRY Antimicrobial Surveillance Program; TRUST, Tracking Resistance in the United States Today; TSN, The Surveillance Network Database, USA.

[b]Ofloxacin = 94.4%.

Abbreviations: BAL, bronchoalveolar lavage; Cdn, Canadian; CA, community acquired; CSF, cerebrospinal fluid; labs, laboratories; LRT, lower respiratory tract; conjunct, conjunctiva; MEF, middle ear fluid; cipro, ciprofloxacin; NP, nasopharyngeal; levo, levofloxacin; NR, not reported; ICU, intensive care unit; RT, respiratory tract, susc., susceptible. *Source*: From Refs. 12–21.

Table 4 Comparison of Selected Pharmacokinetic Parameters

	Ciprofloxacin	Levofloxacin	Gatifloxacin	Moxi-floxacin	Gemifloxacin
Oral dose (mg)	500	500	400	400	320
Bioavailability (%)	70	99	96	86	71
C_{max} (mg/L)	2.3	5.1	3.9	3.3	1.2
Half-life (hr)	3.5	6.9	8.0	12.1	8.0
Dosage adjustment renal	Yes	Yes	Yes	No	Yes
Clcr (mL/min)—recommended dosage	<30—daily	20–49—500 mg day 1, then 250 mg daily; 10–19—500 mg loading dose then 250 mg q 48 hr	< 40–400 mg day 1, then 200 mg daily	NA	≤40–160 mg daily
Dosage adjustment hepatic	No	No	No	No	No

Note: C_{max}, peak plasma concentration; Clcr, creatinine clearance; NA, not applicable.
Source: From Refs. 3,10,32–35.

epithelial lining fluid, and sputum well (3). For example, the concentrations of drug in alveolar macrophages are 26-fold higher than the concentration in serum for gatifloxacin, 90-fold higher for gemifloxacin, and 21-fold higher for moxifloxacin (10). In contrast, the concentrations in CSF are 34–78% of serum levels for moxifloxacin, 36% for gatifloxacin and 22–33% for gemifloxacin (10). The corresponding values for levofloxacin and ciprofloxacin are 16% and 37%, respectively (32).

The elimination half-life of the quinolones ranges from 3.5 hr for ciprofloxacin to 12.1 hr for moxifloxacin (10,32) (Table 4).

Ciprofloxacin is cleared renally (2/3) as well as by hepatic and transintestinal routes (1/3) (33). Gatifloxacin and levofloxacin are excreted in the urine while gemifloxacin is eliminated by both renal (60%) and liver (40%) (10,32). Moxifloxacin undergoes glucuronidation and sulfate conjugation during its elimination by the liver (10). Thus, ciprofloxacin, levofloxacin, gatifloxacin, and gemifloxacin all require dosage adjustment in patients with impaired renal function. It is noteworthy that the pharmacokinetics of levofloxacin, gatifloxacin, gemifloxacin, and moxifloxacin are not altered in the elderly (32).

4.2. Pharmacodynamics

Quinolones exhibit concentration-dependent killing (36). Thus, the 24 hr area under the plasma concentration vs. time curve (AUC_{24})/MIC and peak plasma concentration (C_{max})/MIC ratios have been shown to be predictive of bacteriological eradication and clinical efficacy (37). A C_{max}/MIC ratio of ≥10:1 and an AUC_{24}/MIC ratio in the range of 100–125 results in maximal bacterial

Table 5 Comparison of Selected Pharmacodynamic Parameters

	Ciprofloxacin	Levofloxacin	Gatifloxacin	Moxifloxacin	Gemifloxacin
Oral dosage	500 mg bid	500 mg daily	400 mg daily	400 mg daily	320 mg daily
MIC_{90} S. pneumoniae (mg/L)	2	1	0.5	0.25	0.03
C_{max} (mg/L)	2.3	5.1	3.9	3.3	1.2
C_{max}/MIC_{90}	1.2	5.1	7.8	13.2	40.0
AUC_{24hr} total (mg/L/hr)	20	48	34	34	10
AUC_{24hr} total/ MIC_{90}	10	48	68	136	333
AUC_{24hr} free (mg/L/hr)	14	34	27	18	4
AUC_{24hr} free/ MIC_{90}	7	34	54	72	133

Note: Bid, twice a day; MIC_{90}, minimum inhibitory concentration of 90% of isolates; C_{max}, peak plasma concentration; $AUC_{24\,hr}$, 24 hr area under the plasma concentration time curve.
Source: From Refs. 3,10,32.

eradication in seriously ill patients with nosocomial Gram-negative bacillary infections (38). However, in community-acquired pneumonia due to *S. pneumoniae*, an AUC_{24}/MIC >25 predicts bacterial eradication (39). If one applies this concept to the various quinolones that could be used to treat *S. pneumoniae*, the following AUC_{24}/MIC ratios are obtained with standard doses: 14, 48, 68, 136, and 333 for ciprofloxacin, levofloxacin, gatifloxacin, moxifloxacin, and gemifloxacin, respectively (Table 5). Some authorities feel that the free drug AUC/MIC ratio should be used and that a ratio of >33.7 is adequate for the treatment of Gram-positive infections (40). Thus, ciprofloxacin is not a good agent for the treatment of *S. pneumoniae* infections and levofloxacin is inadequate for isolates with an MIC of ≥ 2 mg/L.

The second pharmacodynamic concept is that of the mutant prevention concentration (MPC) (41). This is the drug concentration at which the selection of resistant mutants is inhibited during antibiotic treatment. The mutational frequency of *S. pneumoniae* for fluoroquinolones is 10^{-7}–10^{-10}. The MPCs for *S. pneumoniae* differ for the different quinolones and vary with different strains. In one study, the MPCs, using standard doses of ciprofloxacin, levofloxacin, gatifloxacin, moxifloxacin, and gemifloxacin, were 16, 2, 1, 1, and 0.13 mg/L, respectively (32). Although not clinically proven, administration of fluoroquinolones to give serum drug levels at or above the MPC may prevent mutant selection.

5. CLINICAL INDICATIONS

Fluoroquinolones are indicated in a wide variety of infections. Perhaps the two most common indications are urinary tract infections (UTIs) and respiratory tract infections (RTIs). Ciprofloxacin is useful for the treatment of cystitis, pyelonephritis, and prostatitis due to a variety of aerobic Gram-negative bacteria. Gatifloxacin and levofloxacin also have Food and Drug Administration approval for cystitis, pyelonephritis, and complicated UTIs. Since moxifloxacin is not renally cleared, it should NOT be used for the treatment of UTIs.

The newer quinolones (levofloxacin, moxifloxacin, gatifloxacin, and gemifloxacin) are useful for the treatment of community-acquired respiratory tract infections, including pneumonia, acute bacterial exacerbations of chronic bronchitis, and acute bacterial sinusitis. Ciprofloxacin is an important antibiotic for the treatment of nosocomial pneumonia but NOT for the treatment of community-acquired pneumonia.

Ciprofloxacin has also proven useful as part of the treatment of diabetic foot infections. It is also useful in osteomyelitis secondary to contiguous spread from pressure ulcers or trauma. In addition, it is useful for Gram-negative prosthetic joint infections and for prosthetic joint infections due to methicillin-susceptible *S. aureus* when used in conjunction with rifampin.

Quinolones have also been used for the empirical treatment of acute infectious diarrhea suspected to be due to *E. coli*, *Salmonella*, *Shigella*, or *Aeromonas*. Fluoroquinolones are especially useful for the treatment of enteric fever due to *Salmonella typhi* or *Salmonella paratyphi*.

Ciprofloxacin can be used in conjunction with an antianaerobic agent in the management of intra-abdominal sepsis. It is noteworthy that because of increasing resistance of *Bacteroides fragilis* to fluoroquinolones, including those with activity against anaerobic bacteria, these agents are not recommended as single therapy of intra-abdominal infections (42). Ciprofloxacin has been used successfully in the treatment of acute cholecystitis and cholangitis.

Quinolones have also been used for the treatment of gonorrhea (ciprofloxacin, ofloxacin, gatifloxacin), *Chlamydia trachomatis* (ofloxacin), chancroid (ciprofloxacin), and donovanosis (granuloma inguinale) due to *Calymmatobacterium granulomatis*. Ofloxacin or ciprofloxacin, in conjunction with other antibiotics, has been used to treat pelvic inflammatory disease.

Quinolones have also been used as part of a multidrug regimen in the empirical treatment of fever in neutropenic patients (43). In addition, quinolones have been prescribed for infection prophylaxis in patients who are rendered neutropenic by cancer chemotherapy (43).

A recent indication for quinolone therapy is as part of a multidrug regimen for the management of infections due to resistant *Mycobacterium tuberculosis* (44). Quinolones can be used to treat tularemia in patients who are intolerant of standard regimens. The recent cases of inhalation anthrax in the United States led to the use of prolonged (60 days) courses of ciprofloxacin as prophylaxis for those exposed (45,46). Ciprofloxacin may also be prescribed for the treatment of anthrax.

Oral ciprofloxacin may also be used as prophylaxis for contacts of patients with *Neisseria meningitidis* meningitis.

Prudent use of these potent broad-spectrum quinolones is essential to minimize the development of resistance and preserve the usefulness of this class of antibiotics.

6. ADMINISTRATION

The usual dosage of ciprofloxacin is 500 or 750 mg twice daily orally (PO), while the intravenous (IV) dosage is 400 mg every 12 hr, or every 8 hr for serious infections. Gatifloxacin is given as 400 mg IV or PO once daily. Levofloxacin is also available in IV and oral formulations. The dosage is 500 or 750 mg once daily. Moxifloxacin is available as an oral and IV formulation in a dosage of 400 mg once daily. Gemifloxacin is available as a 320 mg oral tablet taken once daily.

Table 6 Comparison of the Drug Interactions Associated with Quinolones

Interacting drug(s)-Effect	Ciprofloxacin	Levofloxacin	Gatifloxacin	Moxifloxacin	Gemifloxacin
Drugs that can prolong the QT interval (see text) -Increased risk of cardiotoxicity (QTc prolongation, torsades de pointes, cardiac arrest)	Yes	Yes	Yes	Yes	Yes
Multivalent cations (Al, Fe, Mg, Zn), Sucralfate, Didanosine -Decreased quinolone absorption	Yes (give cipro 2 hr before or 6 hr after)	Yes (give levo 2 hr before or 4 hr after)	Yes (give gati 4 hr before or 4 hr after)	Yes (give moxi 4 hr before or 8 hr after)	Yes (give gemi 2 hr before or 3 hr after)
Calcium -Decreased quinolone absorption	Yes (give cipro 2 hr before or 6 hr after)	No	No	No	No
Antidiabetic agents[a] -Altered blood glucose	Yes	Yes	Yes	Yes	Yes
Theophylline/caffeine -Increased theophylline/caffeine concentration	Yes (monitor levels)	No	No	No	No
Warfarin[b] -Increased effect	Yes (rare)	Yes	No	No	No
Probenecid -Increased quinolone concentration	Yes	No	No	No	Yes
Phenytoin -Reduced metabolism	Yes (rare; monitor phenytoin levels)	—[c]	—	—	—
Digoxin	No	No	No	No	No

[a]Monitor blood glucose closely.
[b]Monitor prothrombin time/INR, and watch for evidence of bleeding.
[c]—, No data available.
Source: From Refs. 3,47,48.

7. DRUG INTERACTIONS

A number of compounds interfere with the absorption of quinolones. These include sucralfate, and anything containing iron, magnesium, aluminium, or zinc (e.g., antacids, vitamin and mineral supplements, didanosine) (49,50). Hence, these compounds should be avoided in patients who are receiving treatment with quinolones. Food does not interfere with the absorption of the quinolones, with the possible exception of ciprofloxacin taken with milk or yogurt alone.

Ciprofloxacin interacts with theophylline, warfarin, and phenytoin (3). The newer fluoroquinolones do not have these interactions, but there is a suggestion that there is an interaction between levofloxacin and warfarin (51). Fluoroquinolones do not interact with digoxin (3) (Table 6).

8. DRUG MONITORING AND ADVERSE REACTIONS

8.1. Drug Monitoring

Monitoring of drug levels is not necessary during therapy with the quinolones. The dosage of quinolones cleared renally should be reduced in patients with impaired renal function. Table 4 summarizes the dosage adjustments required.

8.2. Adverse Effects

At beginning of this chapter the effects of the structure of the quinolones on adverse reactions was indicated.

The most common adverse effects involve the GI and central nervous systems, most notably nausea, vomiting, diarrhea, headache, dizziness, and confusion. Allergic reactions (skin reactions, pruritus) are the next most common adverse drug reaction, although they occur in less than 1% of patients for most of the quinolones. Gemifloxacin, however, appears to have an increased risk of skin rash (3%) (10).

Some quinolones have had such serious adverse effects that they have been restricted or are of no use in clinical medicine. Trovafloxacin use is restricted as it caused hepatotoxicity in 140 patients, 14 of which were severe and eight required transplantation (52). Temafloxacin caused immune hemolytic anemia and multiorgan dysfunction in some patients (53). Two of 114 such affected patients died and 34 required hemodialysis (53). Prolongation of the QTc interval on electrocardiogram by fluoroquinolones is due to blockade of the human cardiac K^+ channel HERG (54). In one study, sparfloxacin was most potent, followed by grepafloxacin and moxifloxacin (54). For levofloxacin, ciprofloxacin, and ofloxacin, inhibition of HERG occurs at concentrations much greater than those achieved clinically (54). However, grepafloxacin was withdrawn from the market because of its effect on the QTc interval (3). Fluoroquinolone therapy should be closely monitored or avoided in patients with known prolongation of the QT interval, predisposition to arrhythmias (hypokalemia, hypomagnesemia, bradycardia), or taking other drugs that can prolong the QT interval such as class Ia (e.g., quinidine, disopyramide, procainamide) or class III (e.g., amiodarone, sotalol) antiarrythmics, cisapride, astemizole, terfenadine, erythromycin, and some psychoactive agents (haloperidol, tricyclic antidepressants, phenothiazines, pimozide) (3).

Phototoxicity is a class effect of the fluoroquinolones. It is related to the dose of the agent but not patient age (3). Mild fluoroquinolone-induced phototoxicity is characterized by erythema, edema, and desquamation while more severe phototoxicity results in blistering (3). Phototoxicity was particularly marked with clinafloxacin resulting in its withdrawal from general use (3). Photoxicity seems to be uncommon (<1%) with ciprofloxacin, levofloxacin, gemifloxacin, moxifloxacin, and gatifloxacin (3).

Tendinopathy has also been associated with fluoroquinolone use (55). In a recent review of 98 case reports of tendinopathy, the Achilles tendon was most commonly involved and not uncommonly, such involvement was bilateral (55). Other sites of involvement included the triceps epicondyle, finger flexor tendon sheath, thumb, patella, supraspinal tendon, quadriceps, subscapularis terrea, and rotator cuff (55). Recovery requires about 2 months and men are affected more commonly than women (55). Just over half the patients with tendon rupture had received corticosteroids.

Gatifloxacin, when given in association with oral hypoglycemic agents, has resulted in severe hypoglycemia (56,57). Health Canada issued an advisory to Canadian physicians based on 28 reports of abnormal glucose metabolism associated with gatifloxacin from February 2001 to February 2003 (58); 19 of the patients had hypoglycemia, 7 had hyperglycemia, and 2 had both hypoglycemia and hyperglycemia. Twenty-five of the patients had type 2 diabetes mellitus. Nineteen of the patients were admitted to hospital and two died. The two patients who died were elderly and had hyperglycemia, no prior history of diabetes mellitus, and decreased renal function at the time of the reaction. In 18 of the 19 reports of hypoglycemia, there was concomitant use of a hypoglycemic agent. It has been postulated that there may be an interaction between glyburide and gatifloxacin or that there is an increase in serum insulin following administration of gatifloxacin (56,59–61). To put this adverse reaction in context it is worth noting that a postmarketing study of gatifloxacin involving more than 15,000 patients reported an incidence of hypoglycemic events of 0.3 per 1000 among nondiabetic patients and 6.4 per 1000 among diabetic patients, and hyperglycemic rates of 0.07 per 1000 among nondiabetic patients and 13 per 1000 among diabetic patients (62). This drug–drug interaction with glyburide/oral hypoglycemics is likely a class effect as product monographs for all marketed quinolones mention this potential interaction (10) and there are case reports of altered blood glucose with antidiabetic agents and ciprofloxacin, ofloxacin, and levofloxacin.

A rare adverse effect that has been reported in patients receiving fluoroquinolones is rhabdomyolysis (63). Anaphylaxis has rarely been reported with quinolones (64). However there are at least 33 such reports involving ciprofloxacin, 10 of which have occurred in human immunodeficiency virus-positive patients. There also have been reports of anaphylaxis with ofloxacin and moxifloxacin (64).

Stahlmann and Lode (33) recently reviewed the safety of quinolones when used in elderly patients. They noted that gatifloxacin adverse events were more common in those patients >74 years of age at 36% compared with 28% for patients in the age range 65–74 years, and 29% for patients 18–64 years old. They also observed that women experienced adverse reactions to quinolones more commonly than men: 33% vs. 24%.

Central nervous system adverse reactions are the second most common adverse reaction to quinolones after GI effects. These adverse reactions include anxiety, restlessness, insomnia, euphoria, nightmares, hallucinations, psychosis, and seizures. Elderly persons are more prone to the neurotoxic complications of the quinolones. However, confusion, weakness, loss of appetite, tremor, and depression are often attributed to old age and hence are underreported as possible adverse drug reactions (33). What is also very important when considering neurotoxicity of quinolones in elderly patients is the potentiation of the neurotoxicity by other drugs (e.g., theophyline, NSAIDs) and by electrolyte disturbance. In particular, hypomagnesemia (65,66) is important in this regard, probably because magnesium modulates the N-methyl-D-aspartate receptor-gated channel. The excitatory effects of the fluoroquinolones may be related to inhibition of brain GABA receptor binding (67). There is clinical and experimental evidence of enhancement of the epileptogenic effect of some quinolones by synergistic inhibition with NSAIDS at the GABA receptor (68). It seems that the seizure-inducing potential of the various quinolones is as follows: levofloxacin = gatifloxacin < ofloxacin < ciprofloxacin < nalidixic acid < moxifloxacin < fleroxacin < lomefloxacin < enoxacin (68,69). However there have been two recent reports of seizures in elderly persons due to gatifloxacin (69,70). The second of these two case reports indicate that myoclonus as well as seizures were induced by gatifloxacin (70).

The best way to put the adverse reactions to the quinolones in perspective is to provide data from population-based surveillance systems. One such system is the spontaneous reporting system database of Emilia Romagna, Lombardy, and the Veneto in Italy (71). These three regions have a population of approximately 18 million persons. The use of quinolones increased with age from about two defined daily doses per 1000 persons in the 31–40 age group to 10 for males >70 years of age and 6 for females in this age group (71). The age-specific adverse reactions reported per 1 million population increased from 4.5 in the 21–30 age group to 23 in the >70 age group (71). It is noteworthy that the quinolones are the most commonly prescribed antibiotics in Italy and of those, levofloxacin is the most commonly used (71). During the study period there were 10,011 reports (a mean annual reporting rate of approximately 185 per million inhabitants): 1920 due to systemic antimicrobials, of which 432 (22.5%) involved fluoroquinolones. Pefloxacin was associated with the highest reporting rate (982 reports/defined daily dose/1000 inhabitants),

Table 7 Comparison of the Incidence of Common Adverse Effects to Selected Quinolones

Adverse effect	Cipro-floxacin	Levofloxacin	Gatifloxacin	Moxi-floxacin	Gemi-floxacin
Gastrointestinal					
Nausea	+++	++	+++	+++	++
Vomiting	++	+	++	++	+
Diarrhea	++	++	++	+++	++
Abdominal pain	++	+	++	++	+
Taste perversion	+	+	+	+	+
Central nervous system					
Dizziness	+	+	++	++	+
Headache	++	+	++	++	++
Dermatologic					
Rash	++	+	+	+	++
Pruritus	+	+	±	+	+
Phototoxicity	+	±	−	−	±

Note: −, adverse effect has not been reported; ±, adverse effect occurs in ≤0.1% of patients; +, adverse effect occurs in >0.1–≤1% of patients; ++, adverse effect occurs in >1–4% of patients; +++, adverse effect occurs in >4–8% of patients. For other adverse effects—QTc prolongation, hepatotoxicity, tendonitis, and tendon rupture, see text.
Source: Refs. 3,34,48,72–76.

followed by moxifloxacin (356), rufloxacin (221), and lomefloxacin (196). The most frequently reported reactions to fluoroquinolones involved the skin, but their percentage (25%) was significantly lower ($p < 0.01$) than that of other systemic antimicrobials (58.5%), whereas the percentages of reactions involving the central nervous (12.2 vs. 3.6%), musculoskeletal (14.7 vs. 0.3%) and psychiatric systems (9.3 vs. 1.8%) were significantly higher ($p < 0.01$). They found some significant differences in the safety profiles of individual fluoroquinolones: ciprofloxacin was more frequently associated with skin reactions ($p < 0.01$), levofloxacin and pefloxacin with musculoskeletal adverse effects ($p < 0.01$), and rufloxacin with psychiatric disorders ($p < 0.05$). Levofloxacin was the fluoroquinolone associated with the highest rate of serious tendon disorders; phototoxic reactions were more frequent with lomefloxacin, and toxic epidermal necrolysis and Stevens–Johnson syndrome were seen only with ciprofloxacin (71).

By way of summary the incidence of common adverse effects to selected quinolones is compared in Table 7.

REFERENCES

1. Lescher GY, Froelich ED, Gruet MD, Bailey JH, Brundage RP. 1–8 naphthyridine derivatives. A new class of chemotherapeutic agents. J Med Pharm 1962; 5:1063–1068.
2. Sheehan G, Chew NSY. The history of quinolones. In: Ronald AR, Low DE, eds. Fluoroquinolone Antibiotics. Basel, Switzerland: Birkhauser Verlag, 2003:1–10.
3. Zhanel GG, Ennis K, Vercaigne L, Walky A, Gin AS, Embil J, Smith H, Hoban DJ. A critical review of the fluoroquinolones. Focus on respiratory tract infections. Drugs 2002; 62:13–59.
4. Ho P-L, Cheng VCC. Epidemiology and mechanisms of resistance. In: Ronald AR, Low DE, eds. Fluoroquinolone Antibiotics. Basel, Switzerland: Birkhauser Verlag, 2003: 49–71.
5. Sable DS, Murakawa GJ. Quinolones in dermatology. Clin Dermatol 2003; 21:56–63.
6. Hooper DC. Quinolones. In: Mandell GL, Bennett JE, eds. Principles and Practice of Infectious Diseases. 5th ed. Philadelphia, PA: Churchill Livingstone, 2000:404–423.
7. Jones RN. Microbiology of newer fluoroquinolones: focus on respiratory pathogens. Diagn Microbiol Infect Dis 2002; 44:213–220.
8. Hurst M, Lamb HM, Scott LJ, Figgitt DP. Levofloxacin. An updated review of its use in the treatment of bacterial infections. Drugs 2002; 62:2127–2167.
9. Wyllie SA, Ridgway GL. The quinolones and sexually transmitted infections. In: Ronald AR, Low DE, eds. Fluoroquinolone Antibiotics. Basel, Switzerland: Birkhauser Verlag, 2003:121–133.
10. Saravoltaz LD, Leggett J. Gatifloxacin, gemifloxacin, and moxifloxacin: the role of 3 newer fluoroquinolones. Clin Infect Dis 2003; 37:1210–1215.
11. Blondeau JM, Hansen G, Metzler KL, Borsos S, Irvine LB, Blanco L. In vitro susceptibility of 4903 bacterial isolates to gemifloxacin—an advanced fluoroquinolone. Int J Antimicrob Agents 2003; 22:147–154.
12. Hoban DJ, Biedenbach DJ, Mutnick AH, Jones RN. Pathogen of occurrence and susceptibility patterns associated with pneumonia in hospitalized patients in North America: results of the SENTRY Antimicrobial Surveillance Study (2000). Diagn Microbiol Infect Dis 2003; 45:279–285.
13. Low DE, de Azavedo J, Weiss K, Mazzulli T, Kuhn M, Church D, Forward K, Zhanel G, Simor A, Canadian Bacterial Surveillance Network, McGeer A. Antimicrobial resistance among clinical isolates of *Streptococcus pneumoniae* in Canada during 2000. Antimicrob Agents Chemother 2002; 46:1295–1301.

14. Zhanel GG, Palatnick L, Nichol KA, Bellyou T, Low DE, Hoban DJ. Antimicrobial resistance in respiratory tract *Streptococcus pneumoniae* isolates: results of the Canadian respiratory organism susceptibility study, 1997–2002. Antimicrob Agents Chemother 2003; 47:1867–1874.

15. Centers for Disease Control and Prevention. Active Bacterial Core Surveillance report, emerging infections program network, *Streptococcus pneumoniae*, 2002. http://www.cdc.gov/ncidod/dbmd/abcs/spneu02.pdf.

16. Doern GV, Heilmann KP, Huynh HK, Rhomberg PR, Coffman SL, Brueggemann AB. Antimicrobial resistance among clinical isolates of *Streptococcus pneumoniae* in the United States during 1999–2000, including a comparison of resistance rates since 1994–1995. Antimicrob Agents Chemother 2001; 45:1721–1729.

17. Karlowsky JA, Thornsberry C, Jones ME, Evangelista AT, Critchley IA, Sahm DF. Factors associated with relative rates of antimicrobial resistance among *Streptococcus pneumoniae* in the United States: results from the TRUST surveillance program (1998–2002). Clin Infect Dis 2003; 36:963–970.

18. Karlowsky JA, Kelly LJ, Thornsberry C, Jones ME, Evangelista AT, Critchley IA, Sahm DF. Susceptibility to fluoroquinolones among commonly isolated Gram-negative bacilli in 2000: TRUST and TSN data for the United States. Int J Antimicrob Agents 2002; 19:21–31.

19. Gordon KA, Jones RN, SENTRY participant groups (Europe, Latin America, North America). Susceptibility patterns of orally administered antimicrobials among urinary tract infection pathogens from hospitalized patients in North America: comparison report to Europe and Latin America. Results from the SENTRY antimicrobial surveillance program (2000). Diagn Microbiol Infect Dis 2003; 45:295–301.

20. Karlowsky JA, Draghi DC, Jones ME, Thornsberry C, Friedland IR, Sahm DF. Surveillance for antimicrobial susceptibility among clinical isolates of *Pseudomonas aeruginosa* and *Acinetobacter baumannii* from hospitalized patients in the United States, 1998 to 2001. Antimicrob Agents Chemother 2003; 47:1681–1688.

21. Sarwal S, Wong T, Sevigny C, Ng L-K. Increasing incidence of ciprofloxacin-resistant *Neisseria gonorrhoeae* infection in Canada. Can Med Assoc J 2003; 168:872–873.

22. Zhanel GG, Palatnick L, Nichol KA, Low DE, the CROSS study group, Hoban DJ. Antimicrobial resistance in *Haemophilus influenzae* and *Moraxella catarrhalis* respiratory tract isolates: results of the Canadian respiratory organism susceptibility study, 1997–2002. Antimicrob Agents Chemother 2003; 47:1875–1881.

23. Thornsberry C, Sahm DF, Kelly LJ, Critchley IA, Jones ME, Evangelista AT, Karlowsky JA. Regional trends in antimicrobial resistance among clinical isolates of *Streptococcus pneumoniae*, *Haemophilus influenzae* and *Moraxella catarrhalis* in the United States: results from the TRUST surveillance program, 1999–2000. Clin Infect Dis 2002; 34(suppl 1):S4–S16.

24. Hoban DJ, Doern GV, Fluit C, Roussel-Delvallez M, Jones RN. Worldwide prevalence of antimicrobial resistance in *Streptococcus pneumoniae*, *Haemophilus influenzae* and *Moraxella catarrhalis* in the SENTRY antimicrobial surveillance program, 1997–1999. Clin Infect Dis 2001; 32(suppl 2):S81–S93.

25. de los Reyes MRA, Pato-Mesola V, Klausner JD, Manalastas R, Wi T, Tuazon CU, Dallabetta G, Whittington WLH, Holmes KK. A randomized trial of ciprofloxacin versus cefixime for treatment of gonorrhea after rapid emergence of gonococcal ciprofloxacin resistance in the Philippines. Clin Infect Dis 2001; 32:1313–1318.

26. Gordon SM, Carlyn CJ, Doyle LJ, Knapp CC, Longworth DL, Hall GS, Washington JA. The emergence of *Neisseria gonorrheae* with decreased susceptibility to ciprofloxacin in Cleveland, Ohio: epidemiology and risk factors. Ann Intern Med 1996; 125:465–470.

27. Smith KE, Besser JM, Hedberg CW, Leano FT, Bender JB, Wicklund JH, Johnson BP, Moore KA, Osterholm MT. Quinolone-resistant *Campylobacter jejuni* infections in Minnesota, 1992–1998. N Engl J Med 1999; 340:1525–1532.

28. Division of Emerging and Other Communicable Disease Surveillance and Control. Use of quinolones in food animals and potential impact on human health: report of a WHO meeting. Geneva, Switzerland, Jun 2–5, 1998. Geneva: World Health Organization, 1998 (Document no. WHO/EMC/ZD/98.10).

29. Perry CM, Barman Balfour JA, Lamb HM. Gatifloxacin. Drugs 1999; 58:683–696.

30. Barman Balfour JA, Wiseman LR. Moxifloxacin. Drugs 1999; 57:363–373.

31. Zervos MJ, Hersberger E, Nicolau DP, Ritchie DJ, Blackner LK, Coyle EA, Donnelly AJ, Eckel SF, Eng RHK, Hiltz A, Kuyumjian AG, Krebs W, McDaniel A, Hogan P, Lubowski TJ. Relationship between fluoroquinolone use and changes in susceptibility to fluoroquinolones of selected pathogens in 10 United States teaching hospitals, 1991–2000. Clin Infect Dis 2003; 37:1643–1648.

32. Zhanel GG, Noreddin AM. Pharmacokinetics and pharmacodynamics (PK/PD) of fluoroquinolones: tools for combating bacteria and preventing resistance. In: Ronald AR, Low DE, eds. Fluoroquinolone antibiotics. Basel, Switzerland: Birkhauser Verlag, 2003:87–105.

33. Stahlmann R, Lode H. Fluoroquinolones in the elderly. Safety considerations. Drugs Aging 2003; 20:289–302.

34. Product monograph Factive® (gemifloxacin). http://www.rxlist.com/cgi/generic3/factive.htm.

35. Gemifloxacin. In: McEvoy GK, Litvak K, Welsh OH, eds. American Hospital Formulary Service Drug Information, Bethesda, MD. http://www.ashp.org/ahfs/.

36. Pickerill KE, Paladino JA, Schentag JJ. Comparison of the fluoroquinolones based on pharmacokinetic and pharmacodynamic parameters. Pharmacotherapy 2000; 20: 417–428.

37. Hyatt JM, McKinnon PS, Zimmer GS, Schentag JJ. The importance of pharmacokinetic/pharmacodynamic surrogate markers to outcome: focus on antibacterial agents. Clin Pharmacokinet 1995; 28:143–160.

38. Forrest A, Nix DE, Ballow CH, Gross TF, Birmingham MC, Schentag JJ. Pharmacodynamics of intravenous ciprofloxacin in seriously ill patients. Antimicrob Agents Chemother 1993; 37:1073–1081.

39. Preston SL, Drusano GL, Berman AL, Fowler CL, Chow AT, Reichl V, Dornseif B, Natarajan J, Wong FA, Corrado M. Pharmacodynamics of levofloxacin: a new paradigm for early clinical trials. J Am Med Assoc 1998; 279:125–129.

40. Schentag JJ, Gilliland KK, Paladino JA. What have we learned from pharmacokinetic and pharmacodynamic theories? Clin Infect Dis 2001; 32(suppl 1):S39–S46

41. Blondeau JM, Xilin A, Hansen G, Drlica K. A mutant prevention concentration of fluroquinolones for clinical isolates of Streptococcus pneumoniae. Antimicrob Agents Chemother 2001; 45:433–438.

42. Solomkin JS, Mazuski JE, Baron JE, Sawyer RG, Nathens AB, Di Piro JJ, Buchman T, Dellinger EP, Jerrigan J, Gorbach S, Chow AW, Bartlett J. Infectious Diseases Society of America. Guidelines for the selection of anti-infective agents for complicated intra-abdominal infections. Clin Infect Dis 2003; 37:997–1005.

43. Giamarellou H, Antoniadou A. The role of fluoroquinolones in the therapy and prophylaxis of neutropenic patients with cancer. In: Ronald AR, Low DE, eds. Fluoroquinolone antibiotics. Basel, Switzerland: Birkhauser Verlag, 2003:219–237.

44. Memish ZA, Mah MW. Less usual indications: mycobacterial, Brucella, Yersinia, Francisella and other infections. In: Ronald AR, Low DE, eds. Fluoroquinolone antibiotics. Basel, Switzerland: Birkhauser Verlag, 2003:239–249.

45. Swartz MN. Recognition and management of anthrax—an update. N Engl J Med 2001; 345:1621–1626.

46. Inglesby TV, Henderson DA, Bartlett JG, Ascher MS, Eitzen E, Friedlander AM, Hauer J, McDade J, Osterholm MT, O'Toole T, Parker G, Perl T, Russell PK, Tonat K. Anthrax as a biological weapon. Medical and public health management. J Am Med Assoc 1999; 281:1735–1745.

47. Oliphant CM, Green GM. Quinolones: a comprehensive review. Am Fam Physician 2002; 65(3):455–464.
48. Fish DN. Fluoroquinolone adverse effects and drug interactions. Pharmacotherapy 2001; 21(10 Pt 2):253S–272S.
49. Allen A, Bygate E, Clark D, Lewis A, Pay V. The effect of food on the bioavailability of oral gemifloxacin in healthy volunteers. Int J Antimicrob Agents 2000; 16:45–50.
50. Allen A, Bygate E, Faessal H, Isaac L, Lewis A. The effect of ferrous sulphate and sucralfate on the bioavailability of oral gemifloxacin in healthy volunteers. Int J Antimicrob Agents 2000; 15:283–289.
51. Jones CB, Fugate SE. Levofloxacin and warfarin interaction. Ann Pharmacother 2002; 36:1554–1557.
52. FDA issues public health advisory on liver toxicity associated with the antibiotic Trovan (FDA talk paper). Rockville, MD: U.S. Department of Health and Human Services, Food and Drug Administration, 1999.
53. Blum MD, Graham DJ, McClosky CA. Temofloxacin syndrome: review of 95 cases. Clin Infect Dis 1994; 18:946–950.
54. Kang J, Wang L, Chen XL, Triggle DJ, Rampe D. Interactions of a series of fluoroquinolone antibacterial drugs with the human cardiac K+ channel HERG. Mol Pharmacol 2001; 59(1):122–126.
55. Khaliq Y, Zhanel GG. Fluroquinolone-associated tendinopathy. A critical review of the literature. Clin Infect Dis 2003; 36:1404–1410.
56. Menzies DJ, Dorsainvil PA, Cunha BA, Johnson DH. Severe and persistent hypoglycemia due to gatifloxacin interaction with oral hypoglycemic agents. Am J Med 2002; 113: 232–234.
57. Baker SE, Hangii MC. Possible gatifloxacin-induced hypoglycemia. Ann Pharmacother 2002; 36:1722–1726.
58. Létourneau G, Morrison H, McMorran M. Gatifloxacin (Tequin™): hypoglycemia and hyperglycemia. Can Adverse React Newslett 2003; 13:1–3.
59. Parilo MA. Gatifloxacin-associated hypoglycemia. J Pharm Technol 2002; 18:319–320.
60. Hussein G, Perkins LT, Sternberg M, Bland C. Gatifloxacin-induced hypoglycemia: a case report and review of the literature. Clin Res Regul Aff 2002; 19(4):333–339.
61. Baker SE, Hangii MC. Possible gatifloxacin-induced hypoglycemia. Ann Pharmacother 2002; 36:1722–1726.
62. Tequin™, gatifloxacin tablets (product monograph). Montreal: Bristol-Myers Squibb Canada Inc., 2002.
63. Petitjeans F, Nadaud J, Perez JP, Debien B, Olive F, Villevieille T, Pats B. A case of rhabdomyolysis with fatal outcome after a treatment with levofloxacin. Eur J Clin Pharmacol 2003; 59:779–780.
64. Ho DY, Song JC, Wang CC. Anaphylactoid reaction to ciprofloxacin. Ann Pharmacother 2003; 37:1018–1023.
65. Kushner JM, Peckman HJ, Snyder CR. Seizures associated with fluoroquinolones. Ann Pharmacother 2001; 35:1194–1198.
66. Schmuck G, Schürmann A, Schlüter G. Determination of the excitatory potencies of fluoroquinolones in the central nervous system by an in vitro model. Antimicrob Agents Chemother 1998; 42:1831–1836.
67. Green MA, Halliwell RF. Selective antagonism of the GABAA receptor by ciprofloxacin and biphenylacetic acid. Br J Pharmacol 1997; 122:584–590.
68. Lode H. Potential interactions of the extended-spectrum fluoroquinolones with the CNS. Drug Safety 1999; 21:123–135.
69. Quigley CA, Lederman JR. Possible gatifloxacin-induced seizure. Ann Pharmacother 2004; 38:235–237.
70. Marinella MA. Myoclonus and generalized seizure associated with gatifloxacin treatment. Arch Intern Med 2001; 161:2261–2262.

71. Leone R, Venegoni M, Motola D, Moretti U, Piazzetta V, Cocci A, Resi D, Mozzo F, Velo G, Burzilleri L, Montanaro N, Conforti A. Adverse drug reactions related to the use of fluoroquinolone antimicrobials. An analysis of spontaneous reports and fluoroquinolone consumption data from three Italian regions. Drug Safety 2003; 26:109–120.

72. Mandell LA. Improved safety profile of newer fluoroquinolones. In: Ronald AR, Low DE, eds. Fluoroquinolone Antibiotics. Basel, Switzerland: Birkhauser Verlag, 2003: 73–85.

73. Hurst M, Lamb HM, Scott LJ, Figgitt DP. Levofloxacin. An updated review of its use in the treatment of bacterial infections. Drugs 2002; 62:2127–2167.

74. Quinolones. In: McEvoy GK, Litvak K, Welsh OH, eds. American Hospital Formulary Service Drug Information. 45th ed. Bethesda, MD, 2003:762–817.

75. Repchinsky C, Welbanks L, Bisson R, eds. Compendium Pharmaceutical Specialties. Ottawa, ON, Canada: Canadian Pharmacists Association, 2003.

76. Anti-infective Drugs Advisory Committee. Factive (gemifloxacin). U.S. Food and Drug Administration briefing document. March 4, 2003. http://www.fda.gov/ohrms/dockets/ac/acmenu.htm.

SUGGESTED READING

Saravoltaz LD, Leggett J. Gatifloxacin, gemifloxacin, and moxifloxacin: the role of 3 newer fluoroquinolones. Clin Infect Dis 2003; 37:1210–1215.

Schentag JJ, Gilliland KK, Paladino JA. What have we learned from pharmacokinetic and pharmacodynamic theories? Clin Infect Dis 2001; 32(suppl 1):S39–S46.

Zhanel GG, Ennis K, Vercaigne L, Walky A, Gin AS, Embil J, Smith H, Hoban DJ. A critical review of the fluoroquinolones. Focus on respiratory tract infections. Drugs 2002; 62:13–59.

14
Aminoglycosides

Dean C. Norman
UCLA Geffen School of Medicine, Veterans Affairs Greater Los Angeles Healthcare System, Los Angeles, California, U.S.A.

Key Points:

- Aminoglycosides are still important antibiotics for the treatment of infections in the elderly because of rapidly emerging microbial resistance to β-lactam drugs and quinolones.
- The pharmacodynamic properties of aminoglycosides differ significantly from β-lactam antibiotics.
- A low therapeutic index limits the use of aminoglycosides.
- Major aminoglycoside toxicities include nephrotoxicity (usually reversible) and ototoxicity (nonreversible).
- Single daily dose aminoglycoside administration is appropriate in most cases.

1. INTRODUCTION

Aminoglycosides continue to be an important class of antibiotics for treating certain infections in the elderly. Their use has been limited due to the availability of less toxic β-lactam and quinolone antibiotics with comparable activity against aerobic Gram-negative bacteria. However, the rapid emergence of microbial resistance to β-lactam and quinolone antibiotics makes the aminoglycosides important therapeutic agents for treating difficult infections due to resistant aerobic Gram-negative bacteria. Furthermore, the combination of an aminoglycoside and a β-lactam antibiotic results in synergistic killing of certain bacterial pathogens. The pharmacodynamic properties of aminoglycosides differ from β-lactam drugs in that the concentration-dependent killing and the postantibiotic effect are observed with aminoglycosides. Aminoglycosides have a low therapeutic index with the major toxicities being oto- and nephrotoxicity. Ototoxicity is usually irreversible and nephrotoxicity, although usually reversible, may cause serious morbidity. Both of these major aminoglycoside-associated toxicities are particularly detrimental to older adults, and it is essential to carefully monitor the therapy to reduce the risk of toxicity.

2. CHEMISTRY AND MECHANISM OF ACTION

Aminoglycosides are composed of two or more amino sugars connected by a glyco-
sidic linkage to a central hexose nucleus (1). They are bactericidal; although it is well
established that aminoglycosides bind to the bacterial 30S and 50S ribosomal subunits and inhibit protein synthesis, the precise mechanisms of bacterial killing are
under investigation. Recent evidence shows that the action is at the outer bacterial
cell membrane, where highly polar cationic antibiotic molecules create fissures by
disrupting magnesium bridges between lipopolysaccharide molecules creating leakage of intracellular contents, and increased antibiotic uptake (2). Transportation of
aminoglycosides across the inner cytoplasmic membrane is active and is dependent
on the availability of oxygen. Once bound to bacterial ribosomes, the inhibition of
protein synthesis further enhances antibiotic influx. The transport of aminoglycosides is enhanced by alkaline environments because less of the drug is ionized. However, there is less transport in acidic environments or anaerobic environments
making aminoglycosides predictably less active against anaerobic bacteria.

3. ANTIMICROBIAL SPECTRUM

Aminoglycosides have broad in vitro activity against many species of aerobic Gram-
negative bacteria. Susceptibly is defined as a minimal inhibitory concentration (MIC)
of <2 µg/mL for gentamicin and tobramycin and <8 µg/mL for amikacin. Generally, most Enterobacteriaceae remain sensitive to aminoglycosides despite the introduction of these drugs many years ago (3). *Pseudomonas* species are not uniformly
sensitive and *Pseudomonas* (now *Burholderia*) *cepacia*, *Haemophilus influenzae*, and
Xanthomonas (now *Stenotrophomonas*) *maltophilia* are generally resistant. Aminoglycosides are not effective against infections caused by either *Salmonella* or *Shigella*
species. These agents do have activity against certain Gram-positive bacteria but,
when used alone, are not adequate for treatment of infections caused by these organisms. *Staphylococcus aureus* and *S. epidermidis* and enteroccoci usually are sensitive
to aminoglycosides. However, a high percentage of enterococci are highly resistant
to these antibiotics. It is important to note that when high-level aminoglycoside resistance occurs, the addition of an aminoglycoside to a β-lactam antibiotic (e.g.,
combined with a penicillin to treat enterococcal endocarditis) does not result in antibacterial synergy. *Streptococcus pneumoniae* and *S. pyogenes* are resistant. Certain
mycobacteria are sensitive to aminoglycosides.

The aminoglycosides approved for clinical use in the United States include
gentamicin, amikacin, kanamycin, tobramycin, neomycin, paromomycin, netilmicin,
streptomycin, and spectinomycin. However, in practice, gentamicin, amikacin, and
tobramycin are the drugs most commonly used in geriatric infections. The
antibacterial spectrum of these three antibiotics is similar although in vitro activity
of tobramycin is more often greater against *Pseudomonas* species and gentamicin
is generally more active against *Serratia* species (3).

3.1. Resistance

Bacteria may become resistant to aminoglycosides through a variety of mechanisms,
but most resistance to aminoglycosides is due to bacterial production of aminoglycoside-modifying enzyme, and the genes that encode for these enzymes may be

passed to other bacteria by exchange of genetic materials. Other less important mechanisms include alterations in bacterial ribosomes that prevent aminoglycosides from binding and loss of bacterial cell permeability to these drugs (2). Amikacin and netilmicin resistance is less common because they are not affected by many types of aminoglycoside-modifying enzymes. As mentioned earlier, Enterobacteriaceae resistance has not significantly changed over the past 10 years, but high-level aminoglycoside resistance now occurs frequently in enteroccoci and especially *E. faecium*, where over 50% of isolates from hospital-acquired infections are resistant (4). *Pseudomonas aeruginosa* aminoglycoside resistance is also a problem, and only 81–94% of strains remain susceptible to aminoglycosides (4). *Pseudomonas* sp. are relatively more resistant than the Enterobacteriaceae because of antibiotic efflux and loss of permeability mechanisms. Resistance patterns for many bacterial species will vary widely and clinical laboratory testing is necessary to confirm susceptibility.

4. CLINICAL PHARMACODYNAMICS AND PHARMACOLOGY

Unlike β-lactam drugs, aminoglycosides have concentration-dependent antibacterial action which means that as antibiotic concentrations increase, the rate of bacterial killing increases (5,6). Therefore, the exposure time of the bacteria to aminoglycosides is not critical. Optimal killing occurs at a value of approximately 8–10 times the MIC, and the goal of therapy should be to achieve the peak concentrations at this level without exceeding concentrations which increase the risk of toxicity. Aminoglycosides also exhibit a postantibiotic effect on bacterial growth against sensitive organisms, and this effect, although variable, is dependent on peak concentration and may persist for several hours. Taken together, these two properties of aminoglycosides mean that the peak concentration achieved is very important and longer dosing intervals are possible even if serum and tissue trough levels fall below the MIC of the target organism for short periods of time. The optimal concentration time profile differs from that for β-lactam antibiotics. Instead of a flat profile where the concentration remains above the MIC of the pathogen throughout the dosing interval, the optimal profile for an aminoglycoside antibiotic is a high peak concentration, but a low trough level to achieve maximal bacterial killing rates and minimal risk for toxicity. There is some evidence to support the positive correlation between the ratio of peak concentration to MIC and the therapeutic outcome (7,8). The latter study (8) demonstrated that the maximum serum concentration achieved to MIC ratio predicted efficacy, and normalization of body temperature and white blood cell counts in a group of patients being treated for nosocomial pneumonia.

Aminoglycosides are poorly absorbed from the gastrointestinal tract. They are distributed primarily in the extracellular fluid but can penetrate bone, synovial fluid, and peritoneal fluid in concentrations high enough to achieve some activity against susceptible pathogens. Intracellular penetration of these antibiotics is poor due to their bipolar structure, with the exception being the renal proximal tubule. Minimal concentrations are achieved in cerebrospinal fluid even when the meninges are inflamed and if aminoglycoside therapy is part of a regimen to treat meningitis, intraventricular or intrathecal injection is usually required. Similarly, subtherapeutic concentrations of the drug occur in the vitreous humor, prostate, and brain (3). Aminoglycosides are not metabolized by the liver but are rapidly excreted by glomerular filtration and concentrations in the urine may be as high as 100-fold to that in the serum. Unfortunately, a portion of these drugs are absorbed by the proximal tubule and the half-life of these antibiotics in the renal cortex is measured in days so that repetitive dosing can result in renal accumulation and toxicity.

Given their propensity to be hydrophilic, and for low protein binding, the volume of distribution for aminoglycosides is approximately the extracellular fluid volume and clearance of aminoglycosides is approximately equal to the glomerular filtration rate (9). Interindividual differences in pharmacology are mostly caused by changes in the volume of distribution and clearance (6). Individual volume of distribution and clearance may vary significantly from the norm with certain conditions such as burns, morbid obesity, and severe dehydration. The pharmacokinetics of aminoglycosides in the elderly will be affected by age-related increases in body fat and declining renal function.

5. CLINICAL INDICATIONS

Newer β-lactam antibiotics including third- and fourth-generation cephalosporins, monobactams, carbapenems, and fluoroquinolones are generally safe to use in infected older persons. Their broad-spectrum activity and safety profile makes them ideal agents for the empirical therapy of infections suspected to be caused by aerobic Gram-negative bacteria. Aminoglycoside therapy for geriatric patients with bacterial infections should be reserved for use as empirical therapy for serious infections in which the risk of death or severe morbidity outweighs the risks of ototoxicity and nephrotoxicity. Aminoglycosides are appropriate first-line drugs for treating infections in the elderly caused by bacteria that are susceptible only to aminoglycosides and in infections in which the addition of an aminoglycoside to another antibiotic provides the needed synergy (e.g., endocarditis caused by aminoglycoside-sensitive Gram-positive streptococci or staphylococci). Some studies cast doubt on the value of adding an aminoglycoside to a β-lactam antibiotic for antimicrobial synergy in patients with sepsis or with neutropenia and fever. A recent meta-analysis of 64 trials including 7586 immunocompetent subjects treated with an aminoglycoside plus β-lactam combination vs. β-lactam monotherapy for sepsis found no difference in mortality between combination and monotherapy. This was true for both Gram-negative infections overall and infections due to *P. aeruginosa*. However, nephrotoxicity was far more common with combination therapy (10). A prior meta-analysis of 29 randomized clinical trials looking at monotherapy with an antipseudomonal penicillin or carbapenem vs. aminoglycoside combinations for empirical therapy of febrile neutropenic patients of all ages found monotherapy to be at least as effective as aminoglycoside-containing combinations (11). Thus, it is clear that if culture results indicate that a less toxic regimen will suffice, then this regimen should be substituted for the aminoglycoside regimen.

6. ADMINISTRATION OF DRUG

Multiple meta-analyses of dozens of studies (12–16) and comprehensive reviews showed (17,18) that single daily dosing of aminoglycosides was as efficacious as "traditional" multidosing and did not lead to increased resistance. There did not appear to be a significant difference in either ototoxicity or nephrotoxicity between the two regimens. In a large study of 2184 patients, including elderly patients, treated with single daily dosing of aminoglycosides, a fixed dose of gentamicin or tobramycin of 7 mg/kg was administered (19). The dosing interval was varied based on estimated creatinine clearance (CrCl) (20). Nephrotoxicity occurred in 1.2% of cases overall when compared with historical nephrotoxicity rates of 3–5% after 7 days of therapy. Ototoxicity occurred in only three subjects in the single daily dose group. Another strong argument for single daily aminoglycoside dosing, also referred to as extended interval aminoglycoside dosing (EIAD), is that it is clearly less costly than traditional dosing; there is a less frequent need to measure serum levels and there is a reduced need for ancillary service time. Of note, the efficacy of aminoglycosides when combined with β-lactam drugs is not diminished with EIAD (21).

EIAD is now in common use in American acute care hospitals. A random sample survey of 500 acute care hospitals in the United States demonstrated that ≈75% of hospitals adopted EIAD (22). Moreover, this survey revealed that monitoring of serum aminoglycoside concentrations shifted to a single concentration level, 6–18 hr after dosing. The rationale cited for extended interval dosing included equal efficacy, equal or less toxicity, and reduced cost of monitoring and administration of drug. Dosing intervals were usually modified using the Hartford hospital once-daily aminoglycoside nomogram (18). Age was not listed as a contraindication in the surveyed institutions, but the use of extended interval dosing occurred in 99.5% of those aged 19–64 vs. 71% of those aged 65 years and older. Of note, very few hospitals (3.2%) in either time period used audiometric testing to monitor for ototoxicity. Finally, the survey reported that EIAD use was related to availability of a pharmacy-based pharmacokinetic service and an infectious disease specialist.

Given all of the previous findings, it is recommended that aminoglycoside dosing for most infections should use EIAD methodology with limited monitoring of antibiotic serum levels. EIAD is not recommended for patients undergoing a change in renal function: those who have ascites, who have morbid obesity or burns, are on dialysis, or have had recent trauma or sepsis syndrome (7,23). Younger trauma patients with high CrCl rates are particularly prone to "fall off the nomogram" with EIAD (23). Patients being treated for infective endocarditis should also be excluded from using EIAD regimens.

Although there are many methods for single daily aminoglycoside dosing of EIAD, the author's acute care hospital employs the following methodology: First, in order to determine the initial or loading dose, ideal body weight (IBW) is calculated as

$$IBW_{male} = 50\,kg + 2.3 \times (\text{height in inches} - 60)$$

$$IBW_{female} = 45.5\,kg + 2.3 \times (\text{height in inches} - 60).$$

Remember that the aminoglycosides penetrate poorly into fat and this will alter the pharmacokinetics of these drugs. Therefore if the actual body weight (ABW) is >20% of the IBW, then use a calculation of obese body weight (OBW) to determine the loading dose:

$$OBW = IBW + 0.4 \times (ABW - IBW)$$

The gentamicin or tobramycin initial recommended dosage is 7 mg/kg body weight given intravenously over 30–60 min. Intramuscular injection is possible but due to diminished muscle mass in the elderly, this route of administration should be reserved for cases in which intravenous access is not possible. For amikacin, the initial dosage is 15 mg/kg body weight.

Table 1 Traditional Dosing of Aminoglycosides

| Dose (mg/kg)[a] | Estimated interval[b] (hr) | Therapeutic serum levels[c] (μg/mL) | |
		Peak	Trough
Gentamicin 1.5–2.5	8	6–10	0.5–2
Tobramycin 1.5–2.5	8	6–10	0.5–2
Amikacin 5–7.5	8[d]	15–30	1–8

[a]Lower doses may be used for urinary tract infections and for synergy. Body weight should be calculated as given earlier.
[b]If creatinine clearance is 40–60 mL/min the interval is increased to every 12 hr; 20–40 mL/min, 24 hr; 10–20 mL/min, 48 hr and if <10 mL/min, the dosing interval is adjusted by frequent determination of peak and trough serum concentrations. Frequent monitoring of levels is strongly recommended (see the following).
[c]Above these levels should be considered toxic.
[d]The dose of amikacin is usually given as 7.5 mg/kg every 12 hr.

The preliminary dosing interval is determined based on the estimation of creatinine clearance by the method of Cockcroft and Gault (20). This method is valid for calculating creatinine clearance in the elderly (24): $CrCl_{male}$ = (140 − age in years) multiplied by ABW divided by serum creatinine × 70. For females, multiply the result by 0.85. For creatinine clearance over 60 mL/min, the interval is 24 hr; 40–59 mL/min, 36 hr; 20–39 mL/min, 48 hr. If the creatinine clearance is <20 mL/min then frequent aminoglycosides levels must be obtained to safely adjust subsequent doses (see later).

When patients are not candidates for single daily dosing and require frequent monitoring of serum concentrations then traditional or individual dosing methodologies should be employed. Traditional dosing methodologies have been extensively reviewed (1). Table 1 gives an example of an acceptable individual dosing strategy.

7. DRUG MONITORING AND ADVERSE EFFECTS

Optimal therapeutic drug monitoring remains controversial (9,25,26). It is recommended that for EIAD aminoglycoside levels be determined between 6 and 14 hr after the start of an aminoglycoside infusion on days 1–3, day 5, and weekly thereafter. More frequent monitoring is necessary for patients whose renal function or fluid status is changing or if at high risk for toxicity. Frequent monitoring of serum creatinine (at least every other day) is recommended. Serum levels should be compared with the Hartford hospital once-daily aminoglycoside nomogram (18), and the dosing interval adjusted accordingly. For traditional aminoglycoside dosing it is recommended that frequent peak levels (30 min after completing the infusion) and trough levels (just before giving the next dose) should be performed in order to adjust the dosage. A recent study suggested that frequent determination of serum levels using traditional dosing methodology was superior to a single daily dosing method in reducing nephrotoxicity (27). The interpretation of levels for traditional aminoglycoside dosing is shown in Table 1.

Routine audiologic monitoring and monitoring of vestibular function is impractical due to the frequency of delirium in seriously ill infected elderly patients (21). However, attempts should be made to monitor hearing (before, after, and during therapy) in cases where administration of aminoglycosides is anticipated to be used beyond 7–10 days.

The major aminoglycoside toxicities are nephrotoxicity and ototoxicity, but occasional hypersensitivity reactions occur. Neuromuscular blockade is very rare, occurring at very high aminoglycoside serum concentration levels which can only occur during rapid administration or during peritoneal administration. This complication is associated with the concomitant administration of anesthesia agents which act on the neuromuscular junction (3).

The incidence of aminoglycoside-induced nephrotoxicity is difficult to accurately assess because of severe underlying disease (e.g., sepsis) and the wide range of definitions of toxicity. However, one study determined that the incidence of nephrotoxicity in the elderly did not differ between single- or multidose aminoglycoside regimens. The incidence of nephrotoxicity in the 86 patients studied was 9.3% (28). Nephrotoxicity usually occurs after at least 5 days after initiating aminoglycoside antibiotics and may progress to nonoliguric renal failure characterized by increasing serum creatinine, blood urea nitrogen concentrations, and decreased renal urinary concentration ability (29). The precise mechanism of nephrotoxicity is not known but aminoglycosides are not metabolized and are eliminated by glomerular filtration.

Nephrotoxicity is clearly related to their partial reabsorption by proximal tubular cell. These drugs bind to acidic phospholipids and inhibit phospholipids' metabolism. Recent experimental data were obtained from intensive care unit patients being treated with aminoglycosides or a glycopeptide antibiotic. Sophisticated proton magnetic resonance spectroscopy of urine was performed, and the data suggested that the damage is not limited to the proximal tubule alone but may involve the Henle loop and collecting duct of the nephron (30). In vivo protein synthesis experiments using a rat model demonstrated reduced renal cellular protein synthesis after just 2 days of treatment with high doses of gentamicin. Moreover, significant alterations in phospholipid metabolism were observed (31).

The risk of nephrotoxicity increases with preexisting renal dysfunction, high peak aminoglycoside concentrations, prolonged therapy (over 1 week), liver disease, and hypoalbuminemia (29,32). Other risk factors include volume depletion and use of potentially nephrotoxic drugs such as amphotericin, nonsteroidal anti-inflammatory agents, and other drugs such as diuretics and angiotensin-converting enzyme inhibitors. Vancomycin may be nephrotoxic (see also the chapter "Glycopeptides") and the combined use with an aminoglycoside may be synergistic in increasing nephrotoxicity. Age in itself is probably not an independent risk factor for nephrotoxicity. Meta-analyses (12–16) have shown no toxicity differences between single or multiple dosing regimens, but prolonged aminoglycoside use was clearly associated with toxicity in the 86 patients studied by Baciewicz et al. (28). One interesting finding in an experimental animal model was that aminoglycoside nephrotoxicity was more likely to occur if the drug is administered during rest periods and was more likely to be efficacious during periods of activity (29).

The incidence of aminoglycoside ototoxicity is difficult to determine because there is no standard definition, and clinical assessment is difficult because it typically affects high-tone hearing loss, not easily detectable at the bedside. Moreover, assessment of vestibular function in ill hospitalized patients is problematical (3). Nevertheless, ototoxicity is thought to range from <1% to as high as 10%. Unlike nephrotoxicity, ototoxicity is not reversible and can be particularly debilitating in geriatric patients. Risk factors include increased age, elevated serum levels, and duration of therapy (1). Gentamicin appears to be more ototoxic than tobramycin or amikacin, and netilmicin appears to be the least ototoxic of the group.

The precise mechanism by which aminoglycosides cause ototoxicity is not clear, but one mechanism by which aminoglycosides damage vestibular and cochlear hair cells is by generating free radicals with resulting apoptosis (33,34). This toxic property has been taken advantage of and intratympanic membrane aminoglycoside injection has been used with success to treat vertigo in patients with Meniere's disease.

REFERENCES

1. Zaske DE. Aminoglycosides. In: Yoshikawa TT, Norman DC, eds. Antimicrobial Therapy in the Elderly Patient. New York: Marcel Dekker, Inc., 1994:183–235.
2. Mingeot-Leclercq MP, Glupczynski Y, Tulkens PM. Activity and resistance. Antimicrob Agents Chemother 1999; 43(4):727–737.
3. Edson R, Terrell CL. The aminoglycosides. Mayo Clin Proc 1999; 74(5):519–528.
4. Jones RN. Hospital acquired infections: realities of risks and resistance. Resistance patterns among nosocomial pathogens. Trends over the past few years. Chest 2001; 119(suppl 2):397S–404S.
5. Lacy MK, Nicolau DP, Nightingale CH, Quintiliani R. The pharmacodynamics of aminoglycosides. Clin Infect Dis 1998; 27:23–27.
6. Turnidge J. Pharmacodynamics and dosing of aminoglycosides. Infect Dis Clin North Am 2003; 17(3):503–528.
7. DiPiro JT, Edmiston CE, Bohnen J. Pharmacodynamics of antimicrobial therapy in surgery. Am J Surg 1996; 171(6):615–622.
8. Kashuba AD, Nafziger AN, Drusano GL, Bertino JS. Optimizing aminoglycoside therapy for nosocomial pneumonia caused by Gram-negative bacteria. Antimicrob Agents Chemother 1999; 43(3):623–629.
9. Begg EJ, Barclay ML, Kirkpatrick CJM. The therapeutic monitoring of antimicrobial agents. Brit J Clin Pharmacol 1999; 47:23–30.
10. Paul M, Benuri-Silbiger I, Soares-Weiser K, Leibovici L. Beta-lactam monotherapy versus beta-lactam aminoglycoside combination therapy for sepsis in immunocompetent patients: systematic review and meta-analysis of randomized trials. Br Med J 2004; 328(7441):668–672.
11. Furno P, Bucaneve G, Del Favero A. Monotherapy or aminoglycoside-containing combinations for empirical antibiotic treatment of febrile neutropenic patients: a meta analysis. Lancet Infect Dis 2002; 2(4):231–242.
12. Ferriols-Lisart R, Alos-Alminana M. Effectiveness and safety of once-daily aminoglycosides: a meta-analysis. Am J Health Syst Pharm 1996; 53(10):1141–1150.
13. Hatala R, Dinh T, Cook DJ. Once-daily aminoglycoside dosing in immunocompetent adults: a meta-analysis. Ann Intern Med 1996; 124(8):717–725.
14. Barza M, Ioannidis JP, Cappelleri JC, Lau J. Single or multiple daily doses of aminoglycosides: a meta-analysis. Br Med J 1996; 312(7027):338–345.
15. Ali MZ, Goetz MB. A meta-analysis of the relative efficacy and toxicity of single daily dosing versus multiple daily dosing of aminoglycosides. Clin Infect Dis 1997; 24(5):796–809.
16. Bailey TC, Little JR, Littenberg B, Reichley RM, Dunagan WC. A meta-analysis of extended-interval dosing versus multiple daily dosing of aminoglycosides. Clin Infect Dis 1997; 24(5):786–795.
17. Anaizi N. Once-daily dosing of aminoglycosides. A consensus document. Int J Clin Pharmacol Ther 1997; 35(6):223–226.

18. Freeman CD, Nicolau DP, Belliveau PP, Nightingale CH. Once-daily dosing of amino-glycosides: review and recommendations for clinical practice. J Antimicrob Chemother 1997; 39(6):677–686.

19. Nicolau DP, Freeman CD, Elliveau PP, Nightingale CH, Ross JW, Quintiliani R. Experience with a once-daily aminoglycoside program administered to 2,184 adult patients. Antimicrob Agents Chemother 1995; 39(3):650–655.

20. Crockcroft DW, Gault MH. Prediction of creatinine clearance from serum creatinine. Nephron 1976; 16:31–41.

21. Gilbert DN, Lee BL, Dworkin RJ, Leggett JL, Chambers HF, Modin G, Tauber MG, Sande MA. A randomized comparison of the safety and efficacy of once-daily gentamicin or thrice-daily gentamicin in combination with ticarcillin-clavulanate. Am J Med 1998; 105(3):182–191.

22. Chuck SK, Raber SR, Rodvold KA, Areff D. National survey of extended-interval aminoglycoside dosing. Clin Infect Dis 2000; 30(3):433–439.

23. Toschlog EA, Blount KP, Rotondo MF, Sagraves SG, Bard MR, Schenarts PJ, Swanson M, Goettler CE. Clinical predictors of subtherapeutic aminoglycoside levels in trauma patients undergoing once-daily dosing. J Trauma-Injury Infect Crit Care 2003; 55(2):255–260.

24. Friedman JR, Norman DC, Yoshikawa TT. Correlation of estimated renal function parameters versus 24-hour creatinine clearance in ambulatory elderly. J Am Geriatr Soc 1989; 37(2):145–149.

25. Winston L, Benowitz N. Once-daily dosing of aminoglycosides: how much monitoring is truly required? Am J Med 2003; 114(3):239–240.

26. Barclay ML, Kirkpatrick CM, Begg EJ. Once daily aminoglycoside therapy. Is it less toxic than multiple daily doses and how should it be monitored? Clin Pharmacokinet 1999; 36(2):89–98.

27. Bartal C, Danon A, Schlaeffer F, Reisenberg K, Alkan M, Smoliakov R, Sidi A, Almog Y. Pharmacokinetic dosing of aminoglycosides: a controlled trial. Am J Med 2003; 114(3):194–198.

28. Baciewicz AM, Sokos DR, Cowan RI. Aminoglycoside-associated nephrotoxicity in the elderly. Ann Pharmacother 2003; 37(2):182–186.

29. Beauchamp D, Labrecque G. Aminoglycoside nephrotoxicity: do time and frequency of administration matter. Curr Opin Crit Care 2001; 7(6):401–408.

30. Le Moyec L, Racine S, Le Toumelin P, Adnet F, Larue V, Cohen Y, Leroux Y, Cupa M, Hantz E. Aminoglycoside and glycopeptide renal toxicity in intensive care patients studied by proton magnetic resonance spectroscopy of urine. Crit Care Med 2002; 30(6):1242–1245.

31. Sundin DP, Sandoval R, Molitoris BA. Gentamicin inhibits renal protein and phospho-lipid metabolism in rats: implications involving intracellular trafficking. J Am Soc Nephrol 2001; 12(1):114–123.

32. Santucci RA, Krieger JN. Gentamicin for the practicing urologist: review of efficacy, single daily dosing, and "switch" therapy. J Urol 2000; 163(4):1076–1084.

33. Rybak LP, Kelly T. Ototoxicity: bioprotective mechanisms. Opin Otolaryngol Head Neck Surg 2003; 11(5):328–333.

34. Nakashima T, Teranishi M, Hibi T, Kobayashi M, Umemura M. Vestibular and cochlear toxicity of aminoglycosides—a review. Acta Oto-Laryngologica 2000; 120(8):904–911.

SUGGESTED READING

Turnidge J. Pharmacodynamics and dosing of aminoglycosides. Infect Dis Clin North Am 2003; 17(3):503–528.

15
Tetracyclines

David R. P. Guay

Department of Experimental and Clinical Pharmacology and Institute for the Study of Geriatric Pharmacotherapy, University of Minnesota, College of Pharmacy and Division of Geriatrics, HealthPartners Inc., Minneapolis, Minnesota, U.S.A.

Key Points:

- Doxycycline is the tetracycline-of-choice in elderly individuals.
- Screen carefully for drug–drug interactions that may compromise tetracycline efficacy by reducing oral drug bioavailability or accelerating drug elimination.
- The tetracyclines are the drugs-of-choice for few of the infection syndromes seen commonly in older individuals.
- Avoid oral tetracyclines, if possible, in older individuals with esophageal dysmotility or other conditions compromising rapid drug transit into the stomach.
- Avoid the intramuscular route of administration as it is painful and may result in lower drug concentrations than the oral or intravenous routes.

1. INTRODUCTION

The first tetracycline, chlortetracycline, was isolated in 1948 from an isolate of *Streptomyces*. This was followed by the semisynthetic derivatives oxytetracycline in 1950 and tetracycline in 1952. In the late 1950s to early 1960s, additional semisynthetic derivatives were marketed (demeclocycline, rolitetracycline, and methacycline) followed by doxycycline in 1966 and minocycline in 1972. Today, there are five tetracyclines available for oral use in the United States. They are oxytetracycline, doxycycline, minocycline (all three available for parenteral administration as well), demeclocycline, and tetracycline (1).

In the past few years, a new class of antimicrobials structurally related to the tetracyclines has entered clinical investigation. They are the glycylcyclines, tetracycline analogues in which a substituted glycyl moiety has been inserted in the C-9 ring position. The only agent to enter clinical investigation as well as be approved by the U.S. Food and Drug Administration (FDA) to date is the 9-*t*-butylglycylamido derivative of minocycline also known as tigecycline (GAR-936) (2).

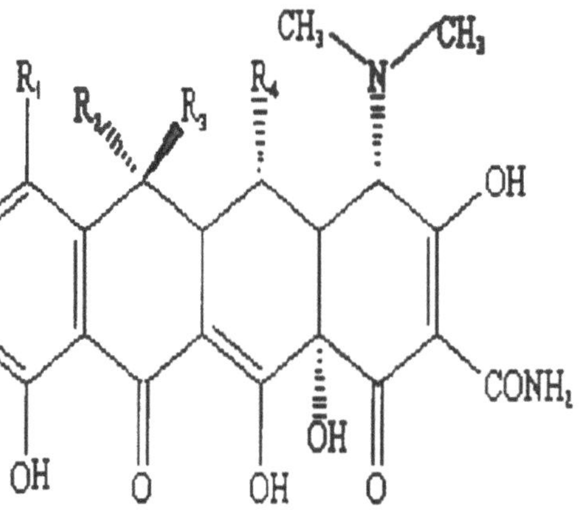

Figure 1 Chemical structure of the tetracycline nucleus.

2. CHEMISTRY AND MECHANISM OF ACTION

All commercially available tetracyclines contain the tetracycline nucleus illustrated in Figure 1. Various substitutions of the tetracycline nucleus resulted in derivatives with different degrees of antimicrobial activity, gastrointestinal (GI) absorption, affinity for multivalent cations, and plasma protein binding. Tetracyclines and their salts generally occur as yellow, crystalline powders. Tetracycline bases are amphoteric and very slightly soluble in water while the salt forms are generally sparingly soluble to freely soluble in water.

The premise for investigating the glycylcycline class was the belief that a peptide substituent would enhance ribosomal permeation and binding. However, later work found that the major effect of 9-glycylation was prevention of recognition of the molecule by the *Tet* A efflux protein, a major effector of tetracycline resistance. Structure–activity studies demonstrated that minocycline was one of the preferred starting points for subsequent modification and that a basic nitrogen must be present in the side chain at C-9 for activity. Also, the nitrogen can be disubstituted with small alkyl groups or part of a ring structure. Further modification of the glycyl substituent led to the discovery of tigecycline (GAR-936), a *t*-butyl substituted glycine derivative. The *t*-butyl substitution provided the best overall activity and was selected for further in vitro and in vivo investigation (2).

Tetracyclines, and presumably tigecycline, inhibit protein synthesis by reversibly binding to the 30S ribosomal subunit, thus preventing access of aminoacyl transfer RNA to the receptor site on the messenger RNA–ribosome complex. They also appear to reversibly bind to the 50S ribosomal subunit. Preliminary evidence suggests that these agents may also alter cytoplasmic membranes, resulting in leakage of nucleotides and other intracellular constituents from the cell. At high concentrations, mammalian protein synthesis is also inhibited (3).

3. ANTIMICROBIAL SPECTRUM

The tetracyclines exhibit broad-spectrum activity against gram-positive and gram-negative aerobic bacteria as well as obligate intracellular bacterial pathogens (e.g.,

Mycoplasma, Ureaplasma, Chlamydia, and *Legionella* species), *Rickettsia* species, spirochetes, and parasites (*Plasmodium* species, filarial nematodes, amebae). In general, these are bacteriostatic agents, although in high concentration or with highly susceptible organisms, they can be bactericidal. Despite their spectrum of activity, their clinical usefulness has been limited by the widespread dissemination of resistance determinants. Table 1 lists the microorganisms against which the tetracyclines exhibit useful in vitro activity (3,4).

Tigecycline, in contrast to the tetracyclines, is much more potent against gram-positive aerobic pathogens, including strains resistant to penicillin, vancomycin, methicillin/oxacillin, erythromycin, and tetracycline/minocycline. It is also unaffected by β-lactamases, including extended-spectrum β-lactamases (ESBL). However, its activity against gram-negative aerobic organisms and anaerobes is quite modest [especially *Proteus* and *Providencia* species, *Morganella morganii*, *Acinetobacter* species, and *Bacteroides fragilis* (group)] and for *Pseudomonas, Burkholderia, Stenotrophomonas,* and many atypical mycobacterial species, it is negligible (2).

Bacterial resistance to the tetracyclines was identified shortly after their introduction to the marketplace (1953). Today, tetracycline (*tet*) resistance can occur by the acquisition of one or more of the 36 known resistance genes which act by reducing cell wall permeability (i.e., drug uptake), enhancing efflux from the cell (via active efflux pumps), altering 16SrRNA sequences (reducing binding to the target site), and generating ribosomal protection proteins (protect ribosomes from the drug effect). Frequently, these resistance determinants are found on mobile elements such as plasmids, transposons, and/or integrons, which facilitate their intra- and interspecies dissemination. For example, *tet* M is the most widely distributed resistance determinant in aerobic gram-positive and nonenteric gram-negative bacteria. *Tet* O, *tet* M, or both together are the major resistance determinants in *Streptococcus pneumoniae*. Fortunately, no acquired tetracycline resistance has been described among obligate intracellular pathogens, protozoa, and other eukaryotic organisms (4).

Novel efflux mutants have already been discovered which confer resistance to the glycylcyclines (*tet* A and B mutants among *Salmonella* species, *Proteus mirabilis,* and *Pseudomonas aeruginosa*) (2).

4. CLINICAL PHARMACOLOGY

Table 2 illustrates the basic pharmacokinetic parameters for the oral tetracyclines and intravenous (IV) tigecycline in normal volunteers (1,5). Oral bioavailability of the tetracyclines is quite variable, ranging from 25–30% (chlortetracycline, no longer available in the United States) to 60–80% (oxytetracycline, demeclocycline, tetracycline) to >90% (doxycycline, minocycline) (1,5). Achlorhydria, a condition frequently occurring in older individuals, does not alter the rate or extent of absorption of a single 250 mg oral dose of tetracycline (6). The presence of bile is necessary for optimal oral bioavailability of tetracycline but not doxycycline (7). Ingestion of food or milk reduces the oral bioavailability of demeclocycline, methacycline, oxytetracycline, and tetracycline by at least 50%. This can be contrasted with the clinically insignificant reduction of <20% seen with food/milk and doxycycline or minocycline (1,5,8). The time to achievement of peak plasma/serum concentrations after oral administration ranges from 1.5 to 4 hr (1,5).

The tetracyclines penetrate various body tissue/fluid compartments reasonably well with the exception of the central nervous system (Table 3) (8). Plasma protein

Table 1 Microorganisms That Are Usually Susceptible or of Intermediate Susceptibility to the Tetracyclines

Gram-positive bacteria
  Bacillus anthracis
  Actinomyces israelii
  Arachnia propionica
  Clostridium perfringens
  Clostridium tetani
  Listeria monocytogenes
  Nocardia
  Propionibacterium acnes
Gram-negative bacteria
  Bartonella bacilliformis
  Bordetella pertussis
  Brucella
  Calymmatobacterium granulomatis
  Campylobacter fetus
  Francisella tularensis
  Haemophilus ducreyi
  H. influenzae
  Legionella
  Leptotrichia buccalis
  Neisseria gonorrhoeae
  Neisseria meningitides
  Pasturella multocida
  Burkholderia pseudomallei
  Burkholderia mallei
  Shigella
  Spirillum minus
  Streptobacillus moniliformis
  Vibrio cholerae
  Vibrio parahaemolyticus
  Yersinia enterocolitica
  Yersinia pestis
Miscellaneous
  Rickettsia
  Coxiella burnetii
  Chlamydia trachomatis
  Chlamydia psittaci
  Mycoplasma hominus
  Mycoplasma pneumoniae
  Ureaplasma urealyticum
  Borrelia recurrentis
  Borrelia burgdorferi
  Leptospira
  Treponema pallidum
  Treponema pertenue
  Mycobacterium fortuitum
  Mycobacterium marinum
  Balantidium coli
  Plasmodium falciparum (asexual erythrocytic forms)

Table 2 Single-Dose Pharmacokinetic Parameters of the Oral Tetracyclines and Intravenous Tigecycline in Normal Volunteers

	F (%)	PPB (%)	$t_{1/2}$ (hr)	C_{max} (mg/L)	t_{max} (hr)	F_e (%)
Demeclocycline	60–80	36–91	10–17		3–4	44
150 mg				0.9–1.2		
300 mg				1.5–1.7		
Oxytetracycline	60–80	10–40	6–10		2–4	60–70
250 mg				1.3–1.4		
500 mg				4.0–4.2		
Tetracycline	60–80	20–67	6–12		2–4	48–60
250 mg				1.5–2.2		
500 mg				3.0–4.3		
Doxycycline	90–100	25–93	14–24			20–26
100 mg[a]				1.5–2.1	1.5–4	
200 mg[a]				2.6–3.0	1.5–4	
200 mg[b]				3.6	2.5	
Minocycline	90–100	55–88	11–26		1–4	4–19
200 mg				2–3.5		
Tigecycline	N/A	71–89	24–36	1.45	N/A	15
100 mg						
150 mg				8.6		
300 mg				17.9		

[a]Hyclate salt.
[b]Monohydrate salt.
Abbreviations: F, oral bioavailability; PPB, plasma protein binding; $t_{1/2}$, terminal disposition half-life; C_{max}, peak plasma concentration; t_{max}, time to C_{max}; F_e, fraction eliminated in urine as parent compound; N/A, not available; ND, not done.

binding varies among the agents from 10% to 93% (Table 2) (1,5). All tetracyclines are distributed into bile and undergo enterohepatic circulation (biliary concentrations are 2–32 times higher than concurrent serum concentrations). Biliary excretion is an important component of doxycycline elimination (1,5,8).

Demeclocycline, oxytetracycline, and tetracycline do not appear to be metabolized and are eliminated principally as parent compounds in the urine. In contrast, minocycline is metabolized, at least in part, to at least six metabolites (all are inactive) (1,5,8). Although it is felt that doxycycline is not metabolized but is inactivated and eliminated via the gut by chelate formation, this is not supported by the results of drug–drug interaction studies with doxycycline and the potent hepatic enzyme inducers phenytoin, carbamazepine, and phenobarbital (vida infra). With the exception of oxytetracycline, the tetracyclines are not dialyzable (via hemodialysis or peritoneal dialysis).

Tigecycline, administered only by IV infusion over at least 1 hr, exhibits a mean volume of distribution at steady state in healthy volunteers of 7–9 L/kg. Metabolism appears to constitute the major route of elimination as the fractional elimination of parent compound in the urine is only about 22% and in the feces is less than 14% in healthy volunteers. Total body clearance in healthy volunteers ranges from 0.3 to 0.5 L/hr/kg. Terminal disposition half-life ranges from 24 to 36 hr in the presence of normal renal function (2).

The effect of renal impairment on the pharmacokinetics of several tetracyclines have been evaluated. One study evaluated doxycycline pharmacokinetics after a

Table 3 Tissue (or Fluid) to Plasma (T/P) Concentration Ratios for Various Tetracyclines

Tissue/fluid compartment	Agent	Mean T/P ratio
Mucous, primary bronchi	PO minocycline	3.06
Mucous, proximal to tumor		1.99
Mucous, distal to tumor		5.16
Lung parencyhyma, healthy		3.78
Lung, tumor		3.16
Bronchial wall		4.40
Arterial wall		3.37
Lung tissue	PO doxycycline	1.74
Bronchial tissue		1.58
Sputum	PO doxycycline	2.4
Bone	IV doxycycline	0.02 (male), 0.02 (female)
Skin		0.21 (male), 0.22 (female)
SC fat		0.18 (male), 0.20 (female)
Tendon		0.18 (male), 0.24 (female)
Muscle		0.63 (male), 0.63 (female)
Sinus secretions	PO minocycline	0.34
Maxillary sinus mucosa	IM tetracycline	1.11
	PO tetracycline	1.52
Sputum	PO tetracycline	0.23
Lung tissue	IV minocycline	3.71
Sputum		0.56

Abbreviations: PO, oral; IV, intravenous; SC, subcutaneous; IM, intramuscular.

single oral 200 mg dose administered to 15 patients with a wide range of renal functional capacity. The only statistically significant intergroup differences occurred with terminal disposition half-life [increased in the group with creatinine clearance (CrCl) 10–50 mL/min vs. the group with CrCl >50 mL/min, mean ± SD, 24.5 ± 6.9 hr vs. 16.0 ± 4.2 hr] and urinary excretion of parent compound (same groups, reduced with reduced CrCl, 29.2 ± 19.1 mg vs. 99.3 ± 45.7 mg). Plasma protein binding was significantly lower in the hemodialysis group compared with the CrCl >50 mL/min group (72.6 ± 6.1% vs. 88.0 ± 6.5%). Significant correlations existed for CrCl with urinary excretion of parent compound, renal clearance, erythrocyte binding, and plasma protein binding (all fell as CrCl fell). Similar findings of reduced urinary excretion of parent compound with reduced renal function after oral and parenteral doxycycline administration have been found in other studies. However, one study did find no significant difference in doxycycline terminal disposition half-life in healthy volunteers ($N = 6$) and hemodialysis patients ($N = 8$), i.e., mean ± SD, 15.5 ± 3.6 hr vs. 19.5 ± 5.5 hr, respectively. The modest effects of renal disease on doxycycline disposition are felt to be due to enhanced biliary (gut) elimination when renal function is reduced. Another study evaluated the single IV and multiple oral dose pharmacokinetics of minocycline in 15 subjects with a wide range of renal functional capacity. In the single-dose portion, the only significant inter-group differences occurred with total body clearance (lower in controls than in the CrCl 20–33 mL/min and CrCl <10 mL/min groups; mean ± SD, 19.6 ± 7.7 vs. 33.5 ± 6.3 or 30.7 ± 4.1 mL/min) and urinary excretion (fell as CrCl fell, with respective values of mean ± SD, 8.3 ± 2.2, 4.1 ± 0.5, and 1.6%). In the multiple-dose portion, virtually identical plasma concentration vs. time curves were seen on all three study days in all three groups. In another study of similar design, similar results were found. In the single-dose portion, only the correlation of renal drug clearance with CrCl was significant (elimination rate constant, total body clearance, volume of distribution were not). Renal clearance was only about 8% of total body clearance. In the multiple-dose portion, elimination rate constant was still independent of the degree of renal functional impairment and the renal clearance–CrCl correlation was still significant (8).

In contrast to doxycycline and minocycline, the other tetracyclines are much more dependent on intact renal function for their elimination, e.g., tetracycline, oxytetracycline, demeclocycline. Evidence for this is readily seen when examining the prolongation of terminal disposition half-life in the presence of severe renal impairment: demeclocycline 10–17 hr prolonged to 42–68 hr, oxytetracycline 6–10 hr prolonged to 47–66 hr, and tetracycline 6–12 hr prolonged to 57–120 hr (1,5). These agents are best avoided in patients with renal impairment although they can be used if dosage intervals are prolonged (e.g., dosage intervals of 3 or 4 days with end-stage renal disease).

In the presence of severe hepatic impairment or common bile duct obstruction, serum concentrations of the tetracyclines may be higher and terminal disposition half-lives slightly prolonged (1,5).

As mentioned previously, the presence of achlorhydria does not alter the rate or extent of single-dose tetracycline absorption. However, in five elders with achlorhydria, mean 72 hr urinary excretion and renal clearance were significantly lower than those in five young controls [39.2 vs. 56.6% of dose, respectively, and 37 (capsule) or 42 (solution) mL/min vs. 64 (capsule) or 69 (solution) mL/min, respectively]. This is probably a result of the reduction in renal function seen with advancing age and nothing to do with achlorhydria (6).

Few studies have evaluated the effect of aging on the pharmacokinetics of tetracyclines. Twenty-five patients 65–80 years old (mean $\pm$ SD, 76 $\pm$ 6) were treated with doxycycline 200 mg IV once or twice daily. After the first dose, the mean $\pm$ SD distribution half-life, terminal disposition half-life, volume of distribution, and total body clearance were 10.1 $\pm$ 7.2 min, 15.1 $\pm$ 8.8 hr, 24.8 $\pm$ 8.9 L, and 1.09 $\pm$ 0.66 L/hr, respectively (9). This may be compared with healthy young volunteer data after the same dose: mean volume of distribution of 52.6 L, terminal disposition half-life of 13.8–15.6 hr, and total body clearance of 2.32 L/hr (8). In a study published in 1960, the serum concentrations of tetracycline after intramuscular (IM) administration (no longer available in the United States) were significantly higher in 27 elderly subjects compared with 26 younger subjects (10). These results can be explained by the known dependence of tetracycline elimination on intact renal function and the fall in renal function with increasing age. Last, the pharmacokinetics of IV minocycline after multiple-dose administration to debilitated elderly patients with acute respiratory tract infections has been evaluated. Study participants, mean $\pm$ SD 82 $\pm$ 6 years old, received minocycline 100 mg IV (over 1 hr) twice daily for at least 10 doses. Blood samples were analyzed for minocycline content after doses 1, 5, and 9. Mean $\pm$ SD terminal disposition half-life, volume of distribution, and total body clearance were 25.0 $\pm$ 16.4 hr, 32.9 $\pm$ 13.4 L, and 1.14 $\pm$ 0.49 L/hr, respectively (11). This may be compared with healthy young volunteer data after the same dose: mean terminal disposition half-life of 12.6–16 hr, volume of distribution of 67.5–115 L, and total body clearance of 3.36–5.7 L/hr (8).

Age, race, and gender do not substantially alter tigecycline pharmacokinetics. In contrast, severe renal impairment (SRI) (CrCl < 30 mL/min) does delay tigecycline elimination. For example, although mean peak plasma concentrations were similar, mean area under the plasma concentration vs. time curve was 40% higher in the SRI group compared with healthy volunteers after a single 100 mg IV dose. As would be expected, urinary recovery of parent compound was less in the SRI group as well (mean 5% vs. 16% of dose). In the hemodialysis compared with healthy volunteer group, mean peak plasma concentration and area under the plasma concentration vs. time curve were 60% and 20% higher, respectively. Tigecycline was not dialyzable (2). Although mild hepatic impairment (Child-Pugh A) does not substantially alter tigecycline pharmacokinetics, moderate (Child-Pugh B), and severe (Child-Pugh C) hepatic impairment dose. Total body clearance is reduced by 25% and 55% and terminal disposition half-life is prolonged 23% and 43% in moderate and severe hepatic impairment, respectively.

5. CLINICAL INDICATIONS

The tetracyclines are active against a wide range of common and uncommon bacterial pathogens as well as some protozoa. Although they are used to treat a variety of infections, including pneumonia, acute exacerbations of chronic bronchitis, infectious diarrhea, sexually transmitted diseases, and prostatitis, their use has declined over the years due to the availability of more effective agents and the dissemination of tetracycline resistance. In addition, the infections due to organisms for which the tetracyclines are considered the drugs-of-choice (Table 4) are not common in the elderly (12). For those infections more common in the elderly, the tetracyclines are frequently just one of the many alternatives (Table 4) (12). Despite this, even the less common but serious infections such as rickettsial diseases, brucellosis, chlamydial infections, melioidosis, cholera, Lyme disease, and atypical pneumonia do occur in older adults. Clinicians providing care to older patients should still be familiar with the clinical role of the tetracyclines.

Although for many years the tetracyclines have been considered among the drugs-of-choice for the treatment of acute exacerbations of chronic bronchitis, the increasing rates of tetracycline resistance among pneumococci and *Haemophilus influenzae* have made these nonpreferred agents. This applies also to bacterial pneumonia, where consensus guidelines have relegated the tetracyclines to lower-tier status except in pneumonias due to a few specific pathogens. Even in atypical pneumonia, the tetracyclines are not considered the drugs-of-choice, having been supplanted by the macrolides and respiratory fluoroquinolones (13,14).

The tetracyclines have some utility in the treatment and prophylaxis of infectious diarrhea. They are useful in treating diarrheal states due to bacterial overgrowth as well as those due to *Campylobacter jejuni* and *Vibrio* species. They are alternatives to trimethoprim–sulfamethoxazole and fluoroquinolones for the prevention of traveller's diarrhea (15).

Tetracyclines also have some utility in the treatment of sexually transmitted infections in sexually active elders. Tetracyclines are among the most effective agents for nongonococcal urethritis and can be used to treat syphilis in those who are penicillin allergic, as well as granuloma inguinale and lymphogranuloma venereum (16).

Despite the availability of tetracyclines for over half a century, the clinical data for these agents in predominantly or exclusively elderly populations are scant, a

Table 4 Indications for Tetracyclines by Organism

Infecting organism (disease)	Drug-of-choice	Alternative
Staphylococcus aureus (methicillin resistant)		X
Streptococcus pneumoniae (penicillin susceptible)		X
Moraxella catarrhalis		X
Bacillus anthracis (anthrax)		X
Clostridium tetani (tetanus)		X
Campylobacter jejuni		X
Citrobacter freundii		X
Acinetobacter spp.		Doxycycline
Bartonella henselae or *quintana* (bacillary angiomatosis)		Doxycycline
Brucella spp.	X (plus rifampin)	X (plus streptomycin or gentamicin)
Burkholderia mallei (glanders)	X (plus streptomycin)	
Burkholderia pseudomallei (melioidosis)		Doxycycline (plus chloramphenicol plus trimethoprim–sulfamethoxazole)
Calymmatobacterium granulomatis (granuloma inguinale)		Doxycycline (with or without gentamicin)
Francisella tularensis (tularemia)		X
H. influenzae		X (URI, bronchitis)
Legionella spp.		Doxycycline (with or without rifampin)
Leptotrichia buccalis		X
Pasturella multocida		X
Spirillum minus (rat bite fever)		X
Stenotrophomonas maltophilia		Minocycline
Streptobacillus moniliformis (rat bite fever, Haverhill fever)		X
Vibrio cholerae	X	
Vibrio vulnificus	X	
Yersinia pestis (plague)	(Streptomycin) with or without a tetracycline	
Mycobacterium fortuitum/chelonae complex		Doxycycline
Mycobacterium marinum	Minocycline	Doxycycline
Mycobacterium leprae (leprosy)		Minocycline
Actinomyces israelii (actinomycosis)		X
Nocardia		X
Tropheryma whippelii (agent of Whipple's disease)		X
Chlamydia psittaci (psittacosis, ornithosis)	X	
Chlamydia trachomatis Trachoma		X (topical + oral)
Lymphogranuloma venereum	X	

(Continued)

Table 4 Indications for Tetracyclines by Organism (*Continued*)

Infecting organism (disease)	Drug-of-choice	Alternative
Chlamydia pneumoniae	X	
Ehrlichia chaffeensis	Doxycycline	
Ehrlichia ewingii	Doxycycline	
Ehrlichia phagocytophila	Doxycycline	
Mycoplasma pneumoniae	X	
Ureaplasma urealyticum		X
Rickettsia (Q fever, trench fever, typhus, Rocky Mountain spotted fever)	Doxycycline	
Borrelia burgdorferi (Lyme disease)	Doxycycline	
Borrelia recurrentis (relapsing fever)	X	
Leptospira		X
Treponema pallidum (syphilis)		X
Treponema pertenue (yaws)		X

Note: X, any tetracycline can be used.
Abbreviation: URI, upper respiratory infection.

mere nine studies (Table 5). Nothing in these nine studies suggest any substantial alteration in tetracycline efficacy or tolerability in older as compared to younger individuals.

Tigecycline in FOA approved for the treatment of complicated skin and skin structure and intrabdomial infections caused by susceptible strains of a variety of specified gram-positive and -negative aerobes and anaerobes.

6. DOSING AND ADMINISTRATION

Demeclocycline is available as 150 and 300 mg tablets. The usual adult dosage is 600 mg daily, in two or four divided doses (1,5).

Oxytetracycline is available as 250 mg capsules and as an injectable for IM use only (50 and 125 mg/mL strengths, both with 2% lidocaine). The usual adult oral dosage is 1 to 2 g daily in four divided doses. The usual adult IM dosage is 250 mg once daily or 300 mg daily in two or three divided doses. Intramuscular administration is rarely indicated as it is painful and usually produces lower serum drug concentrations than does oral administration (1,5).

Tetracycline is available in 250 and 500 mg capsules/tablets. The usual adult dosage is 1 to 2 g daily in four divided doses. Higher daily dosages are indicated in the treatment of psittacosis, melioidosis, and plague (1,5).

Doxycycline is available as 50 and 100 mg capsules/tablets (hyclate salt), oral suspension (50 mg/5 mL) (calcium salt), 50 and 100 mg capsules and oral suspension (25 mg/5 mL) (monohydrate salt), and as an injectable for IV use only (100 and 200 mg doses). The usual oral adult dosage is 100 mg twice daily on day 1 followed by 100 mg daily (in one or two doses). For severe infections, the daily dosage can be increased to 200 mg (in two divided doses). The usual IV adult dosage is 200 mg

Table 5 Tetracycline Efficacy/Tolerability Studies in the Elderly[a,b]

Reference/age data	Study design	Type of infection	N	Treatment regimens	Results	Adverse events
26/means of 68 and 70 years for PIVAMP and TETRA groups, respectively	R, SB	AECB	50	TETRA 500 qid × 10 days	On day 7, clinical cure was noted in 34% of TETRA and 57% of PIVAMP patients ($p < 0.05$) while on day 11, the corresponding rates were 48% vs. 68% ($p < 0.05$); clinical success rates were not significantly different in the TETRA and PIVAMP groups at day 7 (72% vs. 88%) and day 11 (66% vs. 88%); on day 11, 24 hr sputum volume was reduced in a significantly lower proportion of TETRA patients (48%) compared to PIVAMP patients (68%) ($p < 0.05$) while proportions converting purulent to mucoid sputum were not significantly different (66% vs. 72%, respectively); bacteriologic eradication occurred in 53% of PIVAMP and 54% of TETRA recipients; 1-month relapse rates significantly favored PIVAMP (37%) vs. TETRA (62%) ($p < 0.05$)	AE were noted in 12 TETRA recipients (GI only in 5, GI + diarrhea in 5, rash and diarrhea alone in 1 each) and 6 PIVAMP recipients (GI only in 5, GI + diarrhea in 1); these led to three TETRA and five PIVAMP dose changes
			49	PIVAMP 350 qid × 10 days		
27/50–59 y.o., N = 6; 60–69, N = 10; 70–79, N = 7	R	Winter AECB prophylaxis	12	DOXY 100 eod	There were three exacerbations in three DOXY recipients (0.25 exacerbations per patient) and six exacerbations in five OXYTET recipients (0.55 exacerbations per patient); in terms of adherence, for OXYTET, 35% missed > 2 days and 23% missed > 4 days while for DOXY, 4% missed > 2 days and 2% missed > 4 days	Two OXYTET recipients had AE (nausea, epigastric pain in one each) and one DOXY recipient had AE (pruritus)
			11	OXYTET 250 qid (treated × mean 5 months; range, 3–6)		

(Continued)

Table 5 Tetracycline Efficacy/Tolerability Studies in the Elderly[a,b] (*Continued*)

Reference/age data	Study design	Type of infection	N	Treatment regimens	Results	Adverse events
28/all ≥ 60 years old	R, SB	AECB	89 84 86	TETRA 500 qid × 12 days CHLORO 500 qid × 12 days PLACEBO × 12 days	The clinical success rates at day 7 for TETRA, CHLORO, and PLACEBO were 67%, 64%, 47% (NS), while on day 12 they were 65%, 72%, 38% (both active agents vs. placebo, $p < 0.05$); the corresponding resolution rates of purulent to mucoid sputum were 64%, 59%, 34% on day 7 and 68%, 73%, 36% on day 12; the corresponding mean no. of days to achieve mucoid sputum were 6.3, 6.4, 8.2	AE were noted in 28% of TETRA recipients, 10% of CHLORO recipients, and 10% of PLACEBO recipients (TETRA vs. CHLORO and TETRA vs. PLACEBO, both $p = 0.01$); AE were predominately GI in nature, with rash noted in one member of each group
29/mean age 63 years	O	Severe hospital infections	66	DOXY IV 200 qd × 10 days	Overall clinical cure rate was 66% (35% for UTI, 79% for RTI, 75% for SSSI, 100% for sepsis); failures occurred most frequently in infections due to gram-negative bacilli; superinfection occurred in 12%	AE were limited to nausea in a "few" patients, rash and phlebitis in two patients each, and pain during infusion in four patients
30/mean age of 60 years in both groups	DB, R	SSSI	39	DOXY 200 qd × mean ± SD, 9.8 ± 4.9 days ROXI 150 bid × mean ± SD, 10.3 ± 3.7 days	Clinical cure rates were 82% (DOXY) and 92% (ROXI) (NS) and bacteriologic eradication rates were 82% (DOXY) and 92% (ROXI) (NS)	AE occurred in three DOXY recipients (facial edema in one, NorV in two) and no ROXI recipients
31/males: mean age of 66 years; females: mean age of 60 years	O	AECB	39	DOXY 100 bid × 10 days	At 10 days, clinical response was excellent in 67%, good in 8%, moderate in 15%, and bad/failure in 10%; at 17 days, corresponding clinical responses were 56%,	No AE data were provided

					8%, 18%, and 18%; superinfection occurred in four patients with *P. aeruginosa*; one-third of strains of *H. influenzae* were not eradicated	
32/mean age >60 years	R, DB	AECB	36 / 37	DOXY 200 × 1 dose → 100 qd × 6 days / TMP/SMX DS bid × 7 days	Both agents ↓ sputum output to a similar extent and improved patients to a similar extent (improvement in 75% DOXY, 82% TMP/SMX recipients); new exacerbation within 1 month of end of therapy in one TMP/SMX and three DOXY recipients	No AE with DOXY; AE in two TMP/SMX patients (rash in one, glossitis and stomatitis in one)
33/means of 62 and 60 years in the DOXY and MINO groups, respectively	R	RTI, wound infection	67(50 RTI) / 63 (47 RTI)	DOXY 400 × 1 → 200 qd × 8 days / MINO 400 × 1 → 200 qd × 8 days	RTI: For DOXY, favorable clin/ bacteriological responses in 66/66% (excellent in 28%) while for MINO, the corresponding figures were 72/57% and 32%; for pneumococci RTI, the corresponding figures were 73/73% and 31% for DOXY ($N = 26$) and 77/59% and 32% for MINO ($N = 31$); bacterial colonization occurred in 17 DOXY and 16 MINO RTI recipients and clinical superinfection in 2 DOXY and 7 MINO RTI recipients Wound: For DOXY and MINO, clinical cure rates were 76% and 75%, respectively, with corresponding excellent results in 29% and 25%; overall colonization rate was 39% and superinfection rate was 8% (or 19% of colonized patients)	11 AE occurred in DOXY recipients and 6 in MINO recipients (mostly GI)

(Continued)

Table 5 Tetracycline Efficacy/Tolerability Studies in the Elderly[a,b] (*Continued*)

Reference/age data	Study design	Type of infection	N	Treatment regimens	Results	Adverse events
34/means of 60 and 63 years for MINO and AMP groups, respectively	R	UTI	39	MINO 200 qd × mean 9.3 days (range, 4–14)	Clinical cure rates were 85% (MINO) and 73% (AMP)(NS) while bacteriologic erad. rates were 72% (MINO) and 75% (AMP)(NS); excellent responses were noted in 33% of MINO and 30% of AMP recipients (NS); superinfection or colonization occurred in 23% of MINO and 38% of AMP recipients	AE, mainly GI in nature, occurred in 28% of AMP and 18% of MINO recipients
			40	AMP 1000 tid × mean 8.3 days (range, 7–13)		

[a]Note: Where the study populations were predominantly or exclusively over 60 years old ($\geq$ 50%) or mean age was $\geq$ 60 years old (overall or in all groups)
[b]Unless otherwise stated, all drugs were administered by PO route.
Abbreviations: PIVAMP, pivampicillin; TETRA, tetracycline; R, randomized; SB, single (investigator) blind; AECB, acute exacerbations of chronic bronchitis; qid, 4 times daily; AE, adverse events; GI, gastrointestinal; DOXY, doxycycline; OXYTET, oxytetracycline; eod, every other day; CHLORO, chloramphenicol; NS, not statistically-significant; O, open; qd, once daily; DB, double-blind; SSSI, skin and skin-structure infections; bid, twice daily; ROXI, roxithromycin; N, nausea; V, vomiting; TMP/SMX, trimethoprim/sulfamethaxozole; DS, double-strength; $\downarrow$, decrease; RTI, respiratory tract infections; MINO, minocycline; AMP, ampicillin; UTI, urinary tract infection; tid, thrice daily; PO, oral.

on day 1 (in one or two doses) followed by 100–200 mg daily. Intravenous infusions should be given over 1–4 hr. Higher daily dosages are recommended for the treatment of trachoma and syphilis (1,5).

Minocycline is available in 50 and 100 mg capsules/tablets, oral suspension (50 mg/5 mL), and as an injectable for IV use (100 mg dose). The usual adult oral or IV dosage is 200 mg initially followed by 100 mg twice daily or 100–200 mg initially followed by 50 mg four times daily (1,5).

Tigecycline is available soon injectable for IV use only (50 mg vials). The usual dosage regimen is a loading dose of 100 mg followed by 50 mg twice daily. Dosage adjustment is only needed in severe hepatic impairment (Child-Pugh C) wherein the loading done of 100 mg is followed by a reduced maintenance dose of 25 mg twice daily.

7. DRUG MONITORING AND ADVERSE EVENTS

The adverse effects of the tetracyclines have been well characterized due to their extensive use over the past near half-century.

One of the more interesting, although less clinically relevant, adverse effects of the tetracyclines is their linkage to abnormal pigmentation of a wide variety of tissues, due in part to their lipid solubility and the chelation properties with multivalent cations (17). This bluish/black pigmentation, which has been most frequently noted after long-term (years) minocycline therapy, can occur in the skin, sclera, conjunctiva, retina, oral mucosa, ears, thyroid, teeth, nails, and bones. It may not be reversible with drug discontinuation although skin pigmentation may respond to laser therapy. With the exception of the cosmetic consequences of pigmentation in visible skin areas, no clinically important negative consequences of pigmentation have been noted. For example, tetracycline does not alter the results of thyroid function testing.

For years, the tetracyclines have been considered a major factor in drug-induced esophagitis, including complications like esophageal strictures or esophageal–atrial fistula (18). In addition, these agents may rarely be associated with gastric pathology (ulcers). The strongly acidic pH of the tetracyclines in solution (<3) is felt to be directly irritative to GI mucosal tissues. There are several preventive strategies that may reduce the risk and severity of this reaction. Tetracyclines should be avoided in patients with esophageal hypomotility. Patients should be counseled to take each dose with adequate fluid, to not take a dose at bedtime, and to avoid recumbency immediately after drug ingestion.

Drug-associated hypoglycemia has been noted, albeit rarely, with tetracycline, oxytetracycline, and doxycycline. Similarly, these drugs, especially minocycline, have been associated rarely with pneumonitis as well. Pneumonitis was usually of hypersensitive (eosinophilic) origin and occurred with both short- and long-term use. It resolved in all cases after drug discontinuation, whether or not corticosteroids were used, with improvement occurring within 1–3 weeks of discontinuation (19). Rare contact dermatitis and fixed drug eruptions have also been reported. Tetracycline hepatotoxicity, manifested as steatosis caused by inhibition of mitochondrial oxidation of fatty acids in the liver, occurs rarely today due to avoidance of these agents in subjects at high risk (high-dose IV therapy, pregnant females, malnourishment, chronic renal disease) (20). Rare cases of dysosmia and anosmia (all in doxycycline recipients) have been reported.

The tetracyclines have been associated with nephrotoxicity for many years (1,5). One type, associated with the ingestion of outdated tetracycline, results in a

Fanconi-like syndrome, with natriuresis and hypovolemia. This effect reinforces the need to warn patients to take tetracycline therapy to completion and not store a supply for the "next infection." It also supports the need to check the patient's drug supplies and discard any unused tetracycline (prescription labels generally do not include drug expiration dates). A second type of nephrotoxicity is generally manifested by acute renal failure (which may be fatal), metabolic acidosis, hepatorenal syndrome, and severe nausea/vomiting. These agents can worsen preexisting chronic renal failure. The decline in renal function can be irreversible. Risk factors include chronic heart failure, cirrhosis, preexisting renal impairment, dosage too high for the level of renal function, and IV route of administration. This effect can be seen very early in therapy, even with cumulative dosages of only 1–4 g.

The last type of nephrotoxicity is nephrogenic diabetes insipidus, almost exclusively seen with demeclocycline. In fact, this effect is exploited for therapeutic benefit in the treatment of syndrome of inappropriate antidiuretic hormone (SIADH).

Doxycycline does not adversely affect renal function, even in subjects with preexisting renal impairment. All tetracyclines except doxycycline (and perhaps, minocycline) should be avoided in patients with renal insufficiency.

An unusual manifestation of tetracycline intolerance is minocycline vestibulotoxicity, especially in females. In individuals developing this reaction, substitution with tetracycline rarely produces the same result. This syndrome, which appears within 1–2 days after drug initiation, is characterized by nausea, vomiting, weakness, ataxia, anorexia, vertigo, and dizziness (usually in combination). Symptoms are frequently acute and severe. With drug discontinuation, symptoms fully regress (21).

Reactions at the administration site of IV tetracyclines are uncommon (e.g., 6% had induration, swelling, phlebitis, pain, and/or erythema with doxycycline in one large series).

The tetracyclines are well-known phototoxins although the actual risk differs between agents. For example, one placebo-controlled study evaluated the phototoxicity of demeclocycline and methacycline after 7 days of therapy. At the end of the therapy, all subjects went for a 6 hr boat trip in bright sunlight, which resulted in paresthesias and sunburn reactions in 92% and 85% of democlocycline recipients, respectively. In contrast, these reactions occurred in only 6% of placebo and 7% of methacycine recipients (22). Photo-onycholysis has been noted, albeit rarely, with tetracycline and doxycycline.

Tetracyclines are catabolic agents, raising blood urea nitrogen (BUN) especially in the presence of chronic renal impairment. Only doxycycline does not raise BUN. The effect of oxytetracycline and doxycycline on nitrogen balance has been studied in elderly patients maintained on standard total parenteral nutrition. High oxytetracycline doses (0.5–1 g/day IV) led to negative nitrogen balance within 3 days while a lower dose (0.2 g/day IV) had no effect. In contrast, 0.1 g/day of IV doxycycline had no effect on nitrogen balance. In folate-deficient subjects, the antianabolic effect of oxytetracycline was counteracted by folate supplementation (23).

In limited efficacy/tolerability data presented to date, nausea and vomiting have been the major adverse events associated with tigecycline therapy. These events appear to be dose related and can be dose limiting. Administering the drug in the fed state may ameliorate these effects (2).

The most important interacting medications with the tetracycline(s) include antacids, iron, sodium bicarbonate, warfarin, digoxin, phenytoin, carbamazepine, and phenobarbital (24,25).

Divalent and trivalent cations such as calcium, aluminum, magnesium, and iron reduce absorption of the tetracyclines due to the formation of insoluble chelates. The effect of sodium bicarbonate on tetracycline bioavailability is controversial. One study conducted in eight healthy volunteers found that coadministration of sodium bicarbonate 2 g and tetracycline 250 mg (in a capsule formulation from Gyma Labs) resulted in approximately a 50% reduction in tetracycline bioavailability. In contrast, sodium bicarbonate had no significant effect on tetracycline absorption from a solution formulation. However, in another study, 2 g of sodium bicarbonate administered simultaneously with 250 mg tetracycline (in a capsule formulation from Lederle Labs) had no effect on the rate or extent of oral absorption in two volunteers. Perhaps the interaction with sodium bicarbonate is formulation or manufacturer specific.

Metoclopramide, administered orally 15 min prior to tetracycline 500 mg orally, significantly reduced the time to tetracycline peak plasma concentration (from mean $\pm$ SD, 240 ± 34 min to 113 ± 23 min) but had no significant effect on peak plasma concentration (area under the plasma concentration vs. time curve data were unavailable). It would appear that this interaction is of little clinical importance.

Simultaneous administration of zinc sulfate produces different effects on the disposition of different tetracyclines. For example, 200 mg of zinc sulfate (45 mg elemental zinc) given simultaneously with 500 mg of tetracycline reduced serum tetracycline concentrations 2, 4, and 8 hr postdose by 30–40% while area under the serum concentration vs. time curve and 48 hr urinary excretion were reduced approximately 30% compared with tetracycline-only data. In contrast, zinc sulfate coadministration exerted no significant effect on doxycycline diposition.

Although the deleterious effects of multivalent cations on the absorption of the tetracyclines are well known, the opposite effect has seldom been studied, i.e., the effect of the tetracyclines on cation bioavailability. In one study, significant mutual antagonism of absorption was noted for iron (as ferrous sulfate, elemental iron 100 mg) and tetracycline (1 g). Iron absorption fell approximately 50% (from mean $\pm$ SEM, $8.7 \pm 1.4\%$ to $4.4 \pm 1.2\%$ of dose) and tetracycline absorption fell approximately 75% (from 360 ± 37 mg to 91 ± 43 mg excreted in urine over 48 hr postdosing).

Does spacing the administration times of the cation and the tetracycline moderate or eliminate the drug interaction? Unfortunately, the answer is no, at least looking at iron and doxycycline. Even spacing dose administrations by 3 hr did not modify the 20–45% drop in serum doxycycline concentrations induced by iron (as ferrous sulfate, 80 mg elemental iron). It has been hypothesized that iron interferes with the enterohepatic circulation of doxycycline.

Case reports have linked doxycycline use to lithium intoxication and potentiation of warfarin and minocycline and tetracycline use to potentiation of theophylline. In a crossover study involving male patients with chronic obstructive pulmonary disease on maintenance theophylline therapy, the interaction of theophylline and 5 days of oral tetracycline 1 g/day therapy were evaluated. The only significant effects occurred in nonsmokers, wherein steady-state serum theophylline concentrations rose (from mean $\pm$ SD, 9.29 ± 3.04 mg/L to 10.57 ± 3.83 mg/L) and apparent total body clearance fell (from 49.00 ± 11.14 mL/hr/kg to 43.62 ± 10.24 mL/hr/kg) during tetracycline therapy.

Hepatic enzyme inducers such as phenytoin, carbamazepine, phenobarbital, and combinations of these agents appear to accelerate the elimination of doxycycline. Doxycycline terminal disposition half-life falls approximately 50% in recipients of these agents although one study using phenobarbital did not find this. No cases of clinical failure due to accelerated doxycycline metabolism could be found in the literature.

Studies of the interaction of tetracycline and the hepatic enzyme inhibitor cimetidine have yielded conflicting results. In one study, the simultaneous administration of single doses of cimetidine and tetracycline resulted in mean reductions in peak plasma concentration, area under the plasma concentration vs. time curve, and 72 hr urinary excretion of 1.2 mg/L, 40%, and 30%, respectively. In contrast, multiple-dose cimetidine exerted no significant effect on tetracycline disposition. In the second study, 3 days of cimetidine pretreatment reduced tetracycline bioavailability by a mean of 30% (from the capsule formulation only, not the solution formulation). In the third study, simultaneous administration of single doses of cimetidine and tetracycline resulted in no significant alteration in tetracycline pharmacokinetics.

Tigecycline does not affect metabolism mediated by cytochome P450 isozyme 1A2, 2C8, 2C9, 2C19, 2D6, or 3A4 in vitro. It does not interact with digoxin to a clinically-important degree. However, it does reduce R- and S-warfavin clearance by 40% and 23%, respectively. Patients receiving tigecycline and warfavin concurrently should be followed with PT/INR monitoring.

REFERENCES

1. Anonymous. American Hospital Formulary Service Drug Information. Bethesda, MD: American Society of Health-System Pharmacists, 2003.
2. Guay DRP. Oritavancin and tigecycline: investigational antimicrobials for multidrug-resistant bacteria. Pharmacotherapy 2004; 24:58–68.
3. Chopra I, Roberts MC. Tetracycline antibiotics: mode of action, applications, molecular biology, and epidemiology of bacterial resistance. Microbiol Mol Biol Rev 2001; 65: 232–260.
4. Roberts MC. Tetracycline therapy: an update. Clin Infect Dis 2003; 36:462–467.
5. Anonymous. Drug Facts and Comparisons. St. Louis, MO: Wolters Kluwer.
6. Kramer PA, Chapron DJ, Benson J, Mercik SA. Tetracycline absorption in elderly patients with achlorhydria. Clin Pharmacol Ther 1978; 23:467–472.
7. Aukee S, Venho VM, Jussila J, Karjalainen P. Drug absorption in patients with T-tube after cholecystectomy. Ann Clin Res 1975; 7:42–46.
8. Saivin S, Houin G. Clinical pharmacokinetics of doxycycline and minocycline. Clin Pharmacokinet 1988; 15:355–366.
9. Bocker R, Muhlberg W, Platt D, Estler CJ. Serum level, half-life and apparent volume of distribution of doxycycline in geriatric patients. Eur J Clin Pharmacol 1986; 30:105–108.
10. Vartia KO, Leikola E. Serum levels of antibiotics in young and old subjects following administration of dihydrostreptomycin and tetracycline. J Gerontol 1960; 15:392–394.
11. Yamamoto T, Takano K, Matsuyama N, Koike Y, Minshita S, Sanaka M, Kuyama Y, Yamakana M. Pharmacokinetic characteristics of minocycline in debilitated elderly patients. Am J Ther 1999; 6:157–160.
12. Anonymous. The choice of antibacterial drugs. Med Lett Drugs Ther 2001; 43:69–78.
13. Balter M. Just the berries. Management of community-acquired pneumonia, evidence-based update. Can Fam Phys 2002; 48:1773–1775.
14. Finch RG, Low DE. A critical assessment of published guidelines and other decision-support systems for the antibiotic treatment of community-acquired respiratory tract infections. Clin Microbiol Infect 2002; 8(suppl 2):69–91.
15. Slotwiner-Nie PK, Brandt LJ. Infectious diarrhea in the elderly. Gastroenterol Clin North Am 2001; 30:625–635.

16. Miller KE, Ruiz DE, Graves JC. Update on the prevention and treatment of sexually transmitted diseases. Am Fam Phys 2003; 67:1915–1922.

17. Dereure O. Drug-induced skin pigmentation. Epidemiology, diagnosis and treatment. Am J Clin Dermatol 2001; 2:253–262.

18. Bott S, Prakash C, McCallum RW. Medication-induced esophogeal injury: survey of the literature. Am J Gastroenterol 1987; 82:758–763.

19. Toyoshima M, Sato A, Hayakawa H, Taniguchi M, Imokawa S, Chida K. A clinical study of minocycline-induced pneumonitis. Intern Med 1996; 35:176–179.

20. Carson JL, Strom BL, Duff A, Gupta A, Shaw M, Lundin FE, Das K. Acute liver disease associated with erythromycins, sulfonamides, and tetracyclines. Ann Intern Med 1993; 119:576–583.

21. Williams DN, Laughlin LW, Lee YH. Minocycline: possible vestibular side effects. Lancet 1974; 2:744–746.

22. Frost P, Weinstein GD, Gomez EC. Methacycline and demeclocycline in relation to sunlight. J Am Med Assoc 1971; 216:326–329.

23. Korkeila J. Effect of oxytetracycline, doxycycline, and folic acid on nitrogen balance during parenteral nutrition. Ann Clin Res 1974; 6:25–32.

24. Raasch R. Interactions of oral antibiotics and common chronic medications. Geriatrics 1987; 42(1):69–74.

25. D'Arcy PF, McElroy JC. Drug-antacid interactions: assessment of clinical importance. Drug Intell Clin Pharm 1987; 21:607–617.

26. Pines A, Raafat H, Sreedharan KS, Parker P. A comparison of pivampicillin and tetracycline in exacerbations of chronic bronchitis. Chemotherapy 1974; 20:361–369.

27. Ferguson GC. A comparison of oxytetracycline with doxycycline in the winter chemoprophylaxis of chronic bronchitis. Br J Clin Prac 1974; 28:131–133.

28. Pines A, Raafat H, Greenfield JS, Linsell WD, Solari ME. Antibiotic regimens in moderately ill patients with purelent exacerbations of chronic bronchitis. Br J Dis Chest 1972; 66:107–115.

29. Klastersky J, Coppel R, Rens B, Daneau D. Clinical and bacteriological evaluation of intravenous doxycycline in severe hospital infections. Curr Ther Res 1972; 14:49–60.

30. Agache P, Amblard P, Moulin G, Texier L, Beylot C, Bergoend H. Roxithromycin in skin and soft tissue infections. J Antimicrob Chemother 1987; 20(suppl B):153–156.

31. Maesen FP, Davies BI, van Noord JA. Doxycycline in respiratory infections: a reassessment after 17 years. J Antimicrob Chemother 1986; 18:531–536.

32. Renmarker K. A comparative trial of co-trimoxazole and doxycycline in the treatment of acute exacerbation of chronic bronchitis. Scand J Infect Dis 1976; suppl 8:75–78.

33. Klastersky J, Hensgens C, Daneau D. Comparative clinical study of doxycycline and minocycline. Int J Clin Pharmacol Biopharm 1975; 11:19–26.

34. Klastersky J, Daneau D. Comparative study of minocycline and ampicillin in the treatment of urinary tract infections. Int J Clin Pharmacol Ther Toxicol 1974; 9:125–131.

SUGGESTED READING

American Hospital Formulary Service Drug Information. Bethesda, MD: American Society of Health-System Pharmacists, 2003.

Bocker R, Muhlberg W, Platt D, Estler CJ. Serum level, half-life and apparent volume of distribution of doxycycline in geriatric patients. Eur J Clin Pharmacol 1986; 30:105–108.

Guay DRP. Oritavancin and tigecycline: investigational antimicrobials for multidrug-resistant bacteria. Pharmacotherapy 2004; 24:58–68.

16

Macrolides and Ketolides

Charles Huynh and Shobita Rajagopalan
Department of Internal Medicine, Division of Infectious Diseases, Charles R. Drew University of Medicine and Science, Martin Luther King, Jr.–Charles R. Drew Medical Center, Los Angeles, California, U.S.A.

Key Points:

- Macrolide antibiotics (e.g., erythromycin, clarithromycin, and azithromycin) are a widely used class of antimicrobial agents recommended for the treatment of community-acquired pneumonia, genital tract infection, and skin and soft tissue infections, many of which occur in the elderly.
- The newer macrolides clarithromycin and azithromycin are approved by the Food and Drug Administration for the prophylaxis and treatment of *Mycobacterium avium* complex infections.
- As a class, these bacteriostatic antibiotics have the ability to inhibit the growth of gram-positive, gram-negative, and anaerobic bacteria and are the drugs of choice for the "atypical" pneumonia species of *Mycoplasma*, *Chlamydia*, and *Legionella*.
- Common side effects of macrolides include nausea, vomiting, abdominal cramps, indigestion, and diarrhea. Drug interactions of macrolides with other drugs that are metabolized via the hepatic cytochrome system are of particular importance in the elderly in whom polypharmacy is common.
- Ketolides are a new class of antibiotics with improved activity against activity penicillin-resistant gram-positive organisms as well as activity against some gram-negative, anaerobic, and atypical pathogens.

Respiratory infections are among the leading causes of death in older adults in the United States (1,2). Although *Streptococcus pneumoniae* is the most common cause of pneumonia in the elderly, pneumococcal resistance to antibiotics has been increasing in the geriatric population (3). Consequently, alternative agents are constantly being sought to treat serious infections such as pneumonia.

Macrolide and ketolide antibiotics (Table 1) are some of the most commonly prescribed agents used to treat community-acquired respiratory infections in the United States (4). Not surprisingly, the increasing use of these agents has resulted in antibiotic resistance to common community-acquired pathogens such as *S. pneumoniae* (5). In this chapter, we will review current information on the macrolides as well as the new macrolides subclass known as ketolides as they relate to the aging population.

Table 1 Summary of Important Macrolides and Ketolides

Drug name	Mechanism of action	Antimicrobial activity	Indications	Side effects	Drug–drug interaction
Erythromycin	Inhibition of protein synthesis by binding 50S ribosomal subunits by susceptible organism	Gram-positive bacteria *S. pyogenes* *S. pneumoniae* *Listeria monocytogenes* *C. diphtheriae* *Corynebacterium minutissimum* *Staphylococcus aureus* Gram-negative bacteria *B. pertussis* *N. gonorrheae* Others *Chlamydia trachomatis* *Entamoeba histolytica* *Legonella pneumophilia* *Treponena pallidum* *Ureaplasma urealyticum*	Respiratory infection, pharyngitis, tonsillitis, uncomplicated skin infection, eye infection, and erythrasuma, and CAP	Increased LFT, cholestatic hepatitis, nausea, vomiting, abdominal pain, diarrhea and anorexia	Theophylline Digoxin Ergotamine Dihydroergotamine Triazolam HMG-CoA reductase inhibitor Terfenadine Astemizole Pimozide Cisapride Carbazepine Cyclosporine Tacrolimus Phenytoin Bromocriptine Valproate
Azithromycin	Binding to the 50S ribosomal subunit by susceptible microorganism interfering with microbial protein synthesis	Gram-Positive bacteria *S. aureus* *Streptococcus agalactiae* *S. pneumoniae* *S. pyogenes* *Streptococcus* group C, F, G, and viridans group Gram-negative bacteria *H. Influenzae* *Moraxella catarrhalis* *B. pertussis* *Campylobacter jejuni*	Respiratory infection, COPD, CAP, pharyngitis, tonsillitis uncomplicated skin infection, STD-non-gonococcal urethritis and MAC	Angiodema, anaphylaxis, liver abnormalities, cardic arrhythmia, nausea and vomiting	Efavirenz Theophylline Digoxin Ergotamine Triazolam Carbamazepine Cyclosporine Hexobarbital Phenytoin

| | | *Haemophillus ducreyi*
L. pneumophila
Anaerobic bacteria
Bacteroides bovice
Clostridium perfringens
Peptostreptococcus
Other pathogens
Borrelia burgdorferi
Mycoplasma pneumoniae
T. pallidum
U. urealyticum
MAC | | | |
| Clarithromycin | Binding to the 50S ribosomal subunits of susceptible microorganism resulting inhibits of protein synthesis | Gram-negative bacteria
S. agalactiae
S. aureus
S. pneumoniae
S. pyogenes
S. group C, F, G, and viridans group
Gram-negative bacteria
H. influenzae
M. catarrhalis
B. pertussis
L. pneumophila
Pasteurella multocida
Helicobacter pylori
Anaerobes
Clostridium perfringens
Peptococcus niger
Propionibacterium acnes | Peptic ulcer, pharyngitis, tonsillitis, acute sinusitis, acute bronchitis, uncomplicated skin infection, disseminated MAC, CAP and Ottis media | Abdominal pain, headache, diarrhea, dyspepsia flatulence, nausea, vomiting, rash and taste perversion | Cisapride
Astemizole
Terfenadine
Theophylline
Digoxin |

(Continued)

Table 1 Summary of Important Macrolides and Ketolides (*Continued*)

Drug name	Mechanism of action	Antimicrobial activity	Indications	Side effects	Drug–drug interaction

Clarithromycin (*contd.*)		Prevotella
		Melaninogencia
		Others
		  M. pneumoniae
		  C. pneumoniae
		  MAC			

Telithromycin	Binds two sites of the bacterial 50S and if one site is methylated the other site on the ribosome is still presented by the drug and interrupts protein synthesis	Resistant
		  S. pneumoniae from other macrolide
		Others
		  Mycoplasma, *Chlamydia*
		  Legionella
		Anaerobes
		  Peptostreptococcus
		  Prevotella
		  Actinomycetes
		Gram negative
		  H. influenzae
		  M. catarrhalis
		  N. gonorrheae
		  N. meningitidis
			Respiratory infection and CAP	Nausea, vomiting, blurred vision, abnormal LFT, and cardiac arrhythmia	Drugs that interacts with CYP3A4 and CYP2D6
					Paroxatine
					Digoxin
					Theophylline

Abbreviation: CAP, community-acquired pneumonia; LFT, liver function test; COPD, chronic obstructive pulmonary disease; STD, sexually transmitted disease; HMG, 3-hydroxy-3-methylglutaryl; CoA, coenzyme A.

1. MACROLIDES

Macrolides are primarily bacteriostatic antibiotics that are used to treat infections of the respiratory tract, skin and soft tissues, and the genital tract. This group of antimicrobial agents is structurally diverse; biologically active synthetic derivatives have been developed from chemical and microbiological modifications of the basic structure (6). They include erythromycin, clarithromycin, dirithromycin, azithromycin, and spiramycin. The newer macrolide antibiotics represent a significant advance with respect to increased tissue penetration, generally lower minimum inhibitory concentration (MIC) values, better tolerability, and fewer drug interactions.

1.1. Mechanism of Action

Macrolides inhibit the growth of bacteria by inhibiting protein synthesis at the bacterial 50S units of prokaryotic ribosome. These bacteriostatic agents penetrate extensively into mammalian tissue, especially epithelial lining fluid for treatment of intracellular organisms such as *Chlamydia pneumoniae* and *Legionella* sp. (7). These drugs are extremely useful against pathogens that are considered to be extracellular, such as *S. pneumoniae*, *Haemophilus influenzae*, and *Moraxella catarrhalis* that are responsible for infections in the alveolar space and on mucosal surfaces (7).

1.2. Antimicrobial Spectrum

Macrolides, as a class, inhibit the growth of gram-positive, gram-negative, and anaerobic bacteria and species of *Mycoplasma* (6). The newer macrolides have shown activity against nontuberculosis mycobacteria such as *Mycobacterium avium-intracellulare* complex (MAC). The most common side effects of macrolide antibiotics are gastrointestinal (GI), such as nausea, vomiting, abdominal cramps, indigestion, and diarrhea (7) and are seen mostly with the oral administration; however, it can also occur when administered via parenteral routes (8).

1.3. Clinical Pharmacology

Macrolide antibiotics are divided into three families, according to the size of the aglycone ring, which can be a 12-, 14-, or 16-membered ring (6). Erythromycin is the naturally occurring 14-membered macrolide. Its semisynthetic derivatives include erythromycin ethyl succinate, dirithromycin, clarithromycin, and azithromycin. The 16-membered macrolides, such as spiramycin, are divided into leucomycin- and tylosin-related groups, which differ in the substitution pattern of their aglycones (6).

1.4. Emerging Macrolide Resistance

Increasing antibiotic resistance to macrolides has been demonstrated at an alarming rate among respiratory pathogens in the United States (9), such as *S. pneumoniae* (10). During the period of 1993–1999 the number of macrolide prescriptions increased by 13% from ≈17.7 million prescriptions in 1993 to ≈21.2 million prescriptions in 1999 (5). As expected, increased macrolide resistance to *S. pneumoniae* was demonstrated from 10.6% in 1995 to 20.4% in 1999 (5). *S. pneumoniae* can acquire antibiotic resistance gene either through conjugation and phagocytosis or through gene splicing. An efflux transporter, product of *mef* gene, pumps erythromycin out of the bacterial cell resulting in a low-level resistance associated with MICs of 1–8 µg/mL. A second mechanism for macrolide resistance results from methylation of the erythromycin binding sites on the 23S ribosomal RNA of the 50S ribosomal subunit by methylase enzyme, the product of the *erm* gene. The latter mechanism results in a high-level resistance characterized by MICs >16 µg/mL (11). Most macrolide resistance of *S. pneumoniae* in the United States is associated with low-level mechanisms (11).

1.5. Drug Interactions

Because the elderly patients are prescribed many drugs, another problem with macrolide usage in the elderly is its potential interaction with other drugs that are substrates or inhibitors of the CYP3A4 enzymes system (12). Azithromycin and dirithromycin are the exception, because they are not metabolized by the CYP3A4 system. Serious and potentially fatal drug interactions can occur when these CYP3A4 inhibitors, erythromycin and clarithromycin, are combined with substrates of the P4503A4 enzyme system caused by the accumulation of increased plasma levels of the substrate (12). Life-threatening drug interactions have been described with concomitant use of astemizole, cisapride, clozapine, disopyramide, ergotamine, quinidine, and terfenadine (13,14). In addition, close monitoring of possible drug interactions are necessary when macrolides are used in conjunction with drugs such as alprazolam, atorvastatin, buspirone, carbamazepine, cyclosporine, digoxin, lovastatin, methylprednisolone, phenytoin, ritonavir, tacrolimus, theophylline, triazolam, valproic acid, warfarin, and zafirlukast (13–16).

In one study 21,273 drug interactions with erythromycin and clarithromycin were documented among the long-term care Medicaid facility residents in Maryland. In this study, erythromycin was associated with 2.8% of the drug interactions while clarithromycin was associated with 7.4% (12). The combination of erythromycin or clarithromycin with cisapride has been associated with QT interval prolongation on electrocardiogram in 5.0% and 6.3% of patients, respectively (12). Concomitant use of macrolides with digoxin, phenytoin, warfarin, carbamazepine, theophylline, and buspirone—commonly prescribed agents in the elderly—require careful monitoring of levels and observation for evidence of drug toxicity (12).

2. ERYTHROMYCIN

The first macrolide, erythromycin, was isolated in 1952 from a strain of *Streptomyces erythreus* found in the Philippine islands (17). It consists of a 14-membered macrocyclic lactone ring attached to two sugar moieties, desosamine and cladonose (18). Erythromycin is very poorly soluble in water; it is poorly absorbed from the GI tract and is rapidly inactivated by gastric acid. Thus, it is generally recommended with meals (17,18).

2.1. Mechanism of Action

Erythromycin inhibits RNA-dependent protein synthesis from the 50S ribosomal subunit at the step of chain elongation, resulting in the blockage of the transpeptidation and/or translocation reaction within the cell (18).

2.2. Antimicrobial Spectrum

Erythromycin's antimicrobial activity is primarily against gram-positive bacteria and limited number gram-negative bacteria (*H. influenzae*, *Legionella* spp., and *Moraxella* sp.), as well as *Actinomycetes*, mycobacteria, treponemes, mycoplasmas, *Chlamydia*, and rickettsiae (17,18). In the United States, erythromycin had been previously active against the vast majority of pneumococcal and group A streptococcal isolates; however, clinically resistant strains have been steadily increasing worldwide. A study conducted in Spain evaluating resistance of *S. pneumoniae* to erythromycin showed an increase in resistance from 7.6% in 1988 to 15.2% in 1992 (19). In the United States from 1995 to 1998, 10–15% resistance of *S. pneumoniae* to erythromycin has been reported (20).

2.3. Clinical Pharmacology

Erythromycin is a weak base (pK_a 8.8), which makes it vulnerable to destruction by gastric acid, resulting in inconsistent absorption after oral administration (17,18). Hence, several oral preparations have been developed with acid-resistant coating or in esterified forms, with the intent to achieve a delay in dissolution, until it reaches the small bowel for complete absorption (18). In mild to moderate infection, the differences between various oral preparations are not clinically significant (18). A peak serum level of 0.1–1.9 µg/mL is obtained 3–4 hr after single oral dose and a level of 3–10 µg/mL can be achieved 1 hr after a single intravenous (IV) dose (17,18). Erythromycin is 60% protein bound; 45% from an oral dose and 15% from an IV dose are recoverable in the urine and elimination is mainly biliary excretion (17). Some of the drug may be inactivated in the liver by demethylation. The half-life of erythromycin is 1.5 hr (17,18). Little to no data are available on the impact of old age on the pharmacology of erythromycin.

2.4. Clinical Indications

Erythromycin can be used as an alternative drug in documented penicillin- and tetracycline-allergic patients for the treatment of upper respiratory tract, skin and soft tissue, or urinary tract infections caused by susceptible pathogens (17,18). Although erythromycin continued to be used in community-acquired respiratory infections, its use as monotherapy has declined due to the emergence of resistant pneumococci (4). However, erythromycin continues to be useful for the treatment of atypical pneumonia due to *Mycoplasma pneumoniae* and *Legionella* spp. and against most *M. catarrhalis*, *Corynebacterium diphtheriae*, and *Bordetella pertussis*. It has been also shown to be successful in the treatment for Bartonella haemangiomatosis and bacillary peliosis of human immunodeficiency virus (HIV)-infected patients (18).

2.5. Drug Monitoring and Adverse Effects

Erythromycin must be used cautiously in the elderly, especially those who have ventricular arrhythmia, which is associated only with IV form (21). Baseline electrocardiograms should be obtained and examined for arrhythmias and prolonged QT interval. Torsade de pointe occurs when it is used in conjunction with antiarrhythmic agents (21,22). The elderly are at increased risk for adverse events such as transient hearing loss, although rare, which is associated with IV form only. Erythromycin is more likely to evoke GI side effects, largely through stimulation of motility. These side effects include abdominal pain, cramps, nausea, vomiting, diarrhea, and flatulence (24). However, taking erythromycin with food can reduce GI discomfort. It can potentially cause spasm in the sphincter of Oddi in some individuals inducing pancreatitis (25). Erythromycin should not be used for patients with hepatic impairment with or without jaundice; thus, baseline liver function tests should be assessed (26). The dosing range for erythromycin in young and older adults is 250–500 mg, four times per day orally, or 15–50 mg/kg/day divided as four times per day intravenously (17).

2.6. Drug Interactions

Erythromycin can interact with many other drugs, usually by interfering with their hepatic metabolism through the cytochrome P450 (CYP-450) enzyme system (27). Such drug interactions are essential to note in the elderly because of the high numbers of drugs prescribed to this population. Erythromycin can increase blood levels of fentanyl, carbamazepine, clozapine, colchicines, cyclosporine, digoxin, ergotamine, midazolam, nadolol, theophylline, triazolam, valproic acid, vinblastine, and warfarin. This can sometimes lead to serious toxicity. Measurement of blood/serum levels of these drugs (if available) may be warranted when erythromycin is prescribed. The combination of erythromycin with astemizole and terfenadine could lead to serious ventricular arrhythmia, and possible death (28). Thus, erythromycin is contraindicated in patients receiving astemizole or terfenadine.

3.   AZITHROMYCIN AND CLARITHROMYCIN

The newer macrolides, clarithromycin and azithromycin, were developed due to a renewed interest in the mid-1970s to improve the antimicrobial spectrum, pharmacokinetics, and tolerability of erythromycin. All of the macrolides are effective for common respiratory tract and skin and soft tissue infections (SSTI). However, these newer macrolides have better oral absorption, longer half-life, fewer GI side effects, and greater antimicrobial spectrum of activity than erythromycin (17).

3.1. Mechanism of Action

Like erythromycin, both azithromycin and clarithromycin bind to the same receptor on the bacterial 50S ribosomal subunit and inhibit RNA-dependent protein synthesis by the same mechanism (17).

3.2. Antimicrobial Spectrum

Azithromycin and clarithromycin are bacteriostatic, but has bactericidal activity in vitro against *Streptococcus pyogenes*, *S. pneumoniae*, and *H. influenzae* (17). Azithromycin is more active against gram-negative bacteria (*M. catarrhalis* and *H. influenzae*) and it has two- to fourfold higher activity against gram-positive organisms than erythromycin (17). Azithromycin has been used successfully to treat toxoplasmosis in HIV-infected patients.

Clarithromycin has useful additive activity against *H. influenzae* and *M. catarrhalis*, and it is used primarily to treat respiratory infections, including otitis media and sinusitis. It is effective against infection due to MAC, and it is a part of the *Helicobacter pylori* treatment regimen. It is four times more active against gram-positive bacteria than erythromycin (17).

3.3. Clinical Pharmacology

Azithromycin has a 15-membered basic ring with a methyl-substituted nitrogen at the lactone ring. Clarithromycin, however, has a 14-membered ring structure, with a methyl group on the C6 position of the lactone ring of erythromycin (29). This allows for an increase in the stability of these compounds in gastric acid, thus improving oral absorption. Clarithromycin is highly stable in the presence of gastric acid, and undergoes partial hepatic metabolism but is primary excreted in the urine. Although, clarithromycin has a half-life of 5–7 hr, its plasma concentration peaks at 2–4 hr (17). Clarithromycin is well absorbed orally and has ≈50% bioavailability (17). In contrast, azithromycin has ≈37% bioavailability and its plasma concentration peaks at 2–4 hr. It has an extremely long half-life of 68 hr, which makes it possible to be dosed once daily. Food decreases azithromycin's absorption by 50%; therefore, it is must taken 1 hr before or 2 hr after meals. It is metabolized in the liver and excreted in the feces and urine (17).

3.4. Clinical Indications

Azithromycin and clarithromycin are indicated for respiratory tract infection including sinusitis and community-acquired pneumonia, skin infections, and genitourinary infections (30). Emerging pneumococcal resistance to these newer macrolides has been documented; however, they remain highly effective in the management of atypical pneumonia caused by species of *Mycoplasma*, *Chlamydia*, and *Legionella* (17). The usual dose of azithromycin is 500 mg intravenously or orally per day for 3 days (or 500 mg on day 1 and 250 mg on days 2–5), and for clarithromycin 250–500 mg twice a day. Azithromycin's long half-life requires a shorter duration of therapy as the drug is protein-bound and is released over time. The extended release form of clarithromycin can be given 1000 mg once-daily.

3.5. Adverse Effects

Common adverse events include GI symptoms such as diarrhea, nausea, and abdominal pain that rarely require discontinuation of therapy (30). Tinnitus, dizziness, and reversible hearing loss have been reported from patients taking high doses of clarithromycin for MAC. Ventricular tachycardia and "mania" have been reported from anecdotal cases with clarithromycin; reduced clearance of this agent has been documented in patients with renal insufficiency (30).

Due to the differing azalide structure of azithromycin, there is no induction or binding or inactivation of the CYP-450 enzymes (17,30). Clarithromycin, like erythromycin, has been associated with increased concentrations of several drugs that undergo hepatic metabolism by the CYP3A. Clarithromycin may increase the serum concentration of digoxin, while phenytoin, carbamazepine, and rifampin may decrease clarithromycin serum and tissue drug concentration (30). However, the most potent CYP-450 inhibitor is still erythromycin.

4. DIRITHROMYCIN

Dirithromycin became available in the United States in 1995, and it is a synthetic 14-membered macrolide antibiotic. It has an amino group instead of the carbonyl group at the C9 position of the lactone ring (17).

4.1. Mechanism of Activity

Dirithromycin shares the same mechanism of action with the other macrolides. It blocks protein synthesis by binding to the 23S component of the 50S subunit of prokaryotic ribosomes.

4.2. Antimicrobial Spectrum

Its antimicrobial activity is four- to eightfold lower than that of azithromycin and clarithromycin against *S. pneumoniae, H. influenzae,* and *M. catarrhalis* (31,32).

4.3. Clinical Pharmacology

Dirithromycin plasma concentration peaks at 4–5 hr after an oral dose and displays about 10% oral bioavailability (31). It is eliminated via the bile and feces, and has a half-life of 30–44 hr. The bioavailability of dirithromycin is poor, between 6% and 14%, when taken with food or within 1 hr of having a meal (17). The impact of age on the pharmacology of this drug is unknown.

4.4. Clinical Indications

Besides treatment of community-acquired pneumonia, dirithromycin is effective in acute exacerbation of bronchitis, streptococcal pharyngitis, and SSTI (33).

4.5. Adverse Events

The most common side effects of the drug are GI symptoms such as nausea, vomiting, and abdominal pain (17).

The advantage of this drug is its superiority in terms of safety, as compared with select subgroups of the patients taking drugs that would interact with clarithromycin and those with renal impairment and hepatic dysfunction (34,35). Dirithromycin is not widely used due to the low level of antimicrobial activity in vitro (17). The drug is usually given at a dose of 500 mg/day.

5. SPIRAMYCIN

Spiramycin is a 17-membered ring structure and only available in oral form. It has no advantage over the other macrolides other than in treating toxoplasmosis during pregnancy. This drug has shown, although rarely, to cause QT interval prolongation in neonates. It is not available in the United States (36).

5.1. Clinical Indications

Spiramycin is indicated for the treatment of the respiratory tract infections, buccal cavity infections, and SSTI. Previously, when newer agents were unavailable for the treatment of *Neisseria gonorrheae*, it served as an alternative for the treatment of gonorrhea in patients allergic to penicillin (36).

5.2. Adverse Events

Similar to the other macrolides, spiramycin shares the common GI side effects such as nausea, vomiting, and diarrhea, as well as occasional increase in liver enzymes (36).

Spiramycin is a substrate of CYP3A4, and therefore can interact with other drugs that share the same pathway as mentioned earlier with erythromycin and clarithromycin (36).

6. KETOLIDES

Increasingly reported pneumococcal resistance to penicillin (26%) and erythromycin (35%) in recent years (37) has led to the development and approval of a new subclass of macrolide antibiotics known as ketolides for clinical use. The ketolide, telithromycin, shares a 14-membered lactose ring structure like erythromycin with the exception of the replacement of the cladonose sugar by a ketone and substitution of a carbamate derivative at C11–12 (38). These modifications enhance the potency against gram-positive bacteria, which are noted to be resistant to other macrolides. This drug has been specifically designed to treat community-acquired respiratory tract infections (38).

6.1. Mechanism of Action

Ketolides bind two sites of the bacterial 50S and if one site is methylated, the other site on the ribosome is still presented by the telithromycin and interrupts protein synthesis (42).

6.2. Antimicrobial Spectrum

The drug is active against common gram-positive organisms in vitro and potent against erythromycin-sensitive and -resistant *S. pneumoniae* (42,43). Recent data showed that of 169 erythromycin-sensitive isolates of *S. pneumoniae*, telithromycin MIC of 0.06 µg/mL, azithromycin MIC of 0.125 µg/mL, and clarithromycin MIC of 0.25 µg/mL were demonstrated (43,44). Telithromycin also has excellent activity against atypical pneumonia pathogens such as *Mycoplasma*, *Chlamydia*, and *Legionella* as well as anaerobic bacteria, e.g., *Peptostreptococcus* sp., *Prevotella* sp., and *Actinomycetes* (37). In addition, this agent has antimicrobial activity against gram-negative bacteria such as *H. influenzae*, *M. catarrhalis*, *N. gonorhoeae*, and *N. meningitidis* (37).

6.3. Clinical Pharmacology

Telithromycin is given as a single 800 mg dose that can be taken without food, and it has a half-life of 7–11 hr. It has 57% absolute bioavailability, and it is eliminated mainly in the feces (38). There are numerous studies reporting on the ability of ketolides to penetrate into respiratory tract tissues and fluids making it an effective treatment of respiratory tract infections. One study demonstrated that a single 800 mg dose of telithromycin rapidly penetrated bronchopulmonary epithelial lining fluid and bronchial mucosa; this far exceeded the MIC of common respiratory pathogens for 12–24 hr after dosing (39). In a pooled analysis, clinical trials of telithromycin in the treatment of community-acquired pneumonia revealed excellent clinical cure rates for patients with documented infection by *C. pneumoniae* and *L. pneumophila* (40). The advantage of this drug is that it required no dosage adjustment or supplemental dosing in patients with renal or hepatic impairment (38). A study of 12 elderly patients showed an increased maximum concentration for areas under the curve and was well tolerated among the patients. No dose adjustment has been found to be necessary for elderly patients (41). Two-thirds of telithromycin undergo hepatic metabolism and 76% of the drug is eliminated mainly in the feces (38). After absorption, 57% of telithromycin remains unchanged in plasma with complete elimination of the drug within 72 hr.

6.4. Clinical Indications

Telithromycin was introduced as a new class of ketolides for the treatment of respiratory pathogens resistant to other macrolides (37). In a study of 240 low-risk nonhospitalized patients with radiological and clinical signs of community-acquired pneumonia treated with oral telithromycin 800 mg/day for a median of 10 doses (45), 18 (85.7%) of 21 patients aged 65 years and older demonstrated cure. Another study conducted evaluating the efficacy of telithromycin once daily for 5 days for the treatment of acute exacerbation of chronic bronchitis in older individuals demonstrated clinical cure rates of 78–86% (46).

6.5. Adverse Events

Gastrointestinal symptoms such as diarrhea and nausea are more common with telithromycin compared with clarithromycin and azithromycin in clinical trials (37). Pooled data from phase III studies (2045 patients) showed a 4% frequency of diarrhea and 9% for nausea; blurred vision was also frequently reported with telithromycin (47). Other adverse effects include elevated liver enzymes (46) and prolongation of the QT interval (48).

In vitro, telithromycin is a competitive inhibitor of CYP3A4 and CYP2D6 (47). Telithromycin concentrations may increase with concomitant administration of CYP3A4 inhibitors and has the potential to increase the concentration of other drugs metabolized by CYP3A4. Paroxatine, digoxin, and theophylline levels must be closely monitored in all patients, particularly the elderly, when concomitantly administered with telithromycin (47).

REFERENCES

1. Marie TJ. Community-acquired pneumonia in the elderly. Clin Infect Dis 2000; 31: 1066–1078.
2. Mylotte JM. Pneumonia and bronchitis. In: Yoshikawa TT, Ouslander JG, eds. Infection Management for Geriatrics in Long-Term Care Facilities. New York: Marcel Dekker, Inc., 2002:223–243.
3. Yoshikawa TT. Antimicrobial resistance and aging: beginning of the end of the antibiotic era? J Am Geriatr Soc 2002; 50:S226–S229

4. Heffelfinger JD, Dowell SF, Jorgensen JH, Klugman KP, Musher DM, Plouffe JF, Rakowsky A, Schuchat A, Whitney CG. Management of Community-acquired pneumonia in the era of pneumococcal resistance: a report from the drug-resistant *Streptococcus pneumoniae* therapeutic working group. Arch Intern Med 2000; 160:1399–1408.

5. Hyde TB, Gay KV, Stephens DS, Vugia DJ, Barret NL, Schaffner W, Johnson S, Cielat PR, Maupin PS, Zell ER, Jorgensen JH, Facklaus RR, Whitney CG. Macrolide resistance among invasive *Streptococcus pneumoniae* isolates. J Am Med Assoc 2001; 268:1857–1862.

6. Kirk H, Eli Lilly and Company. Abstract: Antibiotics, Macrolides (on-line). Kirk-Othmer Encyclopedia of Chemical Technology. DOI: 10.1002/0471238961.1301031811091819.a01. pub2.

7. File TM Jr. From macrolides to ketolides: innovative solution to resistant respiratory pathogens. Vol. 1, No. 2. www.ket-on-line.com.

8. Canterbury DHB. Macrolide antibiotics. Drug Information Service. Oct 2002, No. 63.

9. Marston BJ, Plouffe JF, File TM Jr, Hackman BA, Saltrom SJ, Lipman HB, Kolczak MS, Brieman RF. Incidence of community-acquired-pneumonia required hospitalization: result of a population-based active surveillance study in Ohio. Arch Intern Med 1977; 157:1709–1718.

10. Doern GV, Plallers MA, Kugler VK, Freeman J, Jones RN. Prevalence of antimicrobial resistance among respiratory isolates of *Streptococcus pneumoniae* in North America: 1997 results from the SENTRY Antimicrobial Surveillance Program. Clin Infect Dis 1998; 27:764–770.

11. Dever LL, Yassin HM. Telithromycin: a new ketolide antimicrobial for treatment of respiratory tract infection. Expert Opin Investig Drugs 2001; 10:353–367.

12. Ammerman DK, Zukerman JH, Hsu VD. Drug interactions with erythromycin and clarithromycin among Maryland medical long-term care facility residents. Am Soc Consult Pharmacist Res Rep 2000; 15:67–73.

13. Mc Evoy GK, ed. American Hospital Formulary Service. Drug Information. Bethesda, MD: American Society of Health-System Pharmacists, 1998.

14. Hansten PD, Horn JR. Drug Interactions Monograph. Vancouver, BC: Applied Therapeutic, Inc., 1996.

15. Kastrup EK. Drug Facts and Comparisons. St Louis, MO: Facts and Comparisons, 1997.

16. U.S. Pharmacopial Convention. Drug Information for the Health Care Professional. Vol. 1. 18th ed. Rockville, MD: USP Convention, Inc., 1998.

17. Stegbigel NH. Macrolides and clindamycin. In: Mandell GL, Bennett JE, Dolin R, eds. Principle and Practice of Infectious Diseases. 5th ed. Philadelphia, PA: Churchill Livingstone, 2000:366–382.

18. Modolfi AA. Erythromycin. Clinical Toxicology Review, Massachusetts Poison Control System, Jun 1995. Vol. 17, No. 9. www.maripoisoncenter.com/ctr/950erythromycin.html.

19. Maruyama S, Yoshioka H, Fujita K, Takimoto M, Satake Y. Sensitivity of group A streptococci to antibiotics. Am J Dis Child 1979; 133:1143–1145.

20. Istre GR, Welch DF, Moyer N, Marks MI. Susceptibility of group A streptococci isolates to penicillin and erythromycin. Antimicrob Agents Chemother 1981; 20:244–246.

21. Gouyon JB, Benoit A, Betremieux P, Sandre D, Sgro C, Baroux F, Beneton C, Badounal J. Cardiac toxicity of intravenous erythromycin lactobronate in pre-term infant. Pediatr Infect Dis J 1994; 13:840–841.

22. Ponsonnaille J, Citron B, Richard A, Troleses JF, Chaperon A, Barrett B, Gras H. Electrophysiological study of pro-arrythogenic effects of erythromycin. Arch Mal Coeur Vaiss 1988; 81:1001–1008.

23. Periti P, Mazzei T, Novelli A, Mini E. Pharmacokinetic drug interaction of macrolides. Clin Pharmacokin 1992; 23:106–131.

24. Seifert CF, Swayney RJ, Bellanger-McCleery RA. Intravenous erythromycin lactobionate-induced severe nausea and vomiting. Ann Pharmacokinet 1989; 23:40–44.

25. Berger TM, Cook WJ, O'Marcaigh AS, Zimmerman D. Acute pancreatitis in 12 years old girl after erythromycin overdose. Pediatrics 1992; 90:624–626.

26. Gholson CF, Wanner GH. Fulminant hepatic failure associated with intravenous erythromycin lactobionate. Arch Intern Med 1990; 150:215–216.

27. Paris DG, Parente TF, Bruschetta HR, Guzman E, Niarcho AP. Torsade de pointes induced by erythromycin and terfenadine. Am J Emerg Med 1994; 12:636–638.

28. Latare PA, Setness PA. Using erythromycin. Some helpful observations. Postgrad Med 1989; 86:55–59.

29. Bahal N, Nahata MC. The new macrolides. Ann Pharmarcother 1992; 26:46–55.

30. Zithromax. www.inhousepharmacy.co.uk/infections/zithromax-information.html.

31. Bryskier A, Butzler JP. Macrolides. In: O'Grady F, Lambert HP, eds. Antibiotic and Chemotherapy: Infective Agents and Their Use in Therapy. 7th ed. Philadelphia, PA: Churchill Livingston, 1997:377–393.

32. Stout JE, Arnold B, Yu VL. Activity of azithromycin, clarithromycin, roxithromycin, dirithromycin, quinupristin/dalfopristin, and erythromycin against Legionella species by intracellular susceptibility testing in HL-60 cells. J Antimicrob Chemother 1998; 41: 289–291.

33. Jacobson K. Clinical efficacy of dirithromycin in pneumonia. J Antimicrob Chemother 1993; 32(suppl C):121–129.

34. Dirithromycin. Med Lett Drugs Ther 1995; 37:109–110.

35. Watkins VS, Polk RE, Stotka JL. Drug interactions of macrolide: emphasis on dithromycin. Ann Pharmacother 1997; 31:349–356.

36. Macrolide. www.dml.co.nz/aguide/Chapter_8_Macrolides.htm.

37. Doern GV, Heilmann KP, Huynh HK, Rhomberg PR, Coffman SL, Brueggemann AB. Antimicrobial resistance among clinical isolates of Streptococcus pneumoniae in the United States during 1999–2000, include comparison of resistance rates since 1994–1995. Antimicrob Agents Chemother 2001; 45:1721–1729.

38. Bearden DT, Neuhausser MM, Garey KW. Telithromycin: an oral ketolide for respiratory infections. Pharmacotherapy 2001; 20:1204–1222.

39. Andrew J, Honeybourne D, Khair O. Penetration of telithromycin into bronchial mucosal, epithelia lining fluid, and alveolar macrophage following multiple oral doses (abstract and poster) In: Program and Abstracts of the 40th Annual ICCAC. Washington, DC: American Society for Microbiology, 2000:20.

40. Harding I, Simpson L. Fluroquinolones: is there a different mechanism of action and resistance against Streptococcus pneumonia? J Chemother 2000; 12(suppl 4):7–15.

41. Sultan E, Lenfant B, Namour F, Mauriac C, Scholtz HE. Pharmacokinetic profile of telithromycin 800 mg once daily in elderly volunteers. Presented at the 5th International Conference on Macrolides, Azalides, Streptogramins, Ketolides, and Oxazolidinones. Seville, Spain, Jan 26–28, 2000.

42. Ackerman G, Rodloff AC. Drugs of the 21st Century: telithromycin—the first ketolide. J Antimicrob Chemother 2003; 51:497–511.

43. Okamoto H, Miyazaki, Tateda K, Ishii Y, Yamaguchi K. Comparative in vitro activity of telithromycin, three macrolides, amoxicillin, cefdinir, and levofloxacin against gram-positive clinical isolates in Japan. J Antimicrob Chemother 2000; 46:797–802.

44. Reinert R, Lutticken R, Bryskier A. In vitro activities of the new ketolide antibiotic HMR 3004 and HMR 3647 against Streptococcus pneumoniae in Germany. Antimicrob Agents Chemother 1998; 42:1059–1061.

45. Carbon C, Moola S, Velancsics I. Telithromycin, a new once-daily ketolide antimicrobial, provides effective treatment of community-acquired pneumonia (abstract and poster). In: Program and Abstract of the 40th ICCAC. Washington, DC: American Society for Microbiology, 2000:490. Press Med 2000; 29(2):2042–2043.

46. Aubier M, Aldons P, Leak A. Efficacy and tolerability of a five day course of a new ketolide antimicrobial, telithromycin, for the treatment of acute exacerbations of chronic bronchitis in patients with COPD (abstract and poster). In: Program and Abstract of the 40th ICCAC. Washington, DC: American Society for Microbiology, 2000:489.

47. Aventis Pharmaceutical. Data on file. Collegeville, PA: Aventis, 2001.

SUGGESTED READING

Ackerman G, Rodloff AC. Drugs of the 21st Century: telithromycin—the first ketolide. J Antimicrob Chemother 2003; 51:497–511.

Periti P, Mazzei T, Novelli A, Mini E. Pharmacokinetic drug interaction of macrolides. Clin Pharmacokinet 1992; 23:106–131.

Stegbigel NH. Macrolides and clindamycin. In: Mandell GL, Bennett JE, Dolin R, eds. Principle and Practice of Infectious Diseases. 5th ed. Philadelphia, PA: Churchill Livingstone, 2000:366–382.

Watkins VS, Polk RE, Stotka JL. Drug interactions of macrolide: emphasis on dithromycin. Ann Pharmacother 1997; 31:349–356.

17
Clindamycin

Jack Wu and Anthony W. Chow
Division of Infectious Diseases, Department of Medicine, University of British Columbia and Vancouver Hospital Health Sciences Center, Vancouver, British Columbia, Canada

Key Points:

- Clindamycin is active against a variety of gram-positive and obligate anaerobic bacteria as well as many protozoa including *Pneumocystis carinii* and *Toxoplasma gondii*.
- The drug is available in both oral and intravenous formulations and is well distributed to most tissues and body fluids except for cerebrospinal fluid.
- Clindamycin is indicated for the treatment of skin and soft tissue infections, diabetic foot infections, infected pressure ulcers, osteomyelitis, oral and pleuropulmonary infections, and intra-abdominal infections caused by susceptible pathogens.
- Diarrhea occurs in up to 20% of patients receiving clindamycin, and 0.1%–10% of patients receiving this drug may experience *Clostridium difficile*-associated diarrhea.
- Antianaerobic antibiotics, including clindamycin, appear to increase the risk of colonization or infection with vancomycin-resistant enterococci.

1. INTRODUCTION

Clindamycin is a derivative of lincomycin, first isolated from *Streptomyces lincolnensis* in the soil near Lincoln, NE, in 1962. It has improved antimicrobial activity and gastrointestinal absorption compared to lincomycin. It has excellent antimicrobial activity against facultative gram-positive bacteria and obligate anaerobes, and is used for a variety of infectious diseases caused by these organisms. However, the consumption of clindamycin has declined significantly in the 1980s because of a severe form of colitis known as "clindamycin-associated colitis." More recently, the emergence of increasing resistance to clindamycin among different clinical isolates, particularly *Staphylococcus aureus* and members of the *Bacteroides fragilis* group, may further diminish its clinical usefulness. Nevertheless, clindamycin remains an important antibiotic in the armamentarium for the treatment of several infectious diseases that are common in the elderly patient population.

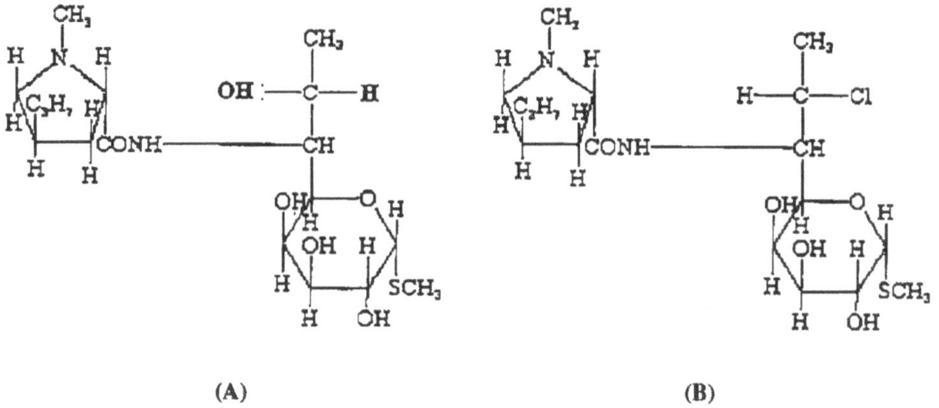

Figure 1 Structure of lincomycin (A) and clindamycin (B).

2. CHEMISTRY AND MECHANISM OF ACTION

Clindamycin, or 7-chloro-7-deoxy-lincomycin, is a lincosamide antibiotic (Fig. 1). Halogenation at the C-7 position in the sugar moiety of lincomycin provides clindamycin with improved antibacterial potency and absorption after oral administration. Its mechanism of action is inhibition of bacterial protein synthesis by binding to the 50S ribosomal subunit, thus interfering with the initiation of peptide chain biosynthesis. Macrolides, streptogramins, and chloramphenicol also act at the same ribosomal binding site, and may compete with clindamycin for the same antimicrobial target. In addition to its antibacterial activity, clindamycin also inhibits exotoxin production by *S. aureus*, group A *Streptococcus* and *Clostridium perfringens*.

3. ANTIMICROBIAL SPECTRUM

Clindamycin has excellent activity against a variety of gram-positive and obligate anaerobic bacteria (Table 1). Most streptococci, including β-hemolytic *Streptococcus* spp. and *Streptococcus pneumoniae*, are susceptible to clindamycin. In a recent study of the antibiotic susceptibility profile among β-hemolytic streptococci collected in the SENTRY Antimicrobial Surveillance Program across North America (1), all Lancefield group C and F *Streptococcus* isolates were uniformly susceptible to clindamycin. Resistance was only rarely detected among Lancefield group A and G isolates (0.8–2.2%), but the rate was higher for group B *Streptococcus* isolates (11.4%). In a nationwide survey of 1531 *S. pneumoniae* isolates, more than 90% were susceptible to clindamycin (2). However, the rate of clindamycin resistance was much higher among penicillin-intermediate and penicillin-resistant *S. pneumoniae* isolates compared to penicillin-susceptible isolates (20.1% and 26.1% vs. 1.5%, respectively). Viridans streptococci are generally susceptible to clindamycin.

Although clindamycin is active against many *S. aureus* strains, a substantial proportion of methicillin-resistant *S. aureus* (MRSA) are resistant to clindamycin. In a recent worldwide surveillance, 63%–88% of MRSA strains were resistant to clindamycin (3). In contrast, the majority (94–98%) of methicillin-sensitive *S. aureus* (MSSA) strains were susceptible to clindamycin (3). Importantly, *S. aureus* isolates that are resistant to erythromycin but appear susceptible to clindamycin may have

Table 1 In Vitro Susceptibility Profile of Clindamycin

Microorganism	Susceptibility
Streptococci	
Group A	+++
Group B	++
Group C	+++
Group F	+++
S. aureus	
Methicillin sensitive	+++
Methicillin resistant	−
Staphylococcus epidermidis	−
Obligate anaerobes	
Peptostreptococcus spp.	+++
Propionibacterium spp.	+++
B. fragilis group	++
Fusobacterium spp.	+++
Porphyromonas spp.	++
Prevotella spp.	++
Eikenella spp.	−

Note: +++, >90% isolates susceptible to clindamycin; ++, 60–90% isolates susceptible to clindamycin; +, 30–59% isolates susceptible to clindamycin; −, <30% isolates susceptible to clindamycin.

inducible resistance to macrolide–lincosamide–streptogramin B (MLSʙ phenotype). This type of resistance is caused by the methylation of an adenine residue of the bacterial 23S ribosomal RNA and is encoded by the *ermB* gene. This resistance phenotype can be selected in vitro by serial subculture of the isolate in the presence of an inducing agent such as erythromycin or clindamycin (4). It may account for the emergence of resistance and treatment failure associated with an apparently clindamycin-susceptible *S. aureus* infection (5). Inducible MLSʙ resistance can be detected in vitro by the double-disk diffusion test (D test) in which the zone of inhibition around the clindamycin disk is distorted in the vicinity of the erythromycin disk (5). Clindamycin has poor activity against enterococci and gram-negative facultative bacteria.

Clindamycin has excellent in vitro activity against both gram-positive and gram-negative obligate anaerobes (Table 1). However, recent susceptibility data have shown increasing resistance to clindamycin among members of the *B. fragilis* group. In a multicenter study of 2673 isolates belonging to the *B. fragilis* group and collected from across the United States during 1997–2000, 23% were resistant to clindamycin (6). Among this group, clindamycin resistance was found in 16% of *B. fragilis*, 29% of *Bacteroides uniformis,* 29% of *Bacteroides thetaiotaomicron*, 30% of *Bacteroides ovatus*, 32% of *Bacteroides distaonis*, and 32% of *Bacteroides vulgatus*. However, all isolates remained susceptible to metronidazole. Clindamycin resistance among members of the *B. fragilis* group is particularly common in hospital-acquired infections. However, other obligate anaerobes such as *Prevotella* spp., *Fusobacterium* spp., *Porphyromonas* spp., and *Peptostreptococcus* spp. remain very susceptible to clindamycin. *Eikenella* spp. is usually resistant while *Clostridium* spp. other than *C. perfringens* is often resistant to clindamycin.

Clindamycin also has activity against many protozoa, including *Plasmodium* spp., *Babesia* spp., *Pneumocystis carinii*, and *Toxoplasma gondii.*

4. CLINICAL PHARMACOLOGY

4.1. Pharmacokinetics

Clindamycin is available for both oral and intravenous administration. The oral preparation is rapidly absorbed from the gastrointestinal tract with approximately 90% bioavailability. The presence of food only slightly delays absorption but does not affect overall bioavailability. The inactive ester forms of clindamycin are rapidly hydrolyzed to the active base after absorption. It is generally well distributed in most tissues and body fluids, except for cerebrospinal fluid (CSF) even in the presence of meningitis. A high bone:serum concentration ratio is achieved, offering an advantage in the treatment of osteomyelitis. Clindamycin is actively concentrated in polymorphonuclear leukocytes, reaching concentrations ~40-fold higher than in the extracellular fluid. It is extensively metabolized in the liver to both active and inactive metabolites that are excreted in the bile. Only a small proportion of clindamycin is excreted in the urine. Dosage reduction may be considered in patients with liver failure, since the half-life of clindamycin is prolonged in such patients. Clindamycin is not removed by hemodialysis or peritoneal dialysis. Generally, the pharmacokinetics of clindamycin is not appreciably altered in elderly patients compared to individuals aged 65 years or younger.

4.2. Pharmacodynamics

Although clindamycin has been used in clinical practice for quite some time, only limited data exist concerning its pharmacodynamic properties. Even though clindamycin is traditionally classified as a bacterostatic agent, it is bactericidal against some organisms such as gram-positive cocci and *Bacteroides* spp. It displays time-dependent killing at concentrations that exceed four times the minimal inhibitory concentration (MIC) and demonstrates a prolonged Post-Antibiotic Effect (PAE) against certain susceptible bacteria. This PAE is dependent on both the concentration and the duration of exposure to clindamycin, and is believed to be due to the persistence of the drug at the ribosomal binding site. At subinhibitory concentrations, clindamycin enhances opsonization of bacteria and their subsequent phagocytosis. Clindamycin has also been shown to inhibit glycocalyx production and bacterial adherence to host cells, In a rabbit model of viridans streptococcal endocarditis, Dall et al. (7) reported that animals receiving clindamycin had smaller vegetations that were sterilized faster than control animals receiving no treatment or penicillin alone. Organisms cultured from clindamycin-treated animals had markedly less glycocalyx formation. Thus, it is believed that clindamycin might lead to improved antimicrobial penetration into infected cardiac vegetations by inhibiting glycocalyx production in vivo (7).

5. CLINICAL INDICATIONS

Elderly patients, especially those residing in long-term care facilities (LTCF), have a substantially increased incidence and severity of many infectious diseases caused by gram-positive cocci or mixed facultative and anaerobic bacteria. The excellence in

Table 2 Clinical Uses of Clindamycin in Elderly Patients

	Preferred therapy	Alternative therapy	Comments
Cellulitis		✓	Penicillinase-resistant penicillin or first-generation cephalosporin is the treatment of choice
Necrotizing fasciitis	✓		Good activity against GAS and anaerobes Antimicrobial activity not affected by "inoculum effect" Inhibits superantigen production Immunomodulating effect Combined with penicillin ± IVIG
Diabetic foot infections and infected pressure ulcers	✓		Activity against GPC and anaerobes Good bone penetration Good bioavailability Combined with other agents for gram-negative coverage
Hematogenous osteomyelitis		✓	Antistaphylococcal penicillin is the treatment of choice of MSSA infections Clindamycin may be suitable for IV–PO sequential therapy
Contiguous osteomyelitis	✓		Good activity against GPC and anaerobes Good bone penetration and bioavailability
Odontogenic and pleuropulmonary infections	✓		Good activity against GPC and oral anaerobes
Intraabdominal infections		✓	Increasing clindamycin resistance among *B. fragilis* group
Prophylaxis for head and neck surgery		✓	First-generation cephalosporin remains the drug-of-choice for surgical prophylaxis
Prophylaxis for infective endocarditis		✓	Amoxicillin is the drug-of-choice for endocarditis prophylaxis

Abbreviation: GAS, group A streptococcus; GPC, gram-positive cocci; IVIG, intravenous immune globulin; IV, intravenous; PO, oral.

vitro activity of clindamycin against these organisms coupled with its favorable tissue penetration and bioavailability following oral administration make clindamycin an attractive antimicrobial agent for the treatment of several common infections in the elderly (Table 2).

5.1. Skin and Soft Tissue Infections

Cellulitis in the elderly is often caused by group A *Streptococcus* (GAS) or *S. aureus*. Most GAS and MSSA isolates are susceptible to clindamycin. Empirical treatment with a penicillinase-resistant penicillin or a first-generation cephalosporin is appropriate. Clindamycin can be used as an alternative for penicillin-allergic patients. However, clindamycin should be avoided in patients infected by MRSA which are frequently associated with high-level clindamycin resistance (4). Failure of clindamycin in patients infected by MRSA strains expressing inducible MLSв resistance has also been reported (5). Thus, vancomycin or linezolid is the treatment of choice for MRSA infections. Daptomycin, a novel lipopeptide, has recently been released for the treatment of complicated skin and soft tissue infections, including GAS and MRSA, but experience in elderly patients is limited (8).

Necrotizing fasciitis is a deep-seated and fulminating infection of subcutaneous tissues, and can be clinically categorized as either type I (caused by mixed, facultative, and anaerobic bacteria) or type II (caused by GAS or other *Streptococcus* spp.). Early and aggressive surgical debridement in combination with appropriate antibiotics is the mainstay of therapy. For type I necrotizing fasciitis, empirical antimicrobial therapy with broad-spectrum agents, such as piperacillin-tazobactam or a carbapenem, is recommended. If clindamycin is used, it should be combined with another agent with gram-negative activity. Type II necrotizing fasciitis is most commonly caused by GAS, but group C and G streptococci have also been reported. Streptococcal pyrogenic exotoxins (SPEs) and M proteins from these organisms are believed to play an important role in the pathogenesis of necrotizing fasciitis and streptococcal toxic shock syndrome (STSS). Management requires aggressive surgical intervention combined with intensive antibiotic treatment. Although GAS continues to be exquisitely susceptible to penicillin, patients with necrotizing fasciitis may respond poorly to penicillin alone. The suboptimal response to penicillin in necrotizing fasciitis associated with GAS has been attributed to the "Inoculum" or "Eagle" effect (9). Penicillin-binding proteins (the primarily target of penicillin) are not expressed well during the stationary phase of growth of GAS. Thus, rapid proliferation of GAS within the infected tissues may allow these organisms to reach the stationary phase of growth when the efficacy of penicillin is diminished due to a slower growth rate. In animal models of streptococcal myositis, Stevens et al. (9) demonstrated that clindamycin was more efficacious than penicillin in achieving improved survival. The enhanced efficacy of clindamycin could be attributed to several reasons. First, the antimicrobial activity of clindamycin is not affected by the inoculum size or the stage of growth of the causative organisms since it acts on target sites (the 50S ribosomal subunit) that are different from penicillin. Second, clindamycin may inhibit the production of exotoxins and M-proteins by GAS in vivo. In an in vitro model that compared the effect of different antibiotics on the growth rate of GAS and release of streptococcal pyrogenic exotoxin A (SPEA), clindamycin alone or combined with penicillin was significantly more effective than penicillin alone in inhibiting the release of SPEA (10). Third, clindamycin has been shown to possess immunomodulating effects by suppressing lipopolysaccharide-induced synthesis of tumor necrosis factor-α by human peripheral blood mononuclear cells (11). For these reasons, the combination of clindamycin plus high-dose penicillin is generally recommended for the treatment of necrotizing fasciitis associated with GAS, with or without STSS (12).

5.2. Diabetic Foot Infection and Infected Pressure Ulcers

Diabetic foot infections can be classified into superficial and limb-threatening. Most superficial infections are caused by gram-positive cocci such as *S. aureus* or streptococci. Outpatient regimens with 2 weeks of oral clindamycin or cephalexin are generally effective. In contrast, severe limb-threatening infections are often polymicrobial, involving both facultative gram-positive and facultative gram-negative bacteria as well as obligate anaerobes. Gram-positive cocci are the most common isolates while *Bacteroides* spp. and *Peptostreptococcus* spp. are the predominant anaerobic isolates. Facultative gram-negative bacteria may also be isolated. As these wounds are always colonized with skin organisms such as *S. epidermidis*, superficial wound swabs should not be used to guide antimicrobial therapy. Specimens obtained from the deep wound during surgical debridement provide a more accurate assessment of the causative organisms. Since limb-threatening infections are frequently associated with chronic osteomyelitis spreading from a contiguous focus, the underlying bone tissue should also be obtained for histopathology and culture if the clinical findings are suggestive of an associated osteomyelitis. Patients with a limb-threatening infection should be admitted to the hospital for intensive and aggressive management as the disease can progress very rapidly. Empirical antibiotics should be administrated immediately after appropriate specimens have been obtained. Antimicrobial therapy without surgical debridement is usually unsuccessful because of poor blood supply to the necrotic tissues. Clindamycin is an effective antibiotic for patients with severe diabetic foot infection, since it has excellent tissue penetration particularly into bone, and provides good coverage of facultative gram-positive bacteria and obligate anaerobes. However, it should be used in combination with another agent, such as a fluoroquinolone or a cephalosporin, for improved gram-negative coverage. Furthermore, prolonged therapy is required if there is underlying osteomyelitis. In one study of 84 hospitalized diabetics with severe lower limb infections, the combination of clindamycin and ciprofloxacin was found to be effective and well tolerated (13). Single agents, such as a β-lactam/β-lactamase-inhibitor or a carbapenem, are also suitable alternatives. Vancomycin or linezolid should be used for MRSA infections.

Similar to diabetic foot infections, infected pressure ulcers are also usually polymicrobial, involving both facultative gram-positive and gram-negative bacteria as well as obligate anaerobes. Contiguous osteomyelitis is also a frequent complication. In contrast to diabetic foot infection, the presence of a nonhealing wound or even exposed bone is not always predictive of underlying bone infection (14). Management of infected pressure ulcers depends on the extent and severity of infection. Superficial infections can be treated locally with wound dressing alone. Patients with clinical sepsis and deep infections, as manifested by the presence of spreading cellulitis or osteomyelitis, should be treated intravenously with broad-spectrum antibiotics, similar to infected diabetic foot infections (14).

5.3. Osteomyelitis

S. aureus is the major causative organism of hematogenous osteomyelitis, while mixed organisms are frequently seen in contiguous osteomyelitis associated with diabetic foot infection and infected pressure ulcers. An antistaphylococcal penicillin (e.g., methicillin or nafcillin) is usually effective for hematogenous osteomyelitis caused by susceptible *S. aureus* isolates (15). Clindamycin is an alternative for penicillin-allergic patients. Clindamycin alone or combined with another antibiotic is recommended in the treatment of contiguous osteomyelitis, such as osteomyelitis of the jaws (15). The role of oral antibiotics in the management of osteomyelitis remains controversial. Although it is common practice to treat acute hematogenous osteomyelitis in children with oral antibiotics after an initial course of intravenous therapy, a full course of intravenous antibiotics (i.e., 4–6 weeks) is generally recommended for adults (15). Clindamycin would be a reasonable drug-of-choice for sequential intravenous–oral therapy for elderly patients with hematogenous or contiguous osteomyelitis.

5.4. Odontogenic and Pleuropulmonary Infections

The organisms associated with odontogenic infections are usually polymicrobial and generally reflect the combined influence of the indigenous oral flora and microhial specificity to dental caries and periodontal disease (16). Streptococcus and obligate anaerobes such as *Peptostreptococcus* spp., *Fusobacterium* spp., *Porphyromonas* spp., *Prevotella* spp., *Veillonella* spp., and *Actinomyces* spp. generally account for more than 95% of odontogenic infections. Penicillin has been the treatment of choice for such infections in the past. However, because of the emergence of β-lactamase production and penicillin resistance among some oral anaerobes, particularly *Bacteroides* spp. and *Prevotella* spp., clindamycin has become the preferred drug of choice (6). Alternative agents, such as a β-lactam/β-lactamase-inhibitor or a carbapenem (such as meropenem), are also appropriate. Metronidazole should not be used alone in treating odontogenic infections as it has poor activity against facultative and microaerophilic streptococci, as well as gram-positive anaerobes in the oral cavity. In immunocompromised patients, such as those undergoing chemotherapy or with neutropenia, it is prudent to administer broad-spectrum agents to cover facultative gram-negative bacilli as well.

Similar to odontogenic infections, the role of penicillin in treating community- or nursing home-acquired aspiration pneumonia has been diminishing because of the emergence of β-lactamase producing oral anaerobes, particularly *Bacteroides* spp. Clindamycin has become a drug-of-choice in treating aspiration pneumonia (17). In a study of 37 adult patients with anaerobic lung infections (27 lung abscesses and 10 necrotizing pneumonias), clindamycin was found to be superior to penicillin (18). A β-lactam/β-lactamase-inhibitor or a carbapenem (such as meropenem) may also be appropriate.

5.5. Intra-abdominal Infections

Mixed anaerobic and facultative gram-negative bacilli are typically found in peritoneal cultures after colonic perforation. Obligate anaerobes, particularly members of the *B. fragilis* group, play a predominant role. Abscess formation is primarily caused by *Bacteroides* spp. Gram-positive organisms can be cultured as well from infections derived from the upper gastrointestinal tract. Antimicrobial therapy of intra-abdominal infections should be directed at both anaerobic and facultative organisms. Historically, clindamycin has been an important antianaerobe agent in the treatment of intra-abdominal infections. However, recent susceptibility surveys have demonstrated substantial resistance to clindamycin among members of the *B. fragilis* group, raising concerns for its empirical use in the treatment of intra-abdominal infections (6). Thus, clindamycin is no longer recommended for the empirical treatment of intra-abdominal infections in which *B. fragilis* is likely to be encountered (19). Combination regimens, such as metronidazole plus either a cephalosporin or a fluoroquinolone, are considered to be appropriate for such infections (19). Monotherapy with a β-lactam/β-lactamase-inhibitor or a carbapenem (such as imipenem or meropenem) has also been shown to be effective (19).

5.6. Prophylaxis for Head and Neck Surgery and Infective Endocarditis

Antibiotic prophylaxis has significantly reduced the rate of postoperative wound infections following major clean–contaminated head and neck surgery. A first-generation cephalosporin is the drug-of-choice for this indication. Clindamycin may be used as an alternative in penicillin-allergic patients.

Elderly patients undergoing dental manipulations may have substantial risk of bacteremia and subsequent seeding to susceptible cardiac valves. Chemoprophylaxis should be provided to patients at risk of bacterial endocarditis. Amoxillin is recommended by the American Heart Association for prophylaxis against bacterial endocarditis. Clindamycin is an alternative agent for patients with a history of penicillin allergy.

5.7. Other Indications

Clindamycin has been shown to be effective, either alone or in combination with other agents, for the treatment of a variety of protozoan infections, including babesiosis, central nervous system toxoplasmosis, pneumocystis carinii pneumonia, and malaria.

6. ADMINISTRATION OF THE DRUG

Clindamycin is available in a number of formulations. Clindamycin hydrochloride is available as capsules with different strengths of 75, 150, and 300 mg, respectively. The usual dosage in adults is 150–600 mg every 6–8 h, depending on the severity of infection. Clindamycin palmite hydrochloride is water soluble and available as an oral suspension for patients who are unable to swallow capsules. Each 5 mL contains the equivalent of 75 mg of clindamycin base. Food does not significantly affect the absorption of clindamycin. The water-soluble ester, clindamycin-2-phosphate, is used for parenteral administration. Each milliliter contains the equivalent of 150 mg of clindamycin. The usual dosage is 20–40 mg/kg/day in three or four divided doses.

There is no formal recommendation for adjusting the dose of clindamycin in patients with hepatic or renal impairment. Patients with liver failure should be closely monitored, and dosage reduction may be considered since the half-life of clindamycin is prolonged in such patients. Clindamycin is not removed by either hemodialysis or peritoneal dialysis.

7. DRUG MONITORING AND ADVERSE EFFECTS

7.1. Clindamycin-Associated Diarrhea

Diarrhea occurs in up to 20% of patients receiving clindamycin. However, the major complication of clindamycin treatment is *Clostridium difficile*-associated diarrhea (CDAD), which is caused by either toxin A or toxin B released by toxigenic strains of *C. difficile* in the gastrointestinal tract. CDAD has been reported to occur in 0.1%–10% of patients receiving clindamycin. Historically, CDAD was also known as "clindamycin colitis" because of its frequent association with clindamycin therapy in the early 1970's. However, CDAD has been associated with numerous other antibiotics, including second- and third-generation cephalosporins, ampicillin, and amoxicillin. Different antibiotics have different propensities to cause CDAD. Based on calculated relative risks among patients receiving different antibiotic regimens, clindamycin and cephalosporins are the most potent causes of CDAD. At present, more cases of CDAD are attributed to β-lactam agents than to clindamycin because of their common usage.

CDAD may begin during or several weeks after discontinuation of clindamycin therapy. It is characterized by the onset of fever, abdominal cramps and frequent diarrhea, often with the passage of blood or mucus in the stool. Some patients may develop toxic megacolon, which carries a very high mortality rate. The diagnosis of CDAD can be made by the presence of pseudomembranes seen at sigmoidoscopy, or by the detection of toxin A or B in the stool using cytotoxicity or immunoassay tests. Culture for the presence of *C. difficile* has a high sensitivity but low specificity for the diagnosis of CDAD, as it cannot distinguish between nontoxigenic and toxigenic *C. difficile* strains. Although in vitro toxin production assays can resolve this issue, most clinical microbiology laboratories are not equipped to perform these tests.

Some patients with CDAD may improve spontaneously after discontinuing the offending antibiotic regimen, but most patients will require specific antimicrobial therapy. Both oral or intravenous metronidazole, and oral vancomycin are equally effective in the treatment of CDAD. Nevertheless, metronidazole is preferable as it is less expensive, and the overuse of vancomycin carries a significant risk for the colonization or infection by vancomycin-resistant enterococcus (VRE), or vancomycin intermediate-resistant staphylococci. Surgical intervention may be considered in cases complicated by toxic megacolon or colonic perforation.

7.2. Vancomycin-Resistant Enterococcus

The prior use of antibiotics including clindamycin, and the presence of a pressure ulcer have been identified as independent risk factors for colonization or infection by vancomycin-resistant enterococcus (VRE) (20). LTCF residents appear to be an important reservoir of VRE. In a recent study, almost half of LTCF residents (14 of 30) were identified by rectal cultures to be colonized with VRE within 72 h after admission (20). In another study of 51 patients colonized with VRE, patients who had received antianaerobe antibiotic regimens, including clindamycin, had a significantly higher density of VRE in their stool specimens compared with those who received minimal antianaerobe antibiotic regimens (21). One possible explanation is that the antibiotics with antianaerobe activity may promote the overgrowth of VRE primarily through the inhibition of normal intestinal anaerobes. Clindamycin may be particularly prone to cause this problem as it has potent antianaerobe activity but minimal effect against other components of the gut flora such as enterococci. Furthermore, clindamycin and its active metabolites are excreted primarily in the bile, leading to prolonged and high-level antimicrobial activity in the gut, causing substantial disturbance of the normal intestinal flora.

7.3. Infection Control Issues

CDAD is the most common cause of nosocomial diarrhea. It is not only endemic in the hospital but also in LTCFs. Direct exposure to healthcare workers or inanimate items, such as commodes, that are contaminated by toxigenic *C. difficile* strains, appear to be an important mode of transmission. Older patients with serious illness, recent abdominal surgery, or gastrointestinal diseases are associated with an increased risk of CDAD. In a prospective study, the incidence of CDAD increased >10-fold among patients in the age range of 60–98 years compared with younger individuals, and was highest in geriatric/rehabilitation wards (22).

Hospital outbreaks of CDAD are not infrequent, and are often caused by a single strain of *C. difficile*. In a study of nosocomial diarrhea caused by a single epidemic strain of *C. difficile* isolated from four hospitals located in different parts of the United States, previous use of clindamycin was found to be a significant risk factor among patients who developed nosocomial diarrhea due to this epidemic strain (odds ratio, 4.35) (23). All of the *C. difficile* isolates were highly resistant to both clindamycin (MIC > 256 μg/mL) and erythromycin. In contrast, only 15% of the nonepidemic strains were resistant to clindamycin, and all other nonepidemic strains were susceptible to both clindamycin and erythromycin. DNA hybridization and polymerase chain reaction analysis demonstrated that all the epidemic isolates harbored the *ermB* gene which encodes a 23S ribosomal RNA methylase that mediates resistance to MLS antibiotics (23). These outbreaks caused by the clindamycin-resistant strain of *C. difficile* were terminated only after removal of clindamycin from the hospital formulary. These findings suggest that the overuse of clindamycin may have dual effects on the development of CDAD: it not only disrupts the normal intestinal flora but may also select for the emergence of clindamycin-resistant strains of *C. difficile*. Thus, infection control measures to reduce the transmission of *C. difficile* from contaminated healthcare workers or inanimate objects and the indiscriminate use of clindamycin as well as other antibiotics are of paramount importance in reducing the incidence of CDAD.

Similar to CDAD, the indiscriminate use of clindamycin may also lead to the selection of VRE within the hospital or LTCF setting. Not surprisingly, patients who are colonized with high-density VRE in the stool are more likely to contaminate the immediate environment than those with low-density colonization (21). This may have a significant impact on infection control measures since the contaminated environment appears to be one of the major routes for the transmission of VRE to other patients. In a recent report, restricting the use of vancomycin and third-generation cephalosporins had little influence on the prevalence of VRE, whereas clindamycin use was significantly correlated with the prevalence of VRE colonization or infection (24), In another study, limiting the use of third-generation cephalosporins, vancomycin as well as clindamycin (because of a concomitant outbreak of CDAD in the same center) decreased the prevalence of fecal VRE colonization rate from 47% to 15% (25).

7.4. Hepatotoxicity

Mild but reversible elevation of hepatic transaminases is frequently seen during clindamycin treatment, particularly in patients receiving intravenous therapy. Severe hepatoxicity, however, has been rarely reported.

7.5. Allergic Reactions

An allergic skin rash has been reported in up to 10% of patients receiving clindamycin therapy. Severe reactions such as the Steven–Johnson syndrome and blood dyscrasias are extremely uncommon.

7.6. Drug Interactions

Concomitant administration of some skeletal muscle relaxants with clindamycin has been reported to cause profound respiratory depression as a result of enhanced neuromuscular blockade. Patients receiving these combinations should be closely monitored and a reduction in the dosage of neuromuscular blocking agents should be considered.

REFERENCES

1. Biedenbach DJ, Stephen JM, Jones RN. Antimicrobial susceptibility profile among beta-haemolytic Streptococcus spp. collected in the SENTRY Antimicrobial Surveillance Program—North America, 2001. Diagn Microbiol Infect Dis 2003; 46(4):291–294.
2. Doern GV, Heilmann KP, Huynh HK, Rhomberg PR, Coffinan SL, Brueggemann AB. Antimicrobial resistance among clinical isolates of Streptococcus pneumoniae in the United States during 1999–2000, including a comparison of resistance rates since 1994–1995. Antimicrob Agents Chemother 2001; 45(6):1721–1729.
3. Diekema DJ, Pfaller MA, Schmitz FJ, Smayevsky J, Bell J, Jones RN, Beach M. Survey of infections due to Staphylococcus species: frequency of occurrence and antimicrobial susceptibility of isolates collected in the United States, Canada, Latin America, Europe, and the Western Pacific region for the SENTRY Antimicrobial Surveillance Program, 1997–1999. Clin Infect Dis 2001; 32(suppl 2):S114–S132.
4. Panagea S, Perry JD, Gould FK. Should clindamycin be used as treatment of patients with infections caused by erythromycin-resistant staphylococci? J Antimicrob Chemother 1999; 44(4):581–582.
5. Siberry GK, Tekle T, Carroll K, Dick J. Failure of clindamycin treatment of methicillin-resistant Staphylococcus aureus expressing inducible clindamycin resistance in vitro. Clin Infect Dis 2003; 37(9):1257–1260.
6. Snydman DR, Jacobus NV, McDermott LA, Ruthazer R, Goldstein E, Finegold S, Harrell L, Hecht DW, Jenkins S, Pierson C, Venezia R, Rihs J, Gorbach SL. National survey on the susceptibility of Bacteroides Fragilis Group: report and analysis of trends for 1997–2000. Clin Infect Dis 2002; 35(suppl 1):S126–S134.
7. Dall L, Keilhofner M, Herndon B, Barnes W, Lane J. Clindamycin effect on glycocalyx production in experimental viridans streptococcal endocarditis. J Infect Dis 1990; 161(6):1221–1224.
8. Daptomycin (Cubicin) for skin and soft tissue infections. Med Lett Drugs Ther 46[1175], 11–12:2004.
9. Stevens DL, Gibbons AE, Bergstrom R, Winn V. The Eagle effect revisited: efficacy of clindamycin, erythromycin, and penicillin in the treatment of streptococcal myositis. J Infect Dis 1988; 158(1):23–28.
10. Coyle EA, Cha R, Rybak MJ. Influences of linezolid, penicillin, and clindamycin, alone and in combination, on streptococcal pyrogenic exotoxin a release. Antimicrob Agents Chemother 2003; 47(5):1752–1755.
11. Stevens DL, Bryant AE, Hackett SP. Antibiotic effects on bacterial viability, toxin production, and host response. Clin Infect Dis 1995; 20(suppl 2):S154–S157.
12. Zimbelman J, Palmer A, Todd J. Improved outcome of clindamycin compared with beta-lactam antibiotic treatment for invasive Streptococcus pyogenes infection. Pediatr Infect Dis J 1999; 18(12):1096–1100.
13. Diamantopoulos EJ, Haritos D, Yfandi G, Grigoriadou M, Margariti G, Paniara O, Raptis SA. Management and outcome of severe diabetic foot infections. Exp Clin Endocrinol Diabetes 1998; 106(4):346–352.

14. Livesley N, Chow AW. Infected pressure ulcers. In: Yoshikawa TT, Ouslander JG, eds. Infection Management for Geriatrics in Long-term Care Facilities. New York: Marcel Dekker, 2002:257–282.
15. Lew DP, Waldvogel FA. Osteomyelitis. N Engl J Med 1997; 336(14):999–1007.
16. Chow AW. Odontogenic infections in the elderly. Infect Dis Clin Pract 1998; 6:587–596.
17. Mandell LA, Bartlett JG, Dowell SF, File TM Jr, Musher DM, Whitney C. Update of practice guidelines for the management of community-acquired pneumonia in immuno-competent adults. Clin Infect Dis 2003; 37(11):1405–1433.
18. Gudiol F, Manresa F, Pallares R, Dorca J, Rufi G, Boada J, Ariza X, Casanova A, Viladrich PF. Clindamycin vs. penicillin for anaerobic lung infections. High rate of peni-cillin failures associated with penicillin-resistant Bacteroides melaninogenicus. Arch Intern Med 1990; 150(12):2525–2529.
19. Solomkin JS, Mazuski JE, Baron EJ, Sawyer RG, Nathens AB, DiPiro JT, Buchman T, Dellinger EP, Jernigan J, Gorbach S, Chow AW, Bartlett J. Guidelines for the selection of anti-infective agents for complicated intra-abdominal infections. Clin Infect Dis 2003; 37(8):997–1005.
20. Elizaga ML, Weinstein RA, Hayden MK. Patients in long-term care facilities: a reservoir for vancomycin-resistant enterococci. Clin Infect Dis 2002; 34(4):441–446.
21. Donskey CJ, Chowdhry TK, Hecker MT, Hoyen CK, Hanrahan JA, Hujer AM, Hutton-Thomas RA, Whalen CC, Bonomo RA, Rice LB. Effect of antibiotic therapy on the density of vancomycin-resistant enterococci in the stool of colonized patients. N Engl J Med 2000; 343(26):1925–1932.
22. Karlstrom O, Fryklund B, Tullus K, Burman LG. A prospective nationwide study of Clostridium difficile-associated diarrhea in Sweden. The Swedish C. difficile Study Group. Clin Infect Dis 1998; 26(1):141–145.
23. Johnson S, Samore MH, Farrow KA, Killgore GE, Tenover FC, Lyras D, Rood JI, DeGirolami P, Baltch AL, Rafferty ME, Pear SM, Gerding DN. Epidemics of diarrhea caused by a clindamycin-resistant strain of Clostridium difficile in four hospitals. N Engl J Med 1999; 341(22):1645–1651.
24. Lautenbach E, LaRosa LA, Marr AM, Nachamkin I, Bilker WB, Fishman NO. Changes in the prevalence of vancomycin-resistant enterococci in response to antimicrobial formulary interventions: impact of progressive restrictions on use of vancomycin and third-generation cephalosporins. Clin Infect Dis 2003; 36(4):440–446.
25. Quale J, Landman D, Saurina G, Atwood E, DiTore V, Patel K. Manipulation of a hospital antimicrobial formulary to control an outbreak of vancomycin-resistant enterococci. Clin Infect Dis 1996; 23(5):1020–1025.

SUGGESTED READING

Chow AW. Infections of the oral cayity, neck and head. In: Mandell GL, Bennett JE, Dolin R, eds. Principles and Practice of Infectious Diseases. New York: Churchill Livingstone, 2000:689–702.
Lamp K, Lacy MK, Freeman C. Metronidazole, Clindamycin, and Streptogramin Pharmaco-dynamics. In: Nightingale CH, Murakawa T, Ambrose PG, eds. Antimicrobial Pharma-codynamics in Theory and Clinical Practice. New York: Marcel Dekker, 2002:221–246.
Lipsky BA. Osteomyelitis of the foot in diabetic patients. Clin Infect Dis 1997; 25(6):1318–1326.
Livesley NJ, Chow AW. Infected pressure ulcers in elderly individuals. Clin Infect Dis 2002; 35(11):1390–1396.

18
Metronidazole in the Elderly

Glenn E. Mathisen
Division of Infectious Diseases, UCLA School of Medicine, Olive View–UCLA Medical Center, Sylmar, California, U.S.A.

Key Points:

- Metronidazole is a nitroimidazole drug with an excellent antimicrobial activity against a wide variety of parasites and obligate anaerobic bacteria.
- The drug is well absorbed, reaches high levels in many tissues, and exhibits bactericidal activity against susceptible organisms; specific dosing adjustments are not required in elderly patients except in those individuals with underlying liver disease.
- Metronidazole has a long half-life ($T_{1/2} = 8$ hr) and exhibits concentration-dependent bacterial killing; these observations suggest that once-daily or twice-daily dosing is effective for most infections.
- Metronidazole—in combination with other antimicrobials—is effective in a wide variety of mixed aerobic–anaerobic infections including intra-abdominal abscess, anaerobic pleuropulmonary infection, diabetic osteomyelitis, and brain abscess.
- Metronidazole is remarkably safe and has few serious adverse effects. Reversible neurological complications (e.g., peripheral neuropathy, encephalitis) may be seen following prolonged, high-dose therapy in selected patients.

1. INTRODUCTION

Originally derived from a natural product excreted by *Streptomyces* species, metronidazole is a nitroimidazole compound with antimicrobial activity against a wide variety of parasites and obligate anaerobic bacteria. A clinical observation that a patient receiving metronidazole for urogenital trichomoniasis experienced an improvement in ulcerative gingivitis suggested that the drug also had antimicrobial activity against anaerobic bacteria. This was confirmed by subsequent studies and metronidazole is now a mainstay in the treatment of infections due to obligate anaerobic bacteria. Geriatric patients have a high incidence of underlying diabetes mellitus, vascular disease, and malignancies; infections associated with these conditions are frequently caused by anaerobes, and metronidazole has come to be widely used in this patient population. In addition to its role in anaerobic bacterial infection, the drug remains an important agent for treatment of parasitic conditions (e.g., trichomoniasis, amebiasis, and giardiasis) and is a key component in antibiotic regimens directed against *Helicobacter pylori*. Metronidazole is well absorbed, reaches high levels in many tissues and exhibits bactericidal activity against susceptible organisms. Although the drug has some recognized toxicities, it is generally quite safe and has become an important drug for management of anaerobic infection in elderly patient populations.

2. CHEMISTRY AND MECHANISM OF ACTION

The nitroimidazole compounds include metronidazole and the related compounds tinidazole and nimorazole. Metronidazole is a small, uncharged molecule whose antimicrobial effect requires activation by bacterial or parasitic enzymes. The chain of events required for drug activity include: (1) uptake of the drug by the bacterial or parasitic cell, (2) reduction of the drug to an active metabolite, (3) interference with cellular elements (DNA, RNA, protein) by short-lived intermediate metabolites, and (4) cellular excretion of inactive end products. Metronidazole enters both aerobic and anaerobic bacteria; however, it has activity only in those organisms possessing anaerobic metabolic pathways able to metabolize it to active end products. This unique feature of the drug accounts for the fact that it has activity against both anaerobic bacteria as well as anaerobic eukaryotes such as *Trichomonas vaginalis* and *Entamoeba histolytica*. Following diffusion into the cell, the nitro side chain of metronidazole is quickly reduced by donation of electrons from ferredoxin-like electron transport proteins (1). This active reduction occurs only in strict anaerobic microorganisms and leads to the formation of short-lived but cytotoxic intermediates including nitroso-free radicals, nitroso- and hydroxylamine derivates. Metronidazole's subsequent mechanism of action is poorly understood; however, it is believed that these cytotoxic intermediates interfere with DNAs of target cells. Subsequent laboratory experiments have shown that reduced metronidazole metabolites interfere with DNA synthesis while unchanged drug does not. The reduced intermediates may attach directly to nucleic acids or cause single-stranded or double-stranded breaks in cellular DNA. Further metabolism of the cytotoxic intermediates of metronidazole leads to the production of acetamide and 2-hydroxyethyl oxamic acid as well as other equally inactive end products.

The mechanism of resistance to metronidazole remains unclear. A decrease in pyruvate:ferredoxin oxidoreductase activity within the cell may lead to decreased activation of the drug and a consequent reduction in the level of active metabolites (2). In addition to altered pyruvate hydrogenase activity, there are two genes—*nim A* and *nim B*—associated with moderate- to high-level metronidazole resistance. These sequences have been found on both chromosome and plasmid elements; however, their function remains unclear and their relation to the pyruvate:ferredoxin oxidoreductase uncertain. Whatever the cause of metronidazole resistance, it is a rare event in clinical practice and surprisingly uncommon considering the widespread use of metronidazole.

3. ANTIMICROBIAL SPECTRUM

Metronidazole exhibits antimicrobial activity against a wide variety of protozoal and bacterial pathogens. Most anaerobic protozoa are susceptible to metronidazole including *T. vaginalis*, *E. histolytica*, *Giardia lamblia*, and *Balantidium coli*. Metronidazole resistance has been reported in *T. vaginalis*, but remains uncommon and can usually be treated with higher and more prolonged dosing (3). Although there are occasional clinical failures, definite metronidazole resistance has not been demonstrated in *E. histolytica* and is rarely a concern for most clinical infections. There is variation in metronidazole sensitivity among isolates of *Giardia* species and this may account for periodic treatment failures seen with the drug (4).

Most commonly encountered obligate anaerobic bacterial pathogens are susceptible to metronidazole (see Table 1). Gram-negative anaerobic bacteria such as *Bacteroides* and *Fusobacterium* species are nearly always sensitive to metronidazole. An early study of *Bacteroides fragilis* susceptibilities exhibited no resistance to metronidazole despite demonstrable antimicrobial resistance to other "anaerobe" agents such as clindamycin (6%) and piperacillin (12%) (5). Recent nationwide studies confirm these findings—metronidazole resistance among *B. fragilis* remains quite uncommon despite widespread use of the drug for the past 20 years (6). Although there are rare reports of resistance to metronidazole among clinical isolates *B. fragilis*, the clinical significance remains uncertain; most of these cases had received prolonged treatment with the drug and the positive cultures may represent colonization rather than active infection (2).

Most obligate gram-positive anaerobic bacteria are also susceptible to metronidazole. These include organisms such as *Peptococcus*, *Peptostreptococcus*, and *Eubacterium* species as well as more common pathogens such as *Clostridium perfringens* and *Clostridium difficile*. Metronidazole resistance is more common among aerotolerant gram-positive anaerobes such as *Proprionibacterium*, *Actinomyces*, and *Lactobacillus* species. In light of these findings, sole use of metronidazole in patients with mixed aerobic–anaerobic infection should be avoided. In this situation,

Table 1 Activity of Metronidazole Against Anaerobic and Microaerophilic Bacteria

Bacteria	No. of strains	Cumulative % susceptible to indicated concentration (μg/mL)			
		4	8	16	32
Bacteroides fragilis[a]	161	90	99	100	—
Prevotella melaninogenica[b]	60	98	100	—	—
Other *Bacteroides* and *Selenomonas* species	154	95	98	100	—
Fusobacterium species	65	199	—	—	—
Anaerobic gram-negative cocci	24	92	96	100	—
Anaerobic gram-positive cocci	124	98	—	—	—
Clostridium perfringens	18	94	100	—	—
Other *Clostridium* species	73	97	99	—	100
Gram-positive nonsporulating bacteria	87	57	60	62	66
Capnocytophaga species	27	52	70	93	—

[a] Includes all species of the *B. fragilis* group.
[b] Includes *P. melaninogenica* (formerly *Bacteroides melaninogenicus*) and *Porphyromonas asaccharolytica* (formerly *Bacteroides asaccharolyticus*).
Source: Modified from Sutter VL. In vitro susceptibility of anaerobic and microaerophilic bacteria to metronidazole and its hydroxy metabolite. In: Finegold SM, George WL, Rolfe RD, eds. Proceedings of the First United States Metronidazole Conference, Tarpon Springs, FL, February 1982. New York: Biomedical Information, 1982:61.

combination therapy (e.g., β-lactam agent + metronidazole) would provide broad coverage for all anaerobes and microaerophilic streptococci that are likely to be present.

4. CLINICAL PHARMACOLOGY

Metronidazole may be administered orally, intravenously, or by rectal suppository; each of these routes appears to be equally efficacious in delivering therapeutic serum concentrations of the drug. Peak serum concentrations (C_{max}) of between 8 and 13 μg/mL are reached within 1–4 hr following oral administration of the drug (500 mg) and similar levels are seen following intravenous (IV) dosing (500 mg). High serum levels (40–50 μg/mL) are achieved following single IV doses of 1500 mg; trough levels measured at 24 hr postdose easily surpass the minimum inhibitory concentrations (MICs) for most susceptible obligate anaerobic bacteria. Metronidazole has a bioavailability of over 90% and absorption does not appear to be altered by food. Although gut motility per se may not affect metronidazole metabolism, some studies have shown higher serum concentrations of the drug in patients with ileostomies and intestinal diseases such as Crohn's disease. One trial demonstrated an increased area under the curve in patients receiving oral therapy after gastrointestinal (GI) surgery (7). GI motility disorders are common in elderly patients; these studies suggest that adequate absorption is likely in this population and standard dosing should lead to appropriate serum levels.

Pharmacokinetic studies reveal that the drug has relatively low serum protein binding (28%) and a corresponding large volume of distribution (≈80% of body weight) as well as an excellent penetration into many tissue/body compartments. Studies demonstrate metronidazole concentrations equivalent to serum levels in polymorphonuclear leucocytes, placenta, pelvic tissue, peritoneal fluid, pancreas, colorectal tissue, and bone. The drug's penetration into central nervous system (CNS) tissue/cerebrospinal fluid is also excellent—brain/CSF levels are equivalent to serum levels and support metronidazole's role as a first-line agent in the management of serious anaerobic CNS infections such as brain abscess.

Metronidazole has two principal routes of metabolism including oxidation by hepatic enzymes and urinary excretion of the parent drug and metabolites. It is metabolized in the liver via oxidation to its primary metabolites, the biologically active hydroxy-metabolite (1-2-hydroxyethyl-2-hydroxymethyl-5-nitroimidazole) and the biologically inactive acid metabolite (1-acetic acid-2-methyl-5-nitroimidazole). Both are subsequently excreted in the urine along with any unaltered drug that may have circumvented hepatic metabolism (≈5–10% of drug is excreted via the bilary tract). Most studies show a drug half-life ($t_{1/2}$) of ≈8–12 hr; this prolonged half-life is further increased in patients with underlying liver disease and impaired oxidation. Although phase I oxidative drug metabolism may be impaired in the elderly, comparative studies of metronidazole elimination in older and younger populations show no age-related differences except for minor alterations in the accumulation of the hydroxy-metabolite (8).

Hepatic and renal dysfunction is commonly encountered in the elderly population and may necessitate dose adjustments in selected populations. Pharmacokinetic studies in patients with liver disease show a reduction in drug elimination and total body clearance as well as an increase in serum half-life of metronidazole and its metabolites. The Child–Pugh criteria for grading patients with liver failure can predict metronidazole elimination in patients with liver disease (9). In one study, patients with

Child–Pugh class C had a $t_{1/2}$ of 21.5 hr compared with normal control patients with a $t_{1/2}$ of 7.4 hr. Another study of metronidazole in critically ill patients demonstrated prolongation of metronidazole half-life ($t_{1/2}$) in individuals with obstructive liver disease compared to those with predominant hepatocellular dysfunction (10). These studies suggest a reduction in metronidazole dosing in patients with severe liver disease—especially in patients whose liver condition demonstrates a prominent component of obstructive liver disease.

Approximately 70% of metronidazole and its metabolites are normally eliminated via the kidney; patients with renal failure demonstrate decreased clearance of metronidazole metabolites and increased metabolite $t_{1/2}$ when compared with normal controls (11). The pharmacokinetics of the parent compound (metronidazole) appears relatively unchanged during renal failure; the increased concentrations of the metabolites seem to have little adverse consequences and most patients do not require alterations in dosing. There is some disagreement regarding dosing and pharmacokinetics of metronidazole during hemodialysis. In one study of patients undergoing hemodialysis for acute renal failure, no demonstrable accumulation of metronidazole occurred with most studies suggesting that the pharmacokinetics of metronidazole during hemodialysis therapy remains relatively unchanged when compared with normal controls (12). Hemodialysis will remove between 25% and 50% of a given dose depending on the length of dialysis and the type of dialysis membrane used. While the majority of patients on dialysis do not require alteration in dosing, patients receiving dialysis with high-flux membranes may require supplementation in order to maintain adequate serum levels in critically ill patients at an early stage of treatment. The limited studies in metronidazole in patients with continuous or intermittent peritoneal dialysis suggest similar pharmacokinetics when compared with normal populations; at the present time, there are no recommendations for dose alterations in chronic ambulatory peritoneal dialysis patients.

Although there are limited studies on the pharmacodynamics of metronidazole, available data suggest that it is rapidly bactericidal and has characteristics associated with concentration-dependent microbial killing. Studies with *Trichomonas vaginalis* demonstrate in vitro concentration-dependent killing at concentrations ranging up to 10 times the minimal lethal concentration of the organism accompanied by a prolonged (6 hr) postantibiotic effect (13). In a study examining once-daily (1.5 g) IV metronidazole, serum trough levels (24 hr postdose) were consistently above the MIC for the majority of obligate anaerobes seen in clinical infections. Another study of 120 patients with serious intra-abdominal infections (e.g., perforated appendicitis or colorectal infection) demonstrated equivalent clinical outcomes when comparing an every (q) 12 hr (750 mg IV q 12 hr) to a q 8 hr (500 mg IV q 8 hr) regimen. A study of 163 patients with gangrenous or perforated appendicitis showed similar outcomes in patients receiving once-daily therapy (1.5 g IV q 24 hr) vs. thrice-daily (500 mg IV q 8 hr) dosing (14). These observations suggest that once-daily or twice-daily metronidazole dosing is an effective approach for most clinical infections. More frequent dosing (e.g., q 6–8 hr) should be reserved for seriously ill patients or those with difficult-to-treat infections such as brain abscess.

Metronidazole's dependence upon hepatic oxidation may interfere with the metabolism of other drugs such as warfarin, theophylline, and quinidine. Since these are drugs commonly encountered in the elderly population, rigorous monitoring of serum levels is warranted when these agents are used in combination with netronidazole.

5. CLINICAL INDICATIONS

5.1. Parasitic Infections

Intestinal parasite infections are a function of exposure and endemicity and therefore may occur in any age group including the elderly (see also chapter "Parasites"). Metronidazole is recognized as an effective agent against many anaerobic protozoa including *T. vaginalis*, *E. histolytica*, *Giardia lamblia*, and *B. coli*. The drug is the treatment of choice for urogenital trichomoniasis and can be given in a once-daily or 7-day regimen depending on patient preference (Table 2). Although standard regimens are usually effective, there are occasional treatment failures due to *T. vaginalis* strains with reduced susceptibility to metronidazole; these patients are usually treated with more prolonged, high-dose therapy or are given tinidazole (available from the Centers for Disease Control and Prevention). Metronidazole is the drug-of-choice for treatment of intestinal amebiasis and amebic liver abscess. The drug is less active against the asymptomatic intraluminal cysts and most experts recommend that patients receive a cysticidal intraluminal agent (e.g., paromomycin, diloxanide, or iodoquinol) to prevent relapse following primary metronidazole therapy. Although considered an "investigational agent" in the United States for the infection, metronidazole is active against and is commonly used for treatment of intestinal giardiasis since it may be better tolerated than other agents such as quinacrine.

5.2. Anaerobic Bacteremia and Endocarditis

Metronidazole is active against most anaerobic bacteria and has demonstrated excellent outcomes in patients with bacteremia due to susceptible strains. In the elderly, the most common cause of anaerobic bacteremia is *Bacteroides fragilis*—this is usually a consequence of underlying gastrointestinal or pelvic infection and the drug

Table 2 Metronidazole Dosing in Management of Common Bacterial and Parasitic Infection

Type of infection	Dose
Bacterial anaerobic infection[a]	
Mild–moderate	500 mg IV/PO q 12 hr
Severe	500 mg IV/PO q 6–8 hr (loading dose of 15 mg/kg IV)
Clostridium difficile pseudomembranous colitis	250 mg PO TID × 7–14 days 500 mg IV q 6 hr[b]
Bacterial vaginosis	2 g PO × 1 dose or 500 mg PO q 12 hr × 7 days or Metronidazole gel (0.075%): one application intravaginal q12 hr × 5 days
Parasitic infection	
Amebic liver abscess and/or dysentery[c]	750 mg PO TID × 10 days
Giardiasis	250 mg PO TID
Trichomoniasis	2 g PO once or 250 mg PO TID × 7 days

[a]Suggested dose for most serious adult infections is 7.5 mg/kg IV q 6 hr. Considering pharmacodynamic factors, this may be modified in selected cases (see text).
[b]Experience with intravenous therapy is anecdotal and variable; use oral therapy whenever possible.
[c]Follow-up therapy with paromomycin, iodoquinol or diloxanide furoate recommended to clear asymptomatic intestinal cysts.
Abbreviations: IV, intravenous; PO, oral; TID, three times a day.

is effective if combined with agents active against other pathogens likely to be involved (15). Although uncommon, anaerobic gram-negative endocarditis is a condition that may be seen in the elderly, especially in patients with underlying gastrointestinal or pelvic infection. Metronidazole has dramatically improved outcomes in the therapy of this condition because of its bactericidal activity organisms such as *B. fragilis* and related species (16). Although uncommon in the elderly population, Lemierre's syndrome (*Fusobacterium necrophorum* bacteremia with underlying pharyngitis and associated internal jugular septic thrombophlebitis) responds to metronidazole and further demonstrates the utility of the drug in anaerobic intravascular infection.

5.3. Intra-abdominal infections

Metronidazole is effective in the treatment of "mixed" aerobic–anaerobic intra-abdominal infection when combined with agents active against facultative or aerobic gram-negative bacilli. Such infections often contain *B. fragilis*—a common intestinal anaerobe that is almost always susceptible to metronidazole. Numerous studies have demonstrated the efficacy of the drug for intra-abdominal infection such as gangrenous appendicitis and related colonic infections (e.g., diverticulitis) (see also chapter "Medical and Surgical Treatment of Intra-abdominal Infections").

5.4. Pulmonary Infection

Lower respiratory infections are a common clinical problem in the elderly and anaerobic bacteria play an important role in lung abscess and aspiration pneumonia (see also chapter "Respiratory Infections: Pneumonia and Bronchitis"). In addition to streptococci and other oral microflora, metronidazole-susceptible anaerobic bacteria such as *Peptococus*, *Peptostreptococcus*, *Fusobacterium nucleatum*, *Porphyromonas*, *Prevotella*, and *Bacteroides* species are frequently seen. *B. fragilis* has been isolated in up to 15% of anaerobic lung infections and is frequently resistant to pencillin due to β-lactamase production. Although metronidazole alone is a poor choice for pulmonary infection, metronidazole in combination with agents active against oral streptococci (e.g., β-lactam antibiotic, vancomycin) provides excellent coverage for serious anaerobic pleuropulmonary infection.

5.5. Pelvic Infection

Bacteroides and *Fusobacterium* sp. are important pathogens in mixed aerobic–anaerobic gynecologic or pelvic infections. Again, metronidazole—in combination with agents providing activity against gram-negative facultative anaerobes and streptococci—provides excellent coverage under these conditions. Metronidazole has poor activity against *Actinomyces* species and should not be used as a single agent in the management of suspected pelvic or intra-abdominal actinomycosis. The drug has activity against *Gardnerella vaginalis* and is an excellent agent for treatment of bacterial vaginosis; in this situation, the drug can be administered as an intravaginal suppository or as an oral medication.

5.6. CNS Infection

Although anaerobic bacteria are a rare cause of meningitis in the elderly but are frequently seen in patients with pyogenic brain abscess and related suppurative intracranial infections. Odontogenic, otitic, and sinusitic sources are important in geriatric patients and necessitate the use of antibiotics active against microaerophilic streptococci as well as anaerobes. Metronidazole penetrates well into CSF and, when used in conjunction with penicillin G or a third-generation cephalosporin such as cefotaxime, provides adequate coverage for most pathogens involved in anaerobic cerebral abscesses. In addition to antimicrobial therapy, surgical drainage is frequently necessary for diagnosis and cure of these infections, especially in patients with large (>3 cm) lesions (17).

5.7. Osteomyelitis

Diabetes mellitus, peripheral vascular disease, osteoarthritis, and the presence of various prosthetic devices may predispose the elderly patient to anaerobic bone infections. Metronidazole has been used successfully in the treatment of osteomyelitis due to *B. fragilis*, *C. difficile*, and other anaerobic pathogens (18). For odontogenic sites, such as mandibular osteomyelitis, it may be used in conjunction with antibiotics active against oral facultative streptococci.

5.8. Pseudomembranous Colitis

C. difficile is a major cause of antibiotic-associated diarrhea and pseudomembranous colitis (PMC). Because of its activity against *C. difficile*, metronidazole is an ideal agent for treatment of this condition and appears to be equal in efficacy to more expensive regimens with oral vancomycin. Recent studies demonstrate metronidazole resistance in 6.3% of isolates from clinical cases, and there are case reports of metronidazole-resistant *C. difficile* leading to clinical failure (19). While oral metronidazole remains the drug-of-choice for PMC, these studies suggest that resistance may become a problem in the future and that a switch to vancomycin is appropriate in patients appearing to fail metronidazole therapy. The treatment of PMC in patients unable to take oral medications remains a problem. Retrospective studies suggest that intravenous metronidazole may be effective in patients unable to take oral medication; however, there are reports of metronidazole failure in this situation and prospective, randomized controlled studies are needed for more definitive recommendations (20).

5.9. *Helicobacter pylori*

Metronidazole is an important component of both three- and four-drug regimens used for treatment of *H. pylori*-associated peptic ulcer disease. Unfortunately, 30–40% of organisms may demonstrate primary resistance to metronidazole and susceptible organisms may develop resistance (secondary resistance) while on therapy leading to drug failure.

5.10. Other Infections

Metronidazole can be used in a wide variety of other infections afflicting the geriatric patient population including anaerobic infections of soft tissues, sinuses, and other head and neck regions. Controversy exists over the role of metronidazole in inflammatory bowel disease. While some studies have shown a decrease in bacterial and inflammatory (e.g., fistula) complications in patients treated with the drug, others have found no significant advantage in adjuvant metronidazole therapy (21). Topical metronidazole is effective in the treatment of rosacea.

5.11. Surgical Prophylaxis

Antibiotic prophylaxis prior to surgical procedures has significantly decreased post-surgical wound infections. Colorectal, gynecologic, and other intra–abdominal procedures are common in the elderly and postoperative abdominal wound infections are most often due to mixed aerobic and anaerobic flora. Metronidazole in conjunction with an agent active against aerobic gram-negative bacteria may decrease the incidence of postoperative infections in elective intra–abdominal surgeries. The benefits of perioperative metronidazole in elective gynecologic surgeries is less certain; one study showed no difference in the incidence of postoperative pelvic infections between patients receiving metronidazole and those who received placebo (22).

6. DOSING AND ROUTES OF ADMINISTRATION

Metronidazole may be administered orally, intravenously, and by rectal suppository. Topical administration can be used for the treatment of rosacea. Standard doses for various infections are listed in Table 1. The high systemic concentrations after oral administration of metronidazole are a particular advantage, allowing for a non-invasive and inexpensive treatment modality. Serious anaerobic infections usually warrant intravenous therapy initially. The standard regimen is 15 mg/kg loading dose, followed by 7.5 mg/kg every 6 hr. Dosage adjustment is probably not warranted in the otherwise healthy elderly patient, but should be considered in patients with underlying renal and/or hepatic disease (see section on Clinical Pharmacology). The maximum daily dose of metronidazole should not exceed 4 g. For most infections, 500–750 mg orally twice a day is appropriate therapy with higher dosing (q 6–8 hr) reserved for individuals with more serious or difficult-to-treat infections. Most infections respond to 7–14 days of therapy although longer courses of therapy may be required in selected cases. Additional recommendations for metronidazole dosing in other conditions including parasitic infections, *C. difficile* pseudomembranous enterocolitis, and bacterial vaginosis are listed in Table 2.

Rectal suppositories can be used when oral administration is not feasible; they are not currently approved for use in the United States but are available in other parts of the world. This form of therapy is a useful modality in nursing home residents or other chronic care patients in whom intravenous or oral therapy is problematic. A 1 g suppository can be inserted every 8 hr for 3 days, followed by every 12 hr for the duration of therapy.

Metronidazole hydrochloride can be reconstituted and diluted with intravenous solution to a concentration not exceeding 8 g/mL; the drug is not compatible with 10% dextrose or sodium lactate solutions. For ease of preparation, a premixed intravenous metronidazole preparation (Flagyl IV RTU) is commercially available.

7. ADVERSE REACTIONS

Metronidazole is a relatively safe and well-tolerated antibiotic. Common adverse reactions are listed in Table 3. Gastrointestinal effects include an unpleasant metallic

Table 3 Adverse Reactions to Metronidazole

Major adverse reactions (rare)
  Seizures, encephalopathy
  Cerebellar dysfunction, ataxia
  Peripheral neuropathy
  Disulfiram reaction with alcohol
  Potentiation of effects of warfarin
  Pseudomembranous colitis
  Pancreatitis
  Aseptic meningitis
  Hepatotoxicity
Minor adverse reactions
  Minor gastrointestinal disturbances
  Reversible neutropenia
  Metallic taste
  Dark or red-brown urine
  Maculopapular rash, urticaria
  Urethral, vaginal burning
  Gynecomastia

taste, furred tongue, stomatitis, and dry mouth. Abdominal pain, nausea, and occasional vomiting may be encountered, especially in cancer patients receiving high-dose metronidazole as adjunctive chemotherapy. Reversible neutropenia, maculopapular rash, urticaria, ototoxicity, and gynecomastia are other minor or uncommon adverse reactions associated with metronidazole use. Although a proven therapy for *C. difficile* infections, rare cases of PMC have been reported with metronidazole use.

Neurologic side effects of metronidazole are of concern, especially in the aged population where preexisting neuropathies and central nervous system disorders are common. Stocking/glove sensory neuropathies are well described with prolonged or high-dose metronidazole use. Dysesthesias usually abate with dose reduction or discontinuation of the drug, though resolution may be slow and there are rare cases of permanent changes. Metronidazole-induced encephalopathy with brain abnormalities found on magnetic resonance imaging has been described in a number of cases, usually associated with high-dose, prolonged treatment (e.g., total dose >50 g) in patients with chronic underlying medical problems such as Crohn's disease (23). Although the mechanism of this toxicity is unclear, magnetic resonance spectroscopy demonstrates elevated brain lactate levels consistent with mitochondrial disorders and suggests the possibility that metronidazole may have mitochondrial toxicity in certain circumstances. In almost all of these patients, clinical resolution occurred following discontinuance of the drug. Such side effects are rare but suggest caution in the use of prolonged metronidazole therapy, especially in patients with underlying neurological conditions.

Metronidazole has been associated with a "disulfiram-like" reaction following alcohol ingestion and the manufacturer recommends against ingesting alcohol for at least 48 hr after taking the drug. This recommendation is based upon clinical observations of symptoms (e.g., abdominal distress, nausea, vomiting, and headache) following ingestion of alcohol while on metronidazole. In one reported case, a patient died following a presumed metronidazole/ethanol reaction (24); at postmortem examination, the blood test was positive for metronidazole although there was no evidence that the patient had been prescribed the drug and a false-positive blood test could not be excluded. More recent authors raise questions about the existence of this reaction and suggest that the concern may be overstated. In one controlled trial, a comparison of patients taking metronidazole with a control group demonstrated no clinical signs of a "disulfiram-like" reaction; neither group showed an increase in serum acetaldehyde—a compound believed to be the "toxic" agent in the reaction (25). The true risk of alcohol ingestion with metronidazole remains unknown. In the meantime, it is probably best to advise against alcohol ingestion in patients receiving metronidazole.

The mutagenic potential of metronidazole is controversial. Bacterial reduction products of the drug may have mutagenic activity in animals; however, data concerning carcinogenicity in humans are less convincing. An increased incidence of colorectal carcinoma has been noted in patients taking metronidazole for Crohn's disease, although it is difficult to separate mutagenicity of drug from that of intrinsic disease. The possible teratogenic effects of the drug during pregnancy add further concern for metronidazole's mutagenic potential. Despite these concerns, a large study of women receiving metronidazole for vaginal trichomoniasis failed to show an association between malignancy and the drug (26). In the elderly, who already have a high incidence of carcinoma, it may be impossible to assess the direct mutagenicity of metronidazole. Pending further investigations, mutagenic concerns should not be the exclusive reason for withholding the drug when treating serious anaerobic infections in older patient populations.

When one compares the serious and occasionally life-threatening side effects associated with other common antibiotics, metronidazole is remarkably safe. Unlike aminoglycosides and other drugs frequently used in geriatric patients, it does not require monitoring of serum levels. Its excellent bioavailability and multiple routes of administrations add to metronidazole's clinical versatility. Finally, and perhaps most importantly, metronidazole's efficacy in treating serious anaerobic infections makes the drug an especially useful antimicrobial agent in the elderly patient population.

REFERENCES

1. Müller M. Mode of action of metronidazole on anaerobic bacteria and protozoa. Surgery 1983; 93:165–177.
2. Rasmussen BA, Bush K, Tally FP. Antimicrobial resistance in anaerobes. Clin Infect Dis 997; 24(suppl 1):S110–S120.
3. Muller M, Meingassner JG, Miller WA, Leder WJ. Three metronidazole resistant strains of *Trichomonas vaginalis* from the United States. Am J Obstet Gynecol 1980; 138: 808–812.
4. Boreham PFL, Phillips RE, Sheperd RW. Heterogeneity in the response of clones of *Giardia intestinalis* to anti-giardial drugs. Trans R Soc Trop Med Hyg 1987; 81:406–407.
5. Tally FP, Cuchural GJ, Jacobus NV, Gorbach SL, Aldridge K, Cleary T, Finegold SM, Hill G, Iannini P, O'Keefe JP, Pierson C. Nationwide study of the susceptibility of the *Bacteroides fragilis* group in the United States. Antimicrob Agents Chemother 1985; 28:674–677.
6. Hedberg M, Nord CE. ESCMID Study Group on Antimicrobial Resistance in Anaerobic Bacteria. Antimicrobial susceptibility of *Bacteroides fragilis* group isolates in Europe. Clin Microbiol Infect 2003; 9:475–488.

7. Thiercelin JF, Diquet B, Levesque C, Ghesquiere F, Simon P, Viars P. Metronidazole kinetics and bioavailability in patients undergoing gastrointestinal surgery. Clin Pharmacol Ther 1984; 35:510–519.

8. Loft S, Egsmose C, Sonne J, Poulsen HD, Døssing M, Andreasen PB. Metronidazole elimination is preserved in the elderly. Hum Exp Toxicol 1990; 9:155–159.

9. Muscara MN, Pedrazzoli J Jr, Miranda EL, Ferraz JG, Hofstatter E, Leite G, Magalhaes AF, Leonardi S, De Nucci G. Plasma hydroxy-metrondiazole/metronidazole ratio in patients with liver disease and in healthy volunteers. Br J Clin Pharmacol 1995; 40:677–680.

10. Plaisance KI, Quintiliani R, Nightingale CH. The pharmacokinetics of metronidazole and its metabolites in critically-ill patients. J Antimicrob Chemother 1998; 21:195–200.

11. Bergan T, Thorsteinsson SB. Pharmacokinetics of metronidazole and its metabolites in reduced renal function. Chemotherapy 1986; 32:305–318.

12. Roux AF, Moirot E, Delhotal B, Leroy JA, Bonmarchand GP, Humber G, Flouvat B. Metronidazole kinetics in patients with acute renal failure on dialysis: a cumulative study. Clin Pharmacol Ther 1984; 36:363–368.

13. Nix DE, Tyrrell R, Muller M. Pharmacodynamics of metronidazole determined by a time-kill assay for *Trichomonas vaginalis*. Antimicrob Agents Chemother 1995; 39:1848–1852.

14. Auger P, Bourgouin J, Bagot C. Intravenous metronidazole in the treatment of abdominal sepsis: once vs. three times daily administration. Curr Ther Res 1988; 43:494–502.

15. Terpenning MS. Anaerobic bacteremia in the elderly. Gerontology 1989; 35:130–136.

16. Bisharat N, Goldstein L, Raz R, Elias M. Gram-negative anaerobic endocarditis: two case reports and review of the literature. Eur J Clin Microbiol Infect Dis 2001; 20: 651–654.

17. Mathisen GE, Johnson P. Brain abscess. Clin Infect Dis 1997; 25:763–781.

18. Templeton WC III, Wawrukiewicz A, Melo JC, Schiller M. Anaerobic osteomyelitis of long bones. Rev Infect Dis 1983; 5:692–712.

19. Peláez T, Alcalá L, Alonso R, Rodriguez-Creixems M, Garcia-Lechuz JM, Bouza E. Reassessment of *Clostridium difficile* susceptibility to metronidazole and vancomycin. Antimicrob Agent Chemother 2002; 46:1647–1650.

20. Friedenberg F, Fernandez A, Kaul V, Niami P, Levine GM. Intravenous metronidazole for the treatment of *Clostridium difficile* colitis. Dis Colon Rectum 2001; 1176–1180.

21. Chapman RW, Selby WS, Jewell DP. Controlled trial of intravenous metronidazole as an adjunct to corticosteroids in severe ulcerative colitis. Gut 1986; 27:1210–1212.

22. Vincelette J, Findelstein F, Aoki FY, Ti TY, Ogilvie RI, Richard GK, Seymour RJ. Double-blind trial of perioperative intravenous metronidazole prophylaxis for abdominal and vaginal hysterectomy. Surgery 1983; 93:185–189.

23. Seok JI, Yi H, Song YM, Lee WY. Metronidazole-induced encephalopathy and inferior olivary hypertrophy. Arch Neurol 2003; 60:1796–1800.

24. Cina SJ, Russell RA, Conradi SE. Sudden death due to metronidazole/ethanol interaction. Am J Forensic Med Pathol 1996; 17:343–346.

25. Visapaa J-P, Tillonen JS, Kaihovaara PS, Salspuro MP. Lack of disulfiram-like reaction with metronidazole and ethanol. Ann Pharmacol 2002; 36:971–974.

26. Beard CM, Noller KL, O'Fallan WM, Kurland LT, Dahlin D. Cancer after exposure to metronidazole. Mayo Clin Proc 1988; 63:147–153.

SUGGESTED READING

Finegold SM, George WL, Rolfe RD, eds. Proceedings of the First United States Metronidazole Conference, Tarpon Springs, FL, February 1982. New York: Biomedical Information, 1982.

Freeman CD, Klutman NE, Lamp KC. Metronidazole: a therapeutic review and update. Drugs 1997; 54:679–708.

Lamp KC, Freeman CD, Klutman NE, Lacy MK. Pharmacokinetics and pharmacodynamics of the nitroimidazole antimicrobials. Clin Pharmacokinet 1999; 36:353–373.

Mathisen GE. Metronidazole. In: Gorbach SL, Bartlett JG, Blacklow NR, eds. Infectious Diseases. 3rd ed. Philadelphia, PA: WB Saunders Co., 2004.

19
Chloramphenicol

Made Sutjita
*Department of Internal Medicine, Division of Infectious Diseases, Charles R. Drew
University of Medicine and Science, Martin Luther King, Jr.–Charles R. Drew Medical
Center, Los Angeles, California, U.S.A.*

Key Points:

- Chloramphenicol is a broad-spectrum antibiotic with activity against a variety of aerobic and anaerobic bacteria as well as spirochetes, rickettsiae, chlamydiae, and mycoplasmas.
- The use of chloramphenicol is limited primarily because of dose-dependent bone marrow suppression and idiosyncratic aplastic anemia.
- Chloramphenicol penetrates well into most body fluids, including cerebrospinal fluid.
- The clinical indications for the drug in the elderly are limited to prescribing as an alternative agent for bacterial meningitis, brain abscess, typhoid fever, and anaerobic infections.
- Hematological abnormalities and neurological deficits (optic neuritis, peripheral neuritis, headache, and ophthalmoplegia) are potential adverse events.

1. INTRODUCTION

Chloramphenicol was first isolated in 1947 from a sample of soil containing *Streptomyces venezuelae*, a species of actinomycetes that originated in Venezuela (1). Chloramphenicol was introduced into clinical use in 1949. Subsequently, reports linked this new broad-spectrum antibiotic with aplastic anemia. Chloramphenicol quickly became an unfavorable antibiotic for clinical use. The availability of other agents has dramatically reduced the need for this antibiotic. It is still used as first-line therapy for enteric fever and other infections in developing countries. In developed countries, chloramphenicol remains a useful antibiotic, but only as alternative therapy in seriously ill young or older patients or for patients infected with very resistant microorganisms.

2. CHEMISTRY AND MECHANISM OF ACTION

The formula of chloramphenicol is $C_{11}H_{12}Cl_2N_2O_5$ (2). Thiamphenicol is an analog in which the *p*-nitro group on the benzene ring is replaced by a methylsulfonyl group. Its spectrum of activity is similar to that of chloramphenicol.

Chloramphenicol enters the cell by an energy-dependent process (3). Inside the bacterial cell, it inhibits protein synthesis by binding to the larger 50S subunit of the 70S ribosome. Mammalian cells contain primarily 80S ribosomes that are supposedly unaffected by chloramphenicol. However, mammalian mitochondria do contain 70S particles. The effect of chloramphenicol on these mitochondrial 70S ribosomes has been suggested as a cause for the dose-related bone marrow suppression of chloramphenicol but not the idiosyncratic aplastic anemia (4). The block in bacterial protein synthesis produces a static effect against susceptible microorganisms. However, chloramphenicol is bactericidal against some pathogens such as *Haemophilus influenzae*, *Streptococcus pneumoniae*, and *Neisseria meningitides* (5,6).

3. ANTIMICROBIAL SPECTRUM

Similar to tetracycline, chloramphenicol has a very broad spectrum. It is active against susceptible aerobic and anaerobic bacteria, spirochetes, rickettsiae, chlamydiae, and mycoplasmas. It is also very active against most anaerobic bacteria such as *Bacteroides fragilis*.

Chloramphenicol resistance is mediated by a bacterial enzyme, acetyltransferase. This enzyme acetylates the antibiotic to an inactive diacetyl derivative (7). Chloramphenicol-resistant *Salmonella typhi* (typhoid fever) and *Shigella* dysentery strains have been reported in Vietnam and India (8,9). The drug is widely used in humans and animals (dairy farms) and thus may contribute to the development of bacterial resistance to chloramphenicol (9,10). Unrestricted use of chloramphenicol in developing countries may result in a resistance pattern similar to that observed with tetracyclines.

4. CLINICAL PHARMACOLOGY

Chloramphenicol is a relatively small lipophilic molecule and is well distributed in the body. Serum protein binding is about 44%. It crosses the blood–brain barrier effectively and reaches the central nervous system. Chloramphenicol also crosses the placenta and is found in breast milk (11). Chloramphenicol is well absorbed by the gastrointestinal tract after oral administration. A chloramphenicol capsule of 1 g results in peak serum levels of 12 μg/mL of active antibiotic (12). In the United States, oral preparations are no longer available.

Chloramphenicol has a serum half-life in adults of 4.1 hr after single intravenous injections. Approximately 25–50% of the drug is bound to protein, and it has an apparent volume of distribution of 100 L (13). The volume of distribution may increase in the elderly because of decreased muscle mass and increase in fat tissue. The antibiotic distributes well into many tissues and body fluids. Levels in the cerebrospinal fluid even without inflamed meninges can achieve 30–50% of serum concentrations, much higher than those of most other antibiotics (14). Chloramphenicol is commonly used to treat conjunctivitis; it is available commercially in the United States as 0.5% sterile ophthalmic solution.

Chloramphenicol is metabolized primarily by the liver. In the liver it is conjugated with glucuronic acid and excreted in this inactive form by the kidney. Aging-related changes in liver function may alter the metabolism of this drug. Only about 5–10% of the administered dose is recovered in the urine as biologically active chloramphenicol. Nonetheless, in the absence of renal disease, concentrations of 150–200 μg/mL of active drug are achieved, which is sufficient to treat urinary tract infections if necessary. In patients with renal failure, chloramphenicol urinary concentrations are markedly reduced (15). Dose adjustment is not routinely necessary in elderly patients with mild or moderate renal dysfunction. Neither peritoneal infusion nor hemodialysis alters serum levels sufficiently to necessitate dose modifications (13,16).

Patients with hepatic failure assimilate chloramphenicol at a slower rate, resulting in serum levels of active chloramphenicol to increase to levels capable of bone marrow suppression (17). It is suggested that in patients with liver dysfunction the course of therapy should be limited, when possible, to 10–14 days and serum drug levels should be monitored (3).

5. CLINICAL INDICATIONS, ADMINISTRATION OF DRUG, DRUG MONITORING, AND ADVERSE EFFECT

Chloramphenicol is toxic and therefore should not be used in the treatment of trivial infections such as common cold, influenza, and sore throat. Because of the availability of less toxic antibiotics (e.g., third-generation cephalosporins, quinolones), chloramphenicol is rarely used nowadays. In developing countries, its cost and availability make it the primary antibiotic to be used in the therapy of typhoid fever. In developed countries, its use is reserved for highly resistant organisms or as an alternative agent for patients, including the elderly, with meningitis due to susceptible organism in severely β-lactam-allergic patients (18). The drug may also be considered as an alternative agent for brain abscess, typhoid fever, and anaerobic infections.

However, a topical ophthalmic solution of chloramphenicol is safe and commonly used to treat superficial eye infection such as conjunctivitis. Such treatment is still effective and comparable in efficacy with newer drugs such as quinolones and fusidic acid (19,20).

Dose-related reversible bone marrow depression can occur in adults given prolonged high doses of more than 4 g/day. The daily dose should not exceed 3 g. If the accumulated dose exceeds 25 g, the reticulocyte count should be checked on a regular basis, i.e., twice weekly until treatment is stopped (3). Idiosyncratic aplastic anemia, which is not related to the dose and duration of treatment, rarely occurs. It occurs with a frequency of 1/25,000–40,000 treatment courses (21).

Optic neuritis resulting in decreased visual acuity is rare but has been described in patients receiving prolonged chloramphenicol therapy (22). Other neurological abnormalities such as peripheral neuritis, headache, confusion, depression, and ophthalmoplegia have also been described.

Chloramphenicol is almost completely metabolized in the liver by cytochrome P450 enzymes. Therefore, there is a possibility that chloramphenicol may affect the level of other drugs that are metabolized by the same enzyme. Chloramphenicol decreases the rate of metabolism of chlorpropamide, phenytoin, and cyclophosphamide (23–26). Rifampin, phenobarbital, and phenytoin may lower chloramphenicol concentrations by induced metabolism (27,28).

REFERENCES

1. Ehrlich J, Bartz QR, Smith RM, Joslyn DA, Burkholder PR. Chloromycetin, a new antibiotic from a soil actinomycete. Science 1947; 106:417.
2. PDR Electronic Library, Thomson PDR 2003 CD-ROM.

3. Stanford HC. Tetracyclines and chloramphenicol. In: Mandell GL, Bennett JE, Dolin R, eds. Principles and Practice of Infectious Diseases. 5th ed. Philadelphia, PA: Churchill Livingstone, Inc., 2000:341–345.

4. Abdel-Sayed S. Transport of chloramphenicol into sensitive strains of *Escherichia coli* and *Pseudomonas aeruginosa*. J Antimicrob Chemother 1987; 19:7–20.

5. Turk DC. A comparison of chloramphenicol and ampicillin as bactericidal agents for *Haemophilus influenzae* type B. J Med Microbiol 1977; 10:127.

6. Rahal JJ, Simberkoff MS. Bactericidal and bacteriostatic action of chloramphenicol against meningeal pathogens. Antimicrob Agents Chemother 1979; 16:13.

7. Okamoto S, Mizuno D. Mechanism of chloramphenicol and tetracycline resistance in *Escherichia coli*. J Gen Microbiol 1964; 35:125.

8. Butler T, Linh NN, Arnold K, Pollack M. Chloramphenicol-resistant typhoid fever in Vietnam associated with R-factor. Lancet 1973; 2:983.

9. Halder KK, Dalal BS, Ghose E, Samyal S. Chloramphenicol resistant *Salmonella typhi*: the cause of recent outbreak of enteric fever in Calcutta. Indian J Pathol Microbiol 1992; 35:11–17.

10. Drug resistance in salmonellas (Editorial). Lancet 1982; 1:1391.

11. Alestig K. Tetracyclines and chloramphenicol. In: Cohen J, Powderly WG, eds. Infectious Diseases. 2nd ed. New York: Mosby Publishers, 2004:1846–1848.

12. Bartelloni PJ, Calia FM, Minchew BH, Beisel WR, Ley HL Jr. Absorption and excretion of two chloramphenicol products in humans after oral administration. Am J Med Sci 1969; 258:203.

13. Kunin CM. A guide to use of antibiotics in patients with renal disease. Ann Intern Med 1967; 67:151.

14. Woodward TE, Wisseman CL. Chloromycetin (chloramphenicol). New York: Medical Encyclopedia, 1958.

15. Lindberg AA, Nilsson LH, Bucht H, Kallings LO. Concentration of chloramphenicol in the urine and blood in relation to renal function. Br Med J 1966; 2:724.

16. Kunin CM, Glazko AJ, Finland M. Persistence of antibiotics in blood of patients with acute renal failure. II. Chloramphenicol and its metabolic products in the blood of patients with severe renal disease or hepatic cirrhosis. J Clin Invest 1959; 38:1498.

17. Suhrland LG, Weisberger AS. Chloramphenicol toxicity in liver and renal disease. Arch Intern Med 1963; 112:161.

18. Reese RE, Betts RF. Antibiotic use. In: Reese RE, Betts RF, eds. A Practical Approach to Infectious Diseases. 4th ed. Boston: Little, Brown and Company, 1996:1268–1272.

19. Power WJ, Collum LM, Easty DL, Bloom PA, Laidlaw DA, Libert J, Sangers D, Wuokko M, Saksela T. Evaluation of efficacy and safety of ciprofloxacin ophthalmic solution versus chloramphenicol. Eur J Ophthalmol 1993; 2:77–82.

20. Horven I. Acute conjunctivitis. A comparison of fusidic acid viscous eye drops and chloramphenicol. Acta Ophthalmol (Copenh) 1993; 2:165–168.

21. Wallerstein RO, Condit PK, Kasper CK, Brown JW, Morrison FR. Statewide study of chloramphenicol therapy and fatal aplastic anemia. J Am Med Assoc 1969; 208:2045–2050.

22. Chloramphenicol blindness (Editorial). Br Med J 1965; 1:1511.

23. Christensen LK, Skovsted L. Inhibition of drug metabolism by chloramphenicol. Lancet 1969; 2:1397.

24. Petitpierre B, Fabre J. Chlorpropamide and chloramphenicol. Lancet 1970; 1:789.

25. Rose JQ, Choi HK, Schentag JJ. Intoxication caused by interaction of chloramphenicol and phenytoin. J Am Med Assoc 1977; 237:2630.

26. Faber OK, Mouridsen HT, Skovsted L. The effect of chloramphenicol and sulphaphenazole on the biotransformation of cyclophosphamide in man. Br J Clin Pharmacol 1975; 2:281.

27. Powell DA, Nahata MC, Durrell DC, Glazer JP, Hilty MD. Interactions among chloramphenicol, phenytoin and phenobarbital in a pediatric patient. J Pediatr 1981; 98:1001.

28. Prober CG. Effect of rifampin on chloramphenicol levels. N Engl J Med 1985; 312:788–789.

SUGGESTED READING

Halder KK, Dalal BS, Ghose E, Samyal S. Chloramphenicol resistant *Salmonella typhi*: the cause of recent outbreak of enteric fever in Calcutta. Indian J Pathol Microbiol 1992; 35:11–17.

Kasten MJ. Clindamycin, metronidazole, and chloramphenicol. Mayo Clin Proc 1999; 74:825–833.

Power WJ, Collum LM, Easty DL, Bloom PA, Laidlaw DA, Libert J, Sangers D, Wuokko M, Saksela T. Evaluation of efficacy and safety of ciprofloxacin ophthalmic solution versus chloramphenicol. Eur J Ophthalmol 1993; 2:77–82.

Rahal JJ, Simberkoff MS. Bactericidal and bacteriostatic action of chloramphenicol against meningeal pathogens. Antimicrob Agents Chemother 1979; 16:13.

20

Trimethoprim–Sulfamethoxazole

Stephen Marer and Shobita Rajagopalan
Department of Internal Medicine, Division of Infectious Diseases, Charles R. Drew University of Medicine and Science, Martin Luther King, Jr.–Charles R. Drew Medical Center, Los Angeles, California, U.S.A.

Key Points:

- Trimethoprim–sulfamethoxazole, a prototype sulfonamide agent that is widely used, interferes with folate metabolism.
- Trimethoprim–sulfamethoxazole is active against a variety of aerobes and certain parasites, but resistance is increasing.
- For the elderly, treatment of urinary tract infection and prostatits as well as *Pneumocystis carinii* pneumonia associated with human immunodeficiency virus infection are the major clinical indications for this drug.
- Elderly patients are more likely to develop drug side effects, i.e., dermatologic and hematologic.
- There are a number of documented drug interactions, which are especially important for older adults.

1. INTRODUCTION

In 1935, Protonsil, a prodrug of sulfanilamide, was the first systemic antibacterial drug used in the United States (1). Modifications of sulfanilamide produced a variety of antibiotics (sulfonamides) that have been widely useful in clinical medicine. All of the sulfonamides act as competitive antagonists of *p*-aminobenzoic acid (PABA) in the folic acid synthesis pathway. The sulfonamides were useful for many years for meningococcal infections and urinary tract infections (UTIs), for example, but resistance has markedly curtailed their use as single agents.

Trimethoprim inhibits dihydrofolate reductase, which converts folic acid into tetrahydrofolic acid, the more active form of folic acid. Trimethoprim potentiates the action of sulfonamides by virtue of its role in inhibiting dihydrofolate reductase. Trimethoprim was first introduced clinically in the late 1960s for use with sulfonamides. Soon after, trimethoprim–sulfamethoxazole (TMP–SMX) became widely used in a fixed drug combination for treatment of a great number of infectious diseases, including bacterial and parasitic diseases. The remainder of this chapter will focus

269

on TMP–SMX, used much more commonly than either component alone with particular emphasis on its application in the elderly.

2. CHEMISTRY AND MECHANISM OF ACTION

The sulfonamides and trimethoprim interfere in the pathway that synthesizes tetra-hydrofolic acid, which leads to thymidine synthesis and eventually DNA synthesis (Fig. 1).

The sulfonamides are structural analogs of PABA, and competitively inhibit dihy-dropteroate synthase, the enzyme that incorporates PABA into dihydropteroic acid, the immediate precursor of folic acid. Bacteria that cannot use preformed folic acid are thus inhibited by sulfonamides. Mammalian cells require preformed folic acid and therefore are unaffected by the action of sulfonamides. Alone, the sulfonamides are generally bacteriostatic.

Trimethoprim is a diaminopyrimidine that competitively inhibits dihydrofolate reductase. Dihydrofolate reductase catalyzes the conversion of folic acid into tetra-hydrofolic acid, the most active form of folic acid. Trimethoprim is highly selective for dihydrofolate reductase of lower organisms, thus leaving the crucial enzymatic step intact in mammalian cells (2). By itself, trimethoprim is bacteriostatic or weakly bactericidal. However, by inhibiting sequential steps in the formation of tetrahyro-folic acid, the combination of sulfonamides with trimethoprim is often synergistic and therefore bactericidal.

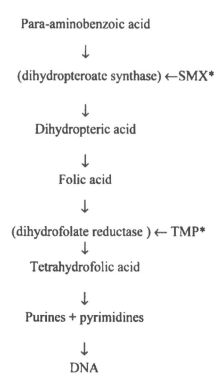

Para-aminobenzoic acid

↓

(dihydropteroate synthase) ←SMX*

↓

Dihydropteric acid

↓

Folic acid

↓

(dihydrofolate reductase) ← TMP*
↓

Tetrahydrofolic acid

↓

Purines + pyrimidines

↓

DNA

Figure 1 Pathway of DNA synthesis and sites of inhibition by trimethoprim (TMP) and sulfamethoxazole (SMX).

Resistance to sulfonamides and trimethoprim have limited their use. There are several possible mechanisms of resistance in both sulfonamides and trimethoprim, and many isolates are resistant to the combination of TMP and SMX. Resistance to sulfonamides and trimethoprim may be chromosomally or plasmid-mediated. Sulfonamide resistance, which is very common, can be caused by overproduction of PABA, mutations in dihydropteroate synthase causing decreased affinity for sulfonamides, or a decrease in the cell permeability to antibacterials. Similar mechanisms can be found in isolates resistant to trimethoprim, but the most important mechanism appears to be plasmid-mediated mutations in the dihydrofolate reductase enzyme (3). Through plasmid transfer of resistance genes, many species of bacteria, including many species of Enterobacteriaceae, have become resistant to one or both antibiotics.

3. ANTIMICROBIAL SPECTRUM

TMP–SMX has activity against a broad spectrum of organisms. These include gram-negative and gram-positive bacteria, *Pneumocystis carinii*, and some protozoa. As previously noted, however, resistance is a growing problem.

Among gram-positive organisms, *Streptococcus pyogenes*, *Staphylococcus saprophyticus*, and *Listeria monocytogenes* are generally susceptible. Importantly, the susceptibility of *Streptococcus pneumoniae*, which correlates with its susceptibility to penicillin, is variable, and resistance is a rapidly increasing problem (4). Similarly, there are increasing numbers of resistant isolates of *Staphylococcus aureus*; although with susceptible strains, TMP–SMX is felt to be an excellent antistaphylococcal agent. TMP–SMX retains activity against *Nocardia* species as well.

Gram-negative organisms that have remained generally susceptible to TMP–SMX include *Yersinia enterocolitica*, *Aeromonas* species, and *Stenotrophomonas maltophila*. Unfortunately, the more clinically relevant gram-negative organisms have variable susceptibility patterns. These include *Escherichia coli*, *Enterobacter* species, *Haemophilus influenzae*, and *Moraxella catarrhalis*.

The spectrum of activity of TMP–SMX is not limited to bacterial organisms. It also has activity against some protozoa, including *Cyclospora cayetensis*, and it is considered the drug of choice for treating *P. carinii*. TMP–SMX does not have activity against *Pseudomonas aeruginosa* or anaerobes.

4. CLINICAL PHARMACOLOGY

The optimal synergistic ratio of trimethoprim to sulfamethoxazole is felt to be 1:20, a ratio achieved best in serum when the drug combination is delivered in a ratio of 1:5(5). Therefore, available preparations are manufactured in a 1:5 trimethoprim-to-sulfamethoxazole ratio. The combination comes in oral and intravenous forms. A single-strength tablet contains 80 mg trimethoprim and 400 mg sulfamethoxazole, whereas a double-strength tablet contains 160 mg trimethoprim and 800 mg sulfamethoxazole. The double-strength tablet is the one more often used.

Both components are well absorbed orally, although trimethoprim is absorbed more rapidly and is more widely distributed throughout the body. Trimethoprim is lipid soluble with a high volume of distribution in the range of 100 L. Sulfamethoxazole, however, is a weak acid and has poor lipid solubility at physiologic pH. Its volume of distribution correlates with that of the extracellular space, in the range of 12–18 L. The volume of distribution in older adults appears unchanged for TMP and SMX . Tissue concentrations of trimethoprim are generally much higher than those of sulfamethoxazole. Both components reach high concentrations in cerebrospinal fluid (CSF), sputum, prostatic fluid, bile, and urine.

Sulfamethoxazole undergoes primarily hepatic metabolism, with about 30% excreted unchanged in the urine. However, trimethoprim is not metabolized very much, only about 10–30% metabolized to inactive components. The remainder is excreted mostly unchanged in the urine. The half-lives of both components are 8–14 hr; therefore, the combination is generally divided in two daily doses. With renal insufficiency, the half-lives can exceed 30 hr; thus adjustment is advised when the creatinine clearance falls below 30 mL/min. Additionally, adults require lower dosages than children, because elimination is faster in children. In limited studies in geriatric patients, it appears that the terminal half-lives and total excretion of TMP and SMX are similar to younger adults; however, the renal clearance of both appear to be reduced by 50% compared with younger patients with comparable renal function.

5. CLINICAL INDICATIONS

In the 1970s, TMP–SMX was effective against a wide range of aerobes, and it was (and is) inexpensive (6). It was therefore a popular agent for use in UTIs, respiratory infections, and gastrointestinal (GI) infections. Unfortunately, bacterial resistance to TMP–SMX has increased over the decades, decreasing its overall usefulness. This may be especially true in the elderly, who, by virtue of previous infections and hospitalizations, are more likely to be colonized with, or infected by, resistant pathogens. However, even in the elderly, TMP–SMX remains a useful agent for certain conditions. Table 1 lists the clinical indications for prescribing TMP–SMX.

5.1. Urinary Tract Infections

TMP–SMX is still active against many Enterobacteriaceae, and therefore remains useful for one of its original indications, acute UTI (see also chapter "Urinary Tract Infection"). It has been the drug of choice for empirical therapy of uncomplicated UTIs in women, but resistance is slowly evicting the drug from that niche. In certain areas, trimethoprim resistance in E. coli can exceed 30%. The Infectious Diseases Society of America (IDSA) recommends TMP–SMX as first-line therapy for uncomplicated cystitis in women provided that local resistance patterns do not exceed 10–20% (7). Risk factors for resistance include recent use of antibiotics, hospitalization and immunosuppression, all of which may be more common in the elderly (8). It would not be unreasonable, then, to favor the use of a fluoroquinolone as first-line therapy in some older adults with uncomplicated UTIs. If, however, susceptibility patterns are favorable, TMP–SMX can be useful in treating uncomplicated UTIs in older women, as well as inpatient or outpatient pyelonephritis, and for prostatic infections. The length of treatment for acute bacterial prostatitis is generally 1 month, and for chronic bacterial prostatitis it is 2–3 months. TMP–SMX also can be useful as a prophylactic agent for recurrent UTIs. The dose for prophylaxis is generally one-half of a single-strength tablet at bedtime.

Table 1 Clinical Indications for Trimethoprim–Sulfamethoxazole

---

Drug of choice[a]
   Uncomplicated urinary tract infection (UTI)
   Acute and chronic bacterial prostatitis
   Prophylaxis for recurrent UTI
   Pneumocystis carinii pneumonia (PCP)
   Prophylaxis against PCP
   Prophylaxis against toxoplasmosis
   Nocardia infections
Alternate drug of choice[a]
   Respiratory tract infections
   Bacterial diarrheas
   Cerebral toxoplasmosis
   Isospora and *Cyclospora* infection
   Methicillin-resistant *Staphylococcus aureus* (limited strains)
   Multidrug-resistant gram-negative bacilli (limited strains)
   Listeria monocytogenes meningitis

---

[a]For susceptible pathogens.

5.2. Respiratory Infections

In previous decades, TMP–SMX had excellent activity against *S. pneumoniae*, *H. influenzae*, and *M. catarrhalis*, which comprise the more common community-acquired respiratory pathogens. It is no surprise, then, that TMP–SMX was a good choice for treating community-acquired pneumonia (CAP), sinusitis, otitis media, and exacerbations of chronic bronchitis. Unfortunately, resistance is increasing to respiratory pathogens as well, making TMP–SMX a less-attractive choice for such infections, particularly among those at risk for resistant pathogens. Most pneumococci that are intermediately or highly resistant to penicillin are also resistant to TMP–SMX. Estimates are that 15–20% of *S. pneumoniae* and *H. influenzae* are resistant to TMP–SMX in the United States. In 1993, the American Thoracic Society (ATS) considered TMP–SMX an option as initial therapy for treatment of outpatient CAP in patients over 60 years old, but this is no longer the case. In their most recent guidelines, both the ATS and the IDSA do not consider TMP–SMX an acceptable primary choice for empirical therapy for CAP (9,10). However, for susceptible pathogens, TMP–SMX remains an excellent drug for respiratory infections.

5.3. Gastrointestinal Infections

The elderly are not generally more prone to GI infections, but the sequelae of such infections can be more severe at the extremes of age. TMP–SMX remains useful in the treatment of many GI infections, with *Shigella* being a notable exception, because of extremely high resistance rates in most parts of the world (11). *Salmonella* species in the United States are often susceptible to TMP–SMX. In the Mexican interior, enterotoxigenic *E. coli* generally are susceptible to TMP–SMX. Other causes of bacterial diarrhea that remain susceptible include *Aeromonas hydrophila*, *Vibrio cholerae*, and *Yersinia enterocolitica*. Although these and certain other organisms retain susceptibility, the fluoroquinolones have generally replaced TMP–SMX for prophylaxis and treatment of traveler's diarrhea. TMP–SMX can be used as an alternative agent for susceptible pathogens.

5.4. Skin Infections

Previously, *S. pyogenes* and *S. aureus* were generally susceptible to TMP–SMX, making the agent a potentially useful drug for skin and soft-tissue infections. However, the resistance patterns now are more variable, and the drug is generally not considered as a primary drug for these infections. With the marked increase in the incidence of community-acquired methicillin resistant *S. aureus* (MRSA) infections, however, it is possible that TMP–SMX may assume a bigger role as a treatment option, as some MRSA isolates retain in vitro susceptibility to the drug. For sensitive strains, TMP–SMX is a very effective antistaphylococcal agent, having been used, for example, in at least one study that included treatment of staphylococcal endocarditis with good results (12). Whether TMP–SMX might assume a role next to vancomycin, linezolid, daptomycin, and others in the treatment of serious MRSA infections is an open question.

5.5. Human Immunodeficiency Virus Infection

TMP–SMX is perhaps best known now for being the drug of choice for *P. carinii* pneumonia (PCP) in immunosuppressed patients, particularly those with the acquired immune deficiency syndrome (AIDS) (13). Given the increase in human immunodeficiency virus (HIV) infections in older adults and the success of highly active antiretroviral therapy, AIDS will likely assume a more prominent role in geriatric medicine (see also chapter "Human Immunodeficiency Virus Infection") and TMP–SMX is considered the drug of first choice for all forms of PCP, from mild to severe. Interestingly, 10–20% of patients with PCP fail to respond to TMP–SMX, and whether this percentage will be higher in the elderly is unknown.

Other common infections in patients with AIDS are the protozoal infections from *Isospora* and *Cyclospora*, and TMP–SMX is effective treatment for both of these infections. TMP–SMX also has activity in cerebral toxoplasmosis, but it is not the drug of first choice (another combination of folate inhibitors, pyrimethamine and sulfadiazine, is the treatment of first choice).

5.6. Other Indications

As is well known, TMP–SMX is used for prophylaxis against PCP and toxoplasmosis in patients with AIDS; it can also be used for prophylaxis in organ transplant patients.

A small number of nonfermentative gram-negative bacilli (primarily hospital acquired) remain susceptible or partially susceptible to TMP–SMX when susceptibility to other broad-spectrum antibiotics is lacking. Such organisms include *Stenotrophomonas maltophilia*, *Pseudomonas cepacia*, *Acinetobacter* spp., and *Alcaligenes* spp. TMP–SMX, with its good CSF penetration, is effective therapy for penicillin-allergic patients with *L. monocytogenes* meningitis. It is usually first-line therapy for *Nocardia* infections; it is used to treat Whipple disease; and it may be useful (for unclear reasons) in Wegener's granulomatosis.

6. ADVERSE REACTIONS

TMP–SMX has a number of well-known side effects, the most common of which are gastrointestinal and dermatologic. Most of the side effects are probably related to the sulfonamide component. It is interesting to note that there is a much higher incidence of side effects in patients with AIDS, and to speculate whether a similar phenomenon can be anticipated in the elderly. A large body of data is lacking, and likely age by itself does not portend a tremendously higher incidence of side effects. Drug interactions and dosages that do not take into account decreased renal function in the elderly are more likely to be associated with adverse reactions. At least one study did implicate age in the incidence of fatal hematologic side effects (2). In the study, the frequency of fatal hematologic reactions was estimated to be 3.7 per million treatments. The mean age of patients who died was 78 years, and only 3 of 18 patients who died were below age 70. Given this finding, one must be careful when prescribing TMP–SMX (and all medications) to the elderly.

GI side effects occur in about 3–8% of patients (5). The effects are usually limited to nausea, vomiting and anorexia. More concerning and fortunately less common side effects are glossitis and stomatitis. Hepatotoxicity can occur but is very rare, perhaps more rare than would be expected given the known potential of sulfonamides in general to cause this reaction (although here again it is a very rare complication of sulfonamide therapy). It is unknown whether age increases the incidence of these GI side effects.

Dermatologic reactions occur in about 4% of patients (5). Many different types of reactions have been described, from urticaria and other relatively minor reactions to the more severe Stevens–Johnson syndrome and toxic epidermal necrolysis (14); the latter severe reactions have been reported in elderly patients (15). These more feared effects are rare but appear to be more commonly related to sulfonamides than to TMP–SMX.

Trimethoprim can also decrease potassium excretion in the distal tubule. This effect may be more common in elderly patients, even those with normal renal function. This potential increase in potassium does not preclude the use of TMP–SMX in the elderly with comorbidities, but does show that the drug should be used judiciously.

Trimethoprim is highly selective for nonhuman dihyrofolate reductase. Estimates are that 50,000 to 100,000 times the normal dose of trimethoprim would be required to inhibit human dihydrofolate reductase (16). Given this selectivity, disturbances in human folate metabolism with the use of trimethoprim should not occur.

Sulfonamides are generally blamed for the variety of hematologic side effects (also rare) seen with TMP–SMX therapy. All types of cytopenias have been described, the rates of which are similar with TMP–SMX as with other sulfonamides. As mentioned previously, the very rare fatal hematologic reactions may be more common in the elderly, but the incidence does not rise to the level to warrant routine testing of blood counts during short courses of therapy.

Interestingly, delirium and psychosis have also been reported with TMP–SMX, especially in the elderly.

As mentioned previously, adverse reactions are more common in patients with immunosuppression, particularly those with AIDS. Hypersensitivity reactions are especially common. Such reactions generally include a rash and fever starting about a week after initiation of treatment. Other reactions, not hypersensitivity reactions, also occur more frequently in those with AIDS, including aseptic meningitis and liver enzyme abnormalities.

6.1. Drug Interactions

TMP–SMX interacts with a number of medications. Drug interactions are of particular concern in the elderly where polypharmacy is common. Importantly, sulfonamides may potentiate the anticoagulant effect of warfarin; trimethoprim may increase serum levels of digoxin; sulfamethoxazole may potentiate the effects of sulfonylureas; and trimethoprim can increase serum levels of procainamide and its metabolite, N acetyl procainamide. As mentioned earlier, TMP–SMX can rarely cause hyperkalemia, an effect that can be exacerbated by the use of angiotensin-converting enzyme (ACE) inhibitors and angiotensin II receptor blockers (ARBs) (17). This effect may occur more commonly in the elderly, the same population more likely to be on ACE inhibitors or ARBs for congestive heart failure, hypertension, and nephropathy.

In contrast to the real potential for hyperkalemia, trimethoprim decreases tubular secretion of creatinine and therefore may falsely elevate serum creatinine levels, without truly increasing the creatinine clearance (18). This may lead to the unnecessary discontinuation of the drug or an exaggerated fear of its use, particularly in the elderly with pre-existing mild elevations in serum creatinine.

7. DESENSITIZATION

For patients allergic to TMP–SMX, there is a method of rapid oral desensitization. It requires use of an oral suspension. At hour 0, 0.004/0.02 mg of TMP–SMX is given. For hours 1–4, the dose is increased by ten times each hour. At hour 5, the equivalent of one double-strength tablet is given.

8. CONCLUSION

The usefulness of TMP–SMX has been severely curtailed by resistance. However, the drug remains useful in a variety of infections in elderly patients. In the elderly, one must be aware of a number of factors when prescribing TMP–SMX. The dose must be adjusted for renal function, there are a number of important drug interactions, and certain side effects may be more prevalent or problematic.

REFERENCES

1. Carithers HA. The first use of an antibiotic in America. Am J Dis Child 1974; 128: 207–211.
2. Norrby SR. Folate inhibitors. In: Cohen J, Powderly WG, eds. Infectious Diseases. 2nd ed. Amsterdam: Elsevier, 2004:1819–1825.
3. Mandell G, Sande M. Antimicrobial agents. In: Gilman AG, Rall TW, Nies AS, Taylor P, eds. Goodman and Gilman's, The Pharmacological Basis of Therapeutics. 8th ed. Elmsford, New York: Pergamon Press, Inc., 1990:1047–1057.
4. Hoban DJ, Doern GV, Fluit AC, Roussel-Delvallez M, Jones RN. Worldwide prevalence of antimicrobial resistance in *Streptococcus pneumoniae*, *Haemophilus influenzae*, and *Moraxella catarrhalis* in the SENTRY Antimicrobial Surveillance Program, 1997–1999. Clin Infect Dis 2001; 32(suppl):S81–S93.
5. Masters PA, O'Bryan TA, Zurlo J, Miller DQ, Joshi N. Trimethoprim–sulfamethoxazole revisited. Arch Intern Med 2003; 163:402–410.
6. Bushby SRM. Trimethoprim–sulfamethoxazole: in vitro microbiological aspects. J Infect Dis 1973; 128(suppl):S442–S462.
7. Warren JW, Abrutyn E, Hebel JR, Johnson JR, Schaeffer AJ, Stamm WE, for the Infectious Diseases Society of America. Guidelines for antimicrobial treatment of uncomplicated acute bacterial cystitis and acute pyelonephritis in women. Clin Infect Dis 1999; 29:745–758.

8. Gupta K, Hooten TM, Stamm WE. Increasing antimicrobial resistance and the management of uncomplicated community-acquired urinary tract infections. Ann Intern Med 2001; 135:41–50.

9. Niederman MS, Mandell LA, Anzueto A, Bass JB, Broughton WA, Campbell GD, Dean N, File T, Fine MJ, Gross PA, Martinez F, Marrie TJ, Plouffe JF, Ramirez J, Sarosi GA, Torres A, Wilson R, Yu VL, for the American Thoracic Society. Guidelines for the management of adults with community-acquired pneumonia: diagnosis, assessment of severity, antimicrobial therapy, and prevention. Am J Respir Crit Care Med 2001; 163:1730–1754.

10. Bartlett JG, Dowell SF, Mandell LA, File TMJ, Musher DM, Fine MJ. Practice guidelines for the management of community-acquired pneumonia in adults. Clin Infect Dis 2000; 31:347–382.

11. Huovinen P. Resistance to trimethoprim–sulfamethoxazole. Clin Infect Dis 2001; 32: 1608–1614.

12. Markowitz N, Quinn EL, Saravolatz LD. Trimethoprim–sulfamethoxazole compared with vancomycin for the treatment of *Staphylococcus aureus* infection. Ann Intern Med 1992; 117:390–398.

13. Klein NC, Duncanson FP, Lenox TH, Forszpaniak C, Sherer CB, Quentzel H, Nunez M, Suarez M, Kawwaff O, Pitta-Alvarez A. Trimethoprim–sulfamethoxazole versus pentamidine for *Pneumocystis carinii* pneumonia in AIDS patients: results of a large prospective randomized treatment trial. AIDS 1992; 6:301–305.

14. Lawson DH, Paice BJ. Adverse reactions to trimethoprim–sulfamethoxazole. Rev Infect Dis 1982; 4:429–433.

15. Fresch JM. Clinical experience with adverse reactions to trimethoprim–sulfamethoxazole. J Infect Dis 1973; 128(suppl):607–611.

16. Zinner SH, Mayer KH. Sulfonamides and trimethoprim. In: In: Mandell GL, Bennett JE, Dolin R, eds. Mandell, Douglas and Bennett's Principles and Practice of Infectious Diseases, 6th ed., Philadelphia, PA: Churchill Livingstone, 2005:440–451.

17. Marinella M. Trimethoprim-induced hyperkalemia: an analysis of reported cases. Gerontology 1999; 45:209–212.

18. Ducharme M, Smythe M, Strohs G. Drug-induced alterations in serum creatinine concentrations. Ann Pharmacother 1993; 27:622–633.

SUGGESTED READING

Mandell G, Sande M. Antimicrobial agents. In: Gilman AG, Rall TW, Nies AS, Taylor P, eds. Goodman and Gilman's, The Pharmacological Basis of Therapeutics. 8th ed. Elmsford, New York: Pergamon Press, Inc., 1990:1047–1057.

Masters PA, O'Bryan TA, Zurlo J, Miller DQ, Joshi N. Trimethoprim–sulfamethoxazole revisited. Arch Intern Med 2003; 163:402–410.

Norrby SR. Folate inhibitors. In: Cohen J, Powderly WG, eds. Infectious Diseases. 2nd ed. New York: Mosby, 2004:1819–1825.

Zinner SH, Mayer KH. Sulfonamides and trimethoprim. In: In: Mandell GL, Bennett JE, Dolin R, eds. Mandell, Douglas and Bennett's Principles and Practice of Infectious Diseases,
6th ed., Philadelphia, PA: Churchill Livingstone, 2005:440–451.

21
Nitrofurans

Sunil Singhania and Thomas T. Yoshikawa
Department of Internal Medicine, Charles R. Drew University of Medicine and Science, Martin Luther King, Jr.–Charles R. Drew Medical Center, Los Angeles, California, U.S.A.

Key Points:

- Nitrofurantoin is prescribed almost exclusively for the treatment of lower urinary tract infection (UTI).
- The antimicrobial spectrum of the drug is primarily gram-negative bacilli; *Proteus* spp. and *Pseudomonas aeruginosa* are generally resistant to nitrofurantoin.
- The standard dose for uncomplicated lower UTI for elderly patients is 100 mg twice a day.
- Nitrofurantoin should not be prescribed for upper UTI or in patients with serum creatinine of less than 60 mL/min.
- Serious adverse effects of the drug include acute pulmonary hypersensitivity reaction (usually reversible with drug discontinuation), hepatic toxicity, and chronic pulmonary fibrosis (usually irreversible).

For nearly 50 years, nitrofurantoin has been used for the treatment of bacterial infections, specifically urinary tract infections (UTIs). During those years, nitrofurantoin was used for the treatment of acute cystitis and prophylactic treatment in the prevention of recurrent UTI in women. This antimicrobial agent accounts for more than 130 million courses of therapy in the United States alone (1). Worldwide, nitrofurantoin has been prescribed more than 220 million times (2). During that time, this drug has maintained its effectiveness with a limited side-effect profile. Given its long history, nitrofurantoin has been well studied and has developed a unique niche in the treatment of UTIs.

1. CHEMISTRY AND MECHANISM OF ACTION

Since it has a long track record of use, the pharmacokinetics of nitrofurantoin has been well documented. Nitrofurantoin is a synthetic, antibacterial agent specific to the urinary tract. It is a nitrofuran derivative, *N*-(5-nitro-2-furfuryliden)-1-amino-hydantoin, that is only slightly water soluble (Fig. 1). However, it is highly soluble in urine, occasionally imparting a brown color to urine.

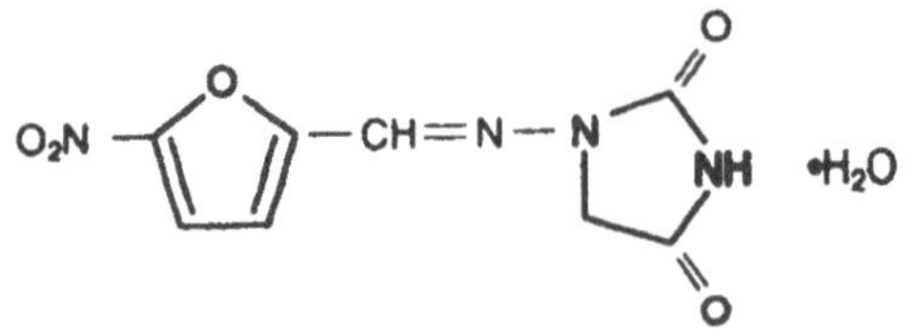

Molecular Weight: 256.17

Figure 1 Chemical structure of nitrofurantoin. *Source*: Adapted from Ref. 3.

Nitrofurantoin is bactericidal in urine at therapeutic doses. The mechanism of action, although not fully understood, involves the use of bacterial flavoproteins. The drug is reduced by the flavoproteins to reactive intermediates, which incapacitates the bacterial ribosomal proteins. The vital biochemical processes of the bacteria, including DNA synthesis, RNA synthesis, protein synthesis, cell wall synthesis, and aerobic energy metabolism are disrupted. Unlike other antibiotics that inhibit one specific process, nitrofurantoin affects several different processes of bacterial duplication. It has been suggested that because of the broad-based nature of the mechanism of action, this drug has met minimal resistance. Indeed, an antibiotic that has been in use for 50 years should have a higher propensity toward resistance. However, there is little evidence of significant resistance despite the abundant use of this antibiotic, making it a formidable choice in cases of acute and recurrent UTI.

2. CLINICAL PHARMACOLOGY

Nitrofurantoin is readily absorbed from the gastrointestinal tract. After ingestion, drug absorption occurs mainly in the small intestine. When nitrofurantoin is taken with food, absorption is delayed. Delayed gastric emptying leads to increased absorption of the drug. When nitrofurantoin is administered with food, bioavailability of the drug increases by 40% (3). A newer form of the drug has a macrocrystalline form that has been available since 1968. This newer formulation, Macrodantin®, retards the absorption and reduces the central nervous system and gastrointestinal side effects (4).

Because of its affinity to the urinary tract, there is minimal plasma concentration of nitrofurantoin following ingestion. Following intake of a single dose of 100 mg of nitrofurantoin, peak concentrations in the plasma are less than 2 µg/mL. Therefore, the antibacterial activity in the plasma is negligible. The plasma half-life is ≈20 min in adults with normal renal function. Because excretion is primarily renal, the urinary concentrations are reduced with impaired renal function and the serum concentration may increase to toxic levels, leading to increased side effects. Peak urine concentrations of 50–150 µg/mL are observed within 30 min of a single dose of 100 mg of the drug as microcrystals (5).

3. ANTIMICROBIAL SPECTRUM

The antimicrobial spectrum of nitrofurantoin includes a variety of gram-positive and gram-negative bacteria; its minimal inhibitory concentration (MIC) is ≤32 µg/mL. However, because of its low plasma concentration (and also low levels in other body fluids and tissues) and high levels in urine, the drug is primarily useful for UTIs. Also, secondary superinfections are relatively infrequent with nitrofurantoin because of its low concentration in sites other than the urinary tract. Most enterobacteriaceae species except *Proteus* spp. and some *Klebscella* spp. are susceptible to the drug. *Pseudomonas aeruginosa* is resistant.

4. CLINICAL INDICATIONS AND ADMINISTRATION OF DRUG

Approximately one-fifth of women in the general population will experience an acute episode of UTI during their lifetime (6), which makes it the most common infection of women in their lifespan. UTIs account for more than eight million office visits in the United States (7). Because of the high prevalence of UTI, many antibiotics have been developed to resolve the problem of antibiotic-resistant uropathogens. Although these newer antibiotics may have broader antimicrobial susceptibility, they often have other disadvantages including increased side effects, higher costs, and higher rates of superinfection. For these reasons and nitrofurantoin's mechanism of action and low incidence of superinfection, nitrofurantoin has remained a useful therapeutic drug against specific uropathogens.

Nitrofurantoin is indicated for the treatment of uncomplicated acute cystitis involving the pathogens *Escherichia coli* and *Staphylococcus saprophyticus*. These two pathogens represent the two most common causes of acute cystitis in women whether in the inpatient or outpatient setting. Several studies have shown *E. coli* to be the primary urinary tract pathogen, accounting for 75–90% of uncomplicated UTIs (8). While this number does decrease to 50–70% in the elderly female population, it still remains the most significant pathogen to affect women of all ages (9). *S. saprophyticus* is one of the most common gram-positive pathogens in UTIs. It accounts for an additional 7–28% of all cases (10). This percentage may be higher in the elderly, especially in males. The difference is not well understood, but may have to do with poorer humoral response in the elderly and increasing resistance of pathogens in patients with recurrent UTI. The standard dose for nitrofurantoin for adults is 200 mg a day either as a single dose or as a divided dose (two to four times per day) depending on the preparation and clinical response. In young women with uncomplicated lower UTI, 3 days of treatment is generally recommended. For men, older patients or more complicated lower UTI, 7–10 days of therapy is preferred.

The choice of antibiotic in a UTI is determined by several factors including the culture and susceptibility of the infecting organism, severity of illness, presence of complication, patient tolerance, and cost. In the outpatient setting, urine cultures are no longer routinely performed on younger women, partially because of cost management and partially based on the narrow spectrum of antimicrobes causing acute cystitis. Typically, the recommended empirical antimicrobial regimen for treating acute uncomplicated bacterial cystitis in a young nonpregnant female is a 3-day course of double-strength trimethoprim–sulfamethoxazole (TMP–SMX). This recommendation is especially true when resistance rates to the empirical use of TMP–SMX are less than 10–20% (11). However, there has been significant new research showing an increasing antimicrobial resistance to TMP–SMX. In such cases, nitrofurantoin, along with other newer antimicrobial agents, has been used with a high success rate (see also chapter "Urinary Tract Infection").

Evidence for the ongoing occurrence of antimicrobial resistance is best seen in The Surveillance Network (TSN) Database—USA. TSN Database—USA assimilates antimicrobial susceptibility testing and patient demographic data from a network of hospitals in the United States (12). The susceptibility to antibiotics followed U.S. Food and Drug Administration approved testing methods and interpretation of the MICs followed the guidelines of the National Committee for Clinical Laboratory Standards. In a study performed by Karlowsky et al. (13), information from this database was analyzed for urinary *E. coli* isolates from female outpatients in 1998–2001. The results of their study are shown in Table 1, wherein it is clearly shown that, based on the susceptibility testing, nitrofurantoin had the highest susceptibility of the most common antimicrobials used in the outpatient setting. Furthermore, their study showed that nitrofurantoin had excellent susceptibility toward *E. coli* isolates that were resistant to TMP–SMX. Moreover, 96.3% of TMP–SMX-resistant isolates were susceptible to nitrofurantoin. This number decreased to 82.5% in ciprofloxacin-resistant isolates and 82.9% in levofloxacin-resistant isolates (13). Nevertheless, nitrofurantoin seems to have excellent susceptibility toward the most common uropathogen, making it a formidable choice as first-line therapy against this isolate.

Further evidence of this trend of resistance was seen in another study performed by Karlowsky et al. (14). This study used the 1998 SENTRY surveillance program, reporting on isolates of *E. coli* collected from 26 centers. The study was conducted to determine national, regional, and institutional in vitro susceptibilities for ampicillin, ciprofloxacin, nitrofurantoin, and TMP–SMX among urine isolates of *E. coli* from female outpatients from across the United States in 2001. The results of this study are shown in Figure 2.

When the scope of the isolates is broadened to include all uropathogens, the pattern of resistance follows a similar trend. One study looked at female patients with acute cystitis during 1992–1996 and excluded patients with a previous episode of acute cystitis in the same month, hospitalization in the 30 days preceding or subsequent to the visit date, or patients with diabetes mellitus. A total of 4342 urine isolates from 4082 patients were obtained. The cultures revealed the causative uropathogens to be *E. coli* (86%), *S. saprophyticus* (4%), *Proteus* species (3%), *Klebsiella* species (3%), and *Enterobacter* (1.4%) (14). The patterns of resistance are shown in Table 2. Here again, there is an increasing trend of resistance of all urinary isolates against TMP–SMX. Conversely, nitrofurantoin has excellent

Table 1 Antimicrobial Susceptibility Testing of Urinary *E. coli* Isolates from Female Outpatients in the United States, 1998–2001

Antimicrobial agent	No. of isolates with results	Susceptible	Intermediate	Resistant
TMP–SMX	416,342	82.4	0.1	17.5
Ampicillin	414,573	61.2	0.7	38.0
Nitrofurantoin	377,852	98.3	0.9	0.8
Ciprofloxacin	350,128	97.7	0.1	2.3
Levofloxacin	255,765	97.3	0.1	2.5
Norfloxacin	149,489	97.8	0.1	2.1
Ofloxacin	79,612	97.7	0.4	1.9
Nalidixic acid	91,005	96.5	<0.1	3.5

Source: Adapted from Ref. 13.

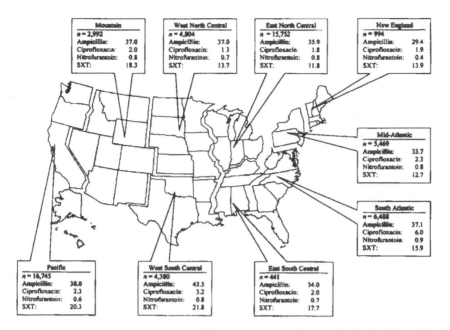

Figure 2 Antimicrobial resistances (%) among urinary isolates in *Escherichia coli* in the nine U.S. Bureau of the Census Regions in 2001. *Abbreviations*: SXT, sulfametheoxazole-trimethoprim. *Source*: Adapted from Ref. 14.

susceptibility against not just *E. coli*, but all isolates. This study did point out that a 3-day regimen was used in the case of TMP–SMX vs. a 7-day regimen of nitrofurantoin. Nevertheless, there is evidence for the use of nitrofurantoin as an empirical medication for acute cystitis in women.

According to the Infectious Diseases Society of America, when the TMP–SMX resistance among urinary pathogens isolated from female outpatients is ≥10–20%, alternative therapies for uncomplicated UTIs should be considered (11). All of these studies show an increasing resistance of *E. coli* and all uropathogens to TMP–SMX (15). More importantly, they show a continued high in vitro susceptibility to nitrofurantoin, even in cases that were resistant to TMP–SMX. Nitrofurantoin then becomes an adequate alternative therapy for uncomplicated cystitis in women when TMP–SMX cannot be used. An example of this might be in a patient who has allergy to sulfa drugs. In this case, fluoroquinolones have often been used, but nitrofurantoin may also be considered. When one additionally factors in that nitrofurantoin has a narrower tissue distribution, narrower spectrum of activity, limited contact with bacteria outside the urinary tract, and nearly undetectable serum concentrations, nitrofurantoin may prove to be an effective treatment in the face of emerging resistance.

4.1. Prophylactic Use

Over the years, nitrofurantoin has developed increasing popularity as a prophylactic drug for patients. Patients with recurrent UTIs, defined as either two or more infections within 6 months or three or more infections within 1 year, are often placed on long-term, low-dose prophylactic treatment. The ideal medication for prophylaxis

Table 2 Percentages of Urinary Isolates from Women with Acute Uncomplicated Cystitis Resistant to Selected Antimicrobial Agents

| | 1992 | | 1993 | | 1994 | | 1995 | | 1996 | |
	E. coli (n = 567)	All (n = 653)	E. coli (n = 931)	All (n = 1081)	E. coli (n = 967)	All (n = 1127)	E. coli (n = 691)	All (n = 807)	E. coli (n = 580)	All (n = 674)
Ampicillin[a]	26	29	29	32	31	33	32	34	34	38
Cephalothin[a]	20	20	25	24	38	37	32	32	28	28
Ciprofloxacin hydrochloride	0.2	0.3	0	0.2	0.1	1	0	0.3	0.2	0.3
Gentamicin	2	2	1	1	1	1	0.4	0.4	1	1
Nitrofurantoin	1	7	1	6	2	9	1	7	0.2	6
Sulfamethoxazole	22	21	25	24	26	24	25	22	27	26
Trimethoprim–sulfamethoxazole[a]	21	8	10	9	9	9	12	12	18	16
Trimethoprim[a]	9	9	10	9	10	9	12	12	18	16

Note: Percentages reflect the number of isolates with each antimicrobial agent; this may be less than the total number for each column. *E. coli* indicates *Escherichia coli.*
[a]There was a significant increasing linear trend in resistance from 1992 to 1996 for *E. coli* and all isolates: ampicillin ($p < 0.002$), cephalothin ($p < 0.001$), trimethoprim ($p < 0.001$), and trimethoprim–sulfamethoxazole ($p < 0.001$), using the χ^2 test for linear trend.
Source: Adapted from Ref. 15.

should be easily ingested, effective against typical pathogens, and well tolerated; have a limited side-effect profile; and be inexpensive. Given the long history of nitrofurantoin, this antimicrobial continues to be one of the most well-studied, time-tested treatment options for prophylaxis against UTI in all age groups.

Unlike in the treatment for acute cystitis, the dose of nitrofurantoin for prevention of UTI is usually a lower dose, i.e., 50 mg once a day, given at bedtime. Treatment periods last from 6 months to 1 year depending on the nature of the problem. Several studies have shown the effectiveness of nitrofurantoin in the prevention of recurrent UTIs. A study by Brumfitt and Hamilton-Miller (16) examined retrospectively all patients treated for recurrent UTIs over an 18-year period. In the study, the average length of time for prophylaxis was 9.9 months. Approximately 50% of patients had no symptomatic episodes during their period of prophylaxis (16). The findings showed that the patients on nitrofurantoin had a 5.4-fold reduction in the mean incidence of symptomatic episodes.

Based on the evaluation of this study and other studies, prophylactic use of nitrofurantoin should be for 12 months (17). Breakthrough infection is reduced when taking prophylactic nitrofurantoin for 1 year. Once-a-day dosing is not a significant factor in terms of compliance. Also, 89% patients who had an adverse reaction had it within the first month (16).

4.2. Special Considerations in the Elderly

Infections in the elderly have always been considered notoriously difficult to manage because of atypical clinical presentation, increased morbidity and mortality, increased rate of recurrence, and increased side-effect profile of treatments. With UTIs in the elderly the problem is complicated by the high prevalence of asymptomatic bacteriuria and a wider variety of uropathogens. All of these aspects of UTIs in the elderly affect clinical management in these specialized patients (see also chapter "Urinary Tract Infection").

As in younger patients E. coli is the most common uropathogen in the elderly. However, studies show that this microbe is the cause of a UTI in only 50–70% of the time in elderly patients (18). Elderly patients are more likely to experience other uropathogens, such as enterobacteriaceae, enterococci, and staphylococci. The diversity of uropathogens mandates that urine cultures be obtained in all older persons with suspected UTI. In such cases, TMP–SMX is still typically given, but at longer periods of time. Given the higher rates of resistance that do exist, the elderly may also benefit from the use of nitrofurantoin. Again, nitrofurantoin has a much lower rate of resistance than TMP–SMX, even in the elderly populations. A 10-day course for elderly should be considered (vs. a 7-day course for younger patients) because of the relatively high rates of failure and relapse. Cure of the infection is defined as resolution of the symptoms (e.g., dysuria, fever) and sterilization of the urine. However, if there are signs of upper urinary tract infection such as flank tenderness or fever >101°F, nitrofurantoin is not recommended.

One of the concerns for nitrofurantoin is the issue of renal clearance. Patients with anuria, oliguria, or significant impairment of renal function (creatinine clearance under 60 mL/min or clinically significant elevated serum creatinine) are contraindications for nitrofurantoin. Treatment in patients with renal impairment carries an increased risk of systemic toxicity, which could lead to a higher likelihood of significant side effects, including pneumonitis and hepatotoxicity. Given the fact that with age there is a physiological decrease in creatinine clearance, there must be some caution of the use of nitrofurantoin in elderly patients. This age-related change of creatinine clearance is best shown in the following formula:

$$\text{Creatinine clearance} = \frac{(140 - \text{age}) \times \text{weight (kg)}}{72 \times \text{serum creatinine}} \times (0.85 \text{ for women})$$

Serum creatinine alone is not a reliable measure of creatinine clearance because it is not only a function of the glomerular filtration rate but also of muscle mass. In an elderly patient, the serum creatinine may appear normal even in the presence of significant renal insufficiency. Given this information, if a typical 110 lb, 75-year-old female has a creatinine of 1.0 mg/dL, her creatinine clearance is 38 mL/min. Based on this calculated creatinine clearance and the contraindications previously explained, this patient would not be a candidate for nitrofurantoin. As with all medications, a physician must be especially concerned with the pharmacodynamics of the nitrofurantoin in older patients.

These concerns are amplified when considering the pharmacodynamics of nitrofurantoin in prophylactic therapies. Previously, it was established that the recommended length of therapy for prophylaxis against recurrent UTIs was 1 year. Given our understanding of the pharmacodynamics of drugs, it stands to reason that long-term therapy may have a higher likelihood of reaching toxic levels in an elderly patient. Indeed, as per the package insert, "spontaneous reports suggest a higher proportion of pulmonary reactions, including fatalities, in elderly patients; these differences appear to be related to the higher proportion of elderly patients receiving long-term therapy." The quote implies both that physicians prescribe long-term therapy to aging patients and that these patients are more likely to develop an adverse event. The insert did emphasize that no clinical studies of Macrobid® had sufficient numbers to indicate a clear difference between younger and older patients. One study concluded that older patients were not more likely to experience an adverse event than younger ones. In this study, adverse events in patients aged 65 years and older were 29% as compared with 38.3% in those less than 65 (16). Although the result was not significant, it does suggest nitrofurantoin is relatively safe for long-term therapy in carefully selected elderly patients. From the data, it seems that monitoring the serum creatinine in aging patients is important when making the decision of long-term use of nitrofurantoin.

In institutionalized patients, aspects of treatment with nitrofurantoin are magnified. Being that dementia is the number one cause of institutionalization of the elderly, communication is particularly difficult with these patients. They may be unable to express symptomatic complaints such as dysuria or foul odor. Furthermore, another one-half of these patients have some urinary incontinence. These debilitating syndromes make the assessment of UTI even more difficult in these patients. Moreover, the rates of bacteriuria in institutionalized patients are very high. In several reports from different developing countries, 17–55% of women and 15–31% of men are bacteriuric. Among incontinent patients, the prevalence rises to 50% for both men and women (19). These complicating factors make the diagnosis of UTI problematic and are why urinary infections remain the most frequent reason for prescribing antibiotics in long-term facilities.

Once the physician decides to treat an institutionalized patient with nitrofurantoin, the physician must be aware of its side effects. As in all elderly patients, having a baseline serum creatinine or creatinine clearance is important. Furthermore, the staff should be aware of clinical manifestations suggesting toxicity such as nausea or shortness of breath, remembering that many institutionalized patients cannot communicate typical complaints. The length of therapy of nitrofurantoin in institutionalized patients is controversial, but a 7–10-day course is usually appropriate. In the case of relapse of UTI, an evaluation for genitourinary abnormalities is indicated before even considering prophylactic therapy in this group (19).

5. DRUG MONITORING AND ADVERSE EFFECTS

Unlike newer medications, nitrofurantoin has a 50-year history, making it one of the oldest antibiotics. One of the advantages of a long history is a well-documented side-effect profile. As per the Physician's Desk Reference, the most common clinical adverse reactions reported are nausea (8%), headache (6%), and flatulence (1.5%) (3). More significant, but rarer adverse events include neuropathy, hemolytic anemia, hepatotoxicity, and pulmonary reactions. Older patients, particularly if there is a decline in renal function, are at higher risk for these side effects. In patients who have a creatinine clearance of less than 60 mL/min, nitrofurantoin is not recommended, because of the increased risk of toxicity. The macrocrystalline form of this medication retards absorption. When taken with food, absorption is improved by 40%. Both of these effects help reduce gastrointestinal side effects and should be recommended to all patients, including the elderly.

The unique pulmonary side effects caused by nitrofurantoin can be acute or chronic in nature. Acute pulmonary hypersensitivity reactions manifest as fever, eosinophilia, respiratory complaints, and pulmonary infiltrates or effusion. Such reactions are typically reversible and subside when the antimicrobial is discontinued. Chronic pulmonary reactions secondary to nitrofurantoin result in pulmonary fibrosis, which is usually nonreversible. These chronic reactions usually occur in patients receiving long-term nitrofurantoin therapy. Again, the elderly are at higher risk. Physicians should use such therapy in the elderly with caution, and educate the patient about the possible, although rare, adverse reactions of nitrofurantoin.

REFERENCES

1. Gait JE. Hemolytic reactions to nitrofurantoin in patients with glucose-6-phosphatase dehydrogenase deficiency: theory and practice. Drug Intell Clin Pharm 1990; 24: 1210–1213.
2. Prescription data. Data on file, Proctor & Gamble Pharmaceuticals..
3. Norwich Eaton Pharmaceuticals, Inc. Macrodantin (nitrofurantoin macocrystals) prescribing information. Physicians' Desk Reference. 46th ed. Montvale, NJ: Medical Economics Company Inc., 1992:1624–1625.
4. Simon C, Stille W, Wilkinson PJ. Antibiotic Therapy in Clinical Practice. 2nd ed. New York: Schattauer, 1993.
5. Conklin JD. The pharmacokinetics of nitrofurantoin and its related bioavailability. Antibiot Chemother 1978; 25:233–252.
6. Soman M, Faulkner S. Urinary tract infections. In: Havens C, Sullivan ND, Tilton P, eds. Manual of Outpatient Gynecology. Boston, MA: Little Brown & Co., 1986:197.
7. Karlowsky JA, Kelly LH, Thornsberry C, Jones ME, Sahm DF. Trends in antimicrobial resistance among urinary tract infection isolates of E. coli from female outpatients in the United States. Antimicrob Agents Chemother 2002; 46:2540–2545.
8. Nicolle LE. Epidemiology of urinary tract infection. Infect Med 2001; 18:153–162.

9. Nicolle LE. Urinary tract infection in the elderly. J Antimicrob Chemother 1994; 33(suppl A):99–107.
10. Latham RH, Running K, Stamm WE. Urinary tract infections in young women caused by *Staphylococcus saprophyticus*. J Am Med Assoc 1983; 250:3063–3066.
11. Warren JW, Abrutyn E, Hebel JR, Johnson JR, Schaeffer AJ, Stamm WE. Guidelines for antimicrobial treatment of uncomplicated acute bacterial cystitis and acute pyelonephritis in women. Clin Infect Dis 1999; 29:745–758.
12. Sahm DF, Marsilio MK, Piazza G. Antimicrobial resistance in key bloodstream bacterial isolates: electronic surveillance with The Surveillance Network Database—USA. Clin Infect Dis 1999; 29:259–263.
13. Karlowsky JA, Thornsberry C, Jones ME, Sahm DF. Susceptibility of antimicrobial-resistant urinary *E. coli* isolates to fluoroquinolones and nitrofurantoin. Clin Infect Dis 2003; 36:183–187.
14. Karlowsky JA, Kelly LH, Thornsberry C, Jones ME, Sahm DF. Trends in antimicrobial resistance among urinary tract infection isolates of *E. coli* from female outpatients in the United States. Antimicrob Agents Chemother 2002; 46:2540–2545.
15. Gupta K, Scholes D, Stamm WE. Increasing prevalence of antimicrobial resistance among uropathogens causing acute cystitis in women. J Am Med Assoc 1999; 281:736–738.
16. Brumfitt W, Hamilton-Miller JMT. Efficacy and safety profile of long-term nitrofurantoin in urinary infections: 18 years' experience. J Antimicrob Chemother 1998; 42: 363–371.
17. Harding GKM, Ronald AR. A controlled study of antimicrobial prophylaxis of recurrent urinary infection in women. N Engl J Med 1974; 291:597–601.
18. Nordenstam G, Sundh V, Lincoln K, Svanborg A, Eden CS. Bacteriuria in representative samples of persons aged 72–79 years. Am J Epidemiol 1989; 130:1176–1186.
19. Yoshikawa TT, Nicolle LE, Norman DC. Management of complicated urinary tract infections in older patients. J Am Geriatr Soc 1996; 44:1235–1241.

SUGGESTED READING

Brumfitt W, Hamilton-Miller MT. Efficacy and safety profile of long-term nitrofurontoin: 18 years experience. J Antimicrob Chemother 1998; 42:363–371.
Karlowsky JA, Kelly LH, Thornsberry C, Jones ME, Sahn DF. Trends in antimicrobial resistance among urinary tract infection isolates of *E. coli* from female outpatients in the United States.. Antimicrob Agents Chemother 2002; 46:2540–2545.

22

Oxazolidinones and Streptogramins

Stephen Marer and Shobita Rajagopalan
Department of Internal Medicine, Division of Infectious Diseases, Charles R. Drew University of Medicine and Science, Martin Luther King, Jr.–Charles R. Drew Medical Center, Los Angeles, California, U.S.A.

Key Points:

- Over the past 15 years, the incidence of resistant gram-positive infections has increased dramatically, highlighting the urgent need for the development of new antimicrobial agents to treat such infections.
- Oxazolidinones and streptogramins are antibiotics approved by the United States Food and Drug Administration (FDA) for the treatment of resistant gram-positive infections.
- Oxazolidinones belong to a new class of antibiotics with a unique mechanism of action. Linezolid, the only clinically available oxazolidinone, is approved for use in skin and skin-structure infections and pneumonia caused by resistant gram-positive bacteria, as well as infections caused by vancomycin-resistant *Enterococcus faecium* infections.
- Quinupristin and dalfopristin are the two streptogramin antibiotics available in a fixed ratio combination (Synercid®) for the treatment of vancomycin-resistant *E. faecium* infections and for skin and skin-structure infections.
- Linezolid is usually bacteriostatic, and quinupristin/dalfopristin is often bactericidal, but the clinical relevance of this pharmacodynamics is unknown. Whether either linezolid or quinupristin/dalfopristin will prove to be inferior, equivalent, or superior to vancomycin for the treatment of more serious infections (such as bacteremia, endocarditis, osteomyelitis, and meningitis) is yet to be elucidated.

1. INTRODUCTION

Antibiotic resistance among gram-positive bacteria is a rapidly growing problem. In the 1980s, methicillin-resistant *Staphylococcus aureus* (MRSA) became a widespread nosocomial pathogen (1). This was followed, in the 1990s, by an exponential increase in the incidence of vancomycin-resistant enterococci (VRE) (2). Throughout this period, drug-resistant *Streptococcus pneumoniae* (DRSP) spread worldwide (3). Unexpectedly, the rate of infections due to community-associated MRSA (CA-MRSA) has begun to increase dramatically in certain areas of the United States and in other parts of the world (4,5). Perhaps equally alarming is the threat of vancomycin-resistant *S. aureus* (VRSA): three such isolates have been discovered thus far in the United States (6).

Glycopeptides (vancomycin and teicoplanin) are no longer an adequate last line of defense against resistant gram-positive infections, for several reasons. First, as discussed earlier, many enterococci are now resistant to glycopeptides. Second, the impending and inevitable emergence of glycopeptide resistance in *S. aureus* is being observed. Third, glycopeptides may be inferior to β-lactam antibiotics for the treatment of certain serious gram-positive infections, such as *S. aureus* endocarditis (7). Fourth, some patients are unable to tolerate glycopeptides (2). Increasing reliance upon glycopeptides, therefore, will likely translate into increasing morbidity and mortality from severe gram-positive infections, as well as further adding to the selection pressure in favor of glycopeptide resistance in general. For these and other reasons, new antibiotics are urgently needed to address the growing threat of resistant gram-positive infections.

The oxazolidinones and streptogramins are two classes of antibiotics that now offer alternatives to glycopeptides for the treatment of gram-positive infections. Thus far, only one agent from each class has been marketed in the United States (Synercid, from the class of streptogramins, is actually a fixed-dose combination of two streptogramins).

In phase III trials, these agents have demonstrated equivalent efficacy, compared with vancomycin, in treating skin and soft tissue infections (SSTI), VRE infections, and certain types of pneumonia (8). The efficacy of these agents in comparison with glycopeptides for a variety of other types of infections is yet unclear.

Elderly patients (both community dwelling and institutionalized) with comorbid illnesses (e.g., diabetes mellitus, cerebrovascular accidents, and pressure ulcers) and common geriatric syndromes (e.g., dementia, falls, urinary incontinence, and frailty) are at particular risk for resistant gram-positive infections. This enhanced risk for resistant gram-positive infections may occur in part as a consequence relative to age-related decline in immune function. In addition, the use of repeated courses of antibiotics to treat genitourinary, respiratory, and SSTI results in the increased potential for selection, colonization, and subsequent infection with these resistant bacteria. This chapter will describe the historical perspective, mechanism of action, antimicrobial spectrum, pharmacokinetics, adverse reactions, and clinical indications of the oxazolidinones and streptogramins with particular emphasis on the elderly. Table 1 provides a general summary comparing the two drugs.

2. HISTORICAL PERSPECTIVES

2.1. Oxazolidinones

The oxazolidinones are a new class of completely synthetic antibiotics. Originally developed as monoamine oxidase (MAO) inhibitors for the treatment of depression, oxazolidinones were later discovered to have antimicrobial activity. In the 1970s, E.I. DuPont de Nemours and Company developed several oxazolidinones for use against microbial infections, initially involving plants. DuPont was successful in producing compounds that had in vitro activity against gram-positive bacteria, some anaerobes, and *Mycobacterium tuberculosis*. One such compound, however, demonstrated lethal activity in animal models, prompting DuPont to abandon further investigation into the oxazolidinones (9).

Upjohn Laboratories then began work on the oxazolidinones, which led to the discovery of two agents, linezolid and eperezolid. Only linezolid was developed clinically because of its superior pharmacokinetics. Linezolid was released in the

Table 1 General Comparisons: Linezolid vs. Quinupristin/Dalfopristin

	Linezolid	Quinupristin/dalfopristin
Principal clinical indications	Resistant gram-positive organisms	Resistant gram-positive organisms
Route of administration	Oral/IV	IV only
Mechanism of action	Ribosomal inhibition	Ribosomal inhibition
Dosing	600 mg twice a day	7.5 mg/kg two to three times/day
Hepatic adjustment	No	Debatable
Renal adjustment	No, but dose adjustment	No
Advantages	Better tolerated with oral bioavailability, more approved indications, and no cross-resistance with other antibiotic classes	Possibly bactericidal and apparent lack of severe or long-term toxicities
Disadvantages	Potential severe toxicities with long-term use central line	Poorly tolerated, no oral form, and requires central line

United States market in 2000. To date, it is the only oxazolidinone antibiotic in clinical use. It is currently marketed by Pfizer under the trade name Zyvox.

2.2. Streptogramins

Streptogramins are antibiotics produced in nature by *Streptomyces pristinaepiralis*. They belong to the antibiotic family of macrolides–lincosamides–streptogramins (10). The streptogramin pristinamycin has been available in Europe for over 25 years for the treatment of gram-positive infections. Because it is water insoluble, it is available only for oral administration. Quinupristin and dalfopristin are both streptogramins that are derived from pristinamycin. Quinupristin is derived from pristinamycin IA, a type B streptogramin. Dalfopristin is derived from pristinamycin IIB, a type A streptogramin. The fixed-ratio 30:70 combination of quinupristin/dalfopristin is now marketed under the trade name Synercid. Because quinupristin and dalfopristin are water-soluble derivatives of pristinamycin, Synercid can be given only by the intravenous (IV) route. Synercid was released in the United States in 1999. For gram-positive organisms, it has essentially the same spectrum of activity as linezolid (with the exception of *E. faecalis*, which is generally resistant to quinupristin/dalfopristin, but sensitive to linezolid), but has fewer approved indications for use.

3. MECHANISM OF ACTION

3.1. Oxazolidinones

Oxazolidinones are protein synthesis inhibitors with a unique mechanism of action. Like certain other protein synthesis inhibitors, including streptogramins, they bind to the 50S ribosome subunit. However, unlike other antibiotics, oxazolidinones block assembly of the initiation complex, thereby preventing the translation of mRNA. Protein synthesis is thus inhibited prior to initiation (11). Other protein synthesis inhibitors, such as lincosamides, tetracyclines, and macrolides, allow mRNA translation to begin but then inhibit peptide elongation. It is widely assumed that the unique action of oxazolidinones precludes cross-resistance with other antibiotics in current use. To date, in fact, there has been no evidence of cross-resistance between linezolid and other antibiotic classes. Additionally, some have speculated that oxazolidinones, by virtue of preventing the translation of mRNA, may be more effective than other protein synthesis inhibitors in preventing the synthesis of certain virulence factors (9).

Like most protein synthesis inhibitors, linezolid is considered primarily bacteriostatic, although it can exhibit bactericidal activity against some bacteria, such as streptococci (including pneumococci) and *Bacteroides fragilis* (9,11). Despite the theoretical disadvantage of bacteriostatic agents compared with bactericidal antibiotics, linezolid has proved as effective as vancomycin in treating several types of infections. Notably, a few cases of infective endocarditis have been treated successfully with linezolid (described in case reports and in the results of compassionate use trials), an infection where bactericidal activity is generally considered mandatory (12). The successful treatment of some cases of infective endocarditis with linezolid should serve as a reminder that the clinical relevance of whether any particular agent is bacteriostatic or bactericidal can be a matter of debate (13). Quinupristin/dalfopristin has also been used, with varying success, in the treatment of infective endocarditis (7).

Linezolid may have a modest postantibiotic effect against certain organisms, but this is unlikely to be important given the fact that, with standard dosing, serum drug levels tend to remain above the minimum inhibitory concentration (MIC) throughout most of the dosing interval (11).

3.2. Quinupristin/Dalfopristin

Quinupristin and dalfopristin, like linezolid, bind to the 50S ribosomal subunit. Unlike linezolid, the two streptogramins inhibit protein synthesis after it begins (2,10). Dalfopristin blocks an early step in protein synthesis, interfering with peptidyl transferase. Quinupristin blocks a later step in the process, preventing the elongation of the peptide chain and causing the release of incomplete chains.

Separately, quinupristin and dalfopristin are generally bacteriostatic. However, the combination, i.e., Synercid, is synergistic and sometimes bactericidal against gram-positive organisms (hence the name Synercid: "synergy" and "cidal"). In addition, quinupristin/dalfopristin sometimes exhibits in vitro synergy in combination with a variety of other antibiotics for certain bacteria (2). In the future, given these in vitro phenomena, quinupristin/dalfopristin might be used in combination with other antibiotics to manage difficult to treat infections. Quinupristin/dalfopristin does have a postantibiotic effect that may have clinical importance.

4. ANTIMICROBIAL SPECTRUM

Linezolid and quinupristin/dalfopristin are primarily used for the treatment of gram-positive infections. The gram-positive organisms of primary clinical interest are staphylococci, streptococci (including pneumococci), and enterococci (Table 2). Both linezolid and quinupristin/dalfopristin are active in vitro against most of these organisms, sharing essentially the same antimicrobial spectrum for gram-positive bacteria. Bacteria that are susceptible to both agents include methicillin-sensitive *S. aureus* (MSSA), MRSA, glycopeptide-intermediate *S. aureus*, vancomycin-susceptible

Table 2 Pathogens Usually Susceptible In Vitro to Linezolid and Quinupristin/Dalfopristin

Coagulase-negative staphylococci
Methicillin-sensitive *Staphylococcus aureus*
Methicillin-resistant *S. aureus*
Glycopeptide-intermediate *S. aureus*
Streptococcus pneumoniae
S. pneumoniae
S. agalactiae
Enterococcus faecium
E. faecalis (linezolid only)

and vancomycin-resistant *E. faecium*, coagulase-negative staphylococci (CNS), and penicillin-susceptible and penicillin-resistant *S. pneumoniae* (2). *E. faecalis* is generally resistant to quinupristin/dalfopristin, due to efflux pumps, but sensitive to linezolid.

Both agents have in vitro activity against a variety of other organisms, including *Legionella* species, *Listeria monocytogenes*, *Neisseria* species, *Moraxella catarrhalis*, *Corynebacterium jeikeium*, and some *Clostridium* species (7). Quinupristin/dalfopristin has demonstrated in vitro activity against *Mycoplasma* species and *Chlamydia pneumoniae*. Linezolid also has good in vitro activity against *Nocardia* species, certain anaerobes, some *Pasturella* species, and has variable activity against *Haemophilus influenzae*. A variety of *Mycobacterium* species, including *M. tuberculosis*, demonstrate in vitro susceptibility to linezolid as well. Gram-negative organisms are generally resistant to linezolid and quinupristin/dalfopristin, due to endogenous efflux pumps.

For the most part, the clinical utility of linezolid and quinupristin/dalfopristin against all but gram-positive organisms remains speculative, despite in vitro susceptibilities. It should be noted, however, that there have been case reports of successful treatment, with linezolid, of tuberculosis, nontuberculous *Mycobacterium* infections, and nocardiosis (7).

4.1. Resistance

Thus far, resistance to linezolid and quinupristin/dalfopristin has been rare among gram-positive organisms. No cross-resistance between other protein synthesis inhibitors and linezolid has been described, as had been predicted by virtue of linezolid's unique mechanism of action. Gram-positive bacteria with de novo resistance to both linezolid and quinupristin/dalfopristin have been described. This has more frequently been the case with quinupristin/dalfopristin, probably because of streptogramin use in livestock in certain parts of the world. More important, it is possible to generate resistance to both linezolid and quinupristin/dalfopristin in the laboratory, and the emergence of resistance to both agents has also occurred in vivo during therapy. The emergence of resistant isolates during therapy can be associated with treatment failure. For linezolid, the emergence of resistance has been more common in enterococci than in staphylococci (11). The mechanism of resistance against linezolid appears to involve mutations in the 23S portion of the ribosomal RNA, which lies within the 50S subunit. The change in the 23S ribosomal RNA presumably alters the oxazolidinone binding site. Clinical conditions that increase the risk of the development of resistant strains include prolonged therapy, sequestered sites of infection, and device-related infections.

There are at least three mechanisms by which bacteria may become resistant to streptogramins. As is the case with linezolid, the most common mechanism is by alteration of the binding site on the 23S portion of the ribosome. Methylation of this area is associated with staphylococcal resistance to macrolides, lincosamides, and group B streptogramins (e.g., quinupristin). This mechanism does not affect group A streptogramins (e.g., dalfopristin), so Synercid may retain some activity against staphylococci despite the presence of group B streptogramin resistance (although the retained activity may be bacteriostatic in nature rather than bactericidal) (2,7).

Enzymatic degradation can produce resistance to quinupristin/dalfopristin. This may be seen in staphylococci or *E. faecium*. Finally, active efflux may confer resistance. As mentioned previously, this appears to be the primary mechanism by which *E. faecalis* is naturally resistant to quinupristin/dalfopristin. Strains of *E. faecium* and CNS may also become resistant via this mechanism.

5. CLINICAL PHARMACOLOGY

One major advantage of linezolid is its near-100% bioavailability, facilitating early transition from the parenteral to the oral form. Peak and trough serum concentrations are ≈18 and 4 µg/mL, respectively, with dosing of 600 mg every 12 hr. These serum concentrations are usually above the MIC for gram-positive organisms throughout most of the dosing interval. The serum half-life with parenteral administration is slightly shorter than with oral administration (4.5 vs. 5.5 hr), but similar area under the curve profiles are observed regardless of the route of administration. When taken with food, there is a minor reduction in peak concentration.

Linezolid is minimally protein bound (30%), with a large volume of distribution of up to 50 L. The drug achieves high concentrations in a variety of tissues, including lung, bone, soft tissues, and central nervous system (14,15). Approximately 30% of the drug is excreted unchanged in the urine, but there is some metabolism via nonenzymatic oxidation in serum and tissue. Two inactive carboxylic acid metabolites are produced by oxidation. Urinary and fecal excretion of inactive metabolites also occurs. Despite significant renal clearance of unchanged drug, there is no recommended dose adjustment for linezolid in those with severe renal impairment. The drug also does not require dose adjustment in elderly patients or for those with hepatic dysfunction. Hemodialysis removes linezolid and its metabolites, so it is suggested that the drug be administered following dialysis.

Quinupristin/dalfopristin is administered intravenously in a fixed ration of 30:70. The half-life of quinupristin is about 1 hr, and that of dalfopristin ≈30 min. However, quinupristin has two active metabolites and dalfopristin has one active metabolite. Additionally, as mentioned previously, there is a postantibiotic effect. This complex pharmacokinetic profile makes it difficult to estimate the effective half-life of Synercid.

Protein binding of quinupristin is over 50%, while protein binding for dalfopristin is between 11% and 26%. Quinupristin/dalfopristin is metabolized in the liver and undergoes biliary excretion. There is no recommended dosing change for patients with renal insufficiency. Some advocate decreasing the dosing frequency for patients with significant liver disease, but there is as yet no firm consensus on this issue (2,7). There is no recommended dose adjustment for elderly patients.

6.   CLINICAL INDICATIONS

6.1.   Skin and Skin-Structure Infections

Table 3 summarizes the FDA-approved indication for these drugs.

Both linezolid and quinupristin/dalfopristin are indicated for the treatment of complicated skin and skin-structure infections (SSSIs), having shown equivalence to a variety of comparator antibiotics in a number of randomized trials (8,9). Quinupristin/dalfopristin is not FDA-approved for MRSA SSSIs, but the available data suggest equivalence to vancomycin in treating such infections (16). Linezolid has also shown equivalence with ampicillin–sulbactam (in one randomized trial) in treating diabetic foot infections (without concomitant osteomyelitis) (17). Arguably, this was a somewhat curious result given the polymicrobial nature of many diabetic foot infections.

6.2.   Nosocomial Pneumonia

Linezolid is approved for use in treating nosocomial pneumonia caused by susceptible pathogens, including MRSA and DRSP. In fact, one posthoc analysis of two trials argues that linezolid is superior to vancomycin in treating MRSA nosocomial pneumonia (18). This conclusion, however, has not been universally accepted.

Quinupristin/dalfopristin is not FDA-approved for treating nosocomial pneumonia, although there are data to suggest equivalence with vancomycin in treating staphylococcal nosocomial pneumonia (19).

6.3.   Vancomycin-Resistant Enterococcal Infections

Linezolid and quinupristin/dalfopristin are both FDA-approved for use in vancomycin-resistant E. faecium infections. Vancomycin-resistant E. faecalis isolates are almost universally susceptible in vitro to linezolid, but the drug is not FDA-approved for treating vancomycin-resistant E. faecalis infections because of the fact that nearly all of the enterococcal isolates involved in clinical trials have been E. faecium.

Table 3   FDA-Approved Indications

Linezolid	Quinupristin/dalfopristin
Complicated SSSIs (from MRSA, MSSA, S. pyogenes, and group B streptococci)	Complicated SSSIs (from MSSA or S. pyogenes) Serious or life-threatening E. faecium infections (including bacteremia)
Diabetic foot infections (from the same organisms listed earlier—without osteomyelitis)	
Serious or life-threatening E. faecium infections (including bacteremia)	
Nosocomial pneumonia (from MSSA, MRSA, S. pneumoniae, including MDRSP)	
Uncomplicated SSTIs (from MSSA or S. pyogenes)	

Abbreviations: FDA, Food and Drug Administration; SSSIs, skin and skin structure infections; MRSA, methicillin-resistant S. aureus; MSSA, methicillin sensitive S. aureus; MDRSP, multidrug-resistant S. pneumoniae.

Before linezolid and quinupristin/dalfopristin were available, there was no standard treatment for VRE infections. The trials that led to the approval of linezolid and quinupristin/dalfopristin for treating VRE infections were therefore, of necessity, open-label without any comparator drug. Each drug has had varying success for a number of different types of VRE infections, including bacteremia, osteomyelitis, endocarditis, and intra-abdominal infections. In a few case reports, linezolid was effective in treating central nervous system infections caused by VRE (20).

6.4. Community-Acquired Pneumonia

Among the two drugs, only linezolid is FDA-approved for treating community-acquired pneumonia (CAP). This approval is based on trials showing linezolid's efficacy of treating CAP caused primarily by susceptible strains of *S. pneumoniae*, although pooled data showed efficacy against DRSP as well. By the definition used in these trials, DRSP are resistant to two or more of the following antibiotics: penicillin, second-generation cephalosporins, macrolides, tetracycline, and trimethoprim–sulfamethoxazole. In these trials, no comparator regimen covered atypical pathogens, and there were no isolates resistant to the third-generation cephalosporins or extended-spectrum penicillins that are commonly used to treat pneumococcal pneumonia. Given these caveats, and given linezolid's inconsistent in vitro activity against atypical pathogens, one might conclude that linezolid does not yet have any obvious advantage over standard therapy in the treatment of CAP, despite its FDA-approved indication. One exception might be in the case of bacteremic pneumococcal pneumonia. In one CAP trial, the subset of bacteremic patients had a better outcome with linezolid than with the comparator drug (21). Regarding quinupristin/dalfopristin, there are no clinical data to support its use in CAP, although as discussed previously, quinupristin/dalfopristin has essentially the same in vitro activity as linezolid (against gram-positive pathogens), so it may well be effective in cases of CAP caused by gram-positive pathogens.

7. ADMINISTRATION OF DRUG

Quinupristin/dalfopristin is only available in the parenteral formulation. It should be administered in nonsaline solution and preferably using a central IV line. The standard dose is 7.5 mg/kg every 8 hr; data are not available to determine if dose adjustment is necessary for elderly patients. However, since a dose change is not recommended for moderate to severe renal failure or moderate hepatic insufficiency, the standard dose of this antibiotic for adults is most likely safe. Linezolid is available in both parenteral and oral preparations. The recommended adult dosage is 600 mg every 12 hr by either parenteral or oral route. Since the drug is eliminated primarily by hepatic metabolism and excretion, dose adjustment is not necessary for renal impairment.

8. DRUG MONITORING AND ADVERSE EFFECTS

8.1. Linezolid

The more commonly reported adverse effects of linezolid include gastrointestinal (GI) tract disturbances and thrombocytopenia. Thrombocytopenia appears to occur more frequently with prolonged use, therefore most authorities recommend weekly monitoring of the complete blood count for patients on linezolid. Linezolid can also cause leukopenia and anemia. Different mechanisms may be responsible for causing cytopenias in different cell lines. For example, one case report suggests an immune-mediated cause for thrombocytopenia, with myelosuppression implicated as the cause of anemia in the same patient (22). In general, the cytopenias have proven reversible, but the bulk of the experience has been with thrombocytopenia. It is interesting to note a small case series (two patients) in which the administration of vitamin B6 had apparently reversed or ameliorated cytopenias associated with long-term linezolid therapy for disseminated *Mycobacterium abscessus* (23). Whether the hematological side effects of linezolid occur more frequently in elderly patients, or other specific groups of patients, is unknown.

Apart from GI side effects and cytopenias, rash and tongue discoloration have been described with linezolid. Perhaps more ominous are reports of peripheral neuropathy and optic neuropathy with longer-term use of linezolid (24,25). Vitamin B_6 was not effective, in the case series described previously, in alleviating peripheral neuropathy (23). So far, there have been few reports of neuropathy, and the mechanisms to account for these neurological effects are unknown. As with the hematological side effects, it is not known whether neuropathies occur more frequently in elderly patients.

8.2. Quinupristin/Dalfopristin

The most bothersome side effects with quinupristin/dalfopristin are phlebitis, arthralgias, and myalgias. Synercid usually needs to be administered through a central venous catheter because of the frequent phlebitis seen when given through a peripheral line. At least 10% of patients (more in some series) experience arthralgias, myalgias, or both. In one study, one-third of the patients had to discontinue Synercid because of bothersome side effects. The mechanism underlying the musculoskeletal side effects of Synercid is unknown.

Other reported side effects include nausea, vomiting, diarrhea, rash, and abnormal liver function tests, i.e., increase in hepatic transaminases and bilirubin. As is true with linezolid, it is not known whether the elderly are more prone to the side effects of quinupristin/dalfopristin.

8.3. Drug Interactions

Quinupristin/dalfopristin inhibits the cytochrome P450 3A4 system, and therefore can increase the levels of a number of important medications. Among these are cyclosporine, quinidine, nifedipine, and certain 3-hydroxyl-3 methyl glutaryl coenzyme A reductase inhibitors (statins). Particular attention should be paid to those drugs metabolized by the P450 3A4 system that have the ability to prolong the QT interval on electrocardiogram. Such interactions are likely to be more problematic in elderly patients, because of polypharmacy and comorbidities (such as cardiomyopathies) that can increase the danger from drug interactions.

Linezolid is not known to affect drug levels in any significant way, but it does have a number of theoretically important drug interactions. Linezolid is a reversible nonselective inhibitor of monoamine oxidase (MAO), which raises the possibility of hypertension reactions and the serotonin syndrome. Pressor responses have been observed when the drug was administered with tyramine. Additionally,

Table 4 Problematic Side Effects/Interactions

Linezolid	Quinupristin/dalfopristin
Cytopenias (especially thrombocytopenia)	Phlebitis
Neuropathy	Arthralgias
Potential for pressor responses with pseudoephedrine or phenyl propanolanime, tyranime-rich foods	Increases levels of nifedipine, statins, quinidine, others
Potential for serotonin syndrome with serotoninergic agents (SSRIs, meperidine)	

Abbreviation: SSRIs, selective serotonin receptor inhibitors.

pseudoephedrine has been shown to induce a pressor response in healthy volunteers. Patients should therefore be advised to avoid tyramine-rich foods and to be cautious when using medications that contain pseudoephedrine. Along similar lines, the use of vasopressors along with linezolid could prove problematic, and must be undertaken with great care. There is no convincing body of evidence, thus far, to suggest that food and drug interactions with linezolid leading to hypertensive responses are more dangerous in the elderly population.

Initially, it was considered safe to use linezolid with serotonergic agents. However, since the release of linezolid, there have been case reports implicating the combination of selective serotonin receptor inhibitors (SSRIs) and linezolid in causing the serotonin syndrome (26). Physicians should therefore carefully weigh the risks and benefits before using linezolid with SSRIs or other agents (such as meperidine) known to have the ability to cause the serotonin syndrome with other MAO inhibitors. In fact, some authorities advocate discontinuation of SSRIs prior to starting linezolid therapy). It is not known whether the polypharmacy often seen in elderly patients could lead to a higher incidence of the serotonin syndrome when using linezolid in this population. Certainly, physicians must be very cautious to ask all patients, including seniors, about the use of any serotonergic drugs prior to prescribing linezolid.

Serotonergic drugs include not just SSRIs, but venlefaxine, trazodone, buspirone, chlomipramine and possibly other tricyclic antidepressants, and dextromethorphan. Additionally, meperidine should be strictly avoided, until more information is available, in patients taking linezolid. Table 4 summarizes side effects and drug interactions for linezolid and quinupristin/dalfopristin.

REFERENCES

1. Panlilio AL, Culver DH, Gaynes RP, Banerjee S, Henderson TS, Tolson JS, Martone WJ. Methicillin-resistant *Staphylococcus aureus* in U.S. hospitals, 1975–1991. Infect Control Hosp Epidemiol 1992; 13:582–586.
2. Rehm S. Two new treatment options for infections due to drug-resistant gram-positive cocci. Cleve Clin J Med 2002; 69:397–413.
3. Whitney CG, Farley MM, Hadler J, Harrison LH, Lexau C, Reingold A, Lefkowitz L, Cieslak PR, Cetron M, Zell ER, Jorgensen JH, Schuchat A. Active bacterial core surveillance program of emerging infections program network. Increasing prevalence of multi-drug-resistant *S. pneumoniae* in the United States. N Engl J Med 2000; 343:1917–1924.

4. Vandenesch F, Naimi T, Enright MC, Lina G, Nimmo GR, Heffernan H, Liassine N, Bes M, Greenland T, Reverdy ME, Etinne J. Community-acquired methicillin-resistant *Staphylococcus aureus* carrying Panton-Valentine leukocidin genes: worldwide emergence. Emerg Infect Dis 2003; 9:978–984.

5. Centers for Disease Control and Prevention. Community-associated methicillin-resistant *Staphylococcus aureus* infections in Pacific Islanders, Hawaii, 2001–2003. Morb Mort Wkly Rep 2004; 53:767–770.

6. Centers for Disease Control and Prevention. Brief report: vancomycin-resistant *Staphylococcus aureus*, New York, 2004. Morb Mort Wkly Rep 2004; 53:322–323.

7. Murray BE, Nannini EC. Glycopeptides (vancomycin and teicoplanin), streptogramins (quinupristin–dalfopristin), and lipopeptides (daptomycin). In: Mandell GL, Bennett JE, Dolin R, eds. Mandell, Douglas and Bennett's Principles and Practice of Infectious Diseases. 6th ed. Philadelphia, PA: Elsevier Churchill Livingstone Inc., 2005:417–434.

8. Eliopoulos GM. Quinupristin–dalfopristin and linezolid: evidence and opinion. Clin Infect Dis 2003; 36:473–481.

9. Moellering RC Jr. Linezolid: the first oxazolidinone antimicrobial. Ann Intern Med 2003; 138:135–142.

10. Manzella J. Quinupristin–dalfopristin: a new antibiotic for severe gram-positive infections. Am Fam Physician 2001; 64:1863–1866.

11. Livermore DM. Linezolid *in vitro*: mechanism and antibacterial spectrum. J Antimicrob Chemother 2003; 51(suppl S2):ii9–ii16.

12. Moise PA, Forrest A, Birmingham MC, Schentag JJ. The efficacy and safety of linezolid as treatment for *Staphylococcus aureus* infections in compassionate use patients who are intolerant of, or who have failed to respond to vancomycin. J Antimicrob Chemother 2002; 50:1017–1026.

13. Pankey GA, Sabath LD. Clinical relevance of bacteriostatic versus bactericidal mechanisms of action in the treatment of gram-positive bacterial infections. Clin Infect Dis 2004; 38:864–870.

14. Lovering AM, Zhang J, Bannister GC, Lankester BJ, Brown JH, Narenda G, MacGowan AP. Penetration of linezolid into bone, fat, muscle, and haematoma of patients undergoing routine hip replacement. J Antimicrob Chemother 2002; 50:73–77.

15. Villani P, Regazzi MG, Marubbi F, Viale P, Pagani L, Cristini F, Cadeo B, Carosi G, Bergomi R. Cerebrospinal fluid linezolid concentrations in postneurosurgical central nervous system infections. Antimicrob Agents Chemother 2002; 46:936–937.

16. Nichols RL, Graham DR, Barriere SL, Rodgers A, Wilson SE, Zervos M, Dunn DL, Kreter B. Treatment of hospitalized patients with complicated gram-positive skin and skin structure infections: two randomized, multicentre studies of quinupristin/dalfopristin versus cefazolin, oxacillin or vancomycin. J Antimicrob Chemother 1999; 44:263–273.

17. Lipsky BA, Itani K, Norden C, Linezolid Diabetic Foot Infections Study Group. Treating foot infections in diabetic patients: a randomized, multicenter, open-label trial of linezolid versus ampicillin-sulbactam/amoxicillin-clavulanate. Clin Infect Dis 2004; 38:17–24.

18. Wunderink RG, Rello J, Cammarata SK, Croos-Dabrera RV, Kollef MH. Linezolid vs vancomycin. Analysis of two double-blind studies of patients with methicillin-resistant *Staphylococcus aureus* nosocomial pneumonia. Chest 2003; 124:1789–1797.

19. Fagon J, Patrick H, Haas DW, Torres A, Gilbert C, Cheadle WG, Falcone RE, Anholm JD, Paganin F, Fabian TC, Lilienthal F. Treatment of gram-positive nosocomial pneumonia. Prospective randomized comparison of quinupristin/dalfopristin versus vancomycin. Nosocomial Pneumonia Group. Am J Respir Crit Care Med 2000; 161:753–762.

20. Steinmetz MP, Vogelbaum MA, De Georgia MA, Andrefsky JC, Isada C. Successful treatment of vancomycin-resistant enterococcus meningitis with linezolid: case report and review of the literature. Crit Care Med 2001; 29:2383–2385.

21. Batts DH, Kollef MH, Lipsky BA, Nicolau DP, Weigelt JA, eds. Creation of a Novel Class: The Oxazolidinone Antibiotics. Tampa, FL: Innova Institute for Medical Education, 2004.

22. Bernstein WB, Trotta RF, Rector JT, Tjaden JA, Barile AJ. Mechanisms for linezolid-induced anemia and thrombocytopenia. Ann Pharmacother 2003; 37:517–520.

23. Spellberg B, Yoo T, Bayer AS. Reversal of linezolid-associated cytopenias, but not peripheral neuropathy, by administration of vitamin B6. J Antimicrob Chemother 2004; 54:832–835.

24. Bressler AM, Zimmer SM, Gilmore JL, Somani J. Peripheral neuropathy associated with prolonged use of linezolid. Lancet Infect Dis 2004; 4:528–531.

25. Lee E, Burger S, Shah J, Melton C, Mullen M, Warren F, Press R. Linezolid-associated toxic optic neuropathy: a report of 2 cases. Clin Infect Dis 2003; 37:1389–1391.

26. Wigen CL, Goetz MB. Serotonin syndrome and linezolid. Clin Infect Dis 2002; 34: 1651–1652.

SUGGESTED READING

Batts DH, Kollef MH, Lipsky BA, Nicolau DP, Weigelt JA, eds. Creation of a Novel Class: The Oxazolidinone Antibiotics. Tampa, FL: Innova Institute for Medical Education, 2004.

Carbon CJ, Rubinstein E. Macrolides, ketolides, lincosamides, and streptogramins. In: Cohen J, Powderly W, eds. Infectious Diseases. 2nd ed. Philadelphia, PA: Elsevier Inc., 2004:1791–1803.

Donowitz GR. Oxazolidinones. In: Mandell GL, Bennett JE, Dolin R, eds. Mandell, Douglas and Bennett's Principles Practice of Infectious Diseases. 6th ed. Philadelphia, PA: Elsevier Churchill Livingstone Inc., 2005:436–440.

Lowy FD. Oxazolidinones. In: Cohen J, Powderly W, eds. Infectious Diseases. 2nd ed. Philadelphia, PA: Elsevier Inc., 2004:1805–1807.

Murray BE, Nannini EC. Glycopeptides (vancomycin and teicoplanin), streptogramins (quinupristin–dalfopristin), and lipopeptides (daptomycin). In: Mandell GL, Bennett JE, Dolin R, eds. Mandell, Douglas and Bennett's Principles and Practice of Infectious Diseases. 6th ed. Philadelphia, PA: Elsevier Churchill Livingstone Inc., 2005:417–434.

23
Antituberculous Drugs

Shobita Rajagopalan
*Department of Internal Medicine, Division of Infectious Diseases, Charles R. Drew
University of Medicine and Science, Martin Luther King, Jr.–Charles R. Drew Medical
Center, Los Angeles, California, U.S.A.*

Key Points:

- In the elderly, chemoprophylaxis and treatment regimens for tuberculosis (TB) are essentially the same as the regimens recommended for younger adults.
- Drugs used for chemoprophylaxis and treatment of TB are often not consistently instituted in the elderly even when indicated because of justifiable concerns regarding polypharmacy and adverse drug reactions.
- Severe and fatal hepatitis with the use of rifampin and pyrazinamide combination therapy recommended for latent TB infection has recently been documented; guidelines for latent TB treatment have been accordingly revised.
- Potential cure can readily be accomplished by careful monitoring for side effects of antituberculous pharmacotherapy.
- Updates from the official joint statement of the American Thoracic Society (ATS), Centers for Disease Control and Prevention (CDC), and the Infectious Diseases Society of America (IDSA) approved in October 2002 are highlighted.

As discussed in the chapter "Tuberculosis," the geriatric population, as a single age group, accounts for the largest reservoir of *Mycobacterium tuberculosis* (*Mtb*) infection, which is also referred to as latent tuberculosis (TB) (asymptomatic infection with potentially viable *Mtb* organisms). Symptomatic TB or TB disease in the elderly may present in an atypical manner with anorexia, chronic fatigue, cognitive impairment, prolonged low-grade fever, unexplained weight loss, loss of appetite, or decline in functional capacity (e.g., activities of daily living) (1). An especially aggressive approach to the prevention, diagnosis, and treatment of TB in older patients is essential to facilitate the national objective of elimination of this potentially curable disease (2).

The chemoprophylaxis and treatment regimens for individuals above 65 years and older are essentially the same as those for younger adults (3). Drug treatment of TB infection and disease is often withheld in the elderly even when indicated because of the legitimate concerns about polypharmacy and adverse drug reactions.

Treatment success can be readily accomplished by careful monitoring of potential drug side effects.

This chapter will review the most recent recommended pharmacotherapy for TB infection and disease provided by the official joint statement of the American Thoracic Society (ATS), the Centers for Disease Control and Prevention (CDC), and the Infectious Diseases Society of America (IDSA) approved in October 2002 (4). Information will also be provided on TB treatment monitoring with particular emphasis on aging.

1. PRINCIPLES OF ANTITUBERCULOUS CHEMOTHERAPY

Antituberculous (anti-TB) chemotherapy consists of three main principles upon which the treatment recommendations are based: (1) regimens for treatment of disease must contain multiple drugs to which the organisms are susceptible, (2) the drugs must be taken regularly, and (3) drug therapy must continue for a sufficient period of time. The goal of treatment must be to provide the safest and most effective therapy in the shortest time frame. There are a large variety of possible combinations of drugs and frequencies of administration. The potential for adverse reactions, particularly in elderly patients who are already burdened with polypharmacy, is an important consideration in selecting treatment regimens.

The first anti-TB drugs were developed in the 1940s. Clinical studies in the 1960s demonstrated that effective TB chemotherapy required the simultaneous use of at least two anti-TB agents. The concept of multidrug regimen for TB was later established consisting of an initial, intensive phase with at least three drugs, followed by a continuation phase of two drugs. The goal of the initial phase of treatment is to rapidly diminish the high bacillary load, thus interrupting transmission and reducing symptoms. A successful first phase of therapy will also prevent the selection of resistant mutants. Continued therapy during the second phase is intended to achieve cure and reduce relapses. Trials conducted in the United States confirmed the efficacy of intermittent regimens, which form the mainstay of current recommendations of the ATS, IDSA, and CDC (4).

Management of TB should combine clinical and public health efforts to deliver a comprehensive control service. All TB cases, diagnosed either in the private or public sectors, must be reported to the public health department. The public health department will monitor the patient's treatment adherence and outcome, conduct an investigation of the patient's contacts, educate patients and their contacts, perform disease surveillance (including drug resistance), and document disease trends.

2. CURRENTLY APPROVED ANTI-TB AGENTS

The anti-TB drugs that are currently approved by the United States Food and Drug Administration (FDA), their doses and adverse effects, are shown in Table 1 (4). In addition, the fluoroquinolones, although not approved by the FDA for TB, are used relatively commonly to treat drug-resistant TB or for patients who are intolerant of some of the first-line drugs. Rifabutin, approved for the prevention of *Mycobacterium avium* complex disease in patients with human immunodeficiency virus (HIV) infection but not approved for TB, is useful in patients concurrently taking drugs that have unacceptable interactions with other rifamycins. Amikacin

Table 1 Currently Approved Anti-TB Drugs in the United States with Doses and Adverse Effects Profile

Drug	Dose	Adverse effects
First-line antituberculosis drugs		
Isoniazid	5 mg/kg (300 mg) daily	Hepatitis, neurotoxicity
Rifampin	10 mg/kg (600 mg) daily	Cholestatic hepatitis, orange discoloration of body fluids, drug interactions
Pyrazinamide	15 mg/kg (1200 mg) daily	Hyperuricemia, skin rash, hepatitis
Ethambutol	15–20 mg/kg (100 mg) daily	Retrobulbar neuritis; decreased color vision
Ethionamide	15–20 mg/kg/day (1.0 g/day), usually 250–500 mg/day in a single daily dose or two divided doses	Gastrointestinal (GI), hepatotoxicity, neurotoxicity, endocrinopathy
Second-line antituberculosis drugs		
Streptomycin	1 g weekly intramuscularly	Nephrotoxicity and neurotoxicity
Amikacin and Kanamycin	15 mg/kg/day (1.0 g/day), intramuscular or intravenous	Ototoxicity and nephrotoxicity
Capreomycin	15–30 mg/kg (1 g/day) as a single daily or twice weekly dose	Nephrotoxicity and neurotoxicity
Paraamino salicylic acid	8–12 g daily in divided doses	Hepatotoxocity, GI intolerance, malabsorption, hypothyroidism, coagulopathy
Fluoroquinolones (levofloxacin used as an example)	500–1000 mg daily	GI, neurological, and cutaneous

Source: Modified from Ref. 44.

and kanamycin, nearly identical aminoglycoside drugs used in treating patients with TB caused by drug-resistant organisms, are not approved by the FDA for TB.

Of the approved drugs isoniazid (INH), rifampin (RIF), ethambutol (EMB), and pyrazinamide (PZA) are considered first-line anti-TB agents and form the core of initial treatment regimens. Rifabutin and rifapentine may also be considered first-line agents under the specific situations described. Streptomycin (SM) was formerly considered to be a first-line agent and, in some instances, is still used in initial treatment; however, an increasing prevalence of resistance to SM in various countries of the world has decreased its overall utility. The remaining drugs are reserved for special situations such as drug intolerance or resistance. Some details regarding the roles in treatment regimens and important adverse reactions of routinely used first-line agents will be highlighted, as follows.

2.1. First-Line Drugs

2.1.1. Isoniazid

INH is a first-line agent for treatment of all forms of TB caused by organisms known or presumed to be susceptible to the drug. It has profound early bactericidal activity against rapidly dividing cells.

Asymptomatic elevation of aminotransferases. Aminotransferase elevations up to five times the upper limit of normal occur in 10–20% of persons receiving INH alone for treatment of latent TB infection. The enzyme levels generally return to normal even with continued administration of the drug.

Clinical hepatitis. Data indicate that the incidence of clinical hepatitis is lower than was previously thought. Hepatitis occurred in only 0.1–0.15% of 11,141 persons receiving INH alone as treatment for latent TB infection in an urban TB control program (5). Prior studies suggested a higher rate, and a meta-analysis of six studies estimated the rate of clinical hepatitis in patients given INH alone to be 0.6% (6–8). In the meta-analysis the rate of clinical hepatitis was 1.6% when INH was given with other agents, not including RIF. The risk was higher when the drug was combined with RIF, an average of 2.7% in 19 reports (8). For INH alone the risk increases with increasing age; it is uncommon in persons <20 years of age but is nearly 2% in persons aged 50–64 years (6). The risk also may be increased in persons with underlying liver disease, in those with a history of heavy alcohol consumption.

Fatal hepatitis. A large survey estimated the rate of fatal hepatitis to be 0.023%, but more recent studies suggest the rate is substantially lower (9,10). Death has been associated with continued administration of INH despite onset of symptoms of hepatitis (11).

Peripheral neurotoxicity. This adverse effect is dose related and is uncommon (<0.2%) at conventional doses. The risk is increased in persons with other conditions that may be associated with neuropathy such as nutritional deficiency, diabetes mellitus, HIV infection, renal failure, and alcoholism. Pyridoxine supplementation (25 mg/day) is recommended for patients with these conditions to help prevent this neuropathy.

2.1.2. Rifampin

RIF is a first-line agent for treatment of all forms of TB. It has activity against organisms that are dividing rapidly (early bactericidal activity) and against semi-dormant bacterial populations, thus accounting for its sterilizing activity. RIF is an essential component of all short-course regimens.

2.2. Important Adverse Effects

Hepatotoxicity. Transient asymptomatic hyperbilirubinemia may occur in as many as 0.6% of patients receiving the drug. More severe clinical hepatitis that typically has a cholestatic pattern may also occur (8). Hepatitis is more common when the drug is given in combination with INH (2.7%) than when given alone (nearly 0%) or in combination with drugs other than INH (1.1%) (8).

Orange discoloration of bodily fluids (sputum, urine, sweat, and tears). This is a universal effect of the drug. Patients should be warned of this effect at the time treatment is begun. Soft contact lenses and clothing may be permanently stained.

Drug interactions due to induction of hepatic microsomal enzymes. There are a number of drug interactions with potentially serious consequences. Of particular concern are reductions, often to ineffective levels, in serum concentrations of common drugs, such as oral contraceptives, methadone, and warfarin. In addition there are important bidirectional interactions between rifamycins and antiretroviral agents. Because information regarding rifamycin drug interactions is evolving rapidly, readers are advised to consult the CDC website www.cdc.gov/nchstp/tb/ to obtain updated information.

2.2.1. Rifabutin

Rifabutin is used as a substitute for RIF in the treatment of TB caused by organisms known or presumed to be susceptible to this agent. The drug is generally reserved for patients who are receiving any medication having unacceptable interactions with RIF or have intolerance to RIF.

Uveitis. This is a rare (<0.01%) complication when the drug is given alone at a standard (300 mg daily) dose. The occurrence is higher (8%) with higher doses or when rifabutin is used in combination with macrolide antimicrobial agents that reduce its clearance (12). Uveitis may also occur with other drugs that reduce clearance such as protease inhibitors and azole antifungal agents.

Hepatotoxity. Asymptomatic elevation of liver enzymes has been reported at a frequency similar to that of RIF (12). Clinical hepatitis occurs in <1% of patients receiving the drug.

Orange discoloration of bodily fluids (sputum, urine, sweat, tears). This is a universal effect of the drug. Patients should be warned of this effect at the time treatment is begun. Soft contact lenses and clothing may be permanently stained.

2.2.2. Rifapentine

Rifapentine may be used once weekly with INH in the continuation phase of treatment for HIV-seronegative patients with noncavitary, drug-susceptible pulmonary tuberculosis who have negative sputum smears at completion of the initial phase of treatment (13).

The adverse effects of rifapentine are similar to those associated with RIF. Rifapentine is an inducer of multiple hepatic enzymes and therefore may increase metabolism of coadministered drugs that are metabolized by these enzymes

2.2.3. Pyrazinamide

Pyrazinamide (PZA) is a first-line agent for the treatment of all forms of tuberculosis caused by organisms with known or presumed susceptibility to the drug. The drug is believed to exert the greatest activity against the population of dormant or semi-dormant organisms contained within macrophages or the acidic environment of caseous foci (14).

Hepatotoxicity. Early studies using doses of 40–70 mg/kg/day reported high rates of hepatotoxicity. However, in treatment trials with multiple other drugs, including INH, liver toxicity has been rare at doses of 25 mg/kg/day or less (15). In one study, however, hepatotoxicity attributable to PZA used in standard doses occurred at a rate of about 1% (16).

Nongouty polyarthralgia. Polyarthralgias may occur in up to 40% of patients receiving daily doses of PZA. This rarely requires dosage adjustment or discontinuation of the drug (17). The pain usually responds to aspirin or other nonsteroidal anti-inflammatory agents. In clinical trials of PZA in the initial intensive phase of treatment, arthralgias were not noted to be a significant problem.

Asymptomatic hyperuricemia. This is an expected effect of the drug and is generally without adverse consequence.

Acute gouty arthritis. Acute gout is rare except in patients with preexisting gout, generally a contraindication to the use of the drug.

2.2.4. Ethambutol

Ethambutol (EMB) is a first-line drug for treating all forms of tuberculosis. It is included in initial treatment regimens primarily to prevent emergence of RIF resistance when primary resistance to INH may be present.

Retrobulbar neuritis. This is manifested as decreased visual acuity or decreased red-green color discrimination that may affect one or both eyes. The effect is dose related, with minimal risk at a daily dose of 15 mg/kg/day (18). No difference was found in the prevalence of decreased visual acuity between regimens that contained EMB at 15 mg/kg and those not containing the drug. The risk of optic toxicity is higher at higher doses given daily (18% of patients receiving more than 30 mg/kg/day) and in patients with renal insufficiency. Higher doses can be given safely for a regimen of twice or three times weekly.

2.2.5. Fixed-Dose Combination Preparations

Two combined preparations, INH and RIF (Rifamate) and INH, RIF, and PZA (Rifater), are available in the United States. These formulations are a means of minimizing inadvertent monotherapy, particularly when directly observed therapy (DOT) is not possible, and, therefore, may decrease the risk of acquired drug resistance (19). The use of fixed-dose formulations may reduce the number of pills that must be taken daily. Constituent drugs are combined in proportions compatible with daily treatment regimens. Formulations for intermittent administration are not available in the United States.

3. TREATMENT OF LATENT TB INFECTION

Table 2 outlines the revised criteria for positive tuberculin skin test reactivity by size of induration requiring drug treatment (20). Drug therapy for latent TB (based on tuberculin skin test reactivity) considerably decreases the risk of progression of TB infection to TB disease. The updated recommended drug treatment of latent TB infection (LTBI) in adults including the elderly is shown in Table 3 (21). Since the LTBI treatment recommendations address adults in general, targeted skin testing and treatment of high-risk populations can be applied to the elderly. The INH daily regimen for 9 months has recently replaced the previously recommended 6-month schedule for treatment of LTBI. Randomized, prospective trials in HIV-negative persons have indicated that a 12-month regimen is more effective than 6 months of treatment; subgroup analyses of several trials indicate that the maximal beneficial effect of INH is likely to be achieved in 9 months, with minimal additional benefit gained by extending therapy to 12 months. Although the 9-month regimen of INH is preferred for the treatment of LTBI, the 6-month LTBI treatment course also provides substantial protection and has been shown to be superior to placebo in both HIV-positive and HIV-negative persons. Hence, clinical judgment must be exercised based on local conditions, health departments or providers' experience, cost and

Table 2   Skin Test Criteria for Positive Tuberculin Reaction (mm Induration)

≥5 mm

   Human immunodeficiency virus positive persons

   Recent contacts of person(s) with infectious tuberculosis

   Persons with chest radiographs consistent with tuberculosis (e.g., fibrotic changes)

   Patients with organ transplants and other immunosuppressed hosts receiving the
   equivalent of >15 mg/day prednisone for >1 month

≥10 mm

   Recent arrivals (<5 years) from high-prevalence countries

   Injection drug users

   Residents and employees of high-risk congregate settings: prisons, jails, nursing homes,
   chronic and residential facilities for acquired immune deficiency syndrome patients, and
   homeless shelters

   Mycobacteriology laboratory personnel

   High-risk clinical conditions: silicosis; gastrectomy; jejunoileal bypass; ≥10% below ideal
   body weight; chronic renal failure; diabetes mellitus; hematological malignancies (e.g.,
   lymphomas, leukemias); other specific malignancies (carcinoma of the head or neck, and
   lung) (alcoholics considered high risk)

≥15 mm

   Persons with no risk factors for tuberculosis

Note: Chemoprophylaxis is recommended for all high-risk persons regardless of age. Persons otherwise low-risk tested at entry into employment; ≥15 mm induration is positive.
Source: American Thoracic Society. Am J Respir Crit Care Med 2000; 161:1376–1395.

compliance issues. In a community-based study conducted in Bethel, AL, persons who took <25% of the prescribed annual dose had a threefold higher risk for TB than those who took more than 50% of the annual dose (22). A more recent analysis of study data indicated that the efficacy decreased significantly if of INH was taken for <9 months (23). In instances of known exposure to drug-resistant organisms, alternative preventive therapy regimens may be recommended. In addition, due to recent reports in 2001 of fatal and severe hepatitis associated with the 2-month RIF and PZA (R-Z) treatment regimen for LTBI, this regimen must be used with caution, especially in patients concurrently taking other medications associated with liver injury and in those with mild liver compromise (24). R-Z is not recommended for persons with known underlying liver disease or for those who have had INH-associated liver injury. Persons being considered for treatment with R-Z should be informed about the potential hepatotoxicity and screened for liver disease or adverse effects from INH. To reduce the risk of liver injury associated with R-Z therapy, the ATS and CDC, with the endorsement of the IDSA, have prepared recommendations that supersede previous guidelines (21).

4. TREATMENT OF TB DISEASE

The recommended treatment regimens are for the most part based on evidence from clinical trials and are rated on the basis of a system developed by the United States Public Health Service (USPHS) and the IDSA. There are four recommended regimens for treating patients with TB caused by drug-susceptible organisms. Although these regimens are broadly applicable, there are modifications that should be made under specified circumstances, described subsequently. Each regimen has an initial phase of 2 months followed by a choice of several options for the continuation

Table 3 Revised Drug Regimens for Treatment of Latent TB Infection in Adults (Including the Elderly)

Drug	Interval and duration	Comments	Ratings HIV negative	(Evidence) HIV infected
Isoniazid	Daily for 9 months	In HIV-infected persons, isoniazid may be administered concurrently with nucleoside reverse transcriptase inhibitors (NRTIs), protease inhibitors, or nonnucleoside reverse transcriptase inhibitors (NNRTIs)	A (II)	A (II)
	Twice weekly for 9 months	DOT must be used with twice-weekly dosing	B (II)	B (II)
Isoniazid	Daily for 6 months	Not indicated for HIV-infected persons, those with fibrotic lesions on chest radiographs, or children.	B (I)	C (I)
	Twice weekly for 6 months	DOT must be used with twice-weekly dosing.	B (II)	C (I)
Rifampin	Daily for 4 months	Used for persons who are contacts of patients with isoniazid-resistant, rifampin-susceptible TB		
		In HIV-infected persons, most protease inhibitors or delavirdine should not be administered concurrently with rifampin. Rifabutin with appropriate dose adjustments can be used with protease inhibitors (saquinavir should be augmented with ritonavir) and NNRTIs (except delavirdine). Clinicians should consult web-based updates for the latest specific recommendations	B (II)	B (III)
Rifampin plus pyrazinamiade (R-Z)	Daily for 2 months	RZ generally should not be offered for treatment of LTBI for HIV-infected or HIV-negative persons	D (II)	D (II)
	Twice weekly for 2–3 months		D (III)	D (III)

Notes: Strength of the recommendation: A. Both strong evidence of efficacy and substantial clinical benefit support recommendation for use. Should always be offered. B. Moderate evidence for efficacy or strong evidence for efficacy but only limited clinical benefit supports recommendation for use. Should generally be offered. C. Evidence for efficacy is insufficient to support a recommendation for or against use, or evidence for efficacy might not outweigh adverse consequences (e.g., drug toxicity, drug interactions) or cost of the treatment or alternative approaches. Optional. D. Moderate evidence for lack of efficacy or for adverse outcome supports a recommendation against use. Should generally not be offered. E. Good evidence for lack of efficacy or for adverse outcome supports a recommendation against use. Should never be offered. Quality of evidence supporting the recommendation: I. Evidence from at least one properly randomized controlled trial. II. Evidence from at least one well-designed clinical trial without randomization for cohort or case-controlled analytic studies (preferably from more than one center), from multiple time-series studies, or from dramatic results form uncontrolled experiments. III. Evidence from opinions of respected authorities based on clinical experience, descriptive studies, or reports of expert committees. The substitution of rifapentine for rifampin is not recommended because rifapentine's safety and effectiveness have not been established for patients with LTBI.
Source: From Refs. 20,21.

phase of either 4 or 7 months. For the TB treatment algorithm, see p. 445. The recommended drug treatment regimens are shown in Table 4.

Because of the relatively high proportion of adult patients with TB caused by organisms that are resistant to INH, four drugs are necessary in the initial phase for the 6-month regimen to be maximally effective. Thus, in most circumstances, the treatment regimen for all adults including the elderly with previously untreated TB should consist of a 2-month initial phase of INH, RIF, PZA, and EMB. If (when) drug susceptibility test results are known and the organisms are fully susceptible, EMB need not be included. If PZA cannot be included in the initial phase of treatment, or if the isolate is resistant to PZA alone (an unusual circumstance), the initial phase should consist of INH, RIF, and EMB given daily for 2 months.

4.1. Baseline and Follow-up Evaluations

It is recommended that all patients with TB have counseling and testing for HIV infection, at least by the time treatment is initiated, if not earlier. For patients with HIV infection, a $CD4^+$ lymphocyte count should be obtained. Patients with risk factors for hepatitis B or C viruses (e.g., injection drug use, foreign birth in Asia or Africa, HIV infection) should have serologic tests for these viruses. For all adult patients baseline measurements of serum aminotransferases [aspartate aminotransferase (AST), alanine aminotransferase (ALT)], bilirubin, alkaline phosphatase, and serum creatinine and a platelet count should be obtained. Testing of visual acuity and red-green color discrimination should be obtained when EMB is to be used.

During treatment of patients with pulmonary TB, a sputum specimen for microscopic examination and culture should be obtained at a minimum of monthly intervals until two consecutive specimens are negative on culture. More frequent acid-fast bacilli (AFB) smears may be useful to assess the early response to treatment and to provide an indication of infectiousness. For patients with extrapulmonary TB the frequency and kinds of evaluations will depend on the site involved. In addition, it is critical that patients have clinical evaluations at least monthly to identify the possible adverse effects of the anti-TB medications and to assess adherence. Generally, patients do not require follow-up after completion of therapy but should be instructed to seek care promptly if symptoms or signs recur.

Routine measurements of hepatic and renal function and platelet count are not recommended during treatment unless patients have baseline abnormalities or are at increased risk of hepatotoxicity (e.g., hepatitis B or C virus infection, alcohol abuse). In the elderly, it may be judicious to thoroughly evaluate patients for clinical evidence of adverse of effects of the anti-TB agents being used. At each monthly visit patients taking EMB should be questioned regarding possible visual disturbances including blurred vision or scotomata; monthly testing of visual acuity and color discrimination is recommended for patients taking doses that exceed 15 mg/kg/day, have renal insufficiency, or are receiving the drug for longer than 2 months.

4.2. Drug-Induced Hepatitis

This is the most serious common adverse effect of anti-TB therapy defined as a serum AST level more than three times the upper limit of normal in the presence of symptoms, or more than five times the upper limit of normal in the absence of symptoms. If hepatitis occurs, INH, RIF, and PZA, all potential causes of hepatic injury, should be stopped immediately. Serologic testing for hepatitis viruses A, B, and C (if not done at baseline) should be performed and the patient questioned

Table 4 Drug Treatment Regimens for Culture-Positive Pulmonary Tuberculosis with Drug-Susceptible Organisms

| Initial phase | | | Continuation phase | | | | Rating[c] (evidence)[d] |
Regimen	Drugs	Intervals and doses[a] (minimal duration)	Regimen	Drugs	Interval and doses[a,b] (minimal duration)	Range of total doses (minimal duration)	HIV− HIV+
1	INH, RIF, PZA, EMB	7 days/week for 56 doses (8 weeks) or days/week for 40 doses (8 weeks)	1a	INH/RIF	7 days/week for 126 doses (18 weeks) or 5 days/week for 90 doses (18 weeks)[e]	182–130 (26 weeks)	A(I) A(II)
			1b	INH/RIF	Twice weekly for 36 doses (18 weeks)	92–76 (26 weeks)	A(I) A(II)[f]
			1c[g]	INH/RPT	Once weekly for 18 doses (18 weeks)	44–58 (26 weeks)	B(I) E(I)
2	INH, RIF, PZA, EMB	7 days/week for 14 doses (2 weeks), then twice weekly for 12 doses (6 weeks) or 5 days/weeks for 10 doses (2 weeks) then twice weekly for 12 doses (6 weeks)	2a	INH/RIF	Twice weekly for 36 doses (18 weeks)	62–58 (26 weeks)	A(II) B(II)[f]
			2b[g]	INH/RPT	Once weekly for 18 doses (18 weeks)	44–40 (26 weeks)	B(I) E(I)
3	INH, RIF, PZA, EMB	Three times weekly for 24 doses (8 weeks)	3a	INH/RIF	Three times weekly for 54 doses (18weeks)	78 (26 weeks)	B(I) B(I)

| 4 | INH, RIF, EMB | 7 days/week for 56 doses (8 weeks) or 5 days/weeks for 40 doses (8 weeks) | 4a | INH/RIF | 7 days/week for 217 doses (31 weeks) or 5 days/week for 155 doses (31 weeks)[e] | 273–195 (39 weeks) | C(I) C(I) |
| | | | 4b | INH/RIF | Twice weekly for 62 doses (31 weeks) | 118–102 (39 weeks) | C(I) C(II) |

[a]When DOT is used, drugs may be given 5 days/week and the necessary number of doses adjusted accordingly. Although there are no studies compare five with seven daily doses, extensive experience indicates this would be an effective practice.

[b]Patients with cavitation on initial chest radiograph and positive cultures at completion of 2 months of therapy should receive a 7-month [31 week; either 217 doses (daily) or 62 doses (twice weekly)] continuation phase.

[c]Definitions of evidence ratings: A = preferred; B = acceptable alternative; C = when A and B cannot be given; E = should never be given.

[d]Definitions of evidence ratings: I = randomized clinical trial; II = data from clinical trials that were not randomized or were conducted in other populations; III = expert opinion.

[e]Five-days-a-week administration is always given by DOT. Rating for 5-days/week regimens is AIII.

[f]Not recommended for HIV-infected patients with CD4 cell counts <100 cells/μL.

[g]Options 1c and 2b should be used only in HIV-negative patients who have negative sputum smears at the time of completion of 2 months of therapy and who do not have cavitation on initial chest radiograph (see text). For patients started on this regimen and found to have a positive culture from the 2-month specimen, treatment should be extended an extra 3 months.

Abbreviations: EMB, ethambutol; INH, isoniazid; PZA, pyrazinamide; RIF, rifampin; RPT, rifapentine.
Source: From Ref. 4.

carefully regarding exposure to other possible hepatotoxins, especially alcohol. Two or more anti-TB medications without hepatotoxicity, such as EMB, SM, amikacin/ kanamycin, capreomycin, or a fluoroquinolone (levofloxacin, moxifloxacin, or gatifloxacin) may be used until the cause of the hepatitis is identified. Once the AST level decreases to less than two times the upper limit of normal and symptoms have significantly improved, the first-line medications should be restarted in sequential fashion. Close monitoring, with repeat measurements of serum AST and bilirubin and symptom review, is essential in managing these patients.

4.3. Treatment in Special Situations

4.3.1. HIV Infection

Recommendations for the treatment of TB in HIV-infected adults are, with a few exceptions, the same as those for HIV-uninfected adults. The paradoxical reaction and details regarding HIV infection are described in a separate chapter on HIV disease.

4.3.2. Extrapulmonary TB

The basic principles that underlie the treatment of pulmonary TB also apply to extrapulmonary forms of the disease. Although relatively few studies have examined treatment of extrapulmonary TB, increasing evidence suggests that 6–9-month regimens that include INH and RIF are effective. Thus, a 6-month course of therapy is recommended for treating TB involving any site with the exception of the meninges, for which a 9–12-month regimen is recommended. Prolongation of therapy also should be considered for patients with TB in any site that is slow to respond. The addition of corticosteroids is recommended for patients with TB pericarditis and meningitis.

4.3.3. Renal Insufficiency and End-Stage Renal Disease

Specific dosing guidelines for patients with renal insufficiency and end-stage renal disease are provided in Table 5. For patients undergoing hemodialysis, administration of all drugs after dialysis is preferred to facilitate DOT and to avoid premature removal of drugs such as PZA and cycloserine. To avoid toxicity it is important to monitor serum drug concentrations in persons with renal failure who are taking cycloserine or EMB. There is little information concerning the effects of peritoneal dialysis on clearance of anti-TB drugs.

4.3.4. Liver Disease

INH, RIF, and PZA all can cause hepatitis that may result in additional liver damage in patients with preexisting liver disease. However, because of the effectiveness of these drugs (particularly INH and RIF), they should be used if at all possible, even in the presence of preexisting liver disease. If serum AST is more than three times normal before the initiation of treatment (and the abnormalities are not thought to be caused by tuberculosis), several treatment options exist. One option is to treat with RIF, EMB, and PZA for 6 months, avoiding INH. A second option is to treat with INH and RIF for 9 months, supplemented by EMB until INH and RIF susceptibility are demonstrated, thereby avoiding PZA. For patients with severe liver disease a regimen with only one hepatotoxic agent, generally RIF plus EMB, could be given for 12 months, preferably with another agent, such as a

Table 5 Dosing Recommendations for Adult Patients with Decreased Renal Function

Drug	Change in frequency	Recommended dose and frequency for patients with creatinine clearance <30 mL/ min or for patients receiving hemodialysis
Isoniazid	No change	300 mg once daily, or 900 mg three times/week
Rifampin	No change	600 mg once daily, or 600 mg three times/week
Pyrazinamide	Yes	25–35 mg/kg/dose three times/week (not daily)
Ethambutol	Yes	15–25 mg/kg/dose three times/week (not daily)
Levofloxacin	Yes	750–1000 mg/dose three times/week (not daily)
Cycloserine	Yes	250 mg once daily,[a] or 500 mg/dose three times/week
Ethionamide	No change	250–500 mg/dose daily
p-aminosalicylic acid	No change	4 g/dose twice daily
Streptomycin	Yes	12–15 mg/kg/dose two or three times/week (not daily)
Capreomycin	Yes	12–15 mg/kg/dose two or three times/week (not daily)
Kanamycin	Yes	12–15 mg/kg/dose two or three times/week (not daily)
Amikacin	Yes	12–15 mg/kg/dose two or three times/week (not daily)

Note: Standard doses are given unless there is intolerance; given after hemodialysis on the day of hemodialysis; monitoring of serum drug concentrations considered to ensure drug absorption and to avoid toxicity; data unavailable for peritoneal dialysis—use a similar regimen for hemodialysis and monitor levels.
[a]The appropriateness of 250 mg daily dose has not been established.
Source: From Ref. 4.

fluoroquinolone, for the first 2 months; however, there are no data to support this recommendation.

In all patients with preexisting liver disease, frequent clinical and laboratory monitoring should be performed to detect drug-induced hepatic injury.

4.4. Management of Relapse, Treatment Failure, and Drug Resistance

4.4.1. Relapse

Relapse is when a patient becomes and remains culture negative while receiving therapy but, at some point after completion of therapy, either becomes culture positive again or has clinical or radiographic deterioration that is consistent with active TB. Most relapses occur within the first 6–12 months after completion of therapy. The selection of empirical treatment for patients with relapse should be based on the prior treatment scheme and severity of disease. For patients with TB caused by drug-susceptible organisms and treated by DOT, initiation of the standard four-drug regimen is appropriate until the results of drug susceptibility tests are available. However, for patients who have life-threatening forms of TB, at least three additional agents to which the organisms are likely to be susceptible should be included. For patients with relapse who did not receive DOT, who were not treated with a rifamycin-based regimen, or who are known or presumed to have had irregular treatment, it is prudent to infer that drug resistance is present and to begin an expanded regimen with INH, RIF, and PZA plus an additional two or three agents based on the probability of in vitro susceptibility. The usual agents to be employed would include a fluoroquinolone (levofloxacin, moxifloxacin, or gatifloxacin), an injectable agent such as SM (if not used previously and susceptibility to SM had been established), amikacin, kanamycin, or capreomycin, with or without an additional oral drug.

4.4.2. Treatment Failure

Treatment failure is continued or recurrently positive cultures during the course of anti-TB therapy. After 3 months of multidrug therapy for pulmonary TB caused by drug-susceptible organisms, 90–95% of patients will have negative cultures and show clinical improvement. Thus, patients with positive cultures after 3 months of presumably effective treatment must be evaluated carefully to identify the cause of the delayed conversion. Patients whose sputum cultures remain positive after 4 months of treatment should be deemed treatment failures.

Possible reasons for treatment failure in patients receiving appropriate regimens include nonadherence to the drug regimen (the most common reason), drug resistance, malabsorption of drugs, laboratory error, and extreme biological variation in response. If failure is likely due to drug resistance and the patient is not seriously ill, an empirical retreatment regimen could be started or administration of an altered regimen could be deferred until results of drug susceptibility testing from a recent isolate are available. If the patient is seriously ill or sputum AFB smears are positive, an empirical regimen should be started immediately and continued until susceptibility tests are available. For patients who have treatment failure, *Mtb* isolates should be sent promptly to a reference laboratory for drug susceptibility testing to both first- and second-line agents.

A basic and well-documented principle in managing patients with treatment failure is never to add a single drug to a failing regimen; acquired resistance is highly likely to develop to the new drug. Instead, a minimum of two, and preferably three, new drugs to which susceptibility could logically be assumed should be added to lessen the probability of further acquired resistance. Empirical retreatment regimens might include a fluoroquinolone, an injectable agent such as SM (if not used previously and the patient is not from an area of the world having high rates of SM resistance), alizarin, kanamycin, or capreomycin, and an additional oral agent such as *p*-aminosalicylic acid (PAS), cycloserine, or ethionamide. Once drug-susceptibility test results are available, the regimen must be modified accordingly.

REFERENCES

1. Rajagopalan S. Tuberculosis. In: Hazzard WR, Blass JP, Ettinger WH Jr., Halter JB, Ouslander JG, eds. Principles of Geriatric Medicine and Gerontology. 5th ed. New York: McGraw Hill, 2003:1099–1105.
2. Geiter L. ed. Institute of Medicine. Ending Neglect: The Elimination of Tuberculosis in the United States. Washington, DC: National Academy Press, 2000:1–269.
3. Rajagopalan S. Tuberculosis. In: Yoshikawa TT, Norman DC, eds. Infectious Disease in the Aging: A Clinical Handbook. Totowa, NJ: Humana Press, 2001:67–77.
4. CDC-ATS-IDSA treatment of tuberculosis. MMWR 2003; 52(RR11); 1–77.
5. Nolan CM, Goldberg SV, Buskin SE. Hepatotoxicity associated with isoniazid preventive therapy: a 7-year survey from a public health tuberculosis clinic. J Am Med Assoc 1999; 281:1014–1018.
6. Kopanoff DE, Snider DE, Caras GJ. Isoniazid-related hepatitis: a US Public Health Service cooperative surveillance study. Am Rev Respir Dis 1979; 117:991–1001.
7. Black M, Mitchell JR, Zimmerman HJ, Ishak KG, Epler GR. Isoniazid associated hepatitis in 114 patients. Gastroenterology 1975; 69:289–302.

8. Steele MA, Burk RF, DesPrez RM. Toxic hepatitis with isoniazid and rifampin. Chest 1991; 99:465–471.

9. Snider DE, Caras GJ. Isoniazid-associated hepatitis deaths: a review of available information. Am Rev Respir Dis 1992; 145:494–497.

10. Salpeter S. Fatal isoniazid-induced hepatitis: its risk during chemoprophylaxis. West J Med 1993; 159:560–564.

11. Moulding TS, Redeker AG, Kanel GC. Twenty isoniazid-associated deaths in one state. Am Rev Respir Dis 1989; 140:700–705.

12. Griffith DE, Brown BA, Girard WM, Wallace RJ Jr. Adverse events associated with high-dose rifabutin in macrolide-containing regimens for the treatment of *Mycobacterium avium* complex lung disease. Clin Infect Dis 1995; 21:594–598.

13. Benator D, Bhattacharya M, Bozeman L, Burman W, Catanzaro A, Chaisson R, et al. Rifapentine and isoniazid once a week versus rifampicin and isoniazid twice a week for treatment of drug-susceptible pulmonary tuberculosis in HIV-negative patients: a randomized clinical trial. Lancet 2002; 360:528–534.

14. Girling DJ. The role of pyrazinamide in primary chemotherapy for pulmonary tuberculosis. Tubercle 1984; 65:1–4.

15. Combs DL, O'Brien RJ, Geiter LJ. USPHS Tuberculosis Short-Course Chemotherapy Trial 21: effectiveness, toxicity and acceptability. Report of the final results. Ann Intern Med 1990; 112:397–406.

16. Døssing M, Wilcke JTR, Askgaard DS, Nybo B. Liver injury during antituberculosis treatment: an 11-year study. Tuber Lung Dis 1996; 77:335–340.

17. Jenner PJ, Ellard GA, Allan WG, Singh D, Girling DJ, Nunn AJ. Serum uric acid concentrations and arthralgia among patients treated with pyrazinamide-containing regimens in Hong Kong and Singapore. Tubercle 1981; 62:175–179.

18. Leibold JE. The ocular toxicity of ethambutol and its relation to dose. Ann NY Acad Sci 1966; 135:904–909.

19. Moulding T, Dutt AK, Reichman LB. Fixed-dose combinations of antituberculous medications to prevent drug resistance. Ann Intern Med 1995; 122:951–954.

20. American Thoracic Society, CDC. Targeted tuberculin testing and treatment of latent tuberculosis infection. Am J Respir Crit Care Med 2000; 161:S221–S247.

21. MMWR Update. Fatal and severe liver injuries associated with rifampin and pyrazinamide for latent tuberculosis infection, and revisions in American Thoracic Society/CDC Recommendations—United States—August 31, 2001; 50(34):733–735.

22. Comstock GW, Livesay VT, Woolpert SF. The prognosis of a positive tuberculin reaction in childhood and adolescence. Am J Epidemiol 1974; 99:131–138.

23. Comstock GW. How much isoniazid is needed for prevention of tuberculosis among immunocompetent adults?. Int Tuberc Lung Dis 1999; 3:847–50.

24. CDC. Update: fatal and severe liver injuries associated with rifampin and pyrazinamide treatment for latent tuberculosis infection. MMWR 2002; 51:998–999.

SUGGESTED READING

CDC-ATS-IDSA treatment of tuberculosis. MMWR 2003; 52 (RR11):1–77.

24
Antiviral Drugs

Ghinwa Dumyati
University of Rochester, Rochester General Hospital, Rochester, New York, U.S.A.

Key Points:

- Viral infections can be treated by two modalities: antiviral drugs, which inhibit viral replication in the host, and immunomodulators, which enhance host immune response to infection.
- Three antivirals are available for treatment of herpes zoster: acyclovir, valcyclovir, and famciclovir. They are equally effective in treating herpes zoster lesions and decreasing viral shedding. Valacylcovir and famciclovir are preferred because of their enhanced oral bioavailability. None affect the frequency or duration of postherpetic neuralgia in elderly patients.
- Interferons are not commonly used in elderly patients. They are recommended for hepatitis C treatment in combination with ribavirin and for treatment of hepatitis B. Newer nucleoside and nucleotide analogues, lamuvidine and adefovir, are now the treatment of choice of hepatitis B chronic carriers.
- Four anti-influenza drugs (amantadine, rimantadine, oseltamivir, and zanamivir) have equal efficacy in treating and preventing influenza A infection, and the later two are also active against influenza B. Because amantadine is commonly associated with central nervous toxicity in the elderly, rimantadine and oseltamivir are preferable.
- Zanamivir and oseltamivir are well tolerated in elderly patients. Amantadine treatment is commonly associated with central nervous toxicity in the elderly patients.

1. INTRODUCTION

Two modalities are available for the treatment of viral infections. One is with the use of antiviral agents that selectively inhibit viral replication in the host cell, and the other is by the use of immunomodulators such as interferon (INF), which enhance the host immune response to infection. These drugs are commonly used in the elderly population for treatment and prophylaxis of influenza and treatment of herpes zoster infections. Less common uses include treatment of hepatitis C, hepatitis B, and human immunodeficiency virus (HIV) infections. Most of the antiviral drugs are well tolerated in the elderly but frequently require dosing adjustment due to altered drug metabolism, decreased renal function or toxicity. Several drugs have only been studied in younger adults, and limited pharmacologic and therapeutic data are available in the elderly patient. This chapter will focus on use of non-HIV antivirals in the elderly (Table 1).

Table 1 Pharmacology and Clinical Indications of Antiviral Drugs

Antiviral	Mechanism of action	Indication in elderly patients	Pharmacology	Pharmacology
Acyclovir	Metabolized to acyclovir triphosphate that inhibits viral DNA polymerase	VZV Herpes simplex	Oral bioavailability 10–20% Half-life 2–3 hr Intracellular half-life 1–2 hr	Plasma concentration higher in elderly patient compared with younger adult in part due to age-related changes in renal function
Valacyclovir	Same as acyclovir	VZV Herpes simplex	Oral bioavailability 54% Plasma half-life 2–3 hr Intracellular half-life 1–2 hr	Same as acyclovir
Famciclovir	Metabolized to penciclovir triphosphate that inhibits viral DNA polymerase	VZV Herpes simplex	Oral bioavailability 77% Plasma half-life 2 hr Intracellular half-life of penciclovir 7–20 hr	Same as acyclovir
Ribavirin	Interfere with viral messenger RNA	Chronic hepatitis C (in combination with interferon) Severe RSV	Oral bioavailability 32% Plasma half-life 30–60 hr Some absorption of aerosolized formulation	Administered cautiously in the elderly
Lamivudine	Inhibition of viral DNA polymerase and reverse transcriptase	Chronic hepatitis B HIV 1	Oral bioavailability 86% Plasma half-life 5–7 hr	No adjustment needed in elderly patients
Adefovir	Inhibition of viral DNA polymerase	Chronic hepatitis B	Oral bioavailability 59% Plasma half-life 7.5 hr Intracellular half-life 16–18 hr	No information available in elderly patients
Amantadine	Blockage of M2 protein ion channel and its ability to modulate intracellular pH	Influenza A (prophylaxis and treatment)	Oral bioavailability >90% Plasma half-life 10–31 hr in adults	Peak concentration higher and plasma half-life longer in patients >50 years old

Drug	Mechanism	Indication	Pharmacokinetics	Elderly
Rimantadine	Same as amantadine	Influenza A (prophylaxis and treatment)	Oral bioavailability >90% Plasma half-life 25–36 hr 75% metabolized in liver	Steady-state concentration in elderly nursing home patients were two- to four-fold higher than those seen in healthy young and elderly adults
Zanamivir	Neuraminidase inhibitors	Influenza A and B (treatment)	13–15% of drug deposited in tracheobronchial tree and lungs Plasma level low (4–17%)	No adjustment needed in elderly patients
Oseltamivir	Neuraminidase inhibitor	Influenza A and B (prophylaxis and treatment)	Oral bioavailability 75% Plasma half-life 1–3 hr (oseltamivir carboxylate half-life 8–10 hr)	No adjustment needed in elderly patients
Interferon-α	Induction of cellular enzymes that interfere with viral protein synthesis	Chronic hepatitis B and C SARS	Oral bioavailability 0% Plasma half-life 2–3 hr	No adjustment needed in elderly patients
Pegylated interferon-α	Same as interferon	Chronic hepatitis C with ribavirin	Oral bioavailability 0% Plasma half-life 40–80 hr	No adjustment needed in elderly patients

Abbreviations: VZV, varicella zoster virus; HIV, human immunodeficiency virus; SARS, severe acute respiratory syndrome.

2. ANTIHERPES VIRUS AGENTS (See Also Chapter 36)

2.1. Acyclovir

Acyclovir is an analog of 2′-deoxyguanosine. It is transformed to the active acyclovir triphosphate form, first by monophosphorylation by the viral thymidine kinase present in infected cells, and then by di- and triphosphorylation by host cell enzymes. The concentration of acyclovir triphosphate is 40–100-fold higher in herpes virus infected cells than noninfected cells. Acyclovir triphosphate competitively inhibits viral DNA polymerase and results in termination of.viral replication. It has minimal effect on human cellular DNA polymerase (1). Acyclovir activity is limited to the herpes virus group; the minimum inhibitory concentration $(MIC)_{50}$ is 0.1 μM for herpes simplex type 1, 0.4 μM for herpes simplex type 2, and 2.6 μM against varicella zoster virus (VZV). The oral bioavailability of acyclovir is low, ≈10–30%, but is adequate for treatment of herpes simplex. Higher and more frequent dosing is needed for the treatment of VZV. Acyclovir is available in both oral (tablet and suspension) and intravenous forms.

2.2. Valacyclovir

Valacyclovir is the L-valyl ester of acyclovir. It is converted to acyclovir in the gastrointestinal tract and liver. The relative bioavailability of acyclovir after oral dosing of valacyclovir is three to five times that of acyclovir and reaches 70% (1). Valacyclovir is only available in the oral (capsule) form.

2.3. Famciclovir

Famciclovir is the diacetyl-6-deoxy analog of penciclovir, a drug with poor oral absorption. Famciclovir is converted to penciclovir in the gastrointestinal tract, blood, and liver. Penciclovir mechanism of action and spectrum of antiviral activity are similar to acyclovir. Its oral bioavailability after intake of famciclovir is 77% (1). Famciclovir is only available in the oral (tablet) form and has the advantage of less frequent dosing because of the long intracellular half-life of penciclovir.

2.4. Clinical Pharmacology

Each of these agents is well tolerated in elderly patients. Since these drugs are excreted by glomerular filtration and tubular secretion, adjustment of the dose is required for renal insufficiency (Table 2). The acyclovir dose for treatment of herpes zoster is 800 mg orally every 4 hr (five times a day) for 7 days. Intravenous acyclovir, 10 mg/kg every 8 hr, is recommended for herpes zoster infection in immunocompromised patients. For valacyclovir, a 2 g dose orally, four times daily, approximates the level achieved with acyclovir 10 mg/kg every 8 hr given intravenously. The dose for VZV is 1000 mg orally every 8 hr for 7 days. The famciclovir dose for herpes zoster treatment is 500 mg every 8 hr for 7 days.

2.5. Clinical Indications

Acyclovir, famciclovir, and valacyclovir are used for herpes simplex and VZV infections. In the elderly, the most common indication is for treatment of herpes zoster.

Table 2 Adverse Effects and Dosages for Antiviral Drugs

Drugs and indications	Adverse effects in the elderly	Dose adjustment for estimated creatinine clearance		
		>50 mL/min	10–50 mL/min	<10 mL/min
Acyclovir (oral) VZV treatment	More frequent nausea, vomiting, dizziness More likely to have renal or central venous systems (CNS) adverse events such as somnolence/hallucinations, confusion, coma	800 mg every 4 hr	800 mg every 4–8 hr	800 mg every 12 hr
Acyclovir (intravenous) VZV treatment	May develop renal insufficiency if inadequately hydrated, rapid rate of infusion and concomitant use of nephrotoxic drugs. More CNS adverse effects	10 mg/kg every 8 hr	10 mg/kg every 12–24 hr	5 mg/kg every 24 hr
Valacyclovir VZV treatment	More likely to have renal or CNS adverse effects (agitation, hallucinations, confusion, delirium, encephalopathy)	1 g every 8 hr	1 g every 12–24 hr	500 mg every 24 hr
Famciclovir VZV treatment	Acute renal failure reported in patients with renal insufficiency who received inappropriate high dose. Hallucinations confusion	500 mg every 8 hr	500 mg every 12–24 hr	250 mg every 24 hr
Ribavirin (used with interferon) Treatment of hepatitis C	No sufficient data available in elderly patients Higher frequency of anemia (67% compared to 28% in young)	Not recommended for creatinine clearance below 50 mL/min Administered cautiously in the elderly starting at a lower end of dosing range (see Table 4)		
Lamuvidine Treatment of hepatitis B	No sufficient data available in elderly patients	100 mg once a day	100 mg first dose then 25–50 mg per day	35 mg first dose then 10–15 mg per day

(Continued)

Table 2 Adverse Effects and Dosages for Antiviral Drugs (*Continued*)

Drugs and indications	Adverse effects in the elderly	Dose adjustment for estimated creatinine clearance		
		>50 mL/min	10–50 mL/min	<10 mL/min
Adefovir Treatment of hepatitis B	No sufficient data available in elderly patients	10 mg per day	10 mg every 48–72 hr	No available data
Amantadine Prophylaxis and treatment of influenza A	More common CNS side effects (dizziness, headaches, anxiety, including seizure). Increase falls in nursing home patients	100 mg per day	100 mg every 48–72 hr	100 mg every 7 days
Rimantadine Prophylaxis and treatment of influenza A	More GI side effects (nausea, vomiting). NLCNS (dizziness, headache, anxiety, fatigue) less frequent than amantadine. Less frequency of seizure	100 mg per day	100 mg per day	100 mg per day
Zanamivir Treatment of influenza A and B	No difference with side effects due to age	Two 5 mg blisters inhaled twice daily		
Oseltamivir Treatment of influenza A and B	No increase frequency of adverse effects	75 mg twice a day	75 mg once a day	No data
Prophylaxis for influenza and B		75 mg once a day	75 mg every other day	No data

Abbreviations: VZV, varicella zoster virus; GI, gastrointestinal.

They are efficacious in decreasing duration of acute pain, decreasing viral shedding and resolution of skin lesions when used within 72 hr of symptom onset. When compared with placebo, acyclovir reduces new vesicle formation by ≈1.5 days and time to crusting of lesions by 2 days. It reduces acute zoster-associated pain but has no effect on the incidence or duration of postherpetic neuralgia (2). Acyclovir also reduces ocular complications of ophthalmic zoster. The combination of acyclovir with corticosteroids results in a moderate acceleration of cutaneous healing and alleviation of acute pain compared with acyclovir alone. The combination also results in improvement in quality of life measures such as shorter time to return to usual activity, uninterrupted sleep, and reduced analgesic use. However, the combination of acyclovir with corticosteroids, as with acyclovir alone, does not affect the incidence or duration of postherpetic neuralgia (2).

Valacyclovir, when compared with acyclovir in immunocompetent patients above the age of 50 years, showed similar effects on cutaneous healing, but patients treated with valacyclovir had a significantly shorter duration of zoster pain (38 vs. 51 days) (3).

In a placebo-controlled study in patients above the age of 50 years, famciclovir reduced the duration of postherpetic neuralgia compared with a placebo (163 days in placebo vs. 63 days in famciclovir groups). Famciclovir is comparable to valcyclovir in treating zoster and reducing associated pain in older adults (4,5). In both groups, 19% of the patients reported residual pain at 6 months.

The choice of agent depends on cost and dosing schedule; valacyclovir and famciclovir are generally preferred because of their improved pharmacokinetics and more convenient dosing regimens.

2.6. Adverse Effects

Side effects are infrequent and include nausea and vomiting, diarrhea, and headaches. In rare cases, renal insufficiency and neurotoxicity can occur with acyclovir, especially when given intravenously. Reversible nephropathy, due to crystallization of the drug in renal tubules, is almost exclusively seen when acyclovir is given intravenously, and occurs in 5% of patients. The risk is increased with rapid infusion, dehydration, and pre-existing renal insufficiency. The nephropathy is prevented by hydration with saline, adjustment of the dose according to creatinine clearance (Table 2), and infusing acyclovir at a constant rate over 1 hr. Neurotoxicity occurs in 1–4% of cases and is manifested by altered sensorium, myoclonus, tremor, seizures, and extrapyramidal signs. It is more likely in renal failure and use with other drugs with central nervous system (CNS) toxicity. On rare occasions, famciclovir causes urticaria rash and, in the elderly, hallucinations and confusional states have been reported (1).

3. INTERFERONS

Natural INFs are glycoproteins produced by cells in response to various inducers such as viral, bacterial, protozoal, mycoplasma infections and various other stimuli. IFNs include INF-β, INF-γ, and IFN-α. IFN-α is the most common form used for treatment of viruses. Commercial preparations of IFN-α are made by recombinant-DNA techniques. Different types are available and approved by Food and Drug Administration in the United States: INF-α2b, INF-α2a, which is different from

IFN-α by one amino acid, and INF alfacon-1. All three have similar efficacy in treating hepatitis C. Pegylated IFN-α is IFN covalently bound to polyethylene glycol, has an extended half-life and duration of therapeutic activity. It is available in two forms, 12 kD pegylated INF-α2b and 40 kD pegylated INF-α2a; both have similar efficacy and side effects in the treatment of hepatitis C. IFN is not directly antiviral but induces the production of cellular proteins that inhibit different stages of viral replication. IFNs are also immunomodulatory and augment cellular immune function.

3.1. Clinical Pharmacology

IFNs are not orally bioavailable and must be given intramuscularly or subcutaneously. IFN activity is usually measured in terms of antiviral effects in cell culture and is expressed as international units (IU) relative to reference standards. After administration, an antiviral state in peripheral mononuclear cells is seen at 1 hr, peaks at 24 hr, and decreases to baseline at 6 days. IFN is cleared from blood by inactivation by various body fluids, cellular uptake, and metabolism by body organs. Little active drug is excreted in urine (1).

IFN-α is administered once daily or three times a week for treatment of hepatitis C or B (see also Chapter 33: Viral Hepatitis). Pegylated IFN is given weekly for the treatment of hepatitis C. No dose adjustment is required for elderly patients, but patients must be able to administer the injections and tolerate the frequent adverse effects. Many will have contraindication to treatment because of comorbidities (Table 3).

3.2. Clinical Indications

IFN is recommended as one of the treatment options for adults with chronic hepatitis C or B infection (see also Chapter 33: Viral Hepatitis). It is used in combinations with other agents such as ribavirin for hepatitis C and possibly in combination with lamivudine in hepatitis B (see details of hepatitis treatment given later). IFNs are also approved for the treatment of papillomavirus and human herpes virus type 8 (Kaposi sarcoma-associated virus) in HIV, multiple sclerosis, and some malignancies. IFN-α is active in vitro against severe acute respiratory syndrome (SARS) coronavirus (CoV), and has been used in uncontrolled studies of human SARS. In a primate model of

Table 3 Contraindications to Treatment with Interferon

Absolute contraindications
  Current psychosis or history of psychosis
  Severe depression
  Neutropenia or thrombocytopenia
  Decompensated cirrhosis
  Uncontrolled seizures
  Organ transplant other than liver

Relative contraindications
  Autoimmune disorders
  Uncontrolled diabetes mellitus

SARS CoV infection, pegylated IFN-α was shown to reduce virus shedding and reduce the severity of lung damage if used shortly after infection (6).

3.2.1. Hepatitis C

Recommendations for hepatitis C treatment have evolved during the past 10 years as more agents and combination treatments have become available. The goal of hepatitis C treatment is prevention of cirrhosis and possible hepatocellular carcinoma and reduction of extrahepatic manifestations such as glomerulonephritis and essential mixed cryoglobulinemia. Several treatment regimens are available with different adverse effects and response rates. When sustained response is defined as undetectable HCV RNA, response rates for a 24-week course of IFN-α are 5% for HCV genotype 1 and 20% for genotypes 2 and 3. Response rates improve with a 48-week treatment duration. The combination of IFN and ribavirin is associated with a 35% and 80% response for genotype 1 and genotypes 2 and 3, respectively. Optimal responses are seen with the combination of pegylated IFN and ribavirin, especially for genotype 1 with a response rate of 48% and for genotypes 2 and 3, 88% (7). The treatment of choice for adult patients with genotype 2 or 3 is presently combination therapy with IFN (standard or pegylated) plus ribavirin for 24 weeks and for genotype 1 pegylated INF with ribavirin for 48 weeks (see Table 4 for doses and duration of treatment).

There is no consensus on treatment of elderly patients with hepatitis C since they are usually excluded from clinical trials. Only four small studies using INF-α2b in patients aged 65 years and older with hepatitis C have been reported (8–11). In these studies response was similar to a younger age group but no sustained virologic response was documented. One Japanese study showed that sustained virologic response to IFN-α was only in 10.6% in men and 8.6% in women above 60 years of age (12). Retrospective subanalysis of large, randomized trials indicated that age greater than 40 years is an independent predictor of nonresponse to an IFN-based regimen. Another study of combination of INF-α2b with ribavirin for 48 weeks was associated with a response rate of 34% in patients older than 40 years compared with 48% in patients under 40 years (13). Of note, patients above the age of 60 years were not included in this study.

Table 4 Treatment of Hepatitis C

Drug	Dose	Duration
Interferon-α 2a or 2b	Three million units subcutaneously three times per week	24–48 weeks depending on response
Interferon-α with ribavirin	Three million units subcutaneously three times a week 1000–1200 mg per day	24–48 weeks depending on response
12 kD Pegylated interferon-α 2b with ribavirin	1.5 µg/kg subcutaneously once a week 11 mg/kg (800–1400 mg/day in two divided doses)	24 weeks for genotype 2 or 3 48 weeks for genotype 1
40 kD Pegylated interferon-α 2a with ribavirin	180 µg subcutaneously per week 1000 mg per day for weight ≤75 kg 1200 mg per day for weight >75 kg	24 weeks for genotype 2 or 3 48 weeks for genotype 1

3.2.2. Hepatitis B

Treatment of hepatitis B with IFN is associated with suppression of hepatitis B virus DNA (HBV DNA), loss of HB-e antigen (HBeAg), and development of anti-HB-e antibody (anti-HBe). Treatment leads to biochemical and histologic improvement on liver biopsy. However, treatment is not curative and many patients do not lose their hepatitis B surface antigen (HBsAg) and HBV DNA is still detectable by sensitive assays such as polymerase chain reaction (PCR). Treatment of adults is recommended for chronic carriers with active infection documented by viremia ($>10^5$ copies/mL) and evidence of liver injury reflected by an increase in alanine aminotransferase (ALT) and necroinflammatory activity on liver biopsy. Treatment has been beneficial in patients with HBe Ag positivity and compensated hepatic cirrhosis. Treatment with IFN, 5–10 million units subcutaneously three times per week for at least 3 months and up to 6 months, results in a 30% successful response defined as loss of HBeAg, development of anti-HBe antibody, and a decline in serum ALT levels (14). IFN treatment has also been associated with a decrease in hepatocellular carcinoma (15). In 20–40% of patients a flare of liver injury due to immune clearance of infected hepatocytes, right before or at the time of clearance of HBeAg, has been reported. It is usually manifested by a transient increase in ALT level to more than twice the base line value (16). Therapy is continued unless symptoms of liver failure are observed. Because of this flare of hepatitis, treatment with IFN is contraindicated in patients with advanced liver disease because it may lead to fulminant liver failure. Patients with cirrhosis often cannot tolerate IFN treatment due to exacerbation of their leukopenia and thrombocytopenia. Treatment of patients with chronic infection with HBV variant, a precore mutant in which synthesis of HBeAg is absent, is of variable benefit because of the heterogeneity of this group and relapse is common (16).

No specific recommendations are available for treatment of elderly patients in a chronic hepatitis B carrier state. However, it should be offered to those with evidence of ongoing viral replication and compensated liver disease. See Table 5 for treatment options and duration.

3.3. Adverse Effects

IFN treatment is commonly associated with influenza-like symptoms beginning several hours after injection. The symptoms include fever, chills, myalgia, headache, arthalgia, nausea, vomiting, and diarrhea. Tolerance improves with repeated treatments. Other side effects include alopecia and CNS effects including depression, somnolence, confusion, and behavioral disturbances. Paranoia or suicidal ideation and seizures occur in less than 1% of patients (17). The principal dose-limiting toxicity is bone marrow

Table 5 Hepatitis B Treatment

Drug	Dose	Duration
Recombinant interferon-α 2b	Five million IU subcutaneously per day or 10 million IU subcutaneous three times per week	HBeAg positive 16 weeks HBeAg negative 1 year
Lamivudine	100 mg per day	One year (see text)
Adefovir dipivoxil	10 mg per day	Unknown

suppression, more commonly thrombocytopenia and less commonly leukopenia. IFN infrequently exacerbates autoimmune diseases such as hypo- or hyperthyroidism, idiopathic thrombocytopenic purpura, and lupus-like syndrome. Other rare toxicities include cardiotoxicity (hypotension and tachycardia), polyneuropathy, proteinuria, and azotemia. With moderate side effects, the dose of IFN is decreased and, if severe, therapy should be withheld.

Adverse effects in patients aged 65 years and older reported in small studies were similar and occurred at a similar rate as in younger patients. None of the elderly patients had severe side effects requiring withdrawal from the study. More severe side effects were seen in a recent study of 23 treated patients aged 65 years and older (11). Treatment was discontinued in 30% of cases. The side effects included severe asthenia, nonspecific digestive complaints, depression, severe leukopenia, thrombocytopenia, and facial paralysis.

4. LAMIVUDINE

Lamivudine is a pyrimidine nucleoside that was originally developed for HIV treatment; it was later found to have activity against hepatitis B virus. It is transformed to lamivudine triphosphate intracellularly and inhibits HIV reverse transcriptase and hepatitis B polymerase. It is only available in the oral (tablets or solution) form.

4.1. Clinical Pharmacology

In healthy elderly volunteers, lamivudine was well tolerated without any significant adverse effects compared with a younger age group. Higher plasma concentrations and lower urinary excretion due to age-associated reduction in renal function was reported. Dose adjustment is unnecessary unless there is evidence of renal insufficiency (Table 2). The dose for treatment of hepatitis B is 100 mg/day (see also Chapter 33: Viral Hepatitis). The duration is 1 year in patients who have persistent HBeAg seroconversion (HBeAg loss, anti-HBe detection, and serum HBV DNA undetectable by non-PCR assays on more than one occasion 2 months apart). Longer duration is considered in patients who did not undergo HBeAg seroconversion or who have breakthrough infection with lamivudine-resistant mutant as long as benefit is maintained. The duration for HBeAg negative carrier is controversial (1).

4.2. Clinical Indications

Lamivudine is recommended for the treatment of chronic hepatitis B infection with evidence of increased serum ALT for more than 6 months and evidence of active viral replication (high HBV DNA levels). Lamivudine is efficacious in patients with HBeAg-positive chronic hepatitis B. In HBeAg-negative chronic hepatitis B, the response is better than placebo but relapse occurs in the majority of patients when treatment is discontinued. It is also beneficial in patients who failed IFN treatment and is effective in patients with decompensated cirrhosis where IFN is contraindicated.

The advantage of lamivudine over IFN is its better tolerability and more rapid loss of HBeAg and seroconversion to anti-HBe positive status (15). It is not immunomodulatory and, therefore, can be used in patients with decompensated cirrhosis. After 1 year of treatment with 100 mg daily, response to treatment is similar to INF with a decrease in HBV DNA, anti-HBe seroconversion in 16–22% of patients, and histologic improvement in 56–60% of patients. Lamivudine reverses fibrosis including cirrhosis. Best responses are seen in patients with elevated pretreatment level of ALT. Some patients experience a transient exacerbation of liver injury when lamivudine is withdrawn and therefore close monitoring for several months after stopping treatment is recommended (16).

The major limitation of lamivudine treatment is the development of drug resistance due to point mutations of the viral reverse transcriptase. After 1 year of treatment, 15–20% of patients have resistant variants, which increase to 40% by the second year and 67% by the fourth year. The clinical significance of resistant virus is unclear as many patients still undergo conversion from HBeAg positive to HBeAg negative status, and 40–50% do so by the fourth year of lamivudine treatment. However, some patients have a rise in their HBV DNA and progression of the liver injury (15).

4.3. Adverse Effects

In studies from China and the United States, which included patients between the ages of 16 and 70 (median 32–40 years), adverse effects were similar in both drug and placebo groups. The most common side effects were malaise, fatigue, nausea, and vomiting (18,19).

5. ADEFOVIR DIPIVOXIL

Adefovir Dipivoxil is a nucleotide analogue; it undergoes cellular phosphorylation to its active form adefovir, which inhibits viral polymerase. Originally developed for treatment of HIV infection but the high dose required to inhibit HIV replication was nephrotoxic. It was recently approved for hepatitis B treatment at a lower dose of 10 mg per day. It is available only in a tablet form.

5.1. Clinical Pharmacology

Adefovir is well absorbed after oral administration with a bioavailability of 59% after a 10-mg oral dose. It is renally excreted by a combination of glomerular filtration and tubular secretion. No pharmacokinetic studies are available in elderly patients. Dose adjustment is recommended in patients with a creatinine clearance below 50 mL/min (Table 2).

5.2. Clinical Indications

Adefovir has been shown to be effective in both HBeAg-positive and HBeAg-negative adult patients with abnormal ALT and elevated viral load. After 48 weeks of adefovir treatment, HBV DNA viral load decreased by 4–5 log. Treatment improves liver histologic findings, normalizes ALT levels, and induces HBeAg loss in 12% of patients. It is effective against lamivudine-resistant strains (15). No significant emergence of adefovir-resistant HBV is seen, an advantage of this drug compared to lamivudine. However, adefovir is twice as expensive as lamivudine.

5.3. Adverse Effects

The safety profile is similar to placebo except for asthenia and diarrhea (20,21). No renal toxicity is reported with the 10-mg dosing, but renal function should be closely monitored.

6. RIBAVIRIN

Ribavirin is a guanosine analog that has activity against RNA and DNA viruses. It is phosphorylated in the cell to ribavirin triphosphate, which interferes with messenger RNA and ribonucleoprotein synthesis. It is available in intravenous, oral, and aerosolized forms, the latter primarily for treatment of infants with respiratory syncytial virus (RSV) infection. The intravenous route is investigational in the United States.

6.1. Clinical Pharmacology

After an oral dose, ribavirin bioavailability varies between 33% and 45%. Ten times higher levels are achieved with intravenous administration. Ribavirin is absorbed after administration by aerosol, and plasma concentration increases with the duration of exposure. The elimination of ribavirin is complex. The plasma half-life is 30–40 hr after a single oral dose but increases to 200–300 hr at a steady state. It concentrates in erythrocytes and is still detectable in plasma up to 4 weeks after cessation of therapy. It is metabolized in the liver and excreted in the urine (1). The drug elimination is decreased in patients with a creatinine clearance <30 mL/min, and it should be used cautiously in patients with a creatinine clearance below 50 mL/min.

In elderly volunteers with chronic obstructive pulmonary disease, aerosolized ribavirin has been found to be safe when given for 6 or 12 hr per day for 4 days (22). In hospitalized elderly patients, a high dose of 60 mg/mL administered over 2 hr three times a day is better tolerated that continuous inhalation of a 20 mg/mL dose (22).

6.2. Clinical Indications

Ribavirin is approved for treatment of hemorrhagic fever viruses, and hepatitis C in combination with IFN-α (described earlier). It is administered by inhalation to high-risk infants with severe RSV infections. It is not usually used in adult patients with RSV infection but could be considered in selected severe cases (22). It has been used for treatment of SARS, but no definite data on benefit are available. Moreover, in vitro studies found that ribavirin lacked activity against SARS CoV, and it is therefore no longer recommended.

Ribavirin is not commonly used in the elderly. Oral and intravenous ribavirin is contraindicated in patients with decompensated heart disease because they are unable to tolerate the ribavirin-associated anemia. Ribavirin is also contraindicated in severe renal insufficiency.

6.3. Adverse Effects

Adverse effects of ribavirin depend on the route of administration. For the inhaled form, adverse effects include deterioration of respiratory function, rarely cardiac arrest, hypotension, and bradycardia. The drug is potentially mutagenic and, therefore, precautions need to be taken by pregnant women during administration by inhalation. Healthcare workers exposed to the drug may develop conjunctivitis and headaches (1).

When ribavirin is used orally for the treatment of hepatitis C together with IFN, 20% of patients withdrew from the study due to adverse effects. The adverse effects included anemia (due to both hemolysis and bone marrow toxicity), fatigue, headaches, anorexia, dyspepsia, and nausea. The combination is not recommended in patients with a creatinine clearance <50 mL/min and in those with unstable or significant cardiac disease. Dose adjustment is recommended for anemia (hemoglobin less than 10 mg/dL or a drop by 2 g/dL in patients with cardiovascular disease) and if severe (hemoglobin less than 8.5 mg/dL) blood transfusion can be considered and treatment discontinued. Intravenous ribavirin is used in hemorrhagic viral diseases such as Lassa fever and hemorrhagic fever with renal syndrome but is not presently licensed in the intravenous form. Intravenous ribavirin has also been used in patients with SARS. A review of the adverse effects seen in the Toronto outbreak in 2003 showed that 61% of patients developed a dose-related hemolytic anemia within the first 6 days of treatment. Almost half of the patients developed hypocalcemia and hypomagnesemia (23).

7. ANTI-INFLUENZA AGENTS

Two classes of antivirals are available for treatment of influenza. The older agents are the M2 channel inhibitors such as amantadine and rimantadine, and the newer neuraminidase inhibitors are zanamivir and oseltamivir.

7.1. Amantadine and Rimantadine

Amantadine and its α-methyl derivative rimantadine are tricyclic amines. They inhibit the replication of influenza A but not influenza B viruses. The mechanism of action is incompletely understood. The primary action is on the M2 protein, a membrane protein that functions as an ion channel. By inhibiting the M2 protein ion channel, these drugs affect pH-dependent viral uncoating in infected cells, which leads to inhibition of viral replication and release (24).

7.2. Clinical Pharmacology

Amantadine and rimantadine are well absorbed in young and healthy elderly subjects after oral administration. The metabolism of amantadine and rimantadine differ. Amantadine is excreted unchanged in the urine by glomerular filtration and tubular secretion. It is recommended to adjust the dose in patients with creatinine clearance below 50 mL/min. In elderly male volunteers, higher levels and longer half-life have been reported after receiving a single dose of amantadine. Thus, it would be best to give half the recommended dose (i.e., 100 mg) in patients aged 65 years and older. Rimantadine is metabolized by the liver and its metabolites are excreted in the urine. There is no need for dose adjustment in patients with renal insufficiency until the creatinine clearance is below 10 mL/min. Dose adjustment is recommended in patients with severe hepatic dysfunction (25). The pharmacokinetics of rimantadine is similar in young and healthy older adults; however, in volunteers aged 71 years and older, plasma concentration and elimination half-life values are 20–30% higher than in subjects between the ages of 50 and 70 years. In elderly nursing home residents, a dose of 200 mg of rimantadine given for several days resulted in high plasma concentrations associated with anxiety and nausea. Some studies showed excess withdrawals compared with placebo at this dose. Thus, the dose for elderly persons is recommended to be 100 mg daily, which is half of the usual adult dose. Both drugs are available in tablet and syrup forms.

Viral resistance to these drugs occurs rapidly and is due to point mutations in the M2 gene with corresponding single amino substitutions in the M2 protein. This results in loss of the ion channel inhibitory effect of these drugs. Resistance develops in 30% of treated patients within 2–3 days after initiation of treatment. The resistant virus is not more virulent but can be transmitted to close contacts such as household members or other nursing home residents and, therefore, prophylaxis or treatment of secondarily infected patients with either amantadine or rimantadine will be ineffective. Transmission of resistance can be prevented by isolation of treated patients. Resistant viruses remain sensitive to the neuraminidase inhibitors.

7.3. Clinical Indications

Amantadine and rimantadine are indicated for the treatment and prophylaxis of influenza A infections.

7.3.1. Treatment of Fever and Symptoms and a Rapid Decline of Virus Shedding

Most efficacy studies with amantadine and rimantadine have been in healthy young adults. Efficacy is equivalent for both drugs when started within 48 hr of influenza symptom onset. In healthy young adults, treatment results in reduction of fever by 1–2 days and in reduction of viral shedding. These drugs have not been extensively studied in the elderly population. One placebo-controlled study of rimantadine in elderly nursing home residents showed a more rapid resolution of fever and symptoms and virus shedding (26). Another study showed decreased use of antibiotics, antipyretics, and antitussive in treated patients (27). The efficacy of treatment in preventing severe complications such as pneumonia is not known. It is also not known if treatment is effective in hospitalized patients with viral pneumonia. One retrospective uncontrolled study in 72 hospitalized patients with influenza showed no difference in duration of fever, rates of intensive care admission, and intubation in patients who received amantadine compared with untreated patients (28).

7.3.2. Prophylaxis

In healthy adults, the use of either drug for seasonal prophylaxis or after exposure to influenza A virus has a protective efficacy of 70–100% (24). Protection against laboratory-documented influenza is lower at 50–60%, which suggests that subclinical infections still occur (29).

In the elderly, influenza prophylaxis is generally used during institutional outbreaks, pending response to vaccination in nonimmune residents at the time of an influenza epidemic. Other uses include seasonal prophylaxis in high-risk people with contraindication to vaccination or when the vaccine virus and epidemic virus antigenic match is poor. Only two double-blind placebo-controlled studies have analyzed rimantadine as seasonal prophylaxis. One showed that the efficacy of rimantadine in reducing risk of influenza-like illness was 58% (30). The other study, in 35 nursing home participants who received either rimantadine or placebo, reported no laboratory-documented influenza in treated patients but two in the placebo group (31). Numerous studies have reported their experience in controlling nursing home outbreaks by initiating either amantadine or rimantadine.

7.4. Adverse Effects

The principal adverse reactions associated with rimantadine and amantadine are gastrointestinal and CNS. Common side effects include nervousness, lightheadedness, difficulty concentrating, insomnia, fatigue, slurred speech, loss of appetite, and nausea. More severe CNS adverse effects include confusion, hallucination, psychosis, and coma. The potential for CNS adverse effect with amantadine is increased by concomitant ingestion of antihistamines and anticholinergic drugs. Patients with a pre-existing seizure disorder develop increased frequency of major seizures during amantadine and rarely during rimantadine therapy. The frequency of adverse effects in elderly nursing home residents receiving 100 mg daily for prophylaxis is 41% and cessation of drug is necessary in 5–35% of patients. The risk of falls also increases (32). The frequency of CNS reaction is less for rimantadine, but gastrointestinal side effects are similar to amantadine.

8. ZANAMIVIR AND OSELTAMIVIR

Zanamivir and oseltamivir are neuraminidase inhibitors. By blocking the activity of the viral neuraminidase, the drugs inhibit spread of influenza virus by preventing budding of the virions, which remain attached to the membrane of the infected cell and to each other. They are active against both influenza A and B viruses.

8.1. Clinical Pharmacology

Zanamivir is mixed with lactose powder and is administered as a dry powder aerosol. After administration, 13–15% of the drug is deposited in the tracheobronchial tree and lungs, and 78% is deposited in the oropharynx. Plasma concentration is low; only 15% of the dose is recovered unchanged in the urine. Elderly patients with poor functional status and dementia might experience difficulty with inhalation of the drug (33).

Oseltamivir is well absorbed after oral administration. It is metabolized quickly to the active form, oseltamivir carboxylate. It is eliminated by glomerular filtration and tubular secretion; however, dose adjustment is not needed in the elderly patients unless advanced renal insufficiency is present. It is available in capsule or oral suspension.

The antiviral activity of both zanamivir and oseltamivir is of long duration; therefore, twice-a-day dosing is recommended for treatment, and once a day for prophylaxis (see Table 2 for dosing).

Oseltamivir resistance is seen in 1.3% of posttreatment isolates from patients aged ≥13 years and in 8.6% among patients aged 1–2 years (25). Zanamivir resistance has not been reported in clinical trials but was described in an immunocompromised child infected with influenza B (34).

8.2. Clinical Indications

8.2.1. Treatment

The neuraminidase inhibitors have similar efficacy as the M2 protein inhibitors. When used within the first 48 hr of illness, they decrease the duration of uncomplicated influenza by 1 day compared with placebo. In patients with fever at enrollment and who began treatment within 30 hr after the onset of symptoms, the median time to alleviation of symptoms was 3 days less in treated patients compared with controls (35,36). The effectiveness of both zanamivir and oseltamivir in the elderly and patients with high risk of complications of influenza is limited. Pooled data from zanamivir studies showed that the greatest effect on duration of illness was in patients aged ≥50 years and in persons with high-risk conditions, with illness reduction of 2.5–3 days (37,38). Treatment of influenza with either drug resulted in a decrease of respiratory complications (acute bronchitis, sinusitis, and lower respiratory tract infection) requiring antibiotic treatment (38,39). A pooled analysis of patients treated with oseltamivir showed that, in the treated group, the incidence of lower respiratory tract infections requiring antibiotic treatment was decreased by 67% in the healthy adult population and by 34% in high-risk patients. No effect was seen in the rate of upper respiratory tract infection such as sinusitis (40). The rate of hospitalization for any cause was decreased by 59% (1.7% in control compared to 0.7% in treated influenza patients).

8.2.2. Prophylaxis

Both drugs were studied for seasonal prophylaxis in healthy adults with a 69–74% relative reduction in laboratory-confirmed symptomatic influenza in treated patients compared with placebo. In postexposure prophylaxis in households, the relative reduction of influenza was between 62% and 96%. One placebo-controlled study in elderly (mostly vaccinated population) in a long-term facility who received prophylaxis with oseltamivir for 6 weeks resulted in a 92% reduction of laboratory-confirmed influenza. Several studies have been published on experiences with either oseltamivir or zanamivir to control nursing home outbreaks due to influenza A/B or both. One reported the control of a nursing home outbreak that failed amantadine control (33).

The decision of which drug to use for prophylaxis of nursing home outbreaks depends on the type of influenza causing the outbreak and on cost constraints and tolerance for adverse effects. During influenza outbreaks, prophylaxis of all nursing home residents, regardless of their vaccination status, should be initiated as soon as possible and should also be given to unvaccinated staff. The drug should be given for at least 2 weeks, or 1 week after the last documented case. The Centers for Disease Control and Prevention recommendations published in 2005 do not specify which agent to use (25). Due to its better safety profile, rimantadine should be considered during influenza A outbreaks. It is, however, more expensive than amantadine and, if monetary constraints are critical, amantadine can be used in patients with no risk factors for seizure, and the dose adjusted according to creatinine clearance. It is important to isolate treated patients from patients receiving prophylaxis because of the potential transmission of resistant virus. During influenza B outbreaks or influenza A outbreaks not controlled by rimantadine or amantadine, oseltamivir should be used.

8.3. Adverse Effects

Zanamivir is well tolerated in high-risk (patients with chronic respiratory disease, significant cardiovascular disease, immunocompromised, and patients with diabetes mellitus) and elderly patients with similar adverse effect reported in placebo recipients (41). In patients with asthma and chronic obstructive pulmonary disease, the zanamivir-treated group had a small but significant increase in peak expiratory flow rate compared with placebo. However, the rate of respiratory effects was not different from the placebo, and none of the patients had to discontinue the study drug due to deterioration in respiratory function. Postmarketing surveillance has reported only rare respiratory adverse effects, including bronchospasm or decline in respiratory function. In many cases, the casuality was difficult to establish since influenza infection can result in respiratory decompensation. Nevertheless, the manufacturer's labeling recommends that zanamivir not be used for treatment of patients with underlying airway disease such as asthma or chronic obstructive pulmonary disease.

Oseltamivir is also well tolerated. The most frequent side effect is nausea and, less commonly, vomiting. These symptoms are usually transient and resolve in 1–2 days. No increase in adverse effect is seen in elderly or high-risk patients (42).

REFERENCES

1. Hayden FG. Antiviral drugs (other than antiretrovirals). In: Mandell GL, Bennett JE, Dolin R, eds. Principles and Practice of Infectious Diseases. 6th ed. Philadelphia, PA: Churchill Livingstone, 2005:514–551.
2. Whitley RJ, Gnann JW. Herpes zoster: focus on treatment in older adults. Antiviral Res 1999; 44:145–154.
3. Beutner KR, Friedman DJ, Forszpaniak C, Andersen PL, Wood MJ. Valacyclovir compared with acyclovir for improved therapy for herpes zoster in immunocompetent adults. Antimicrob Agents Chemother 1995; 39(7):1546–1553.
4. Tyring ST, Beutner KR, Tucker BA, Anderson WC, Crooks RJ. Antiviral therapy for herpes zoster: randomized controlled clinical trial of valacyclovir and famciclovir therapy in immunocompetent patients 50 years and older. Arch Fam Med 2000; 9:863–869.
5. Degreef H. Famciclovir, a new oral antiherpes drug: results of the first controlled clinical study demonstrating its efficacy and safety in the treatment of uncomplicated herpes zoster in immunocompetent patients. Int J Antimicrob Agents 1994; 4:241–246.
6. Haagmans BL, Kuiken T, Martina BE, Fouchier RAM, Rimmelzwaan GF, van Amerongen G, van Riel D, de Jong T, Itamura S, Chan KH, Tashiro M, Osterhaus AD. Pegylated interferon-α protects type 1 pneumocytes against SARS coronavirus infection in macaques. Nat Med 2004; 10(3):290–293.
7. Poynard T, Yuen MF, Ratziu V, Lai CL. Viral hepatitis C. Lancet 2003; 362:2095–2100.
8. Horiike N, Masumoto T, Nakanishi K, Michitaka K, Kurose K, Ohkura I, Onji M. Interferon therapy for patients more than 60 years of age with chronic hepatitis C. J Gastroenterol Hepatol 1995; 10(3):246–249.
9. Bresci G, del Corso L, Romanelli AM, Giuliano G, Pentimone F. The use of recombinant interferon alfa-2b in elderly patients with anti-HCV-positive chronic active hepatitis. J Am Geriatr Soc 1993; 41(8):857–862.
10. van Theiel DH, Friedlander L, Caraceni P, Molloy PJ, Kania RJ. Treatment of hepatitis C virus in elderly persons with interferon α. J Gerontol 1995; 50A(6):M330–M333.
11. Herve S, Savoye G, Riachi G, Capet C, Goria O, Lerebours E, Colin R. Letters to the editor: characteristics of chronic hepatitis C and response to interferon therapy in older patients. Age Ageing 2001; 30:355–356.

12. Hayashi J, Kishihara Y, Ueno K, Yamaji K, Kawakami Y, Furusyo N, Sawayama Y, Kashiwagi S. Age-related response to interferon alfa treatment in women vs men with chronic hepatitis C virus infection. Arch Intern Med 1998; 158(2):177–181.

13. Poynard T, McHutchinson J, Goodman Z, Ling MH, Albrecht J. Is an "a la carte" combination interferon alfa-2b plus ribavirin regimen possible for the first line treatment in patients with chronic hepatitis C? Hepatology 2000; 31(1):211–218

14. Wong DKH, Cheung AM, O'Rourke K, Naylor CD, Detsky AS, Heathcote J. Effect of alpha-interferon treatment in patients with hepatitis B e antigen-positive chronic hepatitis B. Ann Intern Med 1993; 119(4):312–323.

15. Ganem D, Prince AM. Hepatitis B virus infection–natural history and clinical consequences. N Engl J Med 2004; 350(11):1118–1129.

16. Lok A, McMahon B. Chronic hepatitis B. Hepatology 2001; 34(6):1225–1241.

17. Lauer GM, Walker BD. Medical progress. Hepatitis C virus infection. N Engl J Med 2001; 345(1):41–52.

18. Dienstag JL, Schiff ER, Wright TL, Perrillo RP, Hann HWL, Goodman Z, Crowther L, Condreay LD, Woessner M, Rubin M, Brown NA. Lamivudine as initial treatment for chronic hepatitis B in the United States. N Engl J Med 1999; 341(17):1256–1263.

19. Lai CL, Chien RN, Leung NWY, Chang TT, Guan R, Tai DI, Ng KY, Wu PC, Dent JC, Barber J, Stephenson SL, Gray DF. A one-year trial of lamivudine for chronic hepatitis B. N Engl J Med 1998; 339(2):61–68.

20. Hadziyannis SJ, Tassopoulos NC, Heathcote EJ, Chang TT, Kitis G, Rizzetto M, Marcellin P, Lim SG, Goodman Z, Wulfsohn MS, Xiong S, Fry J, Brosgart CL. Adefovir dipivoxil for the treatment of hepatitis B e antigen-negative chronic hepatitis B. N Engl J Med 2003; 348(9):800–807.

21. Marcellin P, Chang TT, Lim SG, Tong MJ, Sievert W, Shiffman ML, Jeffers L, Goodman Z, Wulfsohn MS, Xiong S, Fry J, Brosgart CL. Adefovir dipivoxil for the treatment of hepatitis B e antigen-positive chronic hepatitis B. N Engl J Med 2003; 348(9):808–816.

22. Dumyati G, Falsey AR. Influenza and other respiratory viruses. In: Yoshikawa TT, Ouslander JG, eds. Infection Management for Geriatrics in Long-term Care Facilities. New York: Marcel Dekker, Inc., 2002; 197–222.

23. Knowles SR, Philips EJ, Dresser L, Matukas L. Common adverse events associated with the use of ribavirin for severe acute respiratory syndrome in Canada. Clin Infect Dis 2003; 37:1139–1142.

24. Hayden FG, Aoki FY. Amantadine, rimantadine and related agents. In: Yu VL, Merrigan TC Jr, Barriere SI, Raoult D, eds. Antimicrobial Therapy and Vaccines. Baltimore, MD: Lippincott, Williams & Wilkins, 1999:1344–1365.

25. Centers for Disease Control and Prevention. Prevention and control of influenza: recommendations of the advisory committee on immunization practices. MMWR 2005; 54(July 13):1–40.

26. Betts RF, Treanor J, Graman PS, Bently DW, Dolin R. Antiviral agents to prevent or treat influenza in the elderly. J Resp Dis 1987; (8, suppl):S56–S59.

27. Treanor JJ. Influenza virus. In: Mandell GL, Bennett JE, Dolin R, eds. Principles and Practice of Infectious Diseases. 5th ed. Philadelphia, PA: Churchill Livingston, 2000:1823–1849.

28. Kaiser L, Hayden FG. Hospitalizing influenza in adults. In: Yu VL, Merigan TC, White NJ, Barriere SI, eds. Curr Clin Top Infect Dis 2000:112–134.

29. Tominack RL, Hayden FG. Rimantadine hydrochloride and amantadine hydrochloride use in influenza A virus infections. Infect Dis Clin North Am 1987; 1(2):459–478.

30. Monto AS, Ohmit SE, Hornbuckle K, Pearch CL. Safety and efficacy of long-term use of rimantadine for prophylaxis of type A influenza in nursing homes. Antimicrob Agents Chemother 1995; 39(10):2224–2228.

31. Patriarca PA, Kater NA, Kendal AP, Bregman DJ, Smith JD, Sikes RK. Safety of prolonged administration of rimantadine hydrochloride in the prophylaxis of influenza A virus infections in nursing homes. Antimicrob Agents Chemother 1984; 26:101–103.

32. Stange K, Little DW, Blatnik B. Adverse reactions to amantadine prophylaxis of influenza in a retirement home. J Am Geriatr Soc 1991; 39(7):700–705.
33. Lee C, Loeb M, Phillips A, Nesbitt J, Smith K, Fearon M, McArthur MA, Mazzulli T, Li Y, McGeer A. Zanamivir use during transmission of amantadine-resistant influenza A in a nursing home. Infect Control Hosp Epidemiol 2000; 21:700–704.
34. Gubareva LV, Matrosovich MN, Brenner MK, Bethell RC, Webster RG. Evidence for zanamivir resistance in an immunocompromised child infected with influenza B virus. J Infect Dis 1998; 178:1257–1262.
35. Hayden FG, Osterhaus AD, Treanor JJ, Fleming DM, Aoki FY, Nicholson KG, Bohnen AM, Hirst HM, Keene O, Wightman K. Efficacy and safety of the neuraminidase inhibitor zanamivir in the treatment of influenzavirus infections. N Engl J Med 1997; 337(13):874–880.
36. Monto AS, Fleming DM, Henry D, deGroot R, Makela M, Klein T, Elliott M, Keene ON, Man CY. Efficacy and safety of the neuraminidase inhibitor zanamivir in the treatment of influenza A and B virus infections. J Infect Dis 1999; 180:254–261.
37. Monto AS, Webster A, Keene O. Randomized, placebo-controlled studies of inhaled zanamivir in the treatment of influenza A and B: pooled efficacy analysis. J Antimicrob Chemother 1999; 44(Topic B):23–29.
38. Lalezari J, Campion K, Keene O, Silagy C. Zanamivir for the treatment of influenza A and B infection in high-risk patients. Arch Intern Med 2001; 161:212–217.
39. Kaiser L, Keene ON, Hammond JMJ, Elliott M, Hayden FG. Impact of zanamivir on antibiotic use for respiratory events following acute influenza in adolescents and adults. Arch Intern Med 2000; 160:3234–3240.
40. Kaiser L, Wat C, Mills T, Mahoney P, Ward P, Hayden FG. Impact of oseltamivir treatment on influenza-related lower respiratory tract complications and hospitalizations. Arch Intern Med 2003; 163:1667–1672.
41. Gravenstein S, Davidson HE. Current strategies for management of influenza in the elderly population. Clin Infect Dis 2002; 35:729–737.
42. Gubareva LV, Kaiser L, Hayden FG. Influenza virus neuraminidase inhibitors. Lancet 2000; 355(9206):827–835.

SUGGESTED READING

Gravenstein S, Davidson HE. Current strategies for management of influenza in the elderly population. Clin Infect Dis 2002; 35:729–737.
Hayden FG. Antiviral drugs (other than antiretrovirals). In: Mandell GL, Bennett JE, Dolin R, eds. Principles and Practice of Infectious Diseases. 6th ed. Philadelphia, PA: Churchill Livingstone, 2005:514–551.
Herve S, Savoye G, Riachi G, Capet C, Goria O, Lerebours E, Colin R. Letters to the editor: characteristics of chronic hepatitis C and response to interferon therapy in older patients. Age Ageing 2001; 30:355–356.
Marcellin P, Chang TT, Lim SG, Tong MJ, Sievert W, Shiffman ML, Jeffers L, Goodman Z, Wulfsohn MS, Xiong S, Fry J, Brosgart CL. Adefovir dipivoxil for the treatment of hepatitis B e antigen-positive chronic hepatitis B. N Engl J Med 2003; 348(9):808–816.

25
Antifungal Drugs

Carol A. Kauffman
Division of Infectious Diseases, University of Michigan Medical School, Infectious Diseases Section, Veterans Affairs Ann Arbor Healthcare System, Ann Arbor, Michigan, U.S.A.

Key Points:

- Lipid formulations of amphotericin B should be used for therapy in older adults because they are less nephrotoxic than standard amphotericin B. However, nephrotoxicity still can occur, and infusion reactions remain a common problem with all formulations of amphotericin B.
- All azoles have drug–drug interactions that are often serious and can be life-threatening. Concomitant medications must be carefully assessed before prescribing an azole.
- Itraconazole and terbinafine, the drugs of choice for onychomycosis, both have the potential for hepatotoxicity. The decision to treat onychomycosis must weigh this potential for toxicity against the benefits of treatment.
- Voriconazole, the first second-generation azole, has a broad spectrum of antifungal activity and is fungicidal for molds, but has adverse effects (photopsia and photosensitivity rash) that differ from those noted with other azoles.
- Caspofungin, the first echinocandin antifungal agent, has a narrow spectrum of activity, but is fungicidal for *Candida* species and has very few side effects.

1. AMPHOTERICIN B

1.1. Introduction

Amphotericin B has been the standard treatment for many fungal infections since its introduction in the 1950s. The major drawback to the use of this drug is its inherent toxicity. Some degree of nephrotoxicity occurs in almost every patient receiving the agent, and infusion reactions are common and often severe. Use of amphotericin B has been problematic in older adults, who frequently have underlying renal insufficiency. The introduction of lipid formulations of amphotericin B has ameliorated, but not eliminated, the toxicity of this agent. The introduction of new antifungals has markedly diminished our reliance on amphotericin B.

337

1.2. Chemistry and Mechanism of Action

Amphotericin B is a polyene derived from *Streptomyces nodosus*. It is prepared as a colloidal dispersion with sodium deoxycholate because of its inherent insolubility in water. Three different lipid formulations of amphotericin B are also available: liposomal amphotericin B (AmBisome®), amphotericin B colloidal dispersion (Amphotec®), and amphotericin B lipid complex (Abelcet®). Each of these formulations was developed to diminish the toxicity of amphotericin B. All three differ in their chemical and physical characteristics and their pharmacological attributes, but the active drug in all three remains amphotericin B (1,2).

Amphotericin B acts by binding to ergosterol in the fungal cell membrane resulting in altered membrane permeability, leakage of cell constituents, and cell death. In addition to its effect on ergosterol in fungal cell membranes, amphotericin B also binds, admittedly to a lesser degree, to cholesterol in mammalian cell membranes, accounting for its toxicity.

1.3. Antimicrobial Spectrum

Amphotericin B has a very wide spectrum of activity. It has excellent in vitro activity against the yeasts, including *Candida* species and *Cryptococcus neoformans*, the dimorphic fungi, *Blastomyces dermatitidis*, *Coccidioides immitis*, *Histoplasma capsulatum*, and *Sporothrix schenckii*, and most filamentous fungi, including *Aspergillus* species, the zygomycetes, such as *Rhizopus* and *Mucor*, and many brown-black fungi.

1.4. Clinical Pharmacology

Amphotericin B is not absorbed when given orally and has to be administered by the intravenous (IV) route (3). Peak plasma concentrations occur within the first hour and persist for ≈6–8 hr. Highest tissue concentrations are found in liver and spleen, followed by lungs and kidneys. The drug is highly protein bound to serum lipoproteins. Amphotericin B penetrates poorly into cerebrospinal fluid (CSF) and other body fluids. The metabolism of amphotericin B still has not been elucidated. The half-life is exceedingly long with a terminal half-life of ≥15 days; detectable levels can be recovered from urine for several months after stopping the drug.

1.5. Clinical Indications

Amphotericin B is used less now than previously but remains the drug-of-choice for several fungal infections. These include infection with the zygomycetes, *Rhizopus* and *Mucor*, and initial therapy for cryptococcal meningitis (4). For patients with severe disseminated histoplasmosis, blastomycosis, and coccidioidomycosis, amphotericin B remains the drug-of-choice (5–7). Although used less now, it remains a useful agent for candidemia and invasive candidiasis and for invasive aspergillosis (8,9).

1.6. Administration of Drug

Detailed instructions for administration of amphotericin B are given in Table 1. The manufacturer's specific instructions for administration of the lipid formulations should always be consulted prior to infusion. Sodium loading, as noted in the table, is now routinely employed in an attempt to decrease nephrotoxicity (10). Infusion reactions can be obviated by pretreatment with several medications (11).

Table 1 Guidelines for Administering Amphotericin B Formulations

Mix drug in 5% dextrose in water, not 0.9% saline.
Do not use in-line filters; no need to cover drug while infusing
Dilute drug to concentration suggested by manufacturer
Administer initial portion of drug slowly over 30 min without premedication to look for rare
  instances of anaphylaxis and arrhythmias
Give infusion by central IV line if at all possible
Infuse drug over time specified by manufacturer. For patients with infusion-related reactions,
  slower infusion times are better tolerated
Assess volume status prior to treatment. Stop diuretics if possible. Do not restrict sodium
Prior to each dose, infuse 500 mL 0.9% saline over 1 hr
For subacute or chronic infections, start with lower dosage and increase daily until the
  desired daily dosage is reached. Use pretreatment medications only if required
For life-threatening infections, infuse the desired daily dosage within the first 24 hr.
  Pretreatment medications should be given with the first infusion
Pretreatment medications (if needed): acetaminophen (650 mg), diphenhydramine (50 mg),
  and prochlorperazine (25 mg). Rarely, 25–50 mg hydrocortisone intravenously immediately
  prior to infusion may be required. For rigors, 50 mg meperidine IV or intramuscularly at
  the start of infusion is usually effective
Obtain baseline creatinine/blood urea nitrogen (BUN), electrolytes, magnesium, blood
  count, and liver function tests.
Monitor creatinine/BUN, electrolytes daily until stable, then two to three times weekly;
  monitor blood count weekly; repeat liver function tests if clinically indicated.
If creatinine doubles, reassess volume status and electrolytes, increase sodium supplements; if
  creatinine rises ≥3 mg/dL, hold drug for 1–2 days. When creatinine decreases, reinstitute
  therapy.

1.7. Drug Monitoring and Adverse Effects

Daily monitoring of patients receiving amphotericin B is essential because of the frequent and serious adverse events seen with this agent. Nephrotoxicity occurs in most patients given amphotericin B and is especially problematic in older adults requiring treatment with this agent. Nephrotoxicity is usually seen by the second week of therapy. As many as 60% of patients may have a doubling of creatinine level during amphotericin B therapy. The rate differs in various populations, but patients on other nephrotoxic agents, older adults, and those with preexisting renal failure are at increased risk of amphotericin B-induced nephrotoxicity. Salt restriction and diuretics enhance nephrotoxicity and should be avoided if possible (10). Although amphotericin B-induced renal failure is usually completely reversible, patients who have received many years of this drug suffer irreversible renal failure and may require dialysis.

Renal tubular loss of potassium and magnesium can be quite impressive. Electrolytes should be monitored carefully and replaced as soon as the serum levels show even a slight decrease. In some patients, the renal loss is brisk enough that IV repletion is required.

All of the lipid formulations are less nephrotoxic than amphotericin B deoxycholate (1,2). In older patients, the use of a lipid amphotericin B formulation is strongly advised because of this decreased risk of nephrotoxicity.

Infusion-related reactions are the most common adverse events experienced by patients receiving amphotericin B. Most often, these consist of chills, fever, nausea, headache, and myalgias. In some patients, severe rigors occur, and in rare instances, hypotension and ventricular arrhythmias can occur. One of the lipid formulations, amphotericin B colloidal dispersion, appears to cause as many infusion reactions as amphotericin B deoxycholate. The other two lipid formulations are associated with fewer infusion reactions than standard amphotericin B. Thrombophlebitis at the infusion site is frequent and can be obviated by the use of a central venous catheter.

Anemia is common in patients receiving amphotericin B for an extended period. The anemia, which is due to decreased erythropoietin production, is usually normochromic and normocytic and rarely results in a need for transfusion. Leukopenia, thrombocytopenia, hepatotoxicity, neuropathy, and acute pulmonary edema are other rare adverse effects.

2. AZOLE ANTIFUNGAL AGENTS

There are three first-generation azole antifungal agents, ketoconazole, itraconazole, and fluconazole, currently available for systemic use. There is only one second-generation azole, voriconazole, currently available, but others are likely to be introduced. The second-generation azoles were developed primarily to broaden the spectrum of activity over that seen with the first-generation agents. All azoles act through the same mechanism, inhibition of cytochrome P450 (CYP450)-dependent 14α-lanosterol demethylation, a vital step in cell membrane ergosterol synthesis by fungi. They vary in how selective they are for the fungal cell membrane compared with mammalian cell membranes, and this selectivity predicts toxicity.

As a class, the azoles are relatively safe drugs to use in older adults. However, they do have the potential to produce serious and life-threatening drug–drug interactions through their actions on the CYP450 system. For example, patients receiving cholesterol-lowering "statin" agents [3-hydroxy-3 methyl glutaryl coenzyme A reductase inhibitor] can develop life-threatening rhabdomyolysis, and increased serum levels of warfarin and oral hypoglycemic agents occur when azoles are given. Older adults, who often take many medications, are at increased risk of developing drug–drug interactions. Before prescribing any azole, careful review of the existing drug regimens is essential.

Because each azole differs in regard to antifungal spectrum, pharmacological attributes, and indications for use, each of these aspects will be discussed individually.

3. KETOCONAZOLE

3.1. Introduction

Ketoconazole was the first oral azole and soon found its niche in the treatment of the endemic mycoses and skin and nail infections (12). However, it had a significant number of side effects and drug interactions and was supplanted by itraconazole, with its greater intrinsic activity against many fungi and improved safety profile. Ketoconazole is the least selective azole in regard to its action on cell membrane synthesis and thus the most toxic (13). Currently, ketoconazole is infrequently used, but as the least expensive oral azole, it continues to play a role in the treatment of skin and nail infections and rarely, the endemic mycoses.

3.2. Chemistry and Mechanism of Action

As noted earlier.

3.3. Antimicrobial Spectrum

Ketoconazole has activity against *Candida* species; however, it is not considered appropriate therapy for other than localized mucocutaneous infections. The dermatophytes that cause a variety of tinea infections of skin and nails are susceptible to ketoconazole, as are the endemic fungi, *H. capsulatum*, *B. dermatitidis*, and *C. immitis*. This azole has no activity against *Aspergillus* or the zygomycetes.

3.4. Clinical Pharmacology

Ketoconazole is available only as an oral formulation that requires gastric acid for absorption. The drug is >99% protein-bound and does not penetrate into the CSF, other body fluids, or the eye. Because of its lipophilic characteristics, it accumulates in skin and nails. The drug is metabolized in the liver through the CYP450 system into several inactive metabolites. Active drug is not found in the urine.

3.5. Clinical Indications

There are a few clinical situations in which ketoconazole is the drug-of-choice. The drug is a second-line agent for the endemic mycoses if the patient cannot tolerate itraconazole. It is also a less expensive alternative to itraconazole and terbinafine for treatment of dermatophyte infections.

3.6. Administration of Drug

Ketoconazole is available as 200 mg tablets that should be taken with food. Because it requires gastric acid for absorption, proton pump inhibitors, histamine-2 blockers, and antacids should not be given with ketoconazole. The usual dosage for dermatophyte infections is 200 mg daily and for systemic infections, 400 mg once or twice daily.

3.7. Drug Monitoring and Adverse Effects

At the dosages required for treating systemic infections, ketoconazole can cause nausea, vomiting, and headache. At the dosages used for treatment of dermatophyte infections, these symptoms are uncommon. Hepatitis, which can occur with all azoles, is rare, but can be life-threatening. Liver enzymes should be measured at baseline, after several weeks of therapy, and monthly thereafter. Mild elevations of alanine aminotransferase (ALT) or aspartate aminotransferase (AST) (two- to three-fold increase) do not require stopping the drug, but do require careful follow-up. If the levels increase further, the drug should be discontinued.

A major toxicity associated with the use of ketoconazole, but not other azoles, is that of the interference with synthesis of both androgenic and adrenal steroids. Thus, men can develop impotence, oligospermia, and gynecomastia, and women can become amenorrheic. Adrenal insufficiency has been reported in patients taking higher dosages of ketoconazole. Drug–drug interactions are common, may preclude use of the drug, and are detailed in Tables 2 and 3.

Table 2 Effects of Concomitantly Administered Drugs on Azole Antifungal Drug Levels

Drug affecting azole level	Azole antifungal drug level			
	Ketoconazole	Itraconazole	Fluconazole	Voriconazole
Rifampin	Decreased	Decreased	Decreased	Decreased
Rifabutin	Unknown	Decreased	No effect	Decreased
Isoniazid	Decreased	Decreased	Unknown	Unknown
Phenytoin	Decreased	Decreased	Unknown	Decreased
Carbamazepine	Unknown	Decreased	Unknown	Decreased
Phenobarbital	Unknown	Decreased	Unknown	Decreased
Antacids	Decreased	Decreased	No effect	No effect
Histamine-2 blockers	Decreased	Decreased	No effect	No effect
Proton pump inhibitors	Decreased	Decreased	No effect	No effect
Sucralfate	Decreased	Unknown	No effect	No effect

Table 3 Effects of Azole Antifungal Drugs on Serum Levels of Other Drugs

Drug affected by azole	Azole antifungal drug			
	Ketoconazole	Itraconazole	Fluconazole	Voriconazole
Cyclosporine	Increased[a]	Increased[a]	Increased[a]	Increased[a]
Tacrolimus	Increased[a]	Increased[a]	Increased[a]	Increased[a]
Sirolimus	Unknown	Increased[a]	Unknown	Increased[b]
Warfarin	Increased[a]	Increased[a]	Increased[a]	Increased[a]
Phenytoin	Increased[a]	Unknown	Increased[a]	Increased[a]
Carbamazepine	Increased[a]	Increased[a]	Increased[a]	Increased[a]
Digoxin	Increased[a]	Increased[a]	No effect	No effect
Quinidine	Increased[a]	Increased[b]	Unknown	Increased[b]
Oral hypoglycemics	Increased[a]	Increased[a]	Increased[a]	Increased[a]
Isoniazid	Decreased	Unknown	Unknown	Unknown
Rifampin	Decreased	Unknown	Unknown	Unknown
Rifabutin	Unknown	Increased[a]	Increased[a]	Increased[a]
Ergot alkaloids	Unknown	Unknown	Unknown	Increased[b]
Omeprazole	Unknown	Unknown	Unknown	Increased
Triazolam, alprazolam, midazolam	Increased	Increased[b]	Unknown	Increased[a]
Lovastatin, simvastatin, etc.	Unknown	Increased[b]	Unknown	Increased[a]

[a]Significant interaction: monitor serum levels of drug and/or clinical status.
[b]Life-threatening interaction: avoid the combination.

4. ITRACONAZOLE

4.1. Introduction

Itraconazole has both an enhanced spectrum of activity and an improved safety profile over that of ketoconazole. It has become the drug of choice for the endemic mycoses and for dermatophyte infections of skin and nails (5–7,14–16).

4.2. Chemical Structure and Mechanism of Action

As noted earlier.

4.3. Antimicrobial Spectrum

Itraconazole has activity against most, but not all *Candida* species, *C. neoformans*, most *Aspergillus* species and other filamentous fungi, dermatophytes, and the endemic mycoses. It is not active against the zygomycetes.

4.4. Clinical Pharmacology

Itraconazole is available as both oral and IV formulations. Absorption has been problematic in that both food and gastric acid are required for maximum absorption of the capsule formulation. In older adults, who are more likely to have achlorhydria than younger adults, absorption of itraconazole may be poor. The oral suspension of itraconazole, given on an empty stomach, has ≈30% better absorption than the capsule formulation. The drug is >99% protein-bound. Itraconazole is metabolized in the liver by the CYP450 enzyme system into several metabolites, one of which, hydroxyitraconazole, has antifungal activity. Itraconazole distributes poorly into body fluids, is not excreted as active drug in urine, and is concentrated in nails and skin.

4.5. Clinical Indications

Itraconazole is the drug-of-choice for treatment of the endemic mycoses, *B. dermatitidis*, *C. immitis*, *H. capsulatum*, and *S. schenckii* (5–7,17). Although it has activity against the yeasts, *Candida* and *Cryptococcus*, it is rarely used for serious infections with these organisms. However, the oral suspension is useful for the treatment of refractory thrush and esophagitis caused by *Candida*. Itraconazole has become the treatment of choice for dermatophyte infections of nails and skin (16). The drug is also used for prophylaxis against invasive fungal infections in neutropenic patients.

4.6. Administration of Drug

Itraconazole is available as 100 mg capsules that must be administered with food and require gastric acidity for absorption. Even in the presence of acid and food, absorption is erratic. The oral suspension was developed to increase absorption and is the preferred formulation. The suspension should be given on an empty stomach and does not require gastric acid for absorption. For patients with serious infections, serum concentrations of itraconazole should always be obtained from a reference laboratory in order to ensure adequate absorption of either formulation. An IV formulation that uses a cyclodextrin vehicle is available for use in seriously ill patients. It cannot be used in patients with a creatinine clearance <30 mL/min because of accumulation of the cyclodextrin vehicle, which is cleared through the kidneys.

The usual dosage is 200 mg once or twice daily. Giving more than 200 mg as a single dose does not increase the serum concentrations proportionally; therefore, higher-dosage regimens require twice- or thrice-daily administration of drug. For serious infections, a loading dose of 200 mg thrice daily should be given for the first 2 days to achieve steady state more quickly. For treatment of nail infections, pulse therapy for 1 week out of every month for 3–4 months has proved effective (16).

4.7. Drug Monitoring and Adverse Effects

Nausea, vomiting, headache, and rash have been noted uncommonly with itraconazole. Hepatitis occurs with itraconazole, as it does with all azoles, and serum liver enzymes (ALT, AST) should be obtained routinely during the course of therapy. Two- to three-fold elevation of enzymes does not require a change in therapy, but further elevations should prompt a change to another antifungal class.

Itraconazole is unique among azoles in that it causes a triad of hypertension, edema, and hypokalemia; although uncommon, this complication occurs most often in older adults and requires discontinuing the drug. Itraconazole has also been associated with ventricular dysfunction and should be given with great caution to patients with congestive heart failure.

Drug–drug interactions with itraconazole are more common than with ketoconazole and fluconazole and can be life-threatening. A complete listing of drug–drug interactions is given in Tables 2 and 3.

5. FLUCONAZOLE

5.1. Introduction

Fluconazole has superior pharmacological characteristics, an admirable safety profile, and found widespread use in the treatment of different varieties of yeast infections.

5.2. Chemical Structure and Mechanism of Action

As noted earlier.

5.3. Antimicrobial Spectrum

The antifungal spectrum of fluconazole is narrower than that of other azoles. It has activity against most, but not all, *Candida* species; it has decreased or no activity against *C. glabrata* and *C. krusei*, respectively. It is active against *C. neoformans*, the endemic mycoses, and dermatophytes. It has no activity against *Aspergillus* species, most other filamentous fungi, or the zygomycetes.

5.4. Clinical Pharmacology

Fluconazole is water soluble and available in both IV and oral formulations. The oral formulation is nearly 100% bioavailable. The drug distributes widely into most compartments, including the eye and the CSF, and is only 10% protein-bound. Fluconazole is only partially metabolized through the CYP450 system in the liver; more than 80% of the active drug is excreted into the urine. In patients whose creatine clearance is <50 mL/min, the dose should be decreased to half the normal dose.

5.5. Clinical Indications

Fluconazole has become the drug-of-choice for the treatment of candidemia and invasive *Candida* infections, with the exception of infections due to *C. glabrata* and *C. krusei*, which are resistant to fluconazole (8). It is the first-line agent for *Candida* urinary tract infections, vaginitis, esophagitis, and thrush. It is also the preferred agent for consolidation and maintenance therapy of cryptococcal meningitis after initial induction therapy with amphotericin B (4). Fluconazole has found widespread use as a prophylactic agent to prevent *Candida* infections in highly immunosuppressed patient populations, such as those receiving stem cell transplants (8). It is second-line therapy for dermatophyte infections and most infections with the endemic mycoses. However, it is the drug-of-choice for meningitis caused by *C. immitis* (7).

5.6. Administration of Drug

Fluconazole is available as tablets of varying strengths, an oral suspension, and an IV formulation. A loading dose of twice the daily dose should be given the first day to achieve steady state more quickly. Fluconazole is dosed once daily, and the oral formulations can be given with or without food and do not require acid for absorption. The usual dosage for localized mucocutaneous infections is 100–200 mg daily, and for vaginitis it is simply 1–150 mg tablet. Systemic infections, including meningitis, are treated with 400–800 mg daily, but higher dosages are sometimes used for various infections and have been well tolerated.

5.7. Drug Monitoring and Adverse Effects

Fluconazole is remarkably well tolerated. Nausea, vomiting, headache, and rash can occur, but are uncommon. Chronic administration is often associated with alopecia, which may be mild or profound and is always reversible. Hepatitis can occur, as with all azoles, and liver enzymes should be monitored if the drug is used for more than several weeks. Drug–drug interactions, although less than those noted with itraconazole and voriconazole, can be serious and are listed in Tables 2 and 3.

6. VORICONAZOLE

6.1. Introduction

Voriconazole is the first second-generation azole to become available (18). It was developed primarily to enhance the spectrum of activity compared with the first-generation azoles. The second-generation azoles are fungicidal for filamentous fungi such as *Aspergillus*, a characteristic that sets them apart from the first-generation agents.

6.2. Chemistry and Mechanism of Action

As noted earlier.

6.3. Antimicrobial Spectrum

Voriconazole is active against all species of *Candida*, *C. neoformans*, all species of *Aspergillus*, and appears to be active against the dimorphic fungi *B. dermatitidis*, *C. immitis*, and *H. capsulatum*, but not *S. schenckii*. A variety of other molds, many of which are resistant to amphotericin B, are susceptible to voriconazole in vitro. However, the zygomycetes are not susceptible to voriconazole.

6.4. Clinical Pharmacology

Voriconazole is available as both IV and oral formulations. Absorption of the oral formulation is >90% when given without food. In adults, voriconazole exhibits non-linear pharmacokinetics and there is substantial variability among patients in regard to serum concentrations of voriconazole. Voriconazole is 58% protein-bound and has a large volume of distribution. The drug achieves excellent concentrations in the CSF and the brain tissue. Less than 5% of voriconazole is excreted unchanged in the urine.

The metabolism of voriconazole occurs in the liver via the CYP450 enzyme system (18); CYP2C9, CYP3A4, and CYP2C19 are involved. CYP2C19 is the major metabolic pathway for voriconazole and is highly variable in the population. Persons of Asian lineage may have low activity of this enzyme and thus, elevated voriconazole serum concentrations, which may predict hepatic toxicity.

6.5. Clinical Indications

Voriconazole appears to be more effective than amphotericin B for treatment of invasive aspergillosis and has become the drug-of-choice for that disease (19). It is also indicated for patients who have infection with several uncommon molds, including *Fusarium* species and *Scedosporium apiospermum*, and likely will be increasingly used for other mold infections (20). Voriconazole is efficacious for patients who have esophageal candidiasis, including some who have fluconazole-refractory infection. At this time, voriconazole is not approved for other forms of candidiasis, but it likely will be approved for this indication in the near future.

6.6. Administration of Drug

Voriconazole is available for both IV and oral administration. The IV formulation is infused over 1–2 hr. A loading dose of 6 mg/kg every 12 hr is given the first day so that steady-state concentrations are achieved more quickly. The standard maintenance dosage is 4 mg/kg every 12 hr. The IV formulation should be avoided in patients who have renal insufficiency (creatinine clearance < 50 mL/min) because of accumulation of the cyclodextrin vehicle in which the drug is solubilized.

Both 50 and 200 mg tablets are available, as is an oral suspension. The loading dose is 400 mg every 12 hr for the first day and the standard maintenance dosage is 200 mg every 12 hr. Voriconazole should be administered when the stomach is empty. The oral formulation can be used in patients who have renal insufficiency, and the dosage remains unchanged.

6.7. Drug Monitoring and Side Effects

The most common side effect noted with voriconazole is photopsia, a reversible visual disturbance variously described as altered color discrimination, blurred vision, and the appearance of bright spots and wavy lines (18). Approximately 30% of patients experience this side effect, but few discontinue the drug because of these visual complaints. Patients whose therapy is initiated in the outpatient setting should be cautioned about the danger of visual disturbances while driving. No anatomic changes in the retina have been noted, and this effect decreases over time and stops entirely when the drug is stopped.

Skin rashes are more commonly noted with voriconazole than the other azoles. Most are mild rashes, but severe photosensitivity rashes have also been noted. Other less commonly noted side effects include nausea, vomiting, diarrhea, abdominal pain, headache, and visual hallucinations that are separate from photopsia.

Elevations in hepatic enzymes may occur more frequently with voriconazole than with the other azoles. Although most patients have asymptomatic elevation of hepatic enzymes, several patients have been reported with severe life-threatening hepatitis. The risk of developing hepatitis appears to increase with increased serum voriconazole levels. Thus, increasing the dosage of this agent should be discouraged. Patients on voriconazole should have liver function tests monitored prior to therapy, within the first 2 weeks, and then every 2–4 weeks throughout therapy.

Drug–drug interactions are of major importance with voriconazole because of its multiple CYP450 interactions (Tables 2 and 3).

7. CASPOFUNGIN

7.1. Introduction

Caspofungin is the first echinocandin to be made available for use (21,22). Two other similar compounds will likely be released for use in the next several years. This new class of antifungal agents targets the fungal cell wall. Because mammalian cells do not have cell walls, these are very selective agents and have shown minimal toxicity in humans. The spectrum of activity of the echinocandins is relatively narrow compared with amphotericin B and the second-generation azoles.

7.2. Chemistry and Mechanism of Action

The echinocandins are large lipopeptides that inhibit synthesis of β-(1,3)-D-glucan by interfering with glucan synthase, a UDP-glucosyl-transferase (21). When synthesis of glucan chains that form a large component of the cell wall of certain fungi is inhibited, cell lysis and death of the organism ensues. β-(1,3)-D-glucans are important components of the cell wall of all *Candida* species and *Aspergillus* species, but are not present or occur only in small amounts in other fungi.

7.3. Antimicrobial Spectrum

Caspofungin is fungicidal for all *Candida* species. The drug is not active against *C. neoformans* and other more uncommon yeasts. Most authorities consider the echinocandins to be fungistatic, rather than fungicidal for *Aspergillus* species. Caspofungin is not active against other molds or the endemic fungi, *H. capsulatum*, *B. dermatitidis*, *C. immitis*, and *S. schenckii*.

7.4. Clinical Pharmacology

Caspofungin is available only as an IV formulation. The drug is highly protein-bound (96%) and distributes into liver, spleen, lungs, and kidneys, but very little is found in the brain, eye, and CSF. Active drug is not found in the urine. Caspofungin is hydrolyzed and then acetylated to inactive metabolites. It is neither metabolized by nor an inhibitor of the CYP450 system. However, strong inducers of CYP450, such as rifampin, phenytoin, and carbamazepine, reduce serum concentrations of caspofungin so that a higher daily dosage (70 mg) is needed (21). The drug is administered once daily.

7.5. Clinical Indications

Caspofungin has been shown to be as efficacious as amphotericin B for candidemia and invasive candidiasis in a multicenter, blinded, and randomized trial (22). It is also effective for Candida esophagitis. Caspofungin is approved for the treatment of invasive aspergillosis in patients who are unable to tolerate other antifungal therapy and in those whose infection is refractory to other antifungal therapy. There have been no prospective trials of caspofungin as primary therapy for invasive aspergillosis.

It is possible that the echinocandins will become useful agents when used in combination with either amphotericin B formulations or triazoles. Given its unique mechanism of action on the cell wall, combining an echinocandin with an agent that acts at a different target may produce synergistic killing of the fungal organism. However, no controlled clinical trials have addressed this issue.

7.6. Administration of Drug

Caspofungin is given as an IV infusion once daily over an hour. A loading dosage of 70 mg is given the first day, followed by a daily dosage of 50 mg. Infusion-related reactions, including chills, fever, and flushing have been reported and can be obviated by slowing the infusion time and giving an antihistamine, such as diphenhydramine.

7.7. Drug Monitoring and Adverse Effects

The echinocandins have minimal toxicity. Infusion-related reactions of flushing, fever, and chills occur in <1% of the patients. Rash, pruritus, headache, nausea, vomiting, and phlebitis have been reported, but are uncommon. It is not clear if caspofungin is hepatotoxic; reports vary in regard to this possibility. It seems reasonable to monitor liver enzymes in patients receiving this agent.

8. TERBINAFINE

8.1. Introduction

In contrast to amphotericin B and the azoles, terbinafine is used only for localized dermatophyte infections of skin and nails. It is a relatively safe drug that can be used in older adults with onychomycosis that requires antifungal treatment (23,24).

8.2. Chemistry and Mechanism of Action

Terbinafine is an allylamine derivative that interferes with squalene epoxidase activity and blocks synthesis of ergosterol in the fungal cell membrane.

8.3. Antimicrobial Spectrum

Terbinafine has activity against dermatophytes that cause a variety of skin and nail infections. It has some activity against *C. albicans*, but is not as active as the azoles.

8.4. Clinical Pharmacology

Oral terbinafine is ≈70% absorbed. Terbinafine is >99% protein-bound, concentrates in the stratum corneum, hair follicles, and nails, and is extensively metabolized by CYP450 enzymes in the liver to inactive metabolites. Terbinafine does not inhibit the metabolism of other drugs, such as warfarin, as is noted with the azoles. However, rifampin, a strong inducer of CYP450 enzymes increases the metabolism of terbinafine and markedly decreases serum terbinafine levels.

8.5. Clinical Indications

Terbinafine is indicated for the treatment of onychomycosis and dermatophyte infections of skin that have not responded to application of creams. It is not indicated for any systemic fungal infection.

8.6. Administration of Drug

Terbinafine is available as 250 mg tablets that are given once daily with or without food. The usual dosage for onychomycosis is 250 mg daily for 6–12 weeks. Infected fingernails may respond after 6 weeks, but toenails always require longer therapy. Pulse therapy for 1 week out of each month for 3–4 months also can be used (23).

8.7. Drug Monitoring and Adverse Events

Terbinafine is usually well tolerated. Changes in taste perception can occur and may interfere with appetite. Rash occurs uncommonly, but can manifest as Stevens–Johnson syndrome, which requires immediate discontinuation of the drug. Severe neutropenia also occurs rarely with terbinafine administration. Hepatic dysfunction, cholestatic jaundice, and rarely liver failure have been reported with the use of terbinafine; it is important to obtain liver enzyme tests at baseline, 2 weeks after the start of therapy, and then monthly thereafter, and to warn the patient about the symptoms of hepatotoxicity.

REFERENCES

1. Hiemenz JR, Walsh TJ. Lipid formulations of amphotericin B: recent progress and future directions. Clin Infect Dis 1996; 22(suppl 2):S133–S144.
2. Wong-Beringer A, Jacobs RA, Guglielmo BJ. Lipid formulations of amphotericin B: clinical efficacy and toxicities. Clin Infect Dis 1998; 27:603–618.
3. Kauffman CA, Amphotericin B. Semin Respir Crit Care Med 1997; 18:281–287.
4. Saag MS, Graybill JR, Larsen RA, Pappas PG, Perfect JR, Powderly WG, Sobel JD, Dismukes WE. Practice guidelines for the management of cryptococcal disease. Clin Infect Dis 2000; 30:710–718.

5. Chapman SW, Bradsher RW Jr, Campbell GD Jr, Pappas PG, Kauffman CA. Practice guidelines for the management of patients with blastomycosis. Clin Infect Dis 2000; 30:679–683.

6. Wheat J, Sarosi G, McKinsey D, Hamill R, Bradsher R, Johnson P, Loyd J. Practice guidelines for the management of patients with histoplasmosis. Clin Infect Dis 2000; 30:688–695.

7. Galgiani JN, Ampel NM, Catanzaro A, Johnson RH, Stevens DA, Williams PL. Practice guidelines for the treatment of coccidioidomycosis. Clin Infect Dis 2000; 30:658–661.

8. Pappas PG, Rex JH, Sobel JD, Filler SG, Dismukes WE, Walsh TJ, Edwards JE. Guidelines for the treatment of candidiasis. Clin Infect Dis 2004; 36:161–189.

9. Stevens DA, Kan VL, Judson MA, Morrison VA, Dummer S, Denning DW, Bennett JE, Walsh TJ, Patterson TF, Pankey GA. Practice guidelines for diseases caused by *Aspergillus*. Clin Infect Dis 2000; 30:696–709.

10. Branch RA. Prevention of amphotericin B-induced renal impairment: a review on the use of sodium supplementation. Arch Intern Med 1988; 148:2389–2394.

11. Goodwin SD, Cleary JD, Walawander CA, Taylor JW, Grasela TH. Pretreatment regimens for adverse events related to infusion of amphotericin B. Clin Infect Dis 1995; 20:755–761.

12. National Institute of Allergy and Infectious Diseases Study Group. Treatment of blastomycosis and histoplasmosis with ketoconazole: results of a prospective randomized trial. Ann Intern Med 1985; 103:861–872.

13. Dismukes WE, Stamm AM, Graybill JR, Craven PC, Stevens DA, Stiller RL, Sarosi GA, Medoff G, Gregg CR, Gallis HA, Fields BT Jr, Marier RL, Kerkering TA, Kaplowitz LG, Cloud G, Bowles C, Shadomy S. Treatment of systemic mycoses with ketoconazole: emphasis on toxicity and clinical response in 52 patients. Ann Intern Med 1983; 98:13–20.

14. Dismukes WE, Bradsher RW, Cloud GC, Kauffman CA, Chapman SW, George RB, Stevens DA, Giard WM, Saag MS, Bowles-Patton C. Itraconazole therapy for blastomycosis and histoplasmosis. Am J Med 1992; 93:489–497.

15. Galgiani JN, Catanzaro A, Cloud GA, Johnson RH, Williams PL, Mireles LF, Nassar F, Lutz JE, Stevens DA, Sharkey PK, Singh VR, Larsen RA, Delgado KL, Flanigan C, Rinaldi M. Comparison of oral fluconazole and itraconazole for progressive, nonmeningeal coccidioidomycosis. A randomized, double-blind trial. Ann Intern Med 2000; 133: 676–680.

16. De Doncker P, Gupta AK, Marynissen G, Stoffels P, Heremans A. Itraconazole pulse therapy for onychomycosis and dermatomycoses: An overview. J Am Acad Dermatol 1997; 37:969–974.

17. Kauffman CA, Hajjeh R, Chapman SW. Practice guidelines for the management of patients with sporotrichosis. Clin Infect Dis 2000; 30:684–687.

18. Johnson LB, Kauffman CA. Voriconazole: a new triazole antifungal agent. Clin Infect Dis 2003; 36:630–637.

19. Herbrecht R, Denning DW, Patterson TF, Bennett JE, Greene RE, Oestmann JW, Kern WV, Marr KA, Ribaud P, Lortholary O, Sylvester R, Rubin RH, Wingard JR, Stark P, Duand C, Caillot D, Thiel E, Chandrasekar PH, Hodges MR, Schlamm HT, Troke PF, de Pauw B. Invasive fungal infections group of the European organisation for research and treatment of cancer and the global aspergillus study group. Voriconazole versus amphotericin B for primary therapy of invasive aspergillosis. N Engl J Med 2002; 347(6):408–415.

20. Perfect JR, Marr KA, Walsh TJ, Greenberg RN, DuPont B, de la Torre-Cisneros J, Just-Nubling G, Schlamm HT, Lutsar I, Espinel-Ingraff A, Johnson E. Voriconazole treatment for less-common, emerging, or refractory fungal infections. Clin Infect Dis 2003; 36:1121–1131.

21. Deresinski SC, Stevens DA. Caspofungin. Clin Infect Dis 2003; 36:1445–1457.

22. Mora-Duarte J, Betts R, Rotstein C, Colombo AL, Thompson-Moya L, Smietana J, Lupinacci R, Sable C, Kartsanis N, Perfect J. Caspofungin Invasive Candidiasis Study

Group. Caspofungin vs amphotericin B deoxycholate in the treatment of invasive candidiasis in neutropenic and non-neutropenic patients:a multi-centre, randomized, double-blind study. N Engl J Med 2002; 347:2020–2029.

23. Tosti A, Piraccini BM, Stinchi C, Venturo N, Bardazzi F, Colombo MD. Treatment of dermatophyte infections: an open randomized study comparing intermittent terbinafine therapy with continuous terbinafine treatment and intermittent itraconazole therapy. J Am Acad Derm 1996; 34:595–600.

24. Balfour JA, Faulds D. Terbinafine. A review of its pharmacodynamic and pharmacokinetic properties and therapeutic potential in superficial mycoses. Drugs 1992; 43:259–284.

SUGGESTED READING

Kauffman CA. Fungal infections in older adults. Clin Infect Dis 2001; 33:550–555.

26
Antiparasitic Drugs

Shobita Rajagopalan
Department of Internal Medicine, Division of Infectious Diseases, Charles R. Drew University of Medicine and Science, Martin Luther King, Jr.–Charles R. Drew Medical Center, Los Angeles, California, U.S.A.

Key Points:

- Parasitic infections with protozoa and helminths are important causes of morbidity and mortality worldwide.
- Increasing trends in international travel among the elderly to tropical and subtropical regions wherein such parasitic infections are endemic enhances the risk for disease acquisition.
- Because cell-mediated immune (CMI) responses are largely responsible for the pathogenesis of parasitic infections, age-related relative decline in CMI is likely to result in increased morbidity and mortality in the geriatric population.
- Only a few vaccines are available to prevent human parasitic infections. Hence, chemotherapy in conjunction with public health and vector-control measures plays an important role in prevention and reduction in transmission of parasitic infections as well as in the treatment of individual patients.
- The use of albendazole, fumagilin, trimethoprim–sulfamethoxazole, and paramomycin for the treatment of specific protozoal infections and albendazole, praziquantel, and ivermectin for the treatment of certain helminthic infections is reviewed.

Infections with parasitic protozoa and helminths are common causes of morbidity and mortality in developing countries. Increasing trends in international travel among the elderly to tropical and subtropical destinations, where many parasitic infections are endemic, enhances their risk for disease acquisition. Cell-mediated immune (CMI) responses play a significant role in the pathogenesis of and host resistance to parasitic infections. The age-associated relative decline in CMI is likely to result in increased morbidity and mortality from parasitic infections (1). Few vaccines are available to prevent human parasitic infections. Hence, antiparasitic chemotherapy plays an important role not only in the treatment of individual patients but also, in conjunction with public health and vector-control measures, in preventing and reducing transmission. There are several obstacles to the development of newer antiparasitic agents: limited commercial incentives for the production of drugs designed to combat infections that are mainly endemic in developing countries, sparse scientific knowledge essential to develop antiparasitic drugs, poorly understood mechanisms of action of most antiparasitic agents, and the lack of availability of some of the approved antiparasitic agents in the United States (2). Current recommendations and certain drugs available to prevent and treat particular parasitic infections may be obtained from the Parasitic Disease Branch of the Centers for Disease Control and Prevention in Atlanta (3).

This chapter will focus on the newer antiparasitic drugs with particular emphasis on their use in the elderly, as well as agents that have been recently established to be effective against specific parasites (Table 1). Table 2 shows the newer uses of antiparasitic drugs, their doses and adverse effects. Older, established antiparasitic agents (4,5) are not discussed here.

Table 1 Chemotherapy for Specific Parasitic Infections

Parasite and infection	Standard treatment	Potential new treatment
Helminths		
Intestinal nematodes		
Ascariasis	Mebendazole and pyrantel pamoate	Albendazole and ivermectin
Trichuriasis	Mebendazole	Albendazole[a] and ivermectin[a]
Enterobiasis	Mebendazole and pyrantel pamoate	Albendazole[a] and ivermectin[a]
Hookworm infection	Mebendazole and pyrantel pamoate[a]	Albendozole[a]
Strongyloidiasis	Thiabendazole	Albendazole[a] and ivermectin[a]
Tissue nematodes		
Onchocerciasis	Ivermectin	
Trematodes		
Schistosomiasis	Praziquantel and oxamniquine (*for Schistosoma mansoni*)	
Fascioliasis	Biothionol[a]	Triclabendazole
Other liver, lung and intestinal flukes	Praziquantel[a]	
Cestodes		
Intestinal tapeworms	Praziquantel[a]	
Cysticercosis	Surgery, praziquantel, and albendazole	Albendazole
Echinococcosis	Surgery	
Protozoa		
Giardiasis	Metronidazole, nitazoxanide, and tinidazole	Albendazole
Microsporidiosis in AIDS[b]	None	Albendazole, fumagillin
Cyclosporiasis	Trimethoprim–sulfamethoxazole	Paramomycin
Isosporiasis	Trimethoprim–sulfamethoxazole	
Cryptosporidiosis	Supportive fluid and electrolyte therapy	

[a]Not approved by the Food and Drug Administration.
[b]AIDS denotes acquired immunodeficiency syndrome.

Table 2 Newer Uses of Antiparasitic Drugs

Drug and indication	Dosage	Adverse effects
Albendazole		Abdominal pain, nausea, vomiting, alopecia, increased serum aminotransferase, and neutropenia
Echinococcosis[a]	400 mg twice-daily for 28 days, repeated as necessary	
Cysticercosis	5 mg/kg three times daily for 8–30 days, repeated as necessary	
Ascariasis[a] hookworm infection[a]	400 mg once	
Trichuriasis[a]	400 mg once (repeated for 3 days in heavy infections)	
Enterobiasis[a]	400 mg once, repeated in 2 weeks	
Strongyloidiasis (uncomplicated)[a]	400 mg once, daily for 3 days	
Microspondiosis in AIDS[a,b]	400 mg twice daily for 2–3 weeks	
Ivermectin		Mild pruritus, rash, and dizziness
Onchocerciasis[a]	150 µg/kg once	
Ascariasis,[a] trichuriasis[a]	12 mg once	
Strongyloidiasis[a]	200 µg/kg once daily for 1–2 days	
Paromomycin		Abdominal discomfort
Cryptosporidiosis[a]	500 mg 3–4 times daily for 2 weeks	
Praziquantel		Headache, dizziness, drowsiness, and abdominal discomfort
Schistosorniasis		
S. *mansoni*, S. *haematobium*	20 mg/kg twice daily for 1 day	
S. *japonicum* S. *mekongi*	20 mg/kg three times daily for 1 day	
Fluke infection		
Liver (*Glonorchis sinensis, Opisthorcis viverrini*)[a]	25 mg/kg three times daily for 1 day	
Lung (paragonimus)[a]	25 mg/kg twice daily for 2 days	
Intestine (*fasciolopsis buski, Heterophyes heterophers, Metagonimus yokogawai*)[a]	25 mg/kg three times daily for 1 day	
Nanophygtus salmincola[a]	20 mg/kg three times daily for 1 day	

(*Continued*)

Table 2   Newer Uses of Antiparasitic Drugs (*Continued*)

Drug and indication	Dosage	Adverse effects
Neurocysticercosis[a]	15–20 mg/kg three times daily for 15 days	
Intestinal tapeworm infection		
Fish, beef, pork, and dog[a]	5–10 mg/kg once	
Dwarf *Hymenolepsisnana*[a]	25 mg/kg once	
Oxamniquine		
S. mansoni infection	15 mg/kg once 30 mg/kg in East Africa 30 mg/kg for days in Egypt and South Africa	
Fumagillin		
Microporidial keratoconjunctivitis[a]	Eye drops	

[a]Not approved by the Food and Drug Administration for this indication.
[b]AIDS denotes acquired immunodeficiency syndrome.

1. ANTIPROTOZOAL DRUGS

Protozoan parasites are all unicellular organisms which replicate, often rapidly, in the infected host and belong to four distinct groups: the ameba, the flagellates, the ciliates, and the sporozoa. The drugs albendazole, fumagilin, trimethoprim–sulfamethoxazole (TMP–SMX), and paramomycin will be discussed later.

1.1. Albendazole

1.1.1. Giardiasis

The benzimidazole drugs available for the treatment of parasitic diseases in humans include thiabendazole, mebendazole, and albendazole. The newest benzimidazole, albendazole, has a broad range of activity against certain protozoan and many nematode and cestode parasites. Similar to the other benzimidazole agents, albendazole binds to free β-tubulin and inhibits the polymerization of tubulin and the cytoskeletal microtubule-dependent uptake of glucose (6,7). This property makes it potentially useful in the treatment of protozoan infections such as giardiasis, caused by the flagellated protozoan *Giardia lamblia* (also known as *G. duodenalis*). Although no studies have investigated the effect of age on albendazole pharmacokinetics, data in 26 patients with hydatid cyst (up to 79 years) suggest pharmacokinetics similar to those in young healthy subjects (8).

Giardiasis affects the upper small bowel and is one of the most common parasitic diarrheal infections in the United States and in other countries. Giardiasis is currently treated with metronidazole or tinidazole (the latter drug recently approved for this indication by the Food and Drug Administration), and quinacrine (no longer distributed in the United States) (4,9). In vitro, albendazole inhibits the growth of trophozoites of *G. lamblia* and their adhesion to cultured intestinal epithelial cells and disrupts the activity of microtubules and microribbons in the trophozoite's adhesive disk. The results of treatment of giardiasis with albendazole have been mixed. While demonstrating curative potential in 97% of infections in children in Bangladesh, albendazole was ineffective in a study of adult travelers returning from tropical areas (10,11).

1.1.2. Microsporidiosis

Unlike giardiasis, for which there are effective drugs, the various forms of microsporidiosis have until recently proven a challenge to treat. Microsporidia are small, spore-forming obligate intracellular protozoan parasites that only rarely infect immunocompetent patients but that may cause intestinal, ocular, or disseminated disease in patients with acquired immune deficiency syndrome (AIDS) (12). Five genera of microsporidia, Enterocytozoon, Encephalitozoon, Septata, Pleistophora, and Nosema, and some other unclassified microsporidia cause human disease. Albendazole disrupts the function of tubulin in microsporidia and has antimicrosporidial activity both in vitro and in vivo (13–16). Current clinical trials of albendazole in patients with AIDS who had intestinal microsporidial infections, principally with Enterocytozoon bieneusi and Septata intestinalis, have demonstrated symptomatic improvement with albendazole, with less frequent stools and often decreased fecal excretion of microsporidial spores. However, after the cessation of albendazole therapy, symptomatic illness often recurred; thus, longer-term suppressive treatment may be needed (17–21).

1.2. Fumagillin

1.2.1. Ocular Microsporidiosis

Fumagillin is a water-insoluble antibiotic produced by Aspergillus fumigatus. Over four decades ago, fumagillin was found to inhibit the activity of intestinal protozoa, including Entamoeba histolytica, the causative agent of amebiasis (22). Fumagillin had not been used in human infections, although a water-soluble form of the drug, fumagillin bicyclohexylammonium salt, is used to control microsporidial disease due to Nosema apis in honeybees. Although the mechanism of action of fumagillin has not been established, it suppresses the proliferation of microsporidia in vitro (23). A topical suspension of fumagillin was effective in the treatment of microsporidial keratoconjunctivitis due to Encephalitozoon hellem or Encephalitozoon cuniculi in several patients with AIDS (24,25). Maintenance therapy with twice-daily topical administration of fumagillin was necessary to prevent symptomatic relapses.

1.3. Trimethoprim–Sulfamethoxazole

1.3.1. Cyclosporiasis

Cyclospora, a recently recognized coccidian protozoan parasite, has been reported to cause diarrheal illness, often prolonged, in the United States and other countries (26). TMP–SMX is effective in treating diarrheal disease caused by cyclospora (27). In immunocompetent patients, treatment with a combination of 160 mg of trimethoprim and 800 mg of sulfamethoxazole (i.e., a double-strength tablet) twice daily for 7 days ended diarrheal illness and led to clearance of the parasites (28). In patients infected with the human immunodeficiency virus, treatment with one double-strength tablet of TMP–SMX four times a day for 10 days leads to a rapid resolution of diarrhea (29). Symptomatic cyclosporiasis may recur in the following weeks, but it can be prevented by the administration of TMP–SMX three times weekly.

1.3.2. Isosporiasis

TMP–SMX is also effective in treating enteric infections with *Isospora belli* (30). The double-strength tablet is given orally four times a day for 10 days and then twice a day for 3 weeks. In patients with AIDS, in whom recurrences are common, long-term maintenance therapy with double-strength TMP–SMX tablets given three times a week or a combination of 25 mg of pyrimethamine and 500 mg of sulfadoxine given once a week can be effective (31). Alternatively, for those intolerant of sulfa drugs, pyrimethamine alone (75 mg/day, until the infection is cleared) is effective and can be followed with a maintenance dose of 25 mg/day to prevent relapses (32).

1.4. Paromomycin

1.4.1. Cryptosporidiosis

Cryptosporidium parvum is a common cause of diarrhea in ungulate farm animals and a major cause of waterborne outbreaks of diarrhea among humans. Recent studies suggest that the elderly have an increased risk of severe disease due to *Cryptosporidium* infection with a shorter incubation period than has been previously reported in all adults and with a high risk for secondary person-to-person transmission (33). Cryptosporidiosis is usually a self-limited enteric infection in immunocompetent patients but is a potentially debilitating and chronic diarrheal illness in patients with AIDS or other immunocompromised states (34). An effective antiparasitic drug for cryptosporidiosis in patients with AIDS is greatly needed, but many drugs have proved ineffective. Several recent studies suggest that an older oral aminoglycoside, paromomycin, may be at least partially effective in treating cryptosporidiosis. In both an open trial and a small double-blind trial of paromomycin (in a dose of 500 mg three or four times a day for 2 weeks) in patients with AIDS who had cryptosporidiosis, the drug reduced diarrhea; in the double-blind study the fecal excretion of cryptosporidiosis oocysts was also reduced (35). Paromomycin given orally is not systemically absorbed, even in patients with intestinal cryptosporidiosis. It is not likely to be a definitive antiparasitic therapy, and continued treatment with 500 mg twice daily is needed to prevent relapse (36).

2. ANTHELMINTIC DRUGS

Parasitic helminths, such as nematodes (roundworms), cestodes (e.g., tapeworms), and trematodes (flukes), are complex multicellular organisms with differentiated nervous systems and organs. In contrast to viruses, bacteria, and protozoa, most helminths do not directly replicate in the human body but reproduce sexually, giving rise to eggs or larvae that pass out of the body. Anthelmintic agents often affect some of the more complex systems of cellular physiology, such as microtubule formation or neuromuscular function. The emergence of drug resistance in helminths has been much more gradual and limited than in rapidly replicating protozoa, such as the malarial parasite *Plasmodium falciparum*. (Albendazole, praziquantel, and Ivermectin will be discussed in this section.)

2.1. Albendazole

As mentioned earlier, benzimidazoles (thiabendazole, mebendazole, and albendazole) are highly effective in the treatment of parasitic diseases in humans. Although resistance to benzimidazole develops due to loss of the drug's high affinity for binding to tubulin in intensively treated livestock, resistance has not been documented in humans. This newest benzimidazole, albendazole, has a broad range of activity against many nematode and cestode parasites. The side effects of albendazole usually do not require discontinuation of the drug (Table 2).

2.1.1. Echinococcosis

Albendazole has expanded the therapeutic options for patients with cystic hydatid disease due to *Echinococcus granulosus* (37). Surgery remains the mainstay of treatment for this disease, but it carries the risks of operative morbidity, recurrence of cysts, and spillage of fluid from the cysts, which can lead to anaphylaxis or dissemination of the infection (38). Albendazole reduces the viability of protoscolices and cysts, and its hepatic metabolite, albendazole sulfoxide, is also active against the larval cestodes. The administration of albendazole prior to surgery has been advocated in order to inactivate protoscolices and minimize the likelihood of recurring cysts (39). Drug therapy is also indicated after the spontaneous or operative rupture of cysts, and the spillage of their contents, to prevent secondary dissemination. The usual 4-week course of treatment (Table 2) often needs to be repeated two or more times. The absorption of albendazole is enhanced by taking it with fatty meals.

Albendazole is indicated for patients with inoperable, widespread, or numerous cysts of *E. granulosus* and for patients with complicated medical problems who are unsuitable candidates for surgery. Percutaneous drainage has also been successfully used to treat hepatic hydatid cysts, and when combined with albendazole therapy, further reduces the size of cysts (40,41).

Albendazole is also useful as adjunctive medical therapy for alveolar hydatid disease due to *E. multilocularis* and may be effective against infection with *E. vogeli* (42,43). In infection with either *E. granulosus* or *E. multilocularis*, however, the response to albendazole occurs only after many months. Furthermore, in most treated patients the cystic lesions do not resolve completely, although they cease to enlarge (44). Thus, when feasible, surgical excision of echinococcal cysts remains the definitive therapy and albendazole should be administered in conjunction with surgery or to patients who are not candidates for surgery.

2.1.2. Intestinal Tapeworms and Cysticercosis

Infection with intestinal tapeworms can be treated effectively with available anthelmintic drugs, including praziquantel and niclosamide. However, tissue infection with the larval stage of *Taenia solium* (cysticercosis), and especially neurocysticercosis, the most prevalent helminthic infection of the brain, was for a long time amenable only to surgical therapy. The therapeutic use of praziquantel, and more recently of albendazole, has provided medical treatment for neurocysticercosis (45). For patients with inactive disease and calcified tissue cysts, specific cesticidal therapy is not needed. However, active neurocysticercosis with viable intraparenchymal cysts (which can be seen as low-density cysts on computed tomography with little or no enhancement with contrast medium) requires drug treatment.

The administration of either praziquantel or albendazole results in the reduction or disappearance of cysts in 80–90% of patients. In comparative trials, albendazole (5 mg/kg of body weight three times daily for 28–30 days) was more effective than praziquantel in reducing the number and size of cysts and in inducing overall clinical improvement (46,47). Jung et al. demonstrated that adjunctive therapy with dexamethasone is useful for patients with numerous cysts and for those in whom neurologic symptoms or intracranial hypertension develops after the initiation of therapy against cysticerci (48). Plasma concentrations of albendazole, but not praziquantel, are higher in patients treated with corticosteroids. A shorter course of albendazole (8 days) appears to be as effective as the traditional 28–30-day course. Pharmacokinetic studies suggest that the relatively long half-life of albendazole might allow for twice-a-day dosing for this condition.

Medical therapy is definitely indicated for patients with numerous viable cysts, acute meningitis, or increased intracranial pressure, but it may be effective even in patients with solitary cysts and seizures alone (49–53). However, clinical variability and a tendency toward spontaneous resolution in neurocysticercosis have contributed to continuing uncertainty about the precise indications for anthelmintic therapy and even its overall usefulness in this disease. For patients with giant subarachnoid cysts, albendazole, but not praziquantel, has proved effective. For patients with ventricular, spinal, or intraocular cysts, surgery is the preferred therapy, although concurrent therapy with albendazole is advisable and, on occasion, treatment with albendazole has obviated the need for surgery.

2.1.3. Intestinal Roundworms

Soil-transmitted helminthiases, ascariasis, hookworm infection, and trichuriasis, are among the most prevalent infections in the world (54). In areas in which they are endemic, the efficacy of single doses of albendazole or the older benzimidazole drug mebendazole has made mass chemotherapy feasible. These two drugs have also been used extensively in individualized tailored therapy. Single doses of both albendazole (Table 2) and mebendazole are highly effective against ascariasis, although albendazole appears to be more effective than mebendazole in hookworm infections. Neither drug in a single dose is highly effective in eradicating *Trichuris trichiura*, although in one study, three doses of albendazole resulted in an 80% rate of cure.

2.1.4. Other Roundworms

Albendazole has also proved effective or promising against a number of less common nematode infections of tissue, including cutaneous larva migrans, gnathostomiasis, intestinal capillariasis, clonorchiasis, and infection with lagochilascariasis minor, as well as more recently recognized infections with *Trichinella pseudospiralis* and *Oesophagostomum bifurcum* (55–58). Albendazole (400 mg twice daily for 3 days) is moderately effective for chronic strongyloidiasis, but not as effective as ivermectin (59). The effectiveness of albendazole has not been evaluated in patients with the hyperinfection syndrome of strongyloidiasis for whom thiabendazole, despite its frequent side effects, remains the drug-of-choice. In infections with filarial nematodes, onchocerciasis and loiasis, albendazole has a limited ability to reduce the number of microfilariae, possibly because of an embryotoxic effect on the adult worms (60,61). Albendazole is not active in infections with the filarial parasite *Mansonella perstans* (62).

2.2. Ivermectin

Ivermectin is an extremely potent, broad-spectrum, anthelmintic drug that has been widely used in controlling nematode infections in animals (63). In humans, it has been used most extensively against onchocerciasis (river blindness), through supplies donated by the manufacturer, Merck, to the Onchocerciasis Control Program of the World Bank and the World Health Organization. Ivermectin is a semisynthetic macrocyclic lactone derived from avermectins of the soil mold *Streptomyces avermitilis*. It appears to kill helminths by opening chloride-sensitive channels, and in the free-living nematode *Caenorhabditis elegans* the drug binds to a glutamate-gated chloride channel.

2.2.1. Onchocerciasis

A single oral dose of ivermectin (150 µg/kg) substantially reduces the number of microfilariae in the skin and eyes, thus diminishing the likelihood of disabling onchocerciasis. In areas where the disease is endemic, the dose can be repeated every 6–12 months to maintain suppression of both dermal and ocular microfilariae. After therapy with ivermectin, even severe onchocercal dermatitis is reduced, with amelioration of pruritus but no resolution of depigmentation (64). Ocular disease also responds: damage to the optic nerve is lessened, punctate keratitis and iritis are diminished, and fewer microfilariae are released in the anterior chamber and in the cornea (65). However, there are no effects on sclerosing keratitis or chorioretinitis.

By decreasing the number of microfilariae in the skin of infected persons, mass chemotherapy with ivermectin reduces transmission of this vector-borne disease. Ivermectin may impair the fertility of female onchocerca worms, but it does not kill adult worms. A well-tolerated drug that is effective against adult onchocerca worms has yet to be found. The side effects of ivermectin therapy for patients with onchocerciasis (Table 2) are mainly due to host reactions to the dying microfilariae and include pruritus, papular rash, dizziness, edema in the face and limbs, and, in rare cases, ocular inflammation. These side effects are usually mild and less severe than with diethylcarbamazine.

2.2.2. Other Filariases

The effectiveness of ivermectin in onchocerciasis has led to field trials of the drug for cases of lymphatic filariasis, the other major filarial infection (66). In single doses of between 100 and 440 µg/kg, ivermectin leads to clearance of the microfilariae of *Wuchereria bancrofti* and *Brugia malayi* from the blood, but it is not active against adult filarial worms in the lymphatic system. A single dose of ivermectin is as effective as the traditional 14-day course of diethylcarbamazine in lowering the number of circulating microfilariae and has far fewer side effects. However, the reduction in microfilaremia is not sustained, and a single dose of diethylcarbamazine appears to be as well tolerated and effective as ivermectin in inducing a sustained reduction in microfilaremia. With respect to other filarial parasites, ivermectin is effective against *Mansonella ozzardi* but not *M. perstans* (67,68). In *Loa loa* infections, ivermectin decreases microfilaremia, but because it is not clearly effective against adult worms, the stage of the parasite primarily responsible for human symptoms, diethylcarbamazine remains the drug-of-choice (69).

2.2.3. Other Roundworms

Ivermectin is also effective against several common intestinal parasitic nematodes, including ascaris, trichuris, and enterobius (70). It is ineffective against hookworms in humans, for which mebendazole is the treatment of choice. A single 12 mg dose of ivermectin was more effective than a single 400 mg dose of albendazole for cutaneous larva migrans in one study (71). Ivermectin, in a daily dose of $200\,\mu g/kg$ for 1 or 2 days, is highly effective against chronic intestinal strongyloidiasis, a difficult infection to eradicate. Side effects of treating strongyloidiasis with ivermectin are less frequent than with thiabendazole (72). In one study of strongyloidiasis, ivermectin ($150-200\,\mu g/kg$, given as a single oral dose) cured 83% of patients with the disease, as compared with a rate of 38% with albendazole. Ivermectin has also proved effective for strongyloidiasis in patients with AIDS (73). A series of doses of ivermectin may be effective in the hyperinfection syndrome of strongyloidiasis, but experience with its use in disseminated strongyloidiasis is limited.

2.2.4. Ectoparasites

Scabies is a common problem encountered in elderly residents of long-term care facilities. The severe crusted or "Norwegian" form of scabies is particularly difficult to treat (74,75). The most common treatment for scabies is topical permethrin or lindane (γ-benzene hexachloride). Other treatments include topical benzyl benzoate, crotamiton, or precipitated sulfur. Oral ivermectin is very effective; however, because of occasional deaths being reported in elderly patients, it is best reserved for refractory or extensive infections, such as crusted or Norwegian scabies.

Ivermectin is also effective in treating head lice.

2.3. Praziquantel

Praziquantel is an effective drug against a broad range of trematode and cestode infections (76). Although the drug has been in clinical use for over a decade, its mode of action is still not clearly understood. Praziquantel appears to interfere with calcium homeostasis and causes flaccid paralysis in adult flukes. Studies of parasitic schistosomes indicate that the immune response of the host and the formation of specific antibodies are necessary to create praziquantel's anthelmintic effects (77). Perhaps by disrupting the surface membrane of the parasite, praziquantel causes antigens within the parasite to be exposed to the action of host antibodies.

2.3.1. Schistosomiasis

Praziquantel is the drug of choice for all forms of schistosomiasis (Table 2). Mass treatment with praziquantel has been used as a means of control of the waterborne, snail-transmitted parasites that cause the disease. However, resistance to the drug has been found in infected mice, and the drug was ineffective in a few large-scale campaigns. In some areas of endemic schistosomiasis the low rates of cure attributable to praziquantel might be due to extremely rapid reinfection rather than any intrinsic drug resistance of the parasite. For infection with *Schistosoma mansoni*, oxamniquine (Table 2) is an effective and cheaper alternative to praziquantel.

2.3.2. Other Flukes

Praziquantel is also effective in the treatment of most flukes (Table 2). The only fluke not responsive to praziquantel is *Fasciola hepatica* (sheep-liver fluke), which responds to bithionol (given at a daily dose of 30–50 mg/kg on alternate days for 10–15 doses) and, as seen in a few promising studies, to the veterinary drug triclabendazole.

2.3.3. Cestodes

For infection with intestinal tapeworms, praziquantel in a single dose is effective. Treatment of intestinal *T. solium* infections can lead to neurologic reactions in patients who have occult neurocysticercosis, although patients with neurocysticercosis often have no response to a single dose of praziquantel. As noted earlier, a longer course of praziquantel is effective for neurocysticercosis, although albendazole may be more efficacious. The bioavailability of praziquantel is limited by extensive first-pass metabolism of the drug; this limitation of metabolism is exacerbated by dexamethasone and the antiepileptic drugs that are often given concomitantly with praziquantel for seizure control in patients with neurocysticercosis (79). Phenytoin and carbamazepine induce metabolism of praziquantel by hepatic cytochrome P450 and have contributed to treatment failures (80). Cimetidine, which inhibits hepatic-enzyme metabolism, increases the peak serum concentration of praziquantel and lengthens the drug's elimination half-life.

3. CONCLUSIONS

Although newer drugs such as albendazole and ivermectin have proven to be effective against some common parasitic infections, there remains a need for the continued development of new drugs to counter the many parasitic infections for which there is not yet effective treatment.

REFERENCES

1. Humphreys NE, Grencis RK. Effects of ageing on the immunoregulation of parasitic infection. Infect Immun 2002; 70:5148–5157.
2. White AC. The disappearing arsenal of antiparasitic drugs. N Engl J Med 2000; 343: 1273–1274.
3. Centers for Disease Control and Prevention, Division of Parasitic Diseases. http:// www.dpd.cdc.gov/dpdx/.
4. WHO model prescribing information. Drugs Used in Parasitic Diseases. 2nd ed. Geneva: World Health Organization, 1995.
5. Drugs for parasitic infections. Med Lett Drugs Ther 2004; 46:1–12.
6. Lacey E. Mode of action of benzimidazoles. Parasitol Today 1990; 6:112–115.
7. Lacey E, Gill JH. Biochemistry of benzimidazole resistance. Acta Trop 1994; 56:245–262.
8. Nahmias J, Goldsmith R, Soibelman M, el-On J. Three- to 7-year follow-up after albendazole treatment of 68 patients with cystic echinococcosis (hydatid disease). Ann Trop Med Parasitol 1994; 88:295–304.
9. Tinidazole (Tindamax)—a new antiprotozoal drug. Med Lett Drugs Ther 2004; 46:70–72.
10. Hall A, Nahar Q. Albendazole as a treatment for infections with Giardia duodenalis in children in Bangladesh. Trans R Soc Trop Med Hyg 1993; 87:84–86.
11. Gardner TB, Hill DR. Treatment of giardiasis. Clin Microbiol Rev 2001; 14:114–128.
12. Weber R, Bryan RT. Microsporidial infections in immunodeficient and immunocompetent patients. Clin Infect Dis 1994; 19:517–521.
13. Haque A, Hollister WS, Willcox A, Canning EU. The antimicrosporidial activity of albendazole. J Invertebr Pathol 1993; 62:171–177.
14. Weiss LM, Michalakakis E, Coyle CM, Tanowitz HB, Wittner M. The in vitro activity of albendazole against Encephalitozoon cuniculi. J Eukaryot Microbiol 1994; 41: 65S–65S.

15. Koudela B, Lom J, Vitovec J, Kucerova Z, Ditrich O, Travnicek J. In vivo efficacy of albendazole against Encephalitozoon cuniculi in SCID mice. J Eukaryot Microbiol 1994; 41:49S–50S.

16. Beauvais B, Sarfati C, Challier S, Derouin F. In vitro model to assess effect of antimicrobial agents on Encephalitozoon cuniculi. Antimicrob Agents Chemother 1994; 38: 2440–2448.

17. Blanshard C, Ellis DS, Tovey DG, Dowell S, Gazzard BG. Treatment of intestinal microsporidiosis with albendazole in patients with AIDS. AIDS 1992; 6:311–313.

18. Molina JM, Oksenhendler E, Beauvais B, Sarfati C, Jaccard A, Derouin F, Modai J. Disseminated microsporidiosis due to Septata intestinalis in patients with AIDS: clinical features and response to albendazole therapy. J Infect Dis 1995; 171:245–249.

19. Weber R, Sauer B, Spycher MA, Deplazes P, Keller R, Ammann R, Briner J, Luthy R. Detection of Septata intestinalis in stool specimens and coprodiagnostic monitoring of successful treatment with albendazole. Clin Infect Dis 1994; 19:342–345.

20. Dieterich DT, Lew EA, Kotler DP, Poles MA, Orenstein JM. Treatment with albendazole for intestinal disease due to Enterocytozoon bieneusi in patients with AIDS. J Infect Dis 1994; 169:178–183.

21. Asmuth DM, DeGirolami PC, Federman M, Ezratty CR, Pleskow DK, Desai G, Wanke CA. Clinical features of microsporidiosis in patients with AIDS. Clin Infect Dis 1994; 18:819–825.

22. McCowen MC, Callender ME, Lawlis JF Jr. Fumagillin (H-3), a new antibiotic with amebicidal properties. Science 1951; 113:202–203.

23. Diesenhouse MC, Wilson LA, Corrent GF, Visvesvara GS, Grossniklaus HE, Bryan RT. Treatment of microsporidial keratoconjunctivitis with topical fumagillin. Am J Ophthalmol 1993; 115:293–298.

24. Rosberger DF, Serdarevic ON, Erlandson RA, Bryan RT, Schwartz DA, Visvesvara GS, Keenan PC. Successful treatment of microsporidial keratoconjunctivitis with topical fumagillin in a patient with AIDS. Cornea 1993; 12:261–265.

25. Wilkins JH, Joshi N, Margolis TP, Cevallos V, Dawson CR. Microsporidial keratoconjunctivitis treated successfully with a short course of fumagillin. Eye 1994; 8: 703–704.

26. Ortega YR, Sterling CR, Gilman RH, Cama VA, Díaz F. Cyclospora species—a new protozoan pathogen of humans. N Engl J Med 1993; 328:1308–1312.

27. Madico G, Gilman RH, Miranda E, Cabrera L, Sterling CR. Treatment of Cyclospora infections with co-trimoxazole. Lancet 1993; 342:122–123.

28. Hoge CW, Shlim DR, Ghimire M, Rabold JG, Pandey P, Walsh A, Rajah R, Gaudio P, Echeverria P. Placebo-controlled trial of co-trimoxazole for Cyclospora infections among travellers and foreign residents in Nepal. Lancet 1995; 345:691–693. (Erratum, Lancet 1995; 345:1060.)

29. Pape JW, Verdier RI, Boncy M, Boncy J, Johnson WD Jr. Cyclospora infection in adults infected with HIV: clinical manifestations, treatment, and prophylaxis. Ann Intern Med 1994; 121:654–657.

30. DeHovitz JA, Pape JW, Boncy M, Johnson WD Jr. Clinical manifestations and therapy of Isospora belli infection in patients with the acquired immunodeficiency syndrome. N Engl J Med 1986; 315:87–90.

31. Pape JW, Verdier R-I, Johnson WD Jr. Treatment and prophylaxis of Isospora belli infection in patients with the acquired immunodeficiency syndrome. N Engl J Med 1989; 320:1044–1047.

32. Weiss LM, Perlman DC, Sherman J, Tanowitz H, Wittner M. Isospora belli infection: treatment with pyrimethamine. Ann Intern Med 1988; 109:474–475.

33. Naumova EN, Egorov AI, Morris RD, Griffiths JK. The elderly and waterborne Cryptosporidium infection: gastroenteritis hospitalizations before and during the 1993 Milwaukee outbreak. Emerg Infect Dis 2003; 9:1–15.

34. Bissuel F, Cotte L, Rabodonirina M, Rougier P, Piens MA, Trepo C. Paromomycin: an effective treatment for cryptosporidial diarrhea in patients with AIDS. Clin Infect Dis 1994; 18:447–449.

35. White AC Jr, Chappell CL, Hayat CS, Kimball KT, Flanigan TP, Goodgame RW. Paromomycin for cryptosporidiosis in AIDS: a prospective, double-blind trial. J Infect Dis 1994; 170:419–424.

36. Bissuel F, Cotte L, de Montclos M, Rabodonirina M, Trepo C. Absence of systemic absorption of oral paromomycin during long-term, high-dose treatment for cryptosporidiosis in AIDS. J Infect Dis 1994; 170:749–750.

37. Gil-Grande LA, Rodriguez-Caabeiro F, Prieto JG, Sanchez-Ruano JJ, Brasa C, Aguilar L, Garcia-Hoz F, Casado N, Barcena R, Alvarez AL. Randomised controlled trial of efficacy of albendazole in intra-abdominal hydatid disease. Lancet 1993; 342:1269–1272.

38. Wen H, New RR, Craig PS. Diagnosis and treatment of human hydatidosis. Br J Clin Pharmacol 1993; 35:565–574.

39. Horton RJ. Chemotherapy of Echinococcus infection in man with albendazole. Trans R Soc Trop Med Hyg 1989; 83:97–102.

40. Khuroo MS, Dar MY, Yattoo GN, Shah AH, Jeelani SG. Percutaneous drainage versus albendazole therapy in hepatic hydatidosis: a prospective, randomised study. Gastroenterology 1993; 104:1452–1459.

41. Bastid C, Azar C, Doyer M, Sahel J. Percutaneous treatment of hydatid cysts under sonographic guidance. Dig Dis Sci 1994; 39:1576–1580.

42. Wilson JF, Rausch RL, McMahon BJ, Schantz PM. Parasiticidal effect of chemotherapy in alveolar hydatid disease: review of experience with mebendazole and albendazole in Alaskan Eskimos. Clin Infect Dis 1992; 15:234–249.

43. Ammann RW, Ilitsch N, Marincek B, Freiburghaus AU. Effect of chemotherapy on the larval mass and the long-term course of alveolar echinococcosis: Swiss Echinococcosis Study Group. Hepatology 1994; 19:735–742.

44. Meneghelli UG, Barbo ML, Magro JE, Bellucci AD, Velludo MAL. Polycystic hydatid disease (Echinococcus vogeli): clinical and radiological manifestations and treatment with albendazole of a patient from the Brazilian Amazon region. Arq Gastroenterol 1986; 23:177–183.

45. Del Brutto OH, Sotelo J, Roman GC. Therapy for neurocysticercosis: a reappraisal. Clin Infect Dis 1993; 17:730–735.

46. Takayanagui OM, Jardim E. Therapy for neurocysticercosis: comparison between albendazole and praziquantel. Arch Neurol 1992; 49:290–294.

47. Cruz M, Cruz I, Horton J. Albendazole versus praziquantel in the treatment of cerebral cysticercosis: clinical evaluation. Trans R Soc Trop Med Hyg 1991; 85:244–247.

48. Jung H, Hurtado M, Medina MT, Sanchez M, Sotelo J. Dexamethasone increases plasma levels of albendazole. J Neurol 1990; 237:279–280.

49. Sotelo J, del Brutto OH, Penagos P, Escobedo F, Torres B, Rodríguez-Carbajal J. Comparison of therapeutic regimen of anticysticercal drugs for parenchymal brain cysticercosis. J Neurol 1990; 237:69–72.

50. Jung H, Hurtado M, Sanchez M, Medina MT, Sotelo J. Clinical pharmacokinetics of albendazole in patients with brain cysticercosis. J Clin Pharmacol 1992; 32:28–31.

51. Vazquez V, Sotelo J. The course of seizures after treatment for cerebral cysticercosis. N Engl J Med 1992; 327:696–701.

52. Carpio A, Santillan F, Leon P, Flores C, Hauser WA. Is the course of neurocysticercosis modified by treatment with antihelminthic agents? Arch Intern Med 1995; 155: 1982–1988.

53. Del Brutto OH, Sotelo J, Aguirre R, Diaz-Calderon E, Alarcon TA. Albendazole therapy for giant subarachnoid cysticerci. Arch Neurol 1992; 49:535–538.

54. Albonico M, Smith PG, Hall A, Chwaya HM, Alawi KS, Savioli L. A randomised controlled trial comparing mebendazole and albendazole against Ascaris, Trichuris, and hookworm infections. Trans R Soc Trop Med Hyg 1994; 88:585–589.

55. Davies HD, Sakuls P, Keystone JS. Creeping eruption: a review of clinical presentation and management of 60 cases presenting to a tropical disease unit. Arch Dermatol 1993; 129:588–591.

56. Kollaritsch H, Jeschko E, Wiedermann G. Albendazole is highly effective against cutaneous larva migrans but not against Giardia infection: results of an open pilot trial in travellers returning from the tropics. Trans R Soc Trop Med Hyg 1993; 87:689.

57. Kraivichian P, Kulkumthorn M, Yingyourd P, Akarabovorn P, Paireepai CC. Albendazole for the treatment of human gnathostomiasis. Trans R Soc Trop Med Hyg 1992; 86:418–421.

58. Cross JH, Basaca-Sevilla V. Albendazole in the treatment of intestinal capillariasis. Southeast Asian J Trop Med Public Health 1987; 18:507–510.

59. Archibald LK, Beeching NJ, Gill GV, Bailey JW, Bell DR. Albendazole is effective treatment for chronic strongyloidiasis. QJM 1993; 86:191–195.

60. Klion AD, Massougbodji A, Horton J, Ekoue S, Lanmasso T, Ahouissou NL, Nutman TB. Albendazole in human loiasis: results of a double-blind, placebo-controlled trial. J Infect Dis 1993; 168:202–206.

61. Cline BL, Hernandez JL, Mather FJ, Bartholomew R, De Maza SN, Rodulfo S, Welborn CA, Eberhard ML, Convit J. Albendazole in the treatment of onchocerciasis: double-blind clinical trial in Venezuela. Am J Trop Med Hyg 1992; 47:512–520.

62. Van den Enden E, Van Gompel A, Vervoort T, Van der Stuyft P, Van den Ende J. Mansonella perstans filariasis: failure of albendazole treatment. Ann Soc Belg Med Trop 1992; 72:215–218.

63. Campbell WC. Ivermectin as an antiparasitic agent for use in humans. Annu Rev Microbiol 1991; 45:445–474.

64. Pacqué M, Elmets C, Dukuly ZD, Munoz B, White AT, Taylor HR, Greene BM. Improvement in severe onchocercal skin disease after a single dose of ivermectin. Am J Med 1991; 90:590–594.

65. Whitworth JA, Gilbert CE, Mabey DM, Maude GH, Morgan D, Taylor DW. Effects of repeated doses of ivermectin on ocular onchocerciasis: community-based trial in Sierra Leone. Lancet 1991; 338:1100–1103.

66. Ottesen EA, Vijayasekaran V, Kumaraswami V. A controlled trial of ivermectin and diethylcarbamazine in lymphatic filariasis. N Engl J Med 1990; 322:1113–1117.

67. Nutman TB, Nash TE, Ottesen EA. Ivermectin in the successful treatment of a patient with Mansonella ozzardi infection. J Infect Dis 1987; 156:662–665.

68. Van den Enden E, Van Gompel A, Van der Stuyft P, Vervoort T, Van den Ende J. Treatment failure of a single high dose of ivermectin for Mansonella perstans filariasis. Trans R Soc Trop Med Hyg 1993; 87:90–90.

69. Martin-Prevel Y, Cosnefroy JY, Tshipamba P, Ngari P, Chodakewitz JA, Pinder M. Tolerance and efficacy of single high-dose ivermectin for the treatment of loiasis. Am J Trop Med Hyg 1993; 48:186–192.

70. Naquira C, Jimenez G, Guerra JG, Bernal R, Nalin DR, Neu D, Aziz M. Ivermectin for human strongyloidiasis and other intestinal helminths. Am J Trop Med Hyg 1989; 40:304–309.

71. Caumes E, Carriere J, Datry A, Gaxotte P, Danis M, Gentilini M. A randomised trial of ivermectin versus albendazole for the treatment of cutaneous larva migrans. Am J Trop Med Hyg 1993; 49:641–644.

72. Gann PH, Neva FA, Gam AA. A randomised trial of single- and two-dose ivermectin versus thiabendazole for treatment of strongyloidiasis. J Infect Dis 1994; 169:1076–1079.

73. Torres JR, Isturiz R, Murillo J, Guzman M, Contreras R. Efficacy of ivermectin in the treatment of strongyloidiasis complicating AIDS. Clin Infect Dis 1993; 17:900–902.

74. Aubin F, Humbert P. Ivermectin for crusted (Norwegian) scabies. N Engl J Med 1995; 332:612.

75. Dunne CL, Malone CJ, Whitworth JA. A field study of the effects of ivermectin on ectoparasites of man. Trans R Soc Trop Med Hyg 1991; 85:550–551.

76. Day TA, Bennett JL, Pax RA. Praziquantel: the enigmatic antiparasitic. Parasitol Today 1992; 8:342–344.
77. Brindley PJ, Sher A. Immunologic involvement in the efficacy of praziquantel. Exp Parasitol 1990; 71:245–248.
78. Apt W, Aguilera X, Vega F, Miranda C, Zulantay I, Perez C, Gabor M, Apt P. Treatment of human chronic fascioliasis with triclabendazole: drug efficacy and serologic response. Am J Trop Med Hyg 1995; 52:532–535.
79. Vazquez ML, Jung H, Sotelo J. Plasma levels of praziquantel decrease when dexamethasone is given simultaneously. Neurology 1987; 37:1561–1562.
80. Bittencourt PR, Gracia CM, Martins R, Fernandes AG, Diekmann HW, Jung W. Phenytoin and carbamazepine decreased oral bioavailability of praziquantel. Neurology 1992; 42:492–496.
81. Drugs for parasitic infections. Med Lett Drugs Ther 2004; 46:1–12.
82. White AC. The disappearing arsenal of antiparasitic drugs. N Engl J Med 2000; 343:1273–1274.

SUGGESTED READING

Drugs for parasitic infections. Med Lett Drugs Ther 2004; 46:1–12.
White AC. The disappearing arsenal of antiparasitic drugs. N Engl J Med 2000; 343:1273–1274.

27

Ocular Infections

Richard S. Baker, Charles W. Flowers, Jr., and Richard Casey
Charles R. Drew University of Medicine and Science, Los Angeles, California, U.S.A.

Key Points:

- Age-related degenerative changes in the eye and its adnexal structures predispose the elderly to ocular infections.
- Blepharitis, hordeola, meibomitis, and chalazion are all major eyelid infections and are caused generally by staphylococci.
- Conjunctivitis is caused primarily by bacteria (staphylococci and streptococci) and viruses (herpes simplex and varicella-zoster virus) and generally requires either local antibiotics (bacteria) or symptomatic care (viral).
- Corneal infection (keratitis) can be due to bacteria, virus, or fungi and can be an ocular emergency (bacterial keratitis) as well as be difficult to treat (fungal keratitis).
- Postoperative endophthalmitis is the most significant retinal–vitreal infection encountered by older adults.

Age-related degenerative ocular and adnexal changes predispose older adults to infections of the eye. Alterations in host defenses associated with age-related degenerative changes, which produce tear insufficiency and alter lid–globe apposition, significantly compromise the capacity of eyes of elderly people to withstand prolonged exposure to microbial pathogens. Not surprisingly, the geriatric population has higher rates of eye infection and poorer treatment outcomes. Delays in diagnosis as well as delays in clinical manifestations are, in part, responsible for poorer outcomes.

1. EYELID INFECTIONS

1.1. Epidemiology, Clinical Relevance, Etiologic Pathogens, and Clinical Manifestations

1.1.1. Blepharitis

The eyelid, particularly the lid margin, is a common site of ocular adnexal infection in the elderly. The most common lid infection encountered is staphylococcal blepharitis. Staphylococcal blepharitis is a chronic condition that has periodic exacerbations, which often leads the patient to seek medical attention.

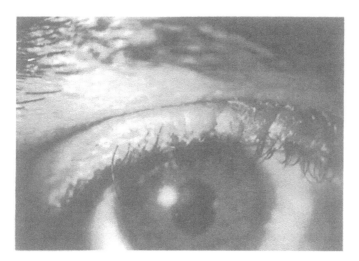

Figure 1 Staphylococcal blepharitis. Notice the lid margin crusting and the dandruff-like flakes adherent to the lashes. *Source*: From Ref. 19.

Blepharitis usually presents with bilateral eye redness, irritation, burning, and tearing. Although these symptoms generally are relatively benign, they can become incapacitating during acute exacerbations. The major clinical features are bilateral lid margin crusting, the accumulation of dandruff-like flakes at the base of the lashes, and lid margin hyperemia (Fig. 1). Because of the chronic nature of this condition, many patients will eventually sustain permanent structural changes to the lid margin, consisting of lid margin thickening, loss of lashes (madarosis), and misdirected lashes.

Meibomitis, a manifestation of blepharitis, is an associated finding in almost every case. Meibomitis is an inflammation of the meibomian glands, which supply the lipid layer of the tear film. The lipid layer of the tear film is the most superficial layer and retards tear evaporation. Inflammation of the meibomian glands disrupts the production and secretion of the tear film lipid layer and, consequently, leads to rapid tear evaporation and ocular surface drying. Thus, patients will also complain of a sandy-gritty foreign body or dry eye sensation.

On slitlamp biomicroscope meibomitis appears as pouting and dilation of the orifices, which lie just posterior to the lashes, and inspissation of the meibomian secretions. Several of the orifices will also display complete occlusion as a result of plugging by congealed meibomian secretions.

1.1.2. Hordeola (Acute Stye)

Hordeola are infections of the lid margin sebaceous glands and manifest in two clinical forms, external (stye) and internal, which are differentiated by the particular group of sebaceous glands infected. An external hordeolum (stye) is an infection of the glands of Zeis, which extend along the base of the eyelash hair follicle. It is by far the most common type of hordeolum, and *Staphylococcus aureus* is the predominant microbial pathogen.

Because of the association with the lash follicle, an external hordeolum, or stye, manifests primarily at the base of an eyelash, with redness, swelling, and micro-abscess formation being the predominant clinical features.

Internal hordeola are caused by infections within the meibomian glands. *S. aureus* is the major microbial pathogen. Internal hordeola typically manifest as red swollen large discrete nodules in the lid a clear distance away from the lid margin. Additionally, these lesions are generally tenderer than styes and point toward the conjunctival surface instead of the external lid surface. There is marked hyperemia of the overlying conjunctiva.

1.1.3. Chalazion

A chalazion is a lid lesion that is often confused with an internal hordeolum. It is a sterile granulomatous reaction to inspissated and impacted meibomian gland secretions. Meibomian gland orifices often become plugged as a result of lid margin inflammation produced by chronic blepharitis. Consequently, meibomian gland secretions accumulate within the gland and eventually leak out into the surrounding lid connective tissue. These lipid secretions are highly inflammatory and incite a granulomatous inflammatory reaction, which leads to the formation of a chalazion.

Chalazia appear as large discrete nontender nodules within the lid a fixed distance away from the lid margin (Fig. 2). Although these lesions look similar to internal hordeola clinically, there are some important differentiating features. Whereas an internal hordeolum represents an acute infectious process, a chalazion is a chronic noninfectious process. Therefore, internal hordeola develop over a much shorter time period (days vs. weeks), manifest signs of acute inflammation such as redness, swelling, and tenderness, and require systemic antibiotic therapy for effective treatment.

1.2. Diagnosis

The diagnosis of all of these infectious processes of the lid is made clinically; consequently, no laboratory or radiological tests exist to aid in the diagnosis of these conditions.

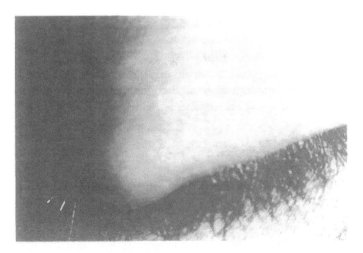

Figure 2 Chalazion. Note the large well-circumscribed lid mass above the lid margin. An internal hordeolum would look similar, except show more intense signs of acute inflammation and manifest exquisite tenderness. *Source*: From Ref. 20.

1.3. Treatment

Treatment of blepharitis consists of lid hygiene and a short course of antistaphylococcal antibiotic therapy. Lid hygiene is achieved by using diluted baby shampoo dissolved in warm water (one or two drops of baby shampoo in a bottle cap full of warm water) and a cotton tip applicator or wash cloth two to three times daily. Commercially prepared eyelid cleansing kits are available over the counter but are generally more expensive. Lid hygienic therapy does not completely eliminate the disease process but simply stabilizes it such that patients are free of symptoms. Consequently, patients must undergo prolonged courses of lid hygiene, usually over several months, and require lifetime maintenance therapy thereafter for disease control. Two- to three-week courses of topical antistaphylococcal antibiotic therapy should be reserved for acute exacerbations or severe, previously untreated disease and should be combined with lid hygiene. Bacitracin or erythromycin ophthalmic ointments are the agents of choice. Systemic tetracycline has been shown to be quite effective in bringing advanced cases of meibomitis under control.

External hordeola often sharply localize and rupture spontaneously within a matter of days after forming; thus, warm compresses four to six times a day more than suffices for treating this condition. Resolution can be hastened if the localizing lesion is decompressed with a fine sterile needle. Antibiotic therapy is of questionable value for a single lesion and is often not indicated. In the case of recurrent or multiple styes, topical antistaphylococcal antibiotic therapy in the form of bacitracin or erythromycin ophthalmic ointment is warranted along with lid hygiene, and depending on the severity, systemic antistaphylococcal antibiotics may be required.

Unlike styes, internal hordeola usually do not rupture and drain spontaneously, and require warm compresses in conjunction with systemic antistaphylococcal antibiotics. If the lesions do not respond to this regimen, incision and drainage is indicated, and the patient should be referred to an ophthalmologist.

Since chalazia develop over a period of weeks to months, are nontender, and have minimal to no associated inflammatory signs, they are effectively treated with lid hygiene and warm compresses in most instances. Table 1 summarizes the key clinical information on eyelid infections.

1.4. Prevention

Lid hygiene is the key to prevention for each of the lid infectious processes. Patients who present with recurrent lid infections should be advised to incorporate twice daily lid cleansing into their daily personal hygiene regimen.

2. LACRIMAL SYSTEM INFECTIONS

2.1. Epidemiology, Clinical Relevance, and Etiologic Pathogens

Lacrimal system infections commonly affecting the elderly predominantly involve the lacrimal outflow system. The lacrimal outflow system is composed of the puncta, which are present on the medial aspect of the upper and lower lid margins, the upper and lower canaliculi, the nasolacrimal sac, and the nasolacrimal duct (Fig. 3). Infections of the lacrimal gland (dacryoadenitis) are uncommon and will not be discussed here.

Table 1 Summary of Eyelid Infections

Eyelid infection	Clinical features			Diagnostic test	Etiology	Treatment options and expected clinical course
	Symptoms	Signs				
Blepharitis	Bilateral Burning Irritated eyes	Injected lid margin "Dandruff-like" flakes on lashes		None clinical	S. epidermidis S. aureus	Chronic disorder, use bacitracin ophthalmic ointment with lid hygiene twice daily May require chronic therapy with systemic doxycycline 100 mg BID
Hordeola (acute stye)	Unilateral Pain Redness Swelling at or adjacent to lid margin	Focal nodular abscess usually single (can be multiple) Can be visible on external lid skin and/or internally with lid eversion		None clinical	S. epidermidis S. aureus	Usually resolves in days Hot compress twice daily Bacitracin ophthalmic ointment twice daily
Chalazion (chronic stye)	Unilateral Painless	Focal nodule usually single Minimal or no obvious inflammation		None clinical	Usually granulomatous inflammation	Usually requires intralesional steroid injection or surgical incision and drainage Resolves in days to weeks

Abbreviations: S., *Staphylococcus;* BID, twice daily.

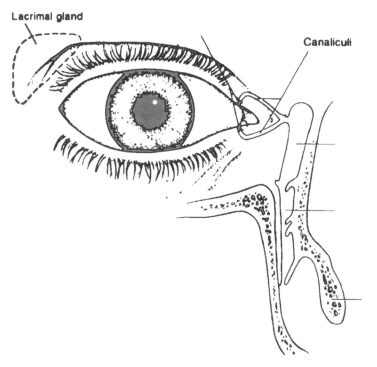

Figure 3 Nasolacrimal system anatomy. *Source*: From Ref. 21.

2.1.1. Canaliculitis

A number of organisms have been found to infect the canaliculi including bacteria (i.e., *Actinomyces israelii*, *Propionibacterium* spp., *Nocardia*, and *Bacteroides*), viruses (i.e., herpes simplex and varicella-zoster), and fungi (i.e., *Candida* and *Aspergillus* spp.).

Despite this seeming variety of potential infectious agents, *A. israelii* causes the overwhelming majority of canalicular infections.

2.1.2. Dacryocystitis

Dacryocystitis refers to an infection of the nasolacrimal sac that often develops as a result of blockage of the nasolacrimal duct. Nasolacrimal duct obstruction causes tear stasis, which leads to ascending bacterial colonization and infection of the naso-lacrimal system from the nasopharynx (1). The cause of acquired lacrimal drainage obstruction may be primary or secondary. Primary acquired nasolacrimal duct obstruction results from inflammation of unknown cause that eventually leads to occlusive fibrosis. Secondary acquired lacrimal drainage obstruction may arise from a wide variety of infectious, inflammatory, neoplastic, traumatic, or mechanical causes. In the elderly, the primary acquired form predominates.

2.2. Clinical Manifestations

2.2.1. Canaliculitis

Canaliculitis clinically manifests with the patient complaining of excessive tearing (epiphora). In addition to the symptom of tearing, the patient will exhibit conjunctival injection, particularly in the nasal area, along with punctal dilation and hyperemia.

Digital pressure applied to over the nasolocrimid sac area will often lead to punctal expression of a yellow-green exudate or yellowish "granules," which is highly characteristic of *A. israelii* infections.

2.2.2. Dacryocystitis

Dacryocystitis may manifest as either an acute or chronic infectious process. The acute infectious process presents with localized pain, swelling, and erythema in the medial canthal area, representing an inflamed and distended nasolacrimal sac. Digital pressure applied to the skin overlying the nasolacrimal sac usually results in the expression of purulent material from the eyelid puncta. Patients will often complain of excessive tearing as well as eye redness and purulent discharge. The most common microbial pathogens in adults are staphylococcal and streptococcal species.

Chronic dacryocystitis typically manifests subtly with patients complaining of chronic or recurrent bouts of excessive tearing. The skin over the lacrimal sac usually appears normal, but digital pressure applied to the medial canthal area often results in the expression of purulent material from the puncta. Additionally, patients may also report intermittent episodes of conjunctivitis in the eye ipsilateral to the chronic dacryocystitis. The conjunctivitis results from the reflux of the bacterial pathogens infecting the nasolacrimal sac into the eye through the puncta. Because of the low-grade activity of this disease process, many patients tolerate the symptoms for an extended period of time before seeking medical attention.

2.3. Diagnosis

2.3.1. Canaliculitis

In cases of canaliculitis, diagnostic confirmation of *Actinomyces* can be obtained by gram-staining the expressed material, which will demonstrate delicate gram-positive branching filaments.

2.3.2. Dacryocystitis

The diagnosis of dacryocystitis is generally made clinically, but culturing any expressed discharge can be helpful in precisely targeting antibiotic therapy to the causative organism.

2.4. Antibiotic Treatment

2.4.1. Canaliculitis

Therapy of canaliculitis consists of mechanical expression of the exudative or granular material from the canaliculi in combination with probing and irrigation of the nasolacrimal system with either a 10% sulfacetamide solution or a penicillin G (100,000 units/mL) eye-drop solution. Referral to an ophthalmologist for definitive therapy of this condition is recommended.

2.4.2. Dacryocystitis

Systemic antibiotic therapy is required in all cases of dacryocystitis and empirical therapy with an antibiotic with good gram-positive activity, such as oral dicloxacillin or cephalexin is usually started while culture specimens are being processed. Systemic antibiotics may be curative in acute disease; however, they are of little benefit in chronic disease. These patients have total nasolacrimal duct obstruction and require surgical decompression for disease eradication. Irrigating the nasolacrimal sac through the puncta with an antibiotic solution, similar to that used to treat canaliculitis, is a good temporizing measure worth instituting in those patients who cannot undergo immediate surgical drainage. However, surgical intervention by an ophthalmologist is necessary to achieve definitive treatment.

2.4.3. Prevention

Currently, there are no known preventive measures that patients can take to avert either of these conditions. Table 2 summarizes the important clinical information on lacrimal system infection.

3. CONJUNCTIVAL INFECTIONS

3.1. Bacteria

3.1.1. Epidemiology, Clinical Relevance, and Etiologic Pathogens

Infectious conjunctivitis is primarily caused by bacteria and viruses, with viruses being the more common offending agent in the United States. Bacterial conjunctivitis may be classified as hyperacute, acute, or chronic based on the rapidity of onset and disease progression. Hyperacute bacterial conjunctivitis is characterized by a very rapid onset (a matter of hours), copious purulent discharge, and intense conjunctival swelling and redness. This form of conjunctivitis is primarily caused by *Neisseria gonorrhoeae* and is uncommon among the elderly population.

3.1.2. Clinical Manifestations

Acute bacterial conjunctivitis, unlike hyperacute bacterial conjunctivitis, evolves over a matter of days and induces a less severe inflammatory response. Patients will manifest a purulent discharge, which is the hallmark feature of all bacterial conjunctivitis, diffuse conjunctival injection, and crusting along the lid margins (Fig. 4). Patients will usually complain of ocular irritation and pain, and experience a decrease in vision due to reflex tearing and the purulent discharge. Staphylococcal and streptococcal species cause the majority of acute bacterial conjunctivitis in adults. Gram-negative bacteria are rare causes of conjunctivitis.

Chronic bacterial conjunctivitis is typically seen in conjunction with one of two conditions: chronic blepharitis and chronic dacryocystitis. Chronic bacterial conjunctivitis associated with blepharitis is generally caused by *S. aureus* and *Moraxella lacunata* and results in prominent lid margin erythema, scaling, and thickening in addition to purulent discharge, which is usually minimal, and conjunctival injection. Lid margin ulcerations may also develop during acute exacerbations. Because of the associated blepharitis, these patients will undoubtedly have some degree of meibomian gland dysfunction resulting in a compromised tear film. The tear film abnormality may intensify the ocular irritation these patients experience, as well as predispose them to corneal epithelial breakdown.

Chronic bacterial conjunctivitis arising from chronic dacryocystitis is predominantly caused by staphylococcal and streptococcal species. These infections cause many of the symptoms and signs noted, but in addition patients will complain of chronic or recurrent bouts of excessive tearing; digital compression of the medial canthal area will result in the expression of purulent material from the puncta.

Table 2 Summary of Lacrimal System Infections

Lacrimal system infection	Clinical features		Diagnostic test	Etiology	Treatment options and expected clinical course
	Symptoms	Signs			
Canaliculitis	Unilateral Swelling Redness	Regional swelling of lids near nasal angle with discharge	Cultures of discharge from puncta	*Actinomyces israelii*	Topical sulfacetamide or penicillin 100,000 u/mL four times per day Resolves in days to weeks
Dacryocystitis	Unilateral Swelling Redness	Regional swelling of lids between nasal bridge and nasal angle of eyelid	Culture discharge from pressure on nasolacrimal sac at puncta	*Staphylococci* or *Streptococci*	Oral dicloxacillin Resolves in days to weeks

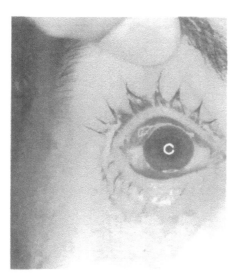

Figure 4 Bacterial conjunctivitis. Note the copious purulent discharge. *Source*: From Ref. 19.

3.1.3. Diagnosis

Culture and sensitivity testing of the conjunctival sac should be performed prior to the initiation of antibiotic therapy in every case of suspected bacterial conjunctivitis. Gram staining of the purulent exudate should also be attempted. The information obtained from either diagnostic maneuver seldom alters the course of therapy; however, in the case of an infection not responding to the standard therapeutic regimen, this diagnostic information proves invaluable.

3.1.4. Antibiotic Treatment

The standard therapy for acute bacterial conjunctivitis consists of topical application of antibiotic drops every 2–4 hr or antibiotic ointment every 4–6 hr for 7–10 days. Repeated saline lavage of the conjunctival sac along with lid hygiene is helpful in rinsing away the bacterial pathogens and removing purulent debris. Cultures should be obtained prior to initiating antibiotic therapy to ensure that the causative organism is sensitive to the empirical antibiotic therapy. Empirical antibiotic therapy should be targeted toward gram-positive organisms, as they are the predominant cause of acute bacterial conjunctivitis (Table 3). In general, aminoglycosides (gentamicin, neomycin, and tobramycin) should be avoided unless culture and sensitivity results indicate that these agents are the most efficacious. Topical aminoglycosides, particularly gentamicin and neomycin, have been found to induce a toxic reaction in a significant percentage of patients.

Treatment for chronic bacterial conjunctivitis in the setting of chronic blepharitis involves combining lid margin hygiene with topical antibiotic therapy. The antibiotics used for chronic bacterial conjunctivitis are no different from those used to treat the acute condition; however, antibiotic ointments are preferred over drops, because they can be easily applied to the lid and conjunctiva simultaneously, as well as aid in combating the ocular surface drying associated with meibomian gland dysfunction. The treatment of dacryocystitis-induced bacterial conjunctivitis involves

Table 3 Commercially Available Antibiotic Eyedrops and Ophthalmic
Ointments Commonly Used to Treat Bacterial Conjunctivitis

Antibiotic	Trade name[a]
Bacitracin ointment	AK-TRACIN®
Ciprofloxacin	Ciloxan®
Ofloxacin	OCUflOX®
Erythromycin ointment	
Sulfacetamide[a]	Bleph-10®, AK-SULF®
Tetracycline ointment	Acromycin®
Trimethoprim, polymyxin B	Polytrim®
Gatifloxacin	Zymar®
Moxifloxacin	Vigamox®

[a]The trade names listed are not all-inclusive.

the same topical antibiotic regimen outlined; however, these patients require surgical intervention for definitive therapy and, thus, should be promptly referred to an
ophthalmologist.

3.1.5. Prevention

Hand-to-eye contact is the primary route of ocular contamination leading to acute
bacterial conjunctivitis. Therefore, patients should be encouraged to avoid frequent
eye rubbing and to engage in diligent handwashing when they come in contact with
individuals with red eyes ("pinkeye"). Moreover, definitive treatment of blepharitis
or dacryocystitis will avert the secondary bacterial conjunctivitis that can develop in
association with these conditions. Table 4 summarizes the relevant clinical information on bacterial conjunctivitis.

3.2. Virus

3.2.1. Epidemiology, Clinical Relevance, and Etiologic Pathogens

Adenovirus is by far the most common cause of viral conjunctivitis and tends to be
the most virulent. Herpes simplex virus (HSV) (usually type 1) primarily causes conjunctivitis in children and usually produces a mild inflammatory response. Other viral
pathogens, which can cause viral conjunctivitis in the elderly, include enterovirus,
coxsackievirus, and varicella-zoster.

3.2.2. Clinical Manifestations

Viral conjunctivitis classically produces a clear watery discharge, a follicular conjunctival reaction, and preauricular lymphadenopathy. A purulent discharge may be seen
on occasion but is usually more characteristic of a bacterial conjunctivitis. Conjunctival follicles represent lymphoid germinal follicles within the conjunctiva and appear
as translucent cobblestones or pebbles with small blood vessels arborizing over the
surface. Follicles are highly characteristic of viral infections, although they can also
be seen in chlamydial infections of the conjunctiva. Because of the highly contagious
nature of viral infections, the majority of patients present with bilateral eye involvement, whereas bacterial conjunctival infections typically present unilaterally.

Epidemic keratoconjunctivitis (EKC) is caused by adenovirus types 8 and 19
and is characterized by severe eye pain, photophobia, diffuse punctate corneal
epithelial defects, and conjunctivitis. The inflammatory reaction produced by this

Table 4 Summary of Conjunctivitis

| Disease | Clinical features | | Diagnostic test | Etiology | Treatment options and expected clinical course |
	Symptoms	Signs			
Bacterial conjunctivitis	Redness Mucous drainage	Conjunctival swelling and injection Mucopurulent discharge	Cultures of conjunctival swab	*Staphylococci,* *Streptococci,* or *Moraxella* *lacunata* Gram negative	Topical fluoroquinolone: Vigamox drops four times per day or Zymar drops four times per day Resolves in <14 days
Viral conjunctivitis	Redness Mucous drainage	Conjunctival swelling and injection Mucopurulent discharge	Cultures to rule out bacterial cause	Adenovirus	Topical fluoroquinolone (for secondary bacterial infection): Vigamox drops four times per day or Zymar drops four times per day Resolves in <14 days

viral organism can be so intense that inflammatory membranes or pseudomembranes and subepithelial corneal infiltrates develop. True membranes are differentiated from pseudomembranes by the presence of bleeding on removal of true membranes. The corneal subepithelial infiltrates do not occur in every patient but typically manifest 10–14 days after the onset of symptoms. These infiltrates are sterile and represent an immune reaction to viral antigens. They usually resolve spontaneously without visual sequelae, but it may take several months for complete resolution. During the acute infiltrative phase, patients may experience a temporary reduction in vision.

EKC typically lasts for 2–4 weeks with contagious viral shedding occurring during the first 2 weeks from the onset of symptoms. Therefore, patients must avoid exposure or contact with others during this infectious period. The virus is extremely contagious and can remain viable on inanimate objects such as equipment, door-knobs, and other fomites for up to 2 months (2). Adenovirus has also been found to be common cause of severe outbreaks of viral conjunctivitis in chronic care facilities (3).

3.2.3. Diagnosis

The diagnosis of viral conjunctivitis is generally made on clinical findings; however, culture and sensitivity testing does prove useful in identifying cases of EKC and excluding a concurrent bacterial conjunctivitis.

3.2.4. Antibiotic Treatment

As with all forms of viral conjunctivitis, there is no specific treatment for adenoviral conjunctivitis. Thus, therapy is aimed at palliation and limiting complications. The use of cool compresses, artificial tears, and analgesics are typically very helpful in easing patients' discomfort. Antibiotics are not indicated, unless the patient develops signs of a superimposed bacterial infection. Topical corticosteroids should be avoided.

3.2.5. Prevention

Hand-to-eye contamination is the primary route of transmission of viral conjunctivitis. Thus, precautions regarding hand-to-eye contact and hand washing should be adhered to regarding this condition. As stated earlier, it is also important to note that adenovirus types 8 and 19 remain infectious for up to 2 months after being deposited on environmental surfaces (2,4). Therefore, contracting EKC does not require direct contact with an infected individual. Table 4 summarizes relevant clinical information on viral conjunctivitis.

4. CORNEAL INFECTIONS

4.1. Bacterial Keratitis

4.1.1. Epidemiology, Clinical Relevance, and Etiologic Pathogens

Infectious keratitis constitutes a sight-threatening ocular emergency that requires prompt recognition and immediate referral to an ophthalmologist. Bacterial keratitis results from a breakdown in the corneal epithelial barrier and subsequent bacterial invasion of the corneal stroma. Bacterial invasion and white cell infiltration of the cornea leads to tissue destruction and may even lead to perforation if therapy is not instituted in a timely manner. Because of the destructive nature of this disease process and the cornea's fragile composition, all bacterial infections of the cornea result in some degree of corneal scarring and opacification, regardless of how soon therapy is instituted. Therefore, the amount of corneal scarring and the extent to which vision is affected is largely determined by the time interval between disease onset and disease control. Staphylococcal and streptococcal species are the predominant corneal pathogens. Table 5 summarizes the relevant clinical information on corneal infections.

The risk factors that appear to be the most important in the elderly include dry eye disease, involutional lid abnormalities, diabetes mellitus, and surgical trauma. All of these conditions predispose the elderly patient to corneal epithelial breakdown and corneal bacterial invasion.

4.1.2. Clinical Manifestations

The major complaints generally are a unilateral decrease in vision, eye redness, pain, light sensitivity (photophobia), tearing, and mucoid discharge. Clinically the eye will manifest marked conjunctival injection, a moderate amount of purulent discharge, corneal clouding, and a well-demarcated corneal white cell infiltrate, which appears as a dense white opacity on direct illumination with a penlight (Fig. 5). There may also be a visible layering of pus in the anterior chamber (hypopyon), which is usually a sterile inflammatory response. Fluorescein staining will demonstrate the size and location of the corneal epithelial defect.

4.1.3. Diagnosis

As was pointed out earlier, prompt antibiotic therapy is crucial for limiting the extent of corneal tissue damage; however, an attempt should be made to obtain diagnostic cultures prior to initiating antibiotic therapy. However, treatment should not be withheld if culturing materials are not readily available. Recent studies have found no significant increase in adverse outcomes when diagnostic scraping and culture are not performed at the outset of therapy (5,6).

4.1.4. Antibiotic Treatment

Although gram-positive organisms cause the majority of community-acquired non-contact lens-related bacterial keratitis, broad-spectrum topical antibiotics are the mainstay of therapy. Most ophthalmologists prescribe specially formulated high-concentration antibiotic eyedrops (i.e., cefazolin 50 mg/mL and tobramycin 14 mg/mL) with an instillation frequency of every 30–60 min around the clock for the first 24–72 hr. The primary care physician's role in these cases will often be to institute temporizing measures, while the patient is en route to the ophthalmologist for definitive therapy. Commercially available fluoroquinolone eyedrops (Ciloxan or Ocuflox) provide the best form of temporizing therapy because of their broad spectrum of antimicrobial activity. Additionally, these agents have been shown to effectively treat bacterial keratitis at their commercially available concentrations (7). Both agents require very frequent instillation (i.e., every 15–30 min for the first 2 hr) at the onset of therapy to provide adequate tissue loading of the antibiotic. Beyond the tissue-loading period, the instillation frequency can be reduced to every hour.

4.1.5. Prevention

Effective prevention for this condition entails ensuring that at-risk individuals are receiving appropriate ophthalmic management of their predisposing conditions. As

Table 5 Summary of Corneal Infections

Keratitis type	Clinical features		Diagnostic test	Etiology	Treatment options and expected clinical course
	Symptoms	Signs			
Bacterial keratitis	Unilateral pain Photophobia Redness Decreased vision "White spot" on cornea	Focal corneal infiltrate Conjunctival injection Lid swelling	Cultures of corneal scrape (essential before starting therapy)	*Staphylococci*, *Streptococci*, or *Pseudomonas aeruginosa*[a]	Emergency referral to ophthalmologist Topical fluoroquinolone[a] Vigamox or zymar every hour Resolves over several weeks
Viral keratitis	Unilateral pain Photophobia Redness Decreased vision	Focal corneal infiltrate Conjunctival injection Lid swelling	"Dendritic" staining pattern with fluorescein and Wood's lamp (or cobalt blue light)	Herpes simplex virus	Emergency referral to ophthalmologist Topical viroptic 1% every 2 hr Resolves over several weeks
Fungal keratitis	Unilateral pain Photophobia Redness Decreased vision "White spot" on cornea Can be multiple	Single or multiple corneal infiltrates	Cultures of corneal scrape	*Fusarium* *Candida* *Aspergillus*	Emergency referral to ophthalmologist Topical natamycin 5% every hour Resolves over several weeks

[a] Ciprofloxacin (Ciloxan®) or ofloxacin (Ocuflox®) should be used if *Pseudomonas aeruginosa* is identified or suspected.

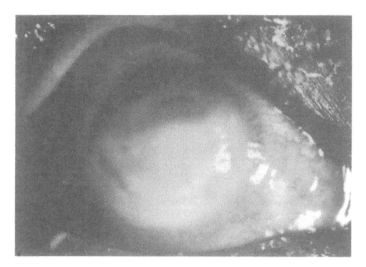

Figure 5 Bacterial keratitis. The white corneal opacity represents white cell infiltration into the corneal stroma. *Source*: From Ref. 19.

stated earlier, in the elderly, dry eye disease and involutional lid malpositions are the most common predisposing risk factors for the development of infectious keratitis. Both predisposing conditions constitute age-related degenerative changes affecting the eye and, thus, have a high prevalence among the elderly. The prevalence of dry eye disease, for example, steadily increases with age, with prevalence rates increasing from 2% in individuals 45 years of age up to 16% in individuals 80 years of age (8). Similarly, the generalized lid laxity and diminution of muscle tone associated with aging result in structural eyelid malpositions that almost exclusively affect the elderly. It is also important to note that several common systemic conditions and a number of over-the-counter and prescription medications predispose elderly patients to developing dry eye disease. Rheumatoid arthritis, Sjogren's syndrome, sarcoidosis, and other autoimmune/collagen-vascular disorders all produce a decrease in tear production as a result of autoimmune-mediated destruction of conjunctival-based lacrimal gland tissue. The systemic medications that adversely affect tear production include adrenergic inhibitors and diuretics used to treat hypertension, tricyclic antidepressants, anti-Parkinsonian agents, and over-the-counter cold or hay fever preparations.

4.2. Viral Keratitis

4.2.1. Epidemiology, Clinical Relevance, and Etiologic Pathogens

HSV and varicella-zoster virus (VZV) are the two most common corneal viral pathogens. HSV is the most common cause of infectious keratitis in the United States, causing an estimated 500,000 cases of infectious keratitis each year (9). Herpes zoster ophthalmicus is the term given to the herpes zoster occurring in the first division of the trigeminal nerve, which innervates the ocular surface. Involvement of the ophthalmic division of the trigeminal nerve accounts for 9–16% of cases of VZV infections occurring annually in the United States and is associated with severe, chronic ocular complications (10). Unlike bacterial keratitis, viral keratitis does not require a breach in the corneal epithelial layer to become established.

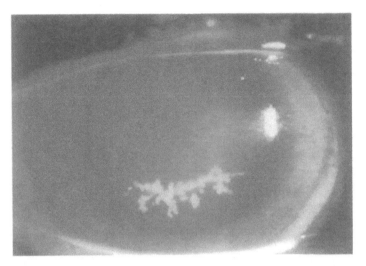

Figure 6 HSV keratitis showing dendritic ulcer highlighted with fluorescein staining. *Source*: From Ref. 19.

4.2.2. Clinical Manifestations

The epithelial keratitis produced by HSV is characterized by thin branching dendritic ulcerations, which are best seen with fluorescein staining (Fig. 6). The lesions are usually centrally or paracentrally located and each linear branch of the dendritic ulcer terminates in bulb-like conglomerations commonly referred to as "terminal bulbs." This infection is predominantly unilateral, with bilateral involvement only rarely seen. Sharp eye pain, light sensitivity, tearing, and blurring of vision are typical symptoms. Curiously, although most patients complain of eye pain, objective testing of corneal sensitivity in the area of the dendritic lesion will demonstrate decreased or absent corneal sensitivity.

VZV epithelial keratitis clinically appears very similar to HSV epithelial keratitis but has several important distinguishing features. First, VZV keratitis is usually accompanied by a vesicular eruption involving the periorbital skin in a dermatomal pattern (Fig. 7). The epithelial keratitis and the rash typically appear together. However, ocular involvement can be delayed, and it is important to note that ocular involvement does not occur in every case of VZV facial dermatitis. Ocular involvement occurs in ≈50–72% of patients with periocular zoster (11). A vesicular eruption extending to the tip of the nose indicates involvement of the nasociliary nerve, which is a branch of the ophthalmic division of the trigeminal nerve. This clinical finding, known as "Hutchinson's sign," has an 85% predictability of eye being involved (12). Other differentiating features of VZV epithelial keratitis include the absence of terminal bulbs, smaller and less branching dendrites, more profound corneal anesthesia, and the lack of recurrences. HSV has been found to recur in ≈33% of patients within 2 years of the initial episode (13).

4.2.3. Diagnosis

The diagnosis of HSV and VZV keratitis is generally made clinically. Because of their unique features, both conditions can be diagnosed in the majority of cases based on the clinical appearance of the lesions, the history of present illness, and

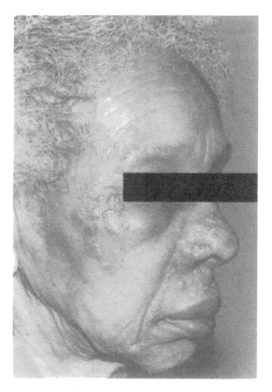

Figure 7 Herpes zoster ophthalmicus. Note the dermatomal pattern of the vesicular eruption. Also note the tip of the nose involvement or "Hutchinson's sign." *Source*: From Ref. 19.

the patient's symptoms. When necessary, confirmation of the diagnosis can be made by culturing a swab or scrape of the corneal epithelium. Alternatively, fluorescent immunoassay of corneal epithelial cells reacting with HSV monoclonal antigen, polyclonal recombinant polymerase chain reaction amplification, and Southern blot analysis of HSV or VZV genomic sequences may be used for diagnosis confirmation.

4.2.4. Antibiotic Treatment

The management of HSV epithelial keratitis consists of the topical administration of antiviral eyedrops. Several agents have been shown to be efficacious in treating this condition; however, at present, only one agent, trifluridine (Viroptic 1%) has been shown to have a greater than 90% cure rate. The recommended dosing regimen is one drop every 2 hr, but no more than nine times a day for the first 3–5 days. The frequency of administration should be decreased to five times a day once the epithelium heals or the fifth day is reached. Topical therapy should be continued for at least 2 weeks, but no more than 3 weeks, because of the risk of drug toxicity. The drop frequency should continue to be tapered over the remainder of the treatment period.

Currently, there are no topical antiviral agents that have been shown to be effective in treating VZV-related epithelial keratitis. Treatment for this condition is aimed at preventing ocular complications and consists of oral acyclovir, 800 mg five times a day for 10 days, if within 72 hr of the appearance of the skin lesions. The epithelial disease is benign and usually resolves spontaneously.

4.3. Fungal Keratitis

4.3.1. Epidemiology, Clinical Relevance, and Etiologic Pathogens

Fungal keratitis is one of the most devastating ocular infections encountered in ophthalmic clinical practice. The destructive nature of these infections is largely due to the lack of effective topical antifungal agents and the organisms' ability to resist host defenses. This fact, coupled with the innate virulence of fungal organisms, makes early detection an absolute requisite for achieving therapeutic success. Fungi, like bacteria, require a breach in the corneal epithelium in order to penetrate the cornea and produce tissue destruction. Fungal infections have been primarily associated with corneal trauma due to vegetable or organic material (e.g., tree branch, nylon lawn trimmer).

The leading corneal pathogens include *Fusarium*, *Aspergillus*, and *Candida*. These organisms cause the overwhelming majority of corneal fungal infections and appear to have climate specificity. *Fusarium* is the predominant corneal pathogen in the warmer southern United States, whereas *Candida* is the predominant corneal pathogen in the cooler northern United States. *Aspergillus* is found both in the northern and southern United States. *Candida* corneal infections are notable for occurring mainly in the setting of a compromised ocular surface (i.e., prolonged topical corticosteroid use, hypesthetic cornea from HZV, severe dry eye disease, and the like).

4.3.2. Clinical Manifestations

Fungal keratitis classically presents as an indolent infection with the infectious process evolving over a matter of days to weeks. In most infections, symptoms and signs typically develop within 1 or 2 days of inoculation, but because of the less fulminant evolution, patients are not motivated to seek medical attention until days or weeks later. The characteristic clinical appearance of a fungal keratitis consists of a gray-white stromal infiltrate with feathery or fluffy borders usually accompanied by several satellite lesions adjacent to the primary focus of infection. The corneal surface often appears to have a dry coarse texture and the epithelium at the margins of the ulcer tends to be heaped up. Keratomycosis is also frequently associated with sterile hypopyon formation.

4.3.3. Diagnosis

The diagnostic evaluation involves culturing for both bacteria and fungi using blood and chocolate agar plates for bacterial isolation and Sabouraud agar for fungal isolation. Smears for Gram and Giemsa stains and potassium hydroxide preparation are obtained as well. Patients should be referred immediately to an ophthalmologist to have definitive culturing performed. If initial cultures are negative, patients often require corneal biopsy and special fungal staining of the biopsied tissue.

4.3.4. Antibiotic Treatment

The treatment of fungal keratitis requires a prolonged course of medical therapy. The antifungal agents currently available are primarily fungistatic and have poor penetration into the cornea. Therefore, protracted courses of therapy are necessary in order to achieve adequate antifungal tissue levels for a sufficient period of time to eradicate the organism. It is generally recommended that therapy for fungal keratitis be continued for at least 12 weeks. Empirical therapy is usually started with natamycin (5%) eyedrops, which is the only ocular antifungal preparation commercially available in the United States. Natamycin belongs to the polyene class of antifungal agents and has been shown to be most effective against filamentous fungi, such as *Aspergillus* and *Fusarium*. This agent is administered every 30–60 min around the clock for the first 24–72 hr.

Unfortunately, natamycin has poor corneal penetration and, therefore, has limited efficacy in those cases in which the organism lies deep within the corneal stroma. Amphotericin B is the drug of choice for treating fungal keratitis produced by yeasts, such as *Candida*. Topical preparations of amphotericin B can be made by a hospital pharmacy. The recommended concentration is 0.15%. Oral flucytosine (150 mg/kg) is often used in combination with amphotericin in treating *Candida* corneal infections because of the demonstrated synergistic effects. Other antifungals commonly used to treat fungal keratitis include clotrimazole 1% vaginal cream, miconazole 1% fabricated from the intravenous preparation, oral fluconazole (400–800 mg/day), and oral ketoconazole (200–400 mg/day). Fungal infections unresponsive to medical therapy require corneal transplantation for disease eradication.

4.3.5. Prevention

Because corneal trauma is the predominant risk factor for the development of fungal keratitis, patients should be strongly encouraged to wear protective eyewear when they are performing yard work. Moreover, patients with severe dry eye disease or hypesthetic corneas require frequent follow-up with an ophthalmologist to monitor the status of their ocular surface.

5. RETINAL AND VITREOUS INFECTIONS: ENDOPHTHALMITIS

5.1. Epidemiology, Clinical Relevance, and Etiologic Pathogens

Postoperative endophthalmitis is the most significant retinal–vitreal infection encountered among the geriatric population. Endophthalmitis is defined as inflammation of the intraocular contents and develops as a result of microbial pathogens or chemical toxins gaining intraocular access. Although several etiologic mechanisms exist for the development of this infection (i.e., penetrating ocular trauma or hematogenous spread from another infectious site), postsurgical infection is the predominant mechanism among the elderly, who undergo the majority of intraocular surgery. Fortunately, it is a rare complication of intraocular surgery. The relative incidence of postoperative endophthalmitis for each of the commonly performed intraocular surgical procedures is listed in Table 6 (14,15).

Studies have shown that postoperative endophthalmitis is primarily caused by organisms that colonize the eyelids, conjunctiva, and nose, with 90% of culture-positive postoperative endophthalmitis cases caused by gram-positive organisms, of which coagulase-negative staphylococci are the most common (16,17). The major host risk factors for the development of postoperative endophthalmitis include bacterial blepharitis, nasolacrimal duct infections, nasolacrimal duct obstruction, active nonocular infections, diabetes mellitus, and immunosuppression from any cause.

Table 6 Incidence of Endophthalmitis Following Intraocular Surgery

Procedure	Incidence (%)
Cataract surgery	0.13
Corneal transplantation surgery	0.11
Glaucoma surgery	0.061
Retinal–vitreous surgery	0.051

5.2. Clinical Manifestations

Postoperative endophthalmitis can manifest early or late in the postoperative period. Early postoperative endophthalmitis typically occurs within the first week after surgery. Patients will typically complain of severe ocular pain and decreased vision. On examination of these patients, intraocular and periocular inflammation in excess of the normal postoperative inflammatory response will be found. Depending on the severity of the infection, patients may also demonstrate frank purulence at the surgical wound site, purulent conjunctival discharge, or a hypopyon in the anterior chamber. Most cases of endophthalmitis following cataract extraction occur early. In the Endophthalmitis Vitrectomy Study (EVS), for example, the median time to presentation was 6 days and about 80% of patients presented within 2 weeks of cataract surgery (16).

Late or delayed-onset postoperative endophthalmitis can occur days to weeks and even years after surgery. The type of surgery appears to have a definite role in the development of these late infections, with glaucoma surgery being more frequently associated with late-onset postoperative endophthalmitis. Late infections can present very subtly or in a fulminant suppurative manner. The type of presentation is primarily determined by the virulence of the infecting organism. The subtle presentation of postoperative endophthalmitis is most commonly associated with postcataract surgery cases. This form of endophthalmitis usually manifests as persistent low-grade postoperative inflammation well beyond the expected time period for normal postoperative inflammation. Patients will complain of persistent photophobia and blurred vision. These patients will typically not manifest any signs of frank purulence and the eyes will often appear white and unremarkable. The etiologic mechanism underlying this form of endophthalmitis has been shown to be colonization of the intraocular lens implant by *Propionibacterium acnes* and coagulase-negative staphylococcal species.

The fulminant presentation of late postoperative endophthalmitis is more frequently associated with streptococcal species and gram-negative organisms, which cause the majority of late endophthalmitis. Glaucoma filtration surgery is the most frequent infection-associated surgical procedure. Patients with this form of the disease will present in similar fashion to patients with acute postoperative endophthalmitis, i.e., severe pain, decreased vision, and marked intraocular and periocular inflammation. Given the strong association of late postoperative endophthalmitis with glaucoma filtration surgery, it is recommended that patients who have undergone glaucoma surgery and present with conjunctivitis be placed on topical antibiotic therapy immediately and referred to an ophthalmologist for a more in-depth evaluation.

5.3. Diagnosis

The diagnosis of endophthalmitis is made primarily on clinical findings. Diagnostic needle aspiration of the anterior chamber or vitreous cavity may be performed to confirm the clinical diagnosis and identify the infecting organism.

5.4. Antibiotic Treatment

The prognosis for postoperative endophthalmitis is largely dependent on the virulence of the infecting organism and the length of time between the onset of infection and the initiation of therapy. The delicate intraocular structures cannot withstand prolonged exposure to destructive bacterial pathogens and inflammatory cells and, therefore, early diagnosis and rapid therapy implementation are the keys to treatment success for this condition. The treatment of endophthalmitis involves intraocular antibiotic injections along with frequent application of topical fortified antibiotics and topical corticosteroids. The antibiotics most commonly used for intraocular injection are amikacin (400 μg) and vancomycin (1 mg). In advanced cases, a vitrectomy is performed in conjunction with the above measures to debulk the infectious debris. One of the key findings of the EVS was that immediate vitrectomy was of use only in patients who presented with visual acuity of light perception or worse (16). Most retinal surgeons will also place patients on a short course of oral corticosteroids following vitrectomy. Diagnostic specimens of the aqueous and vitreous humors are obtained at the time of intraocular antibiotic injection or vitrectomy.

5.5. Prevention

Because of the strong association with lid flora, patients with active blepharitis must be adequately treated prior to undergoing any form of ocular surgery. To further combat this problem ophthalmic surgeons instill preoperative prophylactic broad-spectrum antibiotics in the operative eye. In addition, some surgeons infuse antibiotics in the eye during surgery. A summary of endophthalmitis is given in Table 7.

Table 7 Summary of Endophthalmitis

Clinical features		Diagnostic test	Etiology	Treatment options and expected clinical course
Symptoms	Signs			
Unilateral profound lid swelling Severe brow pain Severe vision loss	Lid swelling Conjunctival injection Hypopyon (layered inflammatory infiltrate in the anterior chamber)	Culture of vitreous aspiration	Patient typically had recent eye surgery Staphylococci *Propionibacterium acne*	Emergency referral to ophthalmologist Intravitreal antibiotics Resolves over several weeks

6. ORBITAL INFECTIONS

6.1. Preseptal Cellulitis

6.1.1. Epidemiology and Clinical Relevance

Preseptal cellulitis represents a superficial cellulitis of the eyelid skin and subcutaneous tissue. This infection can arise from one of three sources: paranasal sinus infections, direct extension from a localized infection of the eyelid or adjacent tissues (i.e., acute dacryocystitis or hordeola), and periorbital trauma (i.e., infected cuts or abrasions to the periorbital facial area). This infectious process is confined to the lid because the orbital septum has not been violated. The orbital septum is a fibrous extension of the bony periosteum attached to the orbital rim that inserts into the upper and lower eyelids and serves as a barrier to the spread of infection from the eyelid posteriorly into the orbit.

6.1.2. Clinical Manifestations

The predominant clinical manifestations of this disease process are lid edema and erythema. There may be associated reactive conjunctival injection, but the ocular globe and visual function are otherwise unaffected. Patients maintain normal visual acuity, normal pupillary responses, and good ocular motility; proptosis does not develop.

6.1.3. Diagnosis

The diagnostic evaluation includes a good history, which specifically ascertains information regarding sinus disease, sinus surgery, trauma, or excessive tearing. In addition, computed tomographic (CT) scans of the orbit and sinuses are important for determining the extent and possible etiology of the disease.

6.1.4. Antibiotic Treatment

Effective therapy is usually obtained with a 10–14-day course of oral antibiotics. Empirical therapy with dicloxacillin or cephalexin is more than adequate in the majority of cases.

6.1.5. Prevention

Localized lid infections and sinus infections should be promptly treated to prevent preseptal cellulitis from developing.

6.2. Orbital Cellulitis

6.2.1. Epidemiology and Clinical Relevance

Orbital or postseptal cellulitis, unlike preseptal cellulitis, is a sight-threatening emergency. Harmful infectious pathogens entering the orbital space have access to the optic nerve, the extraocular muscles, and the principal vasculature of the eye. If left untreated, this condition will surely result in blindness or severe visual impairment.

6.2.2. Clinical Manifestations

Patients present with dull aching pain, eyelid swelling and erythema, decreased vision, proptosis, conjunctival swelling and injection, and ocular motility disturbances.

Table 8 Orbital Infections

| Orbital infections | Clinical features | | Diagnostic test | Etiology | Treatment options and expected clinical course |
	Symptoms	Signs			
Preseptal cellulitis	Unilateral profound lid swelling	Lid swelling Lid redness	None clinical	*Staphylococci* or *Streptococci*	Resolves in days with dicloxicillin or cefuroxime Resolves in <14 days
Orbital cellulitis	Unilateral lid swelling Pain especially with eye movements Diplopia (double vision)	Lid swelling Lid redness Eye bulging forward (proptosis)	Orbital radiograph analysis with CT or MRI	Usually a result of sinus infections or trauma	Emergency referral to ophthalmologist; hospitalization; intravenous aftriaxone Resolves in a few weeks

Abbreviations: CT, computed tomography; MRI, magnetic resonance imaging.

In addition, the patients frequently have constitutional symptoms of fever and malaise. Paranasal sinus infections constitute the most common source of orbital cellulitis, with ethmoid sinusitis being the principal origin. Other important sources include dacryocystitis, dental abscess, and trauma, as well as risk factors such as systemic debilitation. Patients debilitated from advanced diabetic disease, septicemia, systemic malignancy, human immunodeficiency virus disease, chronic diarrhea, and prolonged immunosuppression are particularly at risk for developing fungal orbital infections.

6.2.3. Diagnosis

As with preseptal cellulitis, CT scans of the orbits and sinuses are obtained to determine the extent of disease and look for the presence of orbital abscesses. The presence of an orbital abscess and/or multiple sinus disease is an indication for immediate surgical drainage. Nasopharynx cultures can be helpful in identifying the causative organism, although orbital cellulitis in adults tends to be polymicrobial. It is also important to note that in the elderly intraocular and extraocular tumors can masquerade as orbital cellulitis. Intraocular melanoma extending through the sclera, for example, has been found to induce a significant orbital inflammatory response similar to what one may see with orbital cellulitis (18).

6.2.4. Antibiotic Treatment

Patients diagnosed with orbital cellulitis require hospitalization and the initiation of broad-spectrum intravenous antibiotics. Empirical therapy with ceftriaxone is a regimen frequently employed. Urgent ophthalmology and otolaryngology consultation should be obtained as well.

6.2.5. Prevention

Orbital cellulitis is an infectious process that arises secondarily from extension of a primary infection in a periorbital structure. Thus, appropriate treatment of the primary infectious process will prevent the development of orbital cellulitis in most cases. A summary of clinical infections of the orbit is given in Table 8.

REFERENCES

1. Lundsgard KKK. The Doyne Memorial Lecture. Pneumococcus in connection with ophthalmology. Trans Ophthalmol Soc UK 1927; 47:294–312.
2. Dawson CR, Darrell D. Infections due to adenovirus type 8 in the United States. An outbreak of epidemic keratoconjunctivitis originating in physician's office. N Engl J Med 1963; 268:1031–1034.
3. Buffington J, Chapman LE, Stobierski MG, Hierholzer JC, Gary HE Jr, Guskey LE, Breitenbach RA, Hall WN, Schonberger LB. Epidemic keratoconjunctivitis in a chronic care facility: risk factors and measures for control. J Am Geriatr Soc 1993; 41:1177–1181.
4. Wegman DH, Guinee VF, Millian SJ. Epidemic kertaconjunctivits. Am J Public Health 1970; 60:1230–1237.
5. Kowal VO, Mead MD. Community acquired corneal ulcers: the impact of culture on management. Invest Ophtahlmol Vis Sci 1992; 33:1210.
6. McLeod SD, LaBree LD, Tayyanipour R, Flowers CW, Lee PP, McDonnell PJ. The importance of initial management in the treatment of severe infectious corneal ulcer. Ophthalmology 1995; 102:1943–1948.

7. Leibowitz HM. Clinical evaluation of ciprofloxacin 0.3% ophthalmic solution for treatment of bacterial keratitis. Am J Ophthalmol 1993; 112:34S–47S.
8. Schein OD, Munoz B, Tielsch JM, Bandeen-Roche K, West S. Prevalence of dry eye among the elderly. Am J Ophthalmol 1997; 124:723–728.
9. Mader TH, Stulting RD. Viral keratitis. Infect Dis Clin North Am 1992; 6:831–849.
10. Ragozzino MW, Melton LJ III, Kurland LT, Chu CP, Perry HO. Population-based study of herpes zoster and its sequelae. Medicine 1982; 61:310–316.
11. Chang EJ, Dreyer EB. Herpes virus infection of the anterior segment. Int Ophthalmol Clin 1996; 36:17–28.
12. Jones BD. Herpes zoster ophthalmicus. In: Golden B, ed. Ocular Inflammatory Disease. Springfield, IL: Charles C. Thomas, 1974:198–209.
13. Shuster JJ, Kaufman HE, Nesburn AB. Statistical analysis of the rate of recurrence of herpes virus ocular epithelial disease. Am J Ophthalmol Med 1981; 91:328–331.
14. Kattan HM, Flynn HM, Pflugfelder SC, Robertson C, Forster RK. Nosocomial endophthalmitis survey: current incidence of infection after intraocular surgery. Ophthalmology 1991; 2:227–238.
15. Powe NR, Schein OD, Gieser SC, Tielsch JM, Luthra R, Javitt J, Steinberg EP. Synthesis of the literature on visual acuity and complications following cataract extraction with intraocular lens implantation. Arch Ophthalmol 1994; 112:239–252.
16. Endophthalmitis Vitrectomy Study Group. Results of the endophthalmitis vitrectomy study. Arch Ophthalmol 1995; 113:1479–1496.
17. Speaker MG, Milch FA, Shah MK, Eisner W, Kreiswirth BN. Role of external bacterial flora in the pathogenesis of acute postoperative endophthalmitis. Ophthalmology 1991; 98:639–650.
18. Rumelt S, Rubin PAD. Potential sources for orbital cellulitis. Int Ophthalmol Clin 1996; 36:207–221.
19. Flowers CW. Managing eye infections in older adults. Infect Dis Clin Pract 1998; 7: 447–458.
20. Berson FG. The red eye. In: Berson FG, ed. Basic Ophthalmology for Medical Students and Primary Care Residents. San Francisco, CA: American Academy of Ophthalmology, 1973:57–74.
21. Barza M, Baum J. Ocular infections. Med Clin North Am 1983; 67:131–152.

SUGGESTED READING

Buffington J, Chapman LE, Stobierski MG, Hierholzer JC, Gary HE Jr, Guskey LE, Breitenbach RA, Hall WN, Schonberger LB. Epidemic keratoconjunctivitis in a chronic care facility: risk factors and measures for control. J Am Geriatr Soc 1993; 41: 1177–1181.
McLeod SD, LaBree LD, Tayyanipour R, Flowers CW, Lee PP, McDonnell PJ. The importance of initial management in the treatment of severe infectious corneal ulcer. Ophthalmology 1995; 102:1943–1948.
Powe NR, Schein OD, Gieser SC, Tielsch JM, Luthra R, Javitt J, Steinberg EP. Synthesis of the literature on visual acuity and complications following cataract extraction with intraocular lens implantation. Arch Ophthalmol 1994; 112:239–252.

28

Major Orofacial Infection

Joseph L. McQuirter and Anh Le
Department of Oral and Maxillofacial Surgery, Charles R. Drew University of Medicine and Science, Los Angeles, California, U.S.A.

Key Points:

- Most oral infections are caused by resident oral microbes.
- Rampant or recalcitrant oral infections should alert the clinician to evaluate host immune status.
- Medication-related xerostomia in the elderly is a major risk factor for oral diseases.
- Recurring bacteremia and toxemia from chronic dental infections can adversely affect distant organ systems.
- Routine oral hygiene care for the frail elderly and institutionalized adults is essential in preventing nutritional and pulmonary complications.

1. SPECIAL CONSIDERATIONS IN ORAL INFECTIONS

1.1. Microbial Flora of the Oral Cavity

The oral cavity serves not only as the gateway for the body's nutritional needs but also as the portal entry and resident quarter for a number of microbes. More than 500 bacterial strains have been identified in dental biofilm, also known as plaque, which readily adheres to teeth and other oral structures (1). Most oral infections are caused by organisms that normally reside in the oropharyngeal areas and take advantage of a breach in the body's defense mechanism, especially in the elderly. Diseases produced by these organisms range from localized infections that stimulate pain and affect daily quality of life functions (i.e., eating, swallowing, and speaking) to the systemic dissemination of microbes and their toxic products compromising general health and well-being among the elderly.

1.2. The Elderly Host Defense

Elderly adults are affected adversely by primary immunologic deficiency seen in the aging process, secondary immunologic impairment (due to poor circulation, decrease in salivary function, and allergic response), and emerging resistance to multiple chemotherapeutic agents (2). Locally, other oral factors complement the body's generalized defense system by providing surface barriers (e.g., the highly calcified and smooth surfaces of the tooth's enamel and healthy intact mucosal surfaces) and the cleansing, lubricating and immunological functions of multiple secretory glands (e.g., major and minor salivary glands, gingival crevicular fluids, etc.). Compromise or breakdown of these barriers especially seen in the medically compromised, frail, and institutionalized elderly adult predisposes them to a host of infections predominately caused by the oral microbial inhabitants. Table 1 (3) lists the most common indigenous and colonizing oral flora and microbes, many of which are frequently encountered in oral infections.

1.3. Salivary Function in the Elderly

Xerostomia, a condition of impaired salivary flow commonly found in the elderly aggravates the compromised aging immune system. As many older Americans take both prescription and over the counter drugs (1) they are likely to experience an oral side effect from at least one of the medications; the most common is dry mouth. The inhibited salivary flow increases the risk of oral disease because saliva contains antimicrobial components and minerals that help rebuild tooth enamel after attacked by acid-producing, decay-causing bacteria. When salivary flow is compromised, the gateway can open to local as well as to systemic pathogens (1). As such, the lack of saliva and its protective function further promotes caries, periodontal diseases, odontogenic infections, and traumatic ulceration and inflammation of denture bearing areas.

2. MAJOR ORAL AND OROFACIAL INFECTIONS OF THE ELDERLY

2.1. Odontogenic Infections Limited to Dentoalveolar Structures

2.1.1. Epidemiology and Clinical Relevance

Odontogenic infections, the predominant infections in the orofacial region, usually are caused by dental caries (tooth decay), periodontal diseases (i.e., gingivitis or periodontitis), and infections associated with dental appliances (i.e., partial or complete dentures, tooth-form implants, obturators, etc.). More than 95% of the U.S. population has experienced dental caries during their lifetime (4). In the group of dentate adults of aged ≥75 years, 56% suffered some forms of root decay and 16% experienced untreated coronal decay (1).

Periodontitis, a common disease affecting the periodontal attachments or connective tissues supporting the tooth, has a high prevalence in elderly populations ≥75 years with 97–100% experiencing some forms of acute or chronic disease by the age of 45 (4). The characteristic bone loss in periodontal disease represents the cumulative effect of a lifelong injury (5–8). Increased risk factors for periodontal disease include degree of plaque and calculus accumulation (5), oral hygiene, smoking, low socioeconomic status, male, and race Mexican Americans (9) and non-Hispanic blacks at special risk for periodontal disease (1). Gingival hyperplasia, an overgrowth of the gingival tissues, associated with multiple pharmacotherapeutic agents commonly used in the elderly is also a risk factor for periodontitis. One of the most frequently encountered consequences of unchecked progression of caries and periodontal diseases in the elderly is tooth loss (1), which leads to the need for oral rehabilitation with implants and dental appliances.

Denture stomatitis, a condition in which the mucosa underneath a denture becomes inflamed, affects 25.6% of denture wearers. Additionally, it affects 32% of those with one full denture, 26.7% of those with one or more partial dentures, and

Table 1 Some of the Most Common Indigenous and Colonizing Oral Flora

Aerobic and facultative isolates

Diphtheriods	Spirochetes
Lactobacilli	*Spirochaeta* species
Rothia dentocariosa	Christispira species
Streptococcus faecallis	*Treponema denticola*
Streptococcus milleri	*Treponema orale*
Streptococcus mitis	*Treponema macrodentium*
Streptococcus mutan	*Treponema vincentii*
Streptococcus salivarius	*Borrelia* species
Streptococcus sanguis	*Leptospira* species
	Yeast

Anaerobic isolates

Actinobacillus	Aspergillus species
Actinomycetemcomitans	*Candida albicans*
Actinomyces israelii	Other *Candida* species
Actinomyces naeslundii	*Geotrichum* species
Actinomyces odontolyticus	*Hemispora* species
Actinomyces viscosus	*Penicillium* species
Bacteroides asaccharolyticus	*Scopulariopsis* species
Bacteroides melaninogenicus	Viruses
Bacteroides oralis	Herpes simplex virus
Bacteroides ochraceus	Cytomegalovirus
Bacterionema matruchotii	Protozoa
Branhamella catarrhalis	*Entamoeba gingivalis*
Capnocytophaga gingivalis	*Trichomonas tenax*
Capnocytophaga ochraceus	
Capnocytophaga sputigena	
Eikenella corrodens	
Fusobacterium plauti	
Fusobacterium nucleatum	
Neisseria sicca	
Peptostreptococcus	
Veillonella alcalescens	
Veillonella parvula	

Source: From Ref. 3.

0.87% of those who do not have full or partial dentures (1). Recently, substitution of missing teeth with tooth-form and other implantable devices has revolutionized the practice of modern dentistry. Infection associated with osteo-integrated implants ranges from 1% to 3% immediately after surgical placement to as high as 32% long-term (10). Figure 1 shows the deteriorating oral hygiene that leads to cumulative plaque and calculus buildup, which favors caries, periodontal diseases, odontogenic infection, and, ultimately, tooth loss (11). Maintaining proper oral health is a significant problem for partially incapacitated and institutionalized elderly adults.

2.1.2. Etiologic Pathogens

Mutans streptococci, *Lactobacillus*, *Actinomyces*, and other acid-producing streptococci within dental biofilms have been identified to produce dental caries. More than

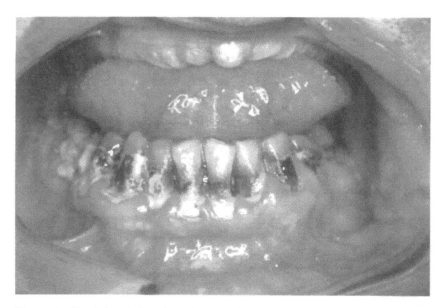

Figure 1 Tooth loss (edentulous) in upper jaw in a patient with heavy plaque and calculus accumulation resulting in root caries in the remaining teeth of the lower jaw.

150 bacterial strains have been isolated from dental pulp infections (1). More than 300 bacterial species are found in the human subgingival plaque samples, but less than 20 of these species play a role in the pathogenesis of destructive periodontal diseases (12,13). Most pathogens seen in periodontal infections are gram-negative anaerobic bacilli, but gram-positive facultative and anaerobic cocci, gram-positive anaerobic bacilli, and other gram-negative facultative bacilli are also isolated. The most common pathogens associated with aggressive periodontitis include *Actinobacillus actinomycetemcomitans*, spirochetes of acute necrotizing gingivitis, and *Porphyromonasgingivalis* (14,15).

2.1.3. Clinical Manifestations

Dental caries presents as a yellowish, dark brown, or black discoloration on the outer surface of the teeth due to demineralization and staining of the calcified tooth structure. In the elderly, interproximal and root caries are more common than those found on the occlusal or biting surfaces of the posterior teeth, which is more commonly seen in younger age groups. Acidogenic and aciduric bacteria colonizes in a biofilm on tooth surfaces as a result of inadequate oral hygiene measures. Arrested caries may occur in response to decreased microbial activity and remineralization with inorganic ions from saliva (4). Upon reaching the tooth's pulp tissues, dental caries usually causes the patient to report the accompanying pain as a toothache. The pain is associated with the inflammatory responses of the pulp (pulpitis) to the invading organisms and their toxins in the severely confined space of the tooth's inner core. The progressive swelling engorges the pulp, constricts the blood supply of the tooth, and causes pulpal necrosis. If the nonvital and infected pulp tissues are not removed by root canal treatment or extraction of the tooth, the suppurative infection will progress into the alveolar bone and subsequently into adjacent anatomical spaces producing additional pain, swelling, fever, chills, and bacteremia.

Periodontal disease ranges from mild gingival inflammation to aggressive loss of tooth and adjacent bone. With gingivitis, the gingival tissues vary in discoloration from a red to dark purple that bleeds with brushing or flossing, marked swelling, and a foul smelling breath. More advanced forms of periodontal disease manifest as gingival inflammation, loss of attachment tissues including gingivae, and alveolar bone and periodontal ligament attachment. Plaque and calculus is frequently abundant both above and below the receding gingival attachment. Halitosis, altered taste, fever, malaise, and lymphadenopathy are seen in more advanced cases (4). Abscess formation from periodontal infections can be localized or diffuse with extremely tender red fluctuant and markedly swollen gingival and alveolar tissues. Pus typically can be expressed from adjacent bony periodontal defects or "pockets." Pyogenic periodontal infections can progress to involve both the apical tissues of the tooth (apical periodontal abscess) and adjacent anatomical spaces; as well, it can affect distant organs by hematogenous spread as seen with dental caries (4).

Most root-formed dental implants enjoy a 5-year survival rate of 90% or better. Although failures are rare, they present as mobile fixtures that can be associated with pain, swelling, bleeding, and adjacent bone loss (implantitis). The role of excessive workload on an implant as a primary cause of failure or infections must be clearly defined. Implants must survive in the same microbe-laden environment as the natural dentition and are subjected to infections similar to those seen in periodontitis.

2.2. Odontogenic Deep Space and Disseminated Infections

2.2.1. Epidemiology and Clinical Relevance

Odontogenic infections progressing beyond the dentoalveolar structures and disseminating into adjacent spaces are rare, especially when proper oral hygiene is maintained and regular dental professional care is provided. When they occur, such complications include propagation of pyogenic infections directly into the sinuses, orbits, brain, and deep spaces of the neck and chest. Pulmonary aspiration, hematogenous and lymphatic spread of oral microbes, can produce systemic complications in response to what may appear to be an innocuous and locally confined dental problem. Oral infections also may represent systemic or more generalized conditions that manifest initially in the oral cavity and alert the clinician or individuals of the need for further investigation. The oral mucosa and its secretory glands can be adversely affected by many pharmaceuticals and other therapies commonly used in medical treatment. Discomfort from such therapies may affect patient compliance with other recommended treatment (1). Odontogenic infections have also been implicated as risk factors for developing atherosclerosis, coronary artery disease, stroke, and premature births (16–19). Poor oral hygiene and periodontal disease have been associated with aspiration pneumonia (16,20,21).

2.2.2. Etiologic Pathogens

The source of the infection can usually be localized by identifying the diseased teeth in the proximity of the involved area. Both odontogenic and non-odontogenic infections have their own characteristic flora (22). Odontogenic infections generally are characterized by a combination of facultative streptococci and oral anaerobes (22).

2.2.3. Clinical Manifestations

Infections located in the more superficial fascial spaces of the orofacial regions include the canine, buccal, masticatory, infratemporal, sublingual, and submandibular spaces. Their anatomic locations serve to localize the potential odontogenic site for the infection. As an example, the roots of the lower second and third molar teeth are frequently located beneath the mylohyoid muscle attached on the medial aspect of the mandible. An abscess at the apex of these teeth typically will erode into the submandibular space in contrast to the apices of the roots of the premolars above the mylohyoid which will produce infections in the sublingual spaces. Orofacial infections are characterized by swelling, asymmetry, loss of anatomic borders and contours, lymphadeopathy, pain, fever, and chills. Masticatory space infections also produce severe trismus and odynophasia. Progression of these infections into the deeper spaces of the neck, including parapharyngeal spaces and spaces surrounding the carotid sheath, produces external fullness, neck rigidity, dysphasia, dysphonia, and trachael deviation. As swelling encroaches on the periglottic region, stridor and progressive airway obstruction occur. Mediastinal spread produces distant heart sounds, murmur or pericardial friction rubs, and heart failure (23).

2.2.4. Diagnosis

Caries not involving the pulpal tissues are typically asymptomatic and are identified clinically by discoloration and softening of the surface enamel or cementum. Sharp edges from partial collapse of the outer tooth structure may serve as a source of irritation to the tongue or cheek tissues. Clinically observed discoloration, probing with a sharp instrument to detect defects and softening of the tooth's calcified tissues are sufficient to institute definitive treatment. When the pulp becomes involved, the tooth may become percussion sensitive, painful to thermal changes, unresponsive to electrical stimulation, and feels as though the tooth contacts prematurely when biting. Chronic pulpal necrosis may result in a grayish to black discoloration of the tooth crown. Clinical observation is sufficient to diagnose gingivitis. Probing the tissue pocket depth immediately adjacent to the tooth measures attachment loss in periodontal disease. A periodontal abscess is present when pus is expressible from tissues surrounding the teeth.

Dental bitewing and periapical x-ray film are used to demonstrate coronal and root caries appearing on the interproximal surfaces of the teeth and loss of interdental bone height due to periodontal disease and periapical abscess producing apical bone destruction. To detect caries radiographically, 30–50% demineralization must have occurred.

The differential diagnosis of infections in the superficial spaces of the head and neck regions must include careful consideration of several other points of origin. Skin, nasal, and paranasal sinuses are all frequent sites of origin for infections. They must be differentiated as the potential source of the infection or merely included as a part of the progression of the odontogenic infection.

Aspirated or swabbed specimens that form the core of the abscess site should be taken to ensure that anaerobic and other microbial growth representative of the infection etiology is cultured. Blood cultures should also be taken when fever peaks and for deep infections that are discontinuous with epithelial surfaces. Gram staining should be performed to observe host inflammatory response and characterize detectable microbial forms.

Computed tomography (CT) and magnetic resonance imaging (MRI) are quick and easy studies to obtain in the hospital setting; each provides unique pieces to the diagnostic picture. MRI is superior to CT in localizing drainable abscesses, in defining the extent and origin of the lesion, and the intracranial extension of infections. CT is better than MRI in detecting intralesional gases, calcifications, and cortical destruction.

2.2.5. Antibiotic Treatment

Although the etiologic agents for dental caries, gingivitis, and periodontitis are microbial, cultures and antibiotic therapy are not routinely necessary for such lesions when not involving the dental pulp and periapical tissues. Removal of the infected tissues and implementing an effective prevention program for removal of plaque and calculus is usually sufficient. In cases where xerostomia contributes to the process, correcting the underlying cause of the xerostomia or salivary replacement therapy may be warranted.

Tetracycline is one of the most commonly used antibiotics in periodontal disease because of its effectiveness against common pathogens and its ability to concentrate in gingival crevicular fluids up to 10 times its serum concentration. Other common antibiotics used in the treatment of periodontal disease include doxycycline, metronidazole, ciprofloxacin, amoxicillin, and clindamycin. Because periodontitis usually is caused by several microbial species, monoantibiotic therapy is unpredictable. Combinations of antibiotics that have been used include metronidazole with amoxicillin and amoxicillin/clavalanate (14).

Once the pulp tissues become infected or an abscess develops at the apex or periodontal areas, drainage and debridement of the infected area are initiated in addition to antibiotic therapy. In the case of pulpal necrosis or irreversible pulpitis, root canal therapy is initiated in conjunction with antibiotic therapy. With a steady rise in resistant bacteria, fungal, and viral strains in patient infections, greater caution has been used in how and when antimicrobials are used during patient care (24). The more fragile state of the elderly may warrant antibiotic use with the presence of an abscess. The more commonly prescribed antibiotics in oral infections are penicillin, amoxicillin, cephalosporins, clindamycin, erythromycin, and tetracycline. These antimicrobial agents usually are well tolerated by most elderly patients and require no dose adjustment. Geriatric patients with renal impairment may require dose adjustment for penicillins, amoxicillins, and some cephalosporins (25).

Empirical choice of antibiotics should be based on a thorough history of the infectious process and knowledge of the indigenous organisms that colonize the infection source (teeth, gums, and mucous membrane). A thorough history should include any antibiotic use within the past 3 months or chronic use of antibiotics during the past 12 months. In the absence of prior antimicrobial therapy that may stimulate the emergence of β-lactamase-producing organisms, penicillin monotherapy is appropriate. The dose and length of therapy should be determined by the severity of the infection (4).

Early identification of the causative organism or group of organisms and the appropriate sensitivity testing allows the clinician the best opportunity to arrive at a definitive diagnosis and make available specific treatment approaches with maximal potential for success. In elderly individuals subjected to frequent episodes of antimicrobial therapy or individuals with hospital-acquired infections, culture and sensitivity testing may disclose antibiotic-resistant bacteria (24). Flynn et al. performed a prospective study of hospitalized patients with odontogenic infections and found a 26% rate of clinical failure with penicillin therapy and a 60% rate of resistance (25).

Antibiotic therapy should be initiated to halt the progression of local and hematogenous spread of odontogenic infections. Immunocompromised patients are at particular risk of spreading unhaulted infections since they may progress without the classic signs of inflammation being present (e.g., marked swelling, tenderness, redness, and regional lymphadenopathy).

2.2.6. Prevention

Several common conditions seen in the elderly can compromise their oral hygiene practices and result in increased bacteria-laden plaque and calculus accumulations. These conditions include diminished motor skills from arthritic joints, neuromuscular movement disorders and convalescence states (16). Also, a number of pharmacological agents used by the elderly may enhance plaque and calculus accumulations including medications causing xerostomia, and gingival hyperplasia. Medication-related ulcerative or reactive lesions can also become secondarily infected in the oral cavity.

Cognitive, visual, and functional motor impairments are conditions seen in the elderly that preclude self-care and increase reliance on others to provide oral hygiene care (26). Instituting good dental hygiene measures typically prevents and arrests the progress of caries and periodontal disease. If xerostomia is a contributing factor, then correcting this underlying problem is warranted.

2.3. Oral Candidiasis

2.3.1. Epidemiology and Clinical Relevance

The oral cavity of older adults, particularly the immunocompromised patients, is susceptible to a variety of bacterial, fungal, and viral soft tissue infections. The most common infection involving oral mucosal tissues in the elderly patient is candidiasis. Rates of candidal infections have been reported from 43% to 93% in human immunodeficiency (HIV) infected patients (27,28). Pharmacotherapeutic agents that alter the normal oral flora, such as long-term antibiotic therapy, and drugs that affect salivary flow frequently associate with an overgrowth of *Candida albicans*.

2.3.2. Etiologic Pathogen

Candida species are normal host saprophyte yeasts commonly found in the gastro intestinal (GI) tract, genitourinary tract, and oropharynx. Seventy percent of nosocomial candidal infection is due to *C. albicans*. Opportunistic overgrowth of *C. albicans* occurs in individuals with impaired immune function, trauma, or induced changes in the oral microbial flora (e.g., prednisone, chemotherapy, and HIV) and xerostomia.

2.3.3. Clinical Manifestations

Clinically, oral candidiasis can be classified into six major types:

1. Pseudomembranous candidiasis, also known as "thrush," manifested as white plaques around the oral cavity. This form is particularly prevalent in HIV infection.
2. Atrophic candidiasis, which is usually presented as generalized depapillation of the tongue following antibiotic therapy, and represents an acute increase in the colonies of *Candida* organisms in the oral cavity. This form is clinically similar to erythematous candidiasis.
3. Chronic atrophic candidiasis, which is manifested as denture stomatitis.

4. Chronic hyperplastic candidiasis, which is also known as candidal leuko-plakia when found on the buccal mucosa and as median rhomboid glossitis when located in the central part of the tongue.
5. Angular cheilitis, also known as perleche, which occurs extraorally at the commissures of the mouth secondary to tooth loss.
6. Chronic mucocutaneous candidiasis, which is the most serious form of candidiasis and manifested as pseudomembranous oral candidiasis, skin, esophageal, and nail involvement.

The two most common forms of oral candidiasis in the elderly are denture stomatitis and angular cheilitis. Mucosal trauma under an ill-fitting denture is a frequent site for candidiasis to develop. Typically, patients may complain of a generalized burning sensation characterized by periodic exacerbation and partial remission. If focal hyperplastic candidiasis is suspected, the differential diagnosis must include hairy leukoplakia, epithelial dysplasia, and squamous carcinoma. It may be secondarily infected with candida. Figure 2 shows an elderly patient with both atrophic candidiasis of the tongue and angular cheilitis.

2.3.4. Diagnosis

When clinical features are insufficient for a definitive diagnosis, the characteristic yeast forms can be identified with an adequate exfoliative cytology smear.

Definitive diagnosis of fungal infection can be obtained from fungus culture of biopsied specimens.

2.3.5. Antibiotic Treatment

The best long-term management is identification and elimination of the local or systemic immunosuppressive factors that cause the opportunistic infection. Local therapy includes topical azoles, clotrimazole troche, miconazole or ketoconazole

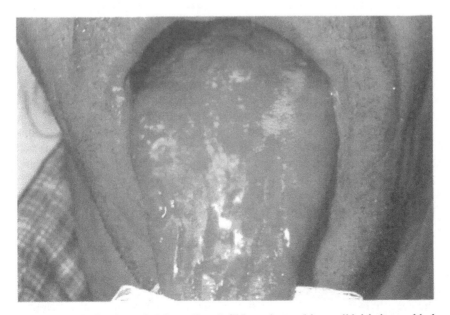

Figure 2   Medication-related angular cheilitis and atrophic candidaisis in an elderly patient.

cream, and nystatin suspension or ointment. Systemic therapy includes oral ketoconazole or fluconazole for severe oral candidasis or for cases poorly responsive to
topical therapy, such as candidial esophagitis.

2.3.6. Prevention

Since oral candidiasis is most likely an opportunistic infection in the elderly, primary
control of the underlying systemic diseases should be emphasized. Cases related to
medication-induced xerostomia may require alteration in medication or supplemental use of sialogogue (pilocarpine).

2.4. Herpes Simplex Viruses

2.4.1. Epidemiology, Clinical Relevance, and Etiologic Pathogen

Herpes simplex is a member of the DNA virus family of herpes virus. Herpes simplex
virus (HSV)-1 infection is common in childhood and usually infects the oral mucosa.
By the fourth decade, ≈90% of individuals will be seropositive for HSV-1. HSV-2 is
less common than HSV-1, predominately affects the genital mucosa, and primary
infections tend to occur in an older age group. The seroprevalence of HSV-2 in
the United States is 10–40%.

The incubation period following exposure to the virus is about a week (range
1–26 days). HSV transmission is the most efficient in individuals with active ulcerations of the mucosal or genital membranes, or in the forms of asymptomatic shedding
of virus.

2.4.2. Clinical Manifestations

Primary herpetic gingivostomatitis in adults is usually more severe than that seen in
children; in such cases infection may be from either HSV-1 or HSV-2. Initially, clear
vesicles develop in the oral cavity, including the pharynx, palate, buccal mucosa, and
tongue. These vesicles rapidly rupture producing shallow ragged painful ulcers that
may coalesce and extend to involve the lips and cheek. Severe primary lesions can be
accompanied by high fever, malaise, cervical lymphadenopathy, and dehydration.
Primary herpetic stomatitis is rare in the elderly and provides immunity from future
attacks but does not prevent reactivation and recurrent mucosal and labial flares (29).

Recurrent herpes labialis and recurrent intraoral herpes for individuals
≥65 years is 88.9% based on positive antibody titers for HSV-1. More than 15%
of individuals in this age group reported at least one episode of recurrent lesions
in the past 12 months (1). Only 33% of individuals initially exposed to the virus will
manifest clinical symptoms characteristic of the disease and 30–40% of those infected
will have recurrences (30,31). Recurrent herpes labialis (cold sores) and recurrent
intraoral herpes develop in response to reactivated latent virus in the regional nerve
ganglia that may be stimulated by stress, irritation, exposure to sunlight, cold, fever,
trauma, and immunosuppression. Prodromal symptoms include burning, tingling,
itching, or pain at the point of eruption. These lesions recur near the point of entry
into the body as small vesicles that quickly erupt and produce ulcerated areas in the
mouth or crusted lesion on skin about the lips. These vesicles and ulcers are laden
with transmissible viruses during the first 2–3 days. Common autoinnoculation sites
include the eyes (herpetic keratitis) and fingers (herpetic whitlow). Transmission of
the virus to others includes interpersonal contact with mucosal surfaces or abraded

skin, or contaminated objects such as cloth, saliva, gloves, medical charts, and other materials (30).

2.4.3. Diagnosis

Diagnosis is usually based on the history and clinical findings. Cultures, cytologic smears that show multinucleation, and special immunofluorescent processing can be helpful when clinical recognition is uncertain. Serologic diagnosis is of value only to determine past exposure. The differential diagnosis of recurrent HSV-1 infections should include herpangina, oral candidiasis, Epstein–Barr virus, Stevens–Johnson syndrome, and recurrent aphthous stomatitis.

2.4.4. Antiviral Treatment

Systemic antiviral agents are used in complicated primary infections, HSV infections in the immunocompromised, prophylaxis for seropositive patients who undergo chemotherapy or transplantation, HSV-associated central nervous system disease, and recurrent erythema multiforme. Precursor antiviral agents, such as valacyclovir and famciclovir, have better oral bioavailability than acyclovir and penciclovir. If not used early in the infection (i.e., the first 3–4 days), antiviral drugs usually are ineffective. Antiseptic, analgesic, and anti-inflammatory medications can be beneficial in reducing pain and transmission of the disease (29). Nephrotoxicity, although rare, is a concern with the use of high-dose systemic acyclovir, valcyclovir and famciclovir, particularly if patients have renal insufficiency (29). For acyclovir-resistant cases, foscarnet (Foscavir) or cidofovir (Vistide) can be used (29).

Recurrent oral and mucosal lesions create a lifetime problem for individuals susceptible to reactivation of latent HSV. The treatment of oral HSV-1 infections by systemic antiviral agents is generally discouraged (30,32) except for serious systemic disease in immunocompromised individuals, where acyclovir may be the drug-of-choice. Antiviral chemotherapy should be essentially reserved for serious mucocutaneous or disseminated HSV infections in immunocompromised hosts and not employed for annoying non-life-threatening infections. Resistance to the azole antiviral agents is increasing and is of serious concern (30,33).

2.4.5. Prevention

Systemic therapeutic and prophylactic antiviral chemotherapy may be considered for people with more than six recurrences per year, a history of erythema multiforme, common exposure to sun or stress, and those undergoing surgery on the trigeminal ganglia for neuralgia (30,34). Oral prophylaxis with acyclovir at 400–800 mg/day may decrease the frequency of HSV-1 recurrences by 50–78% (30,35). Other non-pharmacological preventive measures include avoidance of direct sunlight and use of sunscreen in vulnerable exposed sites.

2.5. Herpes Zoster (Varicella-Zoster Virus; Human Varicella Virus)

2.5.1. Epidemiology, Clinical Relevance, and Etiologic Pathogen

Varicella-zoster virus (VZV) is a neurotropic α-herpes virus that produces two distinct clinical diseases. The first disease, varicella or chickenpox, is predominately seen in children and immunocompromised patients. In adults the disease may be associated with serious morbidity due to pulmonary complications. Varicella is commonly seen in patients with acquired immunodeficiency syndrome (AIDS) and individuals who have undergone bone marrow transplantation. The second form, herpes zoster, is a recurrent infection along the nerve distribution which frequently occurs in elderly patients (30).

VZV as seen with the other α-type herpes virus (HSV-1 and -2) is associated with primary infections, a latency period where the virus resides in the nerve trunk, and a recurrent skin or mucosal eruption along the nerve distribution. VZV is responsible for chickenpox (varicella), as typically seen in children and immunocompromised patients, and shingles (herpes zoster), a reactivation of the latent virus that is seen especially in the elderly. In the U.S. population, >90% of the people are infected with chickenpox virus before 15 years (36,37). The reactivated herpes zoster virus occurs in 0.2% of adults, increasing the incidence with age and immunocompromised states (29).

The virus infects one or more of the sensory ganglia and becomes latent until a recurrence is triggered. Recurrences usually occur in persons aged ≥50 years.

2.5.2. Clinical Manifestations

Triggers can be idiopathic and include a decrease in systemic immunity, medication, or a second virus such as Epstein–Barr, HIV, or debilitating chronic disease (i.e., leukemia and lymphoma). Clinical presentation may be a complaint of toothache when associated with VZV. Prodromes include pain, paresthesia, burning (may last several days), or hypersensitive skin overlying the area of attack. Within days, the classic manifestations are painful vesicles that occur unilaterally along the nerve dermatomes (29). Multiple 1–2 cm clear fluid-filled vesicles are distributed along the path of the sensory nerve(s). Vesicles may coalesce into larger irregular-shaped blisters. Vesicles rupture to produce ulcer that takes 2–3 weeks to heal. This lesion may become secondarily infected by bacteria. The lesions are characterized occasionally by pain that may persist for weeks or months after healing of clinically evident lesions (postherpetic neuralgia).

2.5.3. Diagnosis

Diagnosis is based on history, clinical findings, and serology. Laboratory procedures include exfoliative cytologic examination of vesicular fluid for the presence of multinucleated epithelial giant cells, culture in human or monkey cells. Polymerase chain reaction is used for diagnosis in severe cases that may involve the central nervous system (29,37).

2.5.4. Antiviral Treatment

Early intervention for herpes zoster with acyclovir 800 mg orally five times daily and famciclovir 500 mg three times per day or valacyclovir at 1 g orally three times per day for 7 days can shorten the episode duration in some patients. Famciclovir appears to be effective in shortening the duration of postherpetic neuralgia (30,38). Postherpetic neuralgias have also been treated with nonsteroidal anti-inflammatory medications (i.e., ibuprofen and sulindac), systemic corticosteroid regimens, and tricyclic antidepressants.

Antiviral therapy should be considered for all patients >50 years of age with herpes zoster virus and anyone with herpes zoster associated with ophthalmic complications, peripheral motor neuropathy, cervical dematones, and immunocompromised states. Oral and parenteral antivirals will reduce herpes zoster pain, promote healing, reduce complications, and increase social activity (30,39–41).

Supportive therapy treatment for pain and pruritus should also be instituted. The most painful and discouraging complication is postherpetic neuralgia, which can be debilitating. Early use of corticosteroids along with antiviral treatment may help minimize, or even prevent, the neuropathy. Longer-standing cases benefit from the use of amitriptyline, nortriptyline, topical lidocaine patches, and gabapentin, which should be considered early in the course of treatment (29).

2.5.5. Prevention

Chicken pox vaccine is available for varicella. However, its use is currently under investigation in older adults (see chapter "Herpes Zoster").

2.6. Human Immunodeficiency Virus (HIV)

2.6.1. Epidemiology and Clinical Relevance

Since the appearance of AIDS in 1981, it has created a staggering medical, social, and economic impact. Over 270,000 AIDS cases and 1.5 million carriers were reported in the United States in 1991. More than 10% of these cases were patients aged ≥50 years. Estimates show that 125,000 people aged ≥50 years could be carriers of HIV virus today (42).

While sexual contact and intravenous drug use are the chief causes of transmission in all age groups, blood transfusion is the major route of HIV infection in the elderly (see chapter "Human Immunodeficiency Virus Infection").

2.6.2. Clinical Manifestations and Diagnosis

Recent studies indicated that older patients have a shorter mean HIV incubation period than younger patients (5.8 vs. 7.3 years). HIV is confirmed by serological tests and the disease is followed by measuring viral load. Laboratory values show CD4 cells at <400 mm^3, a CD4/CD8 ratio <1.0, increased serum globulin levels, leukothrombocytopenia, and anemia. Criteria for suspecting AIDS in the elderly include a positive history of transfusion, respiratory distress with typical symptoms of *Pneumocystis carinii*, thrombocytopenic purpura, or cortical dementia. Oral manifestations of HIV infection include a broad spectrum of secondary microbial infections from fungi such as oral candidiasis (e.g., pseudomembranous, erythematous, hyperplastic, and angular cheilitis), oral histoplasmosis, bacterial infections, such as fuso-spirochetal infection (e.g., necrotizing gingivitis), nonspecific infections (e.g., chronic periodontitis), and other infections as well as infections of unknown etiology, such as recurrent aphthous ulcerations, and idiopathic thrombocytopenic purpura.

2.6.3. Antiviral Treatment

For treatment of HIV infection, please refer to the chapter "Human Immunodeficiency Virus Infection." No immunization for HIV infection or AIDS presently exists. Treatment is confined to the various secondary clinical manifestations of the disease related to opportunistic infections.

2.7. Sialadenitis and Suppurative Parotitis

2.7.1. Epidemiology and Clinical Relevance

Acute suppurative sialadenitis is a bacterial infection most commonly associated with the elderly, malnourished, dehydrated, and chronically ill. The parotid gland is most frequently involved with an estimated incidence of ≈0.9% with unilateral involvement in 80% of the cases (43). Nearly 30–40% of hospital-acquired acute sialadenitis occurs postoperatively and is frequently associated with GI surgery (42).

2.7.2. Etiologic Pathogens

Aside from the less common pathogens such as Enterobacteriaceae, oral anaerobes, and other gram-negative bacilli, staphylococci have been the predominant isolates. The organisms most commonly associated with submandibular gland sialadenitis are the same penicillin-resistant *Staphylococcus aureus* (often methicillin resistant) and streptococci species associated with bacterial parotitis.

2.7.3. Clinical Manifestations and Diagnosis

Sialadenitis or infection of salivary glands is relatively common in the elderly and is primarily caused by ductal obstruction. Reduction in salivary flow either by dehydration, polypharmacy, and calculi (sialolithiasis) or by compromised condition of the normal flora could lead to stagnancy and, as a result, ductal obstruction. Most patients will present with a history of recurrent episodes. If the process is chronic, the gland will be palpably firm. Sialadenitis can lead to an acute onset of suppurative parotitis manifested systematically as high fever, chills, and pre- and postauricular swelling and tenderness. Depending on the acuteness and severity of the infection, patients may show varying degrees of leukocytosis and a shift to the left. Most cases undergo periodic acute exacerbations from a baseline of chronic diseases.

Differential diagnosis of sialadenitis should exclude sialolithiasis or a salivary gland tumor using radiographic study such as CT or MRI scan.

The exudates from the inflamed gland should be cultured prior to initiating antibiotic therapy.

2.7.4. Antibiotic Treatment

Patients with a history of only one or two acute episodes of sialadenitis are treated with an intense, 1-month course of culture-specific antibiotics, hydration, and sialagogues. Oral therapy includes amoxicillin/clavulanate (Augmentin), 875 mg twice daily, or dicloxacillin, 500 mg four times daily, for susceptible pathogens. Erythromycin or clindamycin is recommended for penicillin-allergic patients. In refractory cases the affected glands may be evaluated for surgical removal.

2.7.5. Prevention

In the elderly, the precipitating factor appears to be dominantly xerostomia or reduction of salivary flow due to multipharmacy. Hydration and sialagogue therapy are the major preventive measures.

REFERENCES

1. U.S. Department of Health and Human Services. Oral Health in America: A Report of the Surgeon General. Rockville, MD: U.S. Department of Health and Human Services,

National Institute of Dental and Craniofacial Research, National Institute of Health, 2000.

2. Vincent SD, Baker KA. Oral pathology in the aging patient. In: Dembo JB, ed. Surgical Care of the Elderly. Oral Maxillofac Surg Clin North Am. Philadelphia, PA: Saunders, 1996:215–233.

3. Haug RH. The changing microbiology of maxillofacial infections. In: Laskin DM, Strauss RA, eds. Current Concepts in the Management of Maxillofacial Infections. Oral Maxillofac Surg Clin North Am. 2003; 15:1–15.

4. Chow AW. Odontogenic infections. In: Johnson JT, Yu VL, eds. Infectious Diseases and Antimicrobial Therapy of the Ears, Nose, and Throat. Philadelphia, PA: Saunders, 1997:489–499.

5. Holm-Pederson P, Agerbaek N, Theilade E. Experimental gingivitis in young and elderly individuals. J Clin Periodontol 1975; 2:14–24.

6. Horning GM, Hatch CL, Cohen ME. Risk indicators for periodontitis in military treatment population. J Periodontol 1992; 63:297–302.

7. Genco R, Zambon J, Christersson L. The origin of periodontal infections. Adv Dent Res 1988; 2:245–259.

8. Machtei E, Dunford R, Grossi S, Genco R. Cumulative nature of periodontal attachment loss. J Periodontol Res 1994; 29:361–364.

9. Albandar JM, Brunelle JA, Kingman A. Destructive periodontal disease in adults 30 years of age and older in the United States, 1988–1994. J Periodontol 1999; 70:13–29.

10. Ardenkian L, Dobson TB. Complications associated with placement of dental implants. In: Laskin DM, Strauss RA, eds. Current Concepts in the Management of Maxillofacial Infections. Oral Maxillofac Surg Clin North Am. Philadelphia, PA: Saunders, 2003: 243–249.

11. Shou L. Oral health, oral health care, and oral health promotion among older adults. In: Cohen LK, Gift HC, eds. Disease Prevention and Oral Health Promotion: Socio-Dental Sciences in Action. Munksgaard, Denmark: Fe'de'ration Dentaire International, 1995:213–270.

12. Kinane DF. Causation and pathogenesis of periodontal disease. Periodontol 2000, 2001; 25:8–20.

13. Socransky SS, Haffajee AD. Evidence of bacterial etiology: a historical perspective. Periodontol 2000; 1994(5):7–25.

14. Slots J, Feik D, Rams TE. Actinobacillus, actinomycetemcomitans and bacteroides intermedius in human periodontitis—age relationship and mutual association. J Clin Periodontol 1990; 17:659–662.

15. Zambon JJ. Periodontal diseases: microbial factors. Ann Periodontol 1996; 1:879–925.

16. Shenkin JD, Baum BJ. Oral health and the role of the geriatrician. J Am Geriatr Soc 2001; 49:229–230.

17. Holmstrup P, Poulsen AH, Andersen L, Skuldbol T, Fiehn N-E. Oral infections and systemic diseases. Dent Clin North Am 2003; 47:575–598.

18. Beck J, Garcia R, Heiss G, Vokonas PS, Offenbacher S. Periodontal disease and cardiovascular disease. J Periodontol 1996; 67(suppl):1123–1137.

19. Grau AJ, Buggle F, Ziegler C, Schwartz W, Meuser J, Tasman AJ, Buhler A, Benesch C, Becher H, Hacke W. Association between acute cerebrovascular ischemia and chronic and recurrent infection. Stroke 1997; 28:1724–1729.

20. Scannapieco FA, Mylotte JM. Relationships between periodontal disease and bacterial pneumonia. J Periodontol 1996; 67(suppl):1114–1122.

21. Scannapieco FA, Papandonatos GD, Dunford RG. Associations between oral conditions and respiratory diseases in a national sample survey population. Ann Periodontol 1998; 3:252–256.

22. Flynn TR, Halpern LR. Antibiotic selection in head and neck infections. In: Laskin DM, Strauss RA, eds. Current Concepts in the Management of Maxillofacial Infections. Oral Maxillofac Surg Clin North Am. Philadelphia, PA: Saunders, 2003:17–38.

23. Horswell BB. Infections. In: Kwon PH, Laskin DM, eds. Clinician Manual of Oral and Maxillofacial Surgery. 2nd ed. Chicago: Quintessence, 1997:297–311.

24. Molinari JA. Diagnostic modalities for infectious diseases. Dent Clin North Am 2003:605–621.

25. Flynn TR, Wiltz M, Adamo AK, Levi M, McKitrick J, Freeman K, Trieger N. Predicting length of hospital stay and penicillin failure in severe odontogenic infections. Int J Oral Maxillofac Surg 1999; 28(suppl 1):48.

26. Nordenram G, Ljunggren G. Oral status, cognitive and functional capacity versus oral treatment in nursing home residents: a comparison between assessment by dental and ward staff. Oral Dis 2002; 8:296–302.

27. Samaranayake LP. Oral mycoses in HIV infection. Oral Surg Oral Med Oral Pathol 1992; 73:171–180.

28. King GN, Healy CM, Glover MT, Kwan JT, Williams DM, Leigh IM, Thornhill MH. Prevalence and risk factors associated with leukoplakia, hairy leukoplakia, erythematous candiadiasis, and gingival hyperplasia in renal transplant recipients. Oral Surg Oral Med Oral Pathol 1994; 78:718–726.

29. Silverman S, Miller CS. Diagnosis and treatment of viral infections. In: Laskin DM, Strauss RA, eds. Current Concepts in the Management of Maxillofacial Infections. Oral Maxillofac Surg Clin North Am. Philadelphia, PA: Saunders, 2003:79–89.

30. Langenberg AG, Ashley RL, Leong WP, Straus SE. A prospective study of new infections with herpes simpex virus type 1 and type 2. N Engl J Med 1999; 3412:1432–1438.

31. Higgins CR, Tatnall FM, Leigh IM. Natural history, management and complications of herpes labialis. J Med Virol 1993; 1:22–26.

32. Hayden FG. Antiviral drugs (other than antiretrovirals). In: Mandell GL, Bennett JE, Dolin R, eds. Principles and Practice of Infectious Diseases. 5th ed. Philadelphia, PA: Churchill Livingstone, 2000:460–491.

33. Whitley RJ, Lakeman F. Herpes simplex virus. Clin Infect Dis 1998; 26:541–555.

34. Spruance SL. Advances in the treatment of herpes simplex labialis. Antiviral Chem Chemother 1997; 8(suppl 1):69–74.

35. Spruance SL. Prophylactic chemotherapy with acyclovir for recurrent herpes simplex labialis. J Med Virol 1993; 41(suppl 1):27–32.

36. Strauss S, Ostrove JM, Inchaupe G, Felser JM, Freifeld A, Croen KD, Sawyer MH. Varicella-zoster virus infections: biology, natural history, treatment, and prevention. Ann Intern Med 1988; 108:221–237.

37. Markoulatos P, Siafakas N, Plakokefalos E, Tzanakaki G, Kourea-Kremastinou J. Laboratory diagnosis of common herpes virus infections of the central nervous system by a multiplex PCR assay. J Clin Microbiol 2001; 39:426–432.

38. Tyring S, Barbarash RA, Nahlik JE, Cunningham A, Marley J, Heng M, Jones T, Rea T, Boon R, Saltzman R. Famciclovir for the treatment of acute herpes zoster: effects on acute disease and post-herpetic neuralgia. A randomized, double-blind, placebo-controlled trial. Collaborative Famciclovir Herpes Zoster Study Group. Ann Intern Med 1995; 123:89–96.

39. Avin AM. Varicella-zoster virus. Clin Microbiol Rev 1996; 9:361–381.

40. Marley J. Antiviral therapy in herpes zoster: a review. Antiviral Chem Chemother 1997; 8(suppl 1):37–42.

41. Nathwani D. Treatment parameters for the successful management of varicella zoster virus. Antimicrob Agents Chemother 1995; 6(suppl 1):12–16.

42. Blitzer A, Lawson W, Reino A. In: Johnson JT, Yu VL, eds. Infectious Diseases and Antimicrobial Therapy of the Ears, Nose, and Throat. Philadelphia, PA: Saunders, 1997:489–499.

43. Seifert G, Miehlke A, Haubrich J, Chilla R. Sialoadenitis. In: Siefert G, Miehlke A, Haubrich J, Chilla R, eds. Diseases of the Salivary Glands. Pathology, Diagnosis, Treatment, Facial Nerve Surgery. New York: Thieme Medical Publisher, 1986:110–163.

SUGGESTED READING

Flynn TR, Halpern LR. Antibiotic selection in head and neck infections. Laskin DM, Strauss RA, eds. Current Concepts in the Management of Maxillofacial Infections. Oral Maxillofac Surg Clin North Am. Philadelphia, PA: Saunders, 2003:17–38.

Haug RH. The changing microbiology of maxillofacial infections. In: Laskin DM, Strauss RA, eds. Current Concepts in the Management of Maxillofacial Infections. Oral Maxillofac Surg Clin North Am. Philadelphia, PA: Saunders, 2003:1–15.

Holmstrup P, Poulsen AH, Andersen L, Skuldbol T, Fiehn N-E. Oral infections and systemic diseases. Dent Clin North Am 2003; 47:575–598.

Topazian RG, Goldberg MH, Hupp JR. Oral and Maxillofacial Infections. 4th ed. Philadelphia, PA: Saunders, 2002.

29
Sinus and Ear Infections in the Elderly

Lorraine M. Smith
Otolaryngology/Head and Neck Surgery, Charles R. Drew University of Medicine and Science, Los Angeles, California, U.S.A.

Ryan F. Osborne
Head and Neck Oncology, Cedars Sinai Medical Center, Otolaryngology/Head and Neck Surgery, Charles R. Drew University of Medicine and Science, Los Angeles, California, U.S.A.

Key Points:

- Infections of the sinus and ear occur less often in the elderly than in childhood, but the severity of these infections may be increased because of underlying comorbid illness (e.g., diabetes mellitus).
- Acute sinusitis is caused primarily by *Streptococcus pneumoniae*, *Haemophilus influenzae*, and *Moraxella catarrhalis*. However, in chronic sinusitis, anaerobic bacteria predominate with *Staphylococcus aureus* and streptococci occurring less often.
- A severe form of otitis externa called malignant external otitis, necrotizing otitis externa, and skull base osteomyelitis occurs especially in the elderly, diabetic, and immunocompromised, and is caused by *Pseudomonas aeruginosa*.
- Pseudomonas malignant external otitis is life threatening, requires early diagnosis and a multidisciplinary approach to treatment including antibiotics and, in some patients, surgical intervention.
- Elderly patients are predisposed to otitis media because of higher incidences of endotracheal or nasogastric intubation when hospitalized or institutionalized.

1. RHINOSINUSITIS

1.1. Epidemiology and Clinical Relevance

Rhinosinusitis is defined as any mucosal inflammation of the nasal cavity or the paranasal sinuses. The inflammation almost always results from stasis of secretions that provides a culture medium for secondary bacterial infections. Sinusitis represents the fifth most common health care problem for which an antibiotic is prescribed in the United States, and in 2002, $400 million to $600 million was spent on antibiotic prescriptions for sinusitis (1). In addition to the physical symptoms, sinusitis affects individuals functionally and emotionally and has accounted for more than 1 million work days lost annually (1). This is important given the increasing number of elderly still in the workforce and in the population. Despite the relatively high incidence of reported sinus infections in the elderly, little has been reported on the actual incidence or mechanisms of sinus infections in the geriatric population (2).

The sinus mucosa is a pseudostratified ciliated columnar epithelium. This epithelium is composed of columnar cell, basal cells, goblet cells, and submucosal seromucinous glands. The columnar cells have on average between 100 and 200 cilia/cell (3). This mucosa undergoes metaplasia with time. Over the age of 40 years ≈30% of people will undergo mucosal metaplasia (3), resulting in a decrease in the mucosal cilia count and a decline in goblet cell mucous production. As the mucociliary system becomes less functional, the mucosa becomes more susceptible to penetration by microorganisms resulting in cellular damage and inflammation. These events may play a major role in the development of sinusitis in the geriatric patient. Other predisposing factors include a history of gustatory rhinitis, allergic rhinitis, and viral infections, commonly an upper respiratory infection (URI).

1.2. Etiologic Pathogens

1.2.1. Acute Sinusitis

In general the normal nasal mucosa has a bacterial concentration of 10^3–10^6 bacteria/cc with a 5:1 ratio of anaerobes to aerobes (4,5). Despite the preponderance of anaerobes, cultures from antral punctures are overwhelmingly aerobic (Table 1). This is likely due to the extreme difficulty in successfully maintaining the microenvironment needed to grow anaerobes. The commonly identified organisms in acute sinusitis are similar to those in younger patients, i.e., *Streptococcus pneumoniae*, *Haemophilus influenzae*, and *Moraxella catarrhalis* accounting for approximately 75% of infections. Anaerobes account for 4% of acute sinus infections with *Bacteroides* being the most commonly isolated organism (6). The remainder of infections result from various strains of *Streptococcus* and viruses. Rarely, *Staphylococcus aureus* is cultured in acute sinusitis, but it can be quite virulent and should be considered in complicated cases.

1.2.2. Chronic Sinusitis

Poor mucociliary function combined with mechanical obstruction of sinus drainage is a common backdrop for chronic sinusitis. Microbes do not play a major role in these infections; however, the prevalence of anaerobes, gram-negative organisms, and *S. aureus* is notably higher than in acute sinusitis. These infections are typically polymicrobial with anaerobes accounting for more than 50% of the infections

Table 1 Common Pathogens Cultured in Acute Sinusitis and Acute Otitis Media

Pathogens	Sinusitis (%)	Otitis media (%)
Haemophilus influenzae	38	20–30
Streptococcus pneumoniae	37	30–40
Other *Haemophilus* species	8	—
Streptococcus pyogenes	6	—
Moraxella catarrhalis	5	10–15
Alpha-*Streptococcus*	3	—
Gram-negative bacilli/mixed anaerobes	3	—

Table 2 Common Pathogens Involved in Chronic Sinusitis

Aerobic	%	Anaerobic	%
Staphylococcus aureus	4	*Peptostreptococcus* species	22
Streptococcus		*Prevotella* species	15
Hemolytic	6	*Bacteroides* species	8
pyogenes (B-hemo)	3	*Propionibacterium* species	7
pneumoniae	2	*Fusobacterium*	5
Other	4		
Haemophilus species	4		
Moraxella catarrhalis	4		

(Table 2) (7). Also, the same organisms involved in acute sinusitis may be involved, though much less frequently.

1.3. Clinical Manifestations and Diagnosis

Sinusitis is clinically diagnosed based on a constellation of symptoms and physical findings. The early clinical manifestations of acute sinusitis may be difficult to distinguish from those of the common cold (2). Fever, cough, postnasal drainage, hyposmia, and nasal congestion are common to both diseases. Acute rhinosinusitis should be suspected if the symptoms persist for more than 5 days, and as the disease progresses facial pressure/pain and purulent nasal discharge predominate. The sinus involved determines the location of the facial pressure/pain. Periorbital pain usually corresponds to ethmoid involvement. Midface or dental pain is suggestive of maxillary sinusitis. Forehead and retro-orbital discomfort are usually produced by frontal and sphenoid sinusitis, respectively.

The manifestations of chronic sinusitis are similar to those of acute sinusitis with regard to nasal congestion, facial pressure/pain, and hyposmia/anosmia. There are fewer systemic symptoms and often clear rhinorrhea is noted instead of purulence. The duration of symptoms is prolonged (>3 months) and usually associated with physical findings of mechanical obstruction such as polyps, turbinate abnormalities, or septal deviation.

There may be no external physical findings unless there is an associated eye complication, such as orbital cellulitis or abscess. Percussion of the sinuses often elicits tenderness over the involved sinus. Nasal endoscopy may identify pale or erythematous mucosa. In acute sinusitis, purulence may be noted in the nasal cavity or on the posterior pharyngeal wall. No purulence is noted in chronic sinusitis as previously explained. In both processes, cobblestoning may be noted on the posterior pharyngeal wall.

Generally, nasal cultures correlate poorly with sinus cultures and are thus not recommended (8). Middle meatal cultures are notably more sensitive than nasal cultures. Sinus aspirations are required only in refractory cases or in immunocompromised hosts. The computed tomography (CT) scan is the best single-modality imaging method to evaluate the sinuses. Although not part of the standard evaluation for acute sinusitis, in recurrent, acute, chronic, or complicated cases the axial/coronal CT scan is heavily relied upon to assess the involvement of contiguous sinuses and perisinus spaces.

1.4. Antibiotic Treatment

The microbes involved in acute sinusitis are fairly predictable. In uncomplicated or mildly symptomatic cases amoxicillin (2–3 g/day remains the first-line choice for antibiotic therapy). Erythromycin, doxycycline, trimethoprim–sulfamethoxazole, or one of the other macrolides may be used for patients with penicillin allergies. However, up to 50% of *H. influenzae* strains and greater than 90% of *M. catarrhalis* strains are resistant to amoxicillin. In addition, there is an increasing number of amoxicillin-resistant pneumococcal strains that continue to escalate. Therefore, in patients who have acute sinusitis-related complications, subacute sinusitis, or underlying medical conditions which make a treatment failure risky, alternative initial treatment should be utilized.

Also, many geriatric patients have chronic illnesses such as diabetes mellitus, chronic obstructive pulmonary disease, and asthma, which may alter the immune status. These conditions can be severely exacerbated by a suboptimally treated sinus infection. In these cases broader coverage is desired such as with amoxicillin/ clavulanate (Augmentin), the second-generation cephalosporins, or respiratory quinolones (Table 3). Antibiotic therapy should be continued for at least 10–14 days. If no clinical improvement is noted after 2–3 days of therapy, an alternate antibiotic should be considered. High-dose amoxicillin (6 g/day) or amoxicillin/clavulanate is currently being used for recalcitrant or subacute sinusitis in younger patients; however, there have been no reports of use in the geriatric population. The doses of amoxicillin and amoxicillin/clavulanate have to be modified in patients with renal insufficiency and monitored for toxicity for patients on methotrexate. Decongestants—oral and/or nasal—along with saline nasal irrigations may help to decrease nasal congestion, promote sinus drainage and mucociliary flow. The role of antihistamines in acute sinusitis remains controversial.

The role of antibiotic therapy is limited in patients with chronic sinusitis because it often occurs secondary to an anatomic obstruction. Initial therapy usually involves the use of a nasal corticosteroid and/or a topical/systemic decongestant to decrease the inflammatory response and ostial obstruction. The antibiotic treatment of chronic sinusitis should therefore be culture and sensitivity directed. A longer duration of antibiotic therapy is usually required, often >21 days. With the majority of microbes being anaerobic, clindamycin or amoxicillin/clavunate is recommended as a first-line therapy. When *S. aureus* is identified clindamycin is the preferred

Table 3 Recommended Antibiotics for Acute Sinusitis

Primary	Alternatives
Amoxicillin	Amoxicillin with clavulanate
Erythromycin plus trimethoprim– sulfamethoxazole or doxycycline	Levofloxacin
	Gatifloxacin
	Moxifloxacin
	Cefpodoxime
	Cefdinir
	Cefuroxime
	Cefditoren

Note: Primary = mild symptoms or no prior treatment. Alternatives, moderate-severe symptoms or previously treated.

Table 4 Recommended Antimicrobials for Chronic Sinusitis

Primary	Alternatives
Amoxicillin with clavulanate	Metronidazole plus
	A respiratory quinolone, or a
	second-generation cephalosporin or
	second-generation equivalent
	Respiratory quinolones
	Levofloxacin
	Gatifloxacin
	Moxifloxacin
	Second-generation/equivalent cephalosporins
	Cefpodoxime, Cefdinir, Cefuroxime,
	Cefditoren
If Staphylococci: clindamycin	Amoxicillin–clavulanate, cephalexin plus
	metronidazole
If fungi: itraconazole	Voriconazole
If *Pseudomonas aeruginosa*:	IV/irrigation/nebulized
Ciprofloxacin oral, IV	Ceftazidime
Levofloxacin oral, IV	Gentamicin, tobramycin, amikacin

Abbreviation: IV, intravenous.

treatment provided the organism is susceptible. Definitive management of chronic sinusitis often requires surgical intervention (endoscopic sinus surgery) to address the underlying problem. The overall surgical outcomes are similar to those in younger patients, although the elderly are likely to have a few more minor complications and a delay in healing.

Chronic sinusitis may at times result from mycotic infections. Contemporary antifungals such as itraconazole and voriconazole are very affective against aspergillosis including invasive fungal sinusitis (see the following). They can also be administered orally or intravenously (Table 4).

1.5. Prevention

Preventive measures are usually considered in patients with a history of recurrent acute or chronic sinusitis. In these patients saline nasal irrigations as well as nasal corticosteroids are helpful in minimizing the frequency of infections. Nasal decongestants both topical and systemic, and mucolytics have been advocated to assist with resolution of symptoms of the common cold and minimize conversion of a simple upper respiratory tract infection into a frank sinus infection. In addition, avoidance of known antagonists to normal mucociliary function such as chemical fumes, dry climates, and cigarette smoke exposure can assist in preventing the development of sinusitis.

1.6. The Immunocompromised Host and Sinusitis

Many geriatric patients may have compromised immune responses. The etiologies vary widely: diabetes, acquired immunodeficiency syndrome (AIDS), chronic renal disease, immunosuppressive therapy status post organ transplant, poor nutritional states, or chemotherapeutic agents for various malignancies. These patients are at increased risk of developing fungal sinusitis. The most common fungal infection encountered results from the genus *Aspergillus*. The most common species are

Table 5 Common Fungal Pathogens

Aspergillus fumigatus	*Alternaria*
A. flavus	*Candida*
A. niger	*Cryptococcus*
Mucor	*Histoplasma*
Rhizopus	*Blastomyces*
	Coccidioides

Aspergillus fumigatus, *Aspergillus flavus*, and *Aspergillus niger*. Other genera of important pathogenic mycotic organisms are *Mucor*, *Rhizopus*, and *Alternaria* (see Table 5) (9,10). The two most virulent and often rapidly fatal infections are invasive aspergillosis and mucormycosis.

These organisms are highly destructive, causing rapid widespread tissue necrosis that often spreads rapidly to involve the eye and/or brain. Their ability to invade tissue is similar to a high-grade malignancy, hence early suspicion and diagnosis are the key to decreasing the high morbidity and mortality associated with these infections. On physical examination, these patients may have normal, pale, or black mucosa of the nose that may spread to involve the hard palate. Areas of concern should be biopsied to confirm the diagnosis. Biopsy of the middle turbinate is recommended if no obvious necrotic tissue is noted and there is a high index of suspicion. A CT scan of the paranasal sinuses is critical here for early identification of the involved sinus. Bony erosion of the sinus walls, opacification of the nose and or sinus, soft tissue involvement of the perisinus tissues may also be noted.

The treatment for these infections is largely surgical with early wide and aggressive resection of all necrotic tissue followed by early intravenous (IV) antifungal therapy, control of the underlying systemic derangement, and at times hyperbaric oxygen therapy. Since 1955, IV amphotericin B has been the mainstay of treatment, and it remains so in the treatment of mucormycosis in doses of 1–1.5 mg/kg/day (9,10). Although it is still used for invasive aspergillosis, other agents with more acceptable risk profiles and comparable efficacy such as voriconazole and itraconazole have come also into wide practice, along with the liposomal forms of amphotericin B.

2. OTITIS EXTERNA

2.1. Clinical Relevance

Otitis externa (OE) represents an inflammatory process of the external auditory canal (EAC). It may be characterized as acute otitis externa, chronic otitis externa, and fungal otitis externa. The external auditory canal is usually lined by squamous epithelium and contains ceruminous glands that provide a natural lipid layer and an acid environment. Normal EAC bacteria include the nonpathogenic bacteria *Staphylococcus epidermidis* and *Staphylococcus capitis*, as well as *Mycobacterium* (11,12). In the geriatric patient, there is a decrease in the ceruminous glands that leads to a decrease in the lipid layer, with scant and dry cerumen as the outcome. This often leads to pruritus and subsequent digital manipulation with the use of cotton-tipped applicators, fingernails, hairpins, etc. This repetititve instrumentation often leads to a break in the integrity of the skin that allows bacteria to penetrate and grow, especially if there is a warm, humid milieu.

Pseudomonas aeruginosa, Proteus mirabilis, Peptostreptococcus spp., and *S. aureus* are the most common bacteria isolated during culture of the EAC (13–15). Fungal OE occurs in approximately 10% of cases of OE (14,16). *Aspergillus* and *Candida* species are the most common fungal organisms identified. OE also occurs in patients with chronic skin diseases including acne and seborrheic dermatitis. It is more prevalent in the summer months, warm tropical environments, and among those who swim frequently.

2.2. Clinical Manifestations and Diagnosis

Pruritus continues as a major symptom of acute and chronic OE with varying degrees of otorrhea and/or otalgia more commonly found in the acute OE. Aural fullness and hearing loss may also occur; however, systemic symptoms are very uncommon. On physical examination, in acute OE there may be auricular tenderness, edema, and/or erythema of the EAC with a scant to thick, white to green exudate which may obscure the view of the tympanic membrane (TM). In comparison, the discharge is tan-white (*Candida*) or gray (*A. fumigatus*) to black (*A. niger*) with fluffy, hyphal elements if the etiology is fungal (10). In chronic OE, there is no purulence and no edema of the canal. The discharge is often dry and flaky and there is usually a normal TM.

A culture is not initially necessary, unless the infection is not responding to initial therapy since *Pseudomonas aeruginosa* and *S. aureus* are the etiologic agents in >90% of the cases. Roland et al. noted that the incidence of *Pseudomonas* cultured has varied from 12% to 80% and the incidence of *Staphylococcus* has been reported as low as 8.5–29% (12). Involvement of the auricle (perichondritis) or soft tissue of the face (cellulitis) or the presence of granulation tissue in the canal may necessitate a CT scan. Any manipulation of the EAC should be done under direct visualization usually under a microscope after suctioning.

2.2.1. Antibiotic Treatment

OE responds to dry ear precautions, no further aural manipulations, and the administration of otic drops with analgesics as needed. If the EAC is full of discharge or markedly edematous these patients should be seen in the office of an otolaryngologist as soon as possible for debridement and/or wick placement to allow the otic drops to reach the minimum inhibitory concentrations of the antibiotic in the skin of the ear canal. Oral antibiotics are not necessary and may contribute to increasing resistances if used widely.

Otic agents currently on the market for acute bacterial OE are used to acidify the canal or eradicate the *Pseudomonas* organisms. In the presence of an intact TM, they include those containing 2% buffered acetic acid (e.g., Domeboro), the aminoglycoside ophthalmic solutions (e.g., tobramycin 0.3%—Tobrex) and the neomycin–polymyxin B-hydrocortisone solutions/suspensions which may be used three to four times per day for 7–10 days (15). Van Balen et al. have suggested that the corticosteroid/antibiotic or the corticosteroid/acidifying drop combination are equally effective compared with the acidifying drops alone (17). If the integrity of the TM is unknown, suspensions should be used, or the newer otic/ophthalmic quinolone preparations (e.g., ofloxacin 0.3%—Floxin/Oculoflox, ciprofloxacin 0.3%—Cipro HC/Ciloxan) which have no ototoxic effects and have shown similar efficacy.

These newer agents are active against gram-positive and gram-negative organisms, are instilled less frequently (10 drops twice a day for 10–14 days), have no known drug interactions, and therefore have a better compliance (8).

Failure to respond to the above therapy, the presence of systemic symptoms at presentation, immunocompromised status, or an associated middle ear infection, cellulitis or perichondritis may necessitate the use of oral antibiotics (10,14,15). The oral quinolones, ofloxacin or levofloxacin, are used though any other antipseudomonal antibiotic is likely to be effective. If the acute OE is not adequately treated especially in those immunocompromised, necrotizing OE or skull base osteomyelitis may occur.

For otomycosis, the following ototopic agents may be used three to four times per day for 1 week: 2% buffered acetic acid (e.g., Domeboro), clotrimazole 1%—Lotrimin, thimerosal-merthiolate, M-cresyl acetate-cresylate are effective. Tolnaftate 1% solution (Tinactin) may be used when the TM is perforated (10,14,15). Topical corticosteroid ointments and creams (hydrocortisone 1%) and dandruff shampoos are commonly used for chronic OE and those associated with dermatologic conditions. If the acute OE is not adequately treated especially in those immunocompromised, necrotizing OE or skull base osteomyelitis (SBO) may occur.

3. SKULL BASE OSTEOMYELITIS

3.1. Epidemiological and Clinical Relevance

In 1968, Chandler described "malignant external otitis" as a virulent, invasive infection of the EAC that was responsible for multiple cranial nerve palsies, meningitis, and death. The disease affects the skin, cartilage, and in severe cases the temporal bone and often was associated with a poor outcome, i.e., high mortality (8,13,18). Recently, this spectrum of disease also known as necrotizing otitis externa (NOE) has been more clearly described as a SBO. SBO is a spectrum of diseases initially described and now commonly found in the elderly, and immunocompromised patients (diabetic, human immunodeficiency virus infection, chemotherapy, etc.) (9,13,14). The small vessel disease characteristic of diabetes mellitus and aging results in vascular damage with poor perfusion and oxygenation with devitalized tissue that increases the susceptibility to the infection (18,19).

3.2. Etiologic Pathogen

P. aeruginosa remains the most common causative organism in >98% of cases although *Mucor* may also cause this infection. *Pseudomonas* is a known obligate gram-negative aerobic bacillus that prefers a warm humid environs and has a propensity to invade soft tissue and bone through the secretion of enzymes (10,20). Other organisms noted include *S. aureus*, *Proteus mirabilis*, and *Klebsiella oxytoca*.

3.3. Clinical Manifestations and Diagnosis

Patients present with a history of OE or a chronic draining ear with pain out of proportion to clinical findings. They may also present with facial paralysis, hearing loss, hoarseness, and/or dysphagia as the inflammatory process involves the periauricular tissue and cranial nerves V–XII. Characteristically, one also finds granulation tissue on otoscopic examination in the floor of the canal at the bony-cartilaginous junction. Rarely, altered mental status may be noted when the infection has spread to the intracranial cavity. This may result in meningitis or an otogenic abscess each with significant morbidity and mortality. Usually there are no other systemic symptoms.

A high index of suspicion is necessary to make this diagnosis with early involvement of an otolaryngologist. Blood analysis often reveals a normal white blood cell (WBC) count with an altered differential. The erythrocyte sedimentation rate (ESR) is often elevated and can be used to monitor the infection and response to antibiotics. Radiologically, CT and magnetic resonance imaging (MRI) scans have been used in addition to gallium-67 (Ga-67), bone and single photon emission computed tomography (SPECT) scans (19). The CT scan of the temporal bone with contrast is used to determine bony erosion and extension into the petrous apex; this may be negative early in the disease process. An MRI scan with gadolinium is useful to determine soft tissue (periauricular and parotid) and bone marrow involvement. Absorption of Ga-67 directly into granulocytes and bacteria allows for early detection and monitoring of the disease as it reverts to normal once the acute infectious process is controlled. This is often complemented by a technetium-99 bone scan which is absorbed at the sites of osteoblastic activity but remains persistently positive. The performance of the combined Ga-67–SPECT scan has increased sensitivity over the gallium scan alone. Biopsy of the granulation tissue is necessary to exclude aural malignancies (squamous cell carcinoma or metastatic carcinomas), which may also present as a chronic draining ear.

3.4. Antibiotic Treatment

The key to managing SBO lies in treating the underlying disorder and often a multidisciplinary physician approach to the care of the patient is needed. Dry ear precautions, frequent surgical aural debridement, use of otic drops, and 4–6 weeks of IV antipseudomonal antibiotics are needed. Culture and sensitivity results from aural cultures and/or debrided tissue may be used with individualized appropriate antibiotic therapy after the first few days. Most *P. aeruginosa* strains respond to tobramycin and amikacin; however, 10–15% of *Pseudomonas* strains are resistant to gentamicin (10,15). Hence, the aminoglycosides are combined with the antipseudomonal penicillins (e.g., ticarcillin or piperacillin), third-generation cephalosporins, and other β-lactam agents (e.g., imepenem) which may have a synergistic effect.

The broad-spectrum IV quinolones, levofloxacin and ciprofloxacin, are now the drugs-of-choice for SBO. These agents may be used in patients with penicillin allergies, are very efficacious, have few side effects, and no associated ototoxicity, unlike the aminoglycosides. Additionally, they have had a low level of resistance, which is increasing (20). The fluoroquinolones are effective against *P. aeruginosa*, *H. influenzae*, and *M. catarrhalis*. Levofloxacin is also effective against penicillin-resistant and sensitive strains of *S. pneumoniae* (10). With the development of the fluoroquinolones and earlier suspicions with diagnosis by primary care physicians, many otherwise healthy patients may now be treated as an outpatients. Oral ciprofloxacin, and now levofloxacin, may be used for early cases of SBO in an outpatient setting or more commonly in the convalescent stage once the acute infectious process has resolved (10). Surgical debridement often is necessary to remove granulation tissue or other necrotic areas in the temporal bone or periauricular soft tissue. Antibiotic therapy is usually continued for 4–6 weeks or until resolution of disease is noted on the gallium scan. The need for topical quinolone drops has been questioned. The authors recommend use of any of the otic drops described in acute otitis externa. Once symptoms have resolved or the gallium scan has reverted to negative, IV therapy may be switched to oral quinolones for two more weeks of therapy.

4. OTITIS MEDIA

4.1. Epidemiology and Clinical Relevance

Otitis media (OM) represent an inflammation of the middle ear space. Although, OM remains rather common among children there is a decreased incidence as one ages, leading to few cases in the elderly. The microbiologic profile and antibiotic therapy are similar to those of acute sinusitis since these spaces are linked via the eustachian tube. No studies have documented the prevalence of acute or serous otitis media or the change in the function of the eustachian tube that occurs with aging. However, brainstem-stroke patients and those who are hospitalized/institutionalized with endotracheal or nasogastric tubes are predisposed to OM because of modifications of the eustachian airway as a result of neurologic or mechanical obstruction.

4.2. Etiologic Pathogens, Clinical Manifestations, and Diagnosis

Patients may present with otalgia, aural fullness, and occasionally otorrhea because of TM perforation. On physical examination, the EAC is normal. The TM is bulging and erythematous with the middle ear structures obscured in acute OM. The TM is normal in color, and may be in a neutral or retracted position with clear honey-colored fluid in the middle ear. The presence of altered mental status, facial or sixth nerve palsy represents a complication of OM, mastoiditis, intracranial abscess, or acute petrositis. Predisposing factors also include withholding antimicrobials in the treatment of OM, use of suboptimal therapy, or shortened periods of antibiotic use (15). *S. pneumoniae* is the most significant pathogen associated with complications of OM (10). Institutionalized patients may be difficult to diagnose because they cannot communicate the pain, aural fullness, or hearing loss that is characteristic. A rising ESR and WBC count that cannot otherwise be explained should prompt further examination of the ears and/or sinuses. Pneumatic otoscopy and/or tympanometry are also useful adjuncts in the diagnosis. The CT scan of the temporal bone may also be useful in institutionalized patients, and in the presence of any complication of otitis media.

4.3. Antibiotic Treatment

The treatment of acute OM is similar to that of acute sinusitis with amoxicillin as the first-line therapeutic agent. Erythromycin or another macrolide may be used in patients with penicillin allergies. Amoxicillin/clavulanate, second-generation cephalosporins, or ceftriaxone may be used as second-line therapies. Otitis media with effusion does not usually require antibiotic therapy but should prompt a nasopharyngeal examination to examine the eustachian tube orifice and exclude the presence of a nasopharyngeal mass especially if unilateral. In the presence of a complication of otitis, treatment includes surgical intervention (insertion of a ventilation tube and/or debridement) combined with IV antibiotics (vancomycin and a third-generation cephalosporin) that cross the blood–brain barrier. The incidence of these complications has decreased with antibiotic therapy.

5. LABYRINTHITIS

Suppurative labyrinthitis is now rare, but may be suspected in a patient with antecedent OM who acutely develops severe vertigo and a profound hearing loss. The most common form is viral labyrinthitis, which is usually preceded by an URI. Nausea, vomiting, nystagmus, past-pointing, and falling toward the opposite side may occur. The diagnosis is mainly clinical but may be aided by evidence of enhancement of the semicircular canals on an MRI scan with gadolinium. Treatment is symptomatic in viral labyrinthitis. High-dose corticosteroids, antiviral agents, and vestibular suppressants such as meclizine are the mainstays of therapy. Antibiotic therapy (intravenously) is necessary if suppurative labyrinthitis is suspected.

6. CONCLUSION

While no studies have elucidated the prevalence or etiology of sinus and ear infections in the elderly, these infections continue to occur and are more likely to be seen by physicians given the increasing elderly population. Rhinosinusitis and chronic otitis externa occur more commonly than the other infections mentioned; yet the uncommon invasive fungal sinusitis and skull base osteomyelitis have devastating morbidities and mortalities. The development of antibiotics has in general led to a decrease in the prevalence, morbidity, and mortality associated with these complications. A complete head and neck examination along with a high level of suspicion is required especially in the care of the institutionalized and/or immunocompromised geriatric patient. These diagnoses may often be confirmed with a CT scan. Early and judicious use of antibiotic therapy along with other adjunctive therapies mentioned is often curative.

REFERENCES

1. Sinus and Allergy Health Partnership. Otolaryngol Head Neck Surg 2004; 130:S1–S45.
2. Knutson JW, Slavin RG. Sinusitis in the aged: optimal management strategies. Drugs Aging 1995; 7:310–316.
3. Boysen M. The surface structure of human nasal mucosa: I. Ciliated and metaplastic epithelium in normal individuals. A correlated study by scanning transmission electron and light microscopy. Virchows Arch B Cell Pathol 1982; 40:279.
4. Gorbach SL, Bartlett JG, Tally FP. Biology of anaerobes. Kalamazoo, MI: Upjohn Company, 1981.
5. Gwaltney JM, Sydnor A, Sande MA. Etiology and antimicrobial treatment of acute sinusitis in adults. Ann Otol Rhinol Laryngol 1981; 90:68–71.
6. Frederich J, Braude AI. Anaerobic infection of the paranasal sinuses. N Engl J Med 1974; 290:135.
7. Gwaltney JM, Scheld WM, Sande MA, Sydnor A. The microbial etiology and antimicrobial therapy of adults with acute community acquired sinusitis: a 15-year experience at the University of Virginia and review of selected studies. J Allergy Clin Immunol 1992; 90:457–461.

8.   Chandler JR, Langer DJ, Stevens JR. The pathogenesis of orbital complications in acute sinusitis. Laryngoscope 1970; 80:1414–1428.

9.   Calvet H, Yoshikawa TT. Infections in diabetics. Infect Dis Clin North Am 2001; 15(2):407–411.

10. Fairbanks D. Pocket Guide to Antimicrobial Therapy on Otolaryngology—Head and Neck Surgery 10th ed. American Academy of Otolaryngology—Head and Neck Surgery Foundation Inc, 2001.

11. Cassisi N, Cohn A, Davidson T. Diffuse otitis externa: clinical and microbiologic findings in the course of a multicenter study on a new otic solution. Ann Otol Rhinol Laryngol 1977; 86(suppl 39):1–16.

12. Roland PS, Stroman DW. Microbiology of acute otitis externa. Laryngoscope 2002; 112(7 Pt 1):1166–1177.

13. Balkany T, Ress B. Infections of the external ear. In: Cummings C, Frederickson J, Harker L, eds. Otolaryngology Head and Neck Surgery. 3rd ed. St. Louis, MO: Mosby-Yearbook Inc, 1998:2979–2986.

14. Sander R. Otitis externa: a practical guide to treatment and prevention. Am Fam Physician 2001; 63(5):941–942.

15. Smith L, Osborne R. Infections of the head and neck. Top Emerg Med 2003; 25: 106–116.

16. Dibb WL. Microbial etiology of otititis externa. J Infect Dis 1991; 22:233–239.

17. van Balen FA, Smith WM, Zuithoff NP, Verheij TJ. Clinical efficacy of three common treatments in acute otitis externa in primary care: randomised controlled trial. Br Med J 2003; 327(7425):1201–1205.

18. Lucente FE, Parisier SC, Chandler JR. Malignant external otitis. (Laryngoscope 1968; 78:1257–1294.) Laryngoscope 1996; 106(7):805–807.

19. Rubin Grandis J. The changing face of malignant (necrotising) external otitis: clinical, radiological, and anatomic correlations. Lancet Infect Dis 2004; 4(1):34–39.

20. Berenholz L, Katzenell U, Harell M. Evolving resistant pseudomonas to ciprofloxacin in malignant otitis externa. Laryngoscope 2002; 112(9):1619–1622.

SUGGESTED READING

Knutson JW, Slavin RG. Sinusitis in the aged: optimal management strategies. Drugs Aging 1995; 7:310–316.

Lucente FE, Parisier SC, Chandler JR. Malignant external otitis. (Laryngoscope 1968; 78: 1257–1294.) Laryngoscope 1996; 106(7):805–807.

Pichichero ME. Acute otitis media: part II. Treatment in an era of increasing antibiotic resistance. Am Fam Physician 2000; 61(8):2410–2416.

Pinheiro A, Facer G, Kern E. Rhinosinusitis: current concepts and management. In: Bailey B, ed. Neck Surgery—Otolaryngology. 3rd. Philadelphia, PA: Lippincott, Williams and Wilkins, 2001:345–358.

30
Pneumonia

Mutsuo Yamaya and Hidetada Sasaki
*Department of Geriatric and Respiratory Medicine, Tohoku University
School of Medicine, Sendai, Japan*

Key Points:

- Pneumonia is the fifth leading cause of death in the elderly.
- Silent aspiration associated with impaired coughing and swallowing reflexes is the most important pathogenetic mechanism for causing pneumonia in the elderly.
- Clinical manifestations of pneumonia in older patients may be atypical with fever, cough and sputum production being minimal or absent.
- Microbial causes of pneumonia in the elderly will vary depending on whether it is community, hospital or nursing home acquired. Antibiotic therapy should be pathogen specific whenever possible.
- Preventive interventions are the most important method of reducing the mortality and morbidity associated with pneumonia.

1. INTRODUCTION

Pneumonia is a leading cause of infectious disease in the United States, including community-acquired pneumonia (CAP) and hospital-acquired pneumonia (HAP). Despite the availability of adequate antimicrobial agents to treat pneumonia, pneumonia in the elderly is currently the fifth most common cause of death. Whereas the death rate from pneumonia in younger adults has declined substantially, pneumonia mortality of older adults has remained very high over the past 100 years. The majority of deaths due to pneumonia are in people aged ≥65 years (1). Moreover, the risk of HAP increases with age and with the length of hospital stay. Risk factors for the development of pneumonia in older adults can be broadly classified into factors that alter host defenses and factors that increase exposure to bacteria. Silent aspiration of oropharyngeal secretions is an important risk factor of pneumonia in the elderly. Therefore, pharmacological agents to prevent aspiration pneumonia as well as antibiotics are recommended for the management of pneumonia in older patients. Here, we review the pathogenesis and management for pneumonia in geriatric patients, including risk factors, clinical manifestations and diagnostic procedures, microbial causes, choice of antibiotics, and pharmacokinetics and pharmacodynamics of antibiotics. We also describe a new strategy to prevent and treat pneumonia in older people.

2. RISK FACTORS FOR PNEUMONIA IN OLDER PEOPLE

Risk factors for the development of pneumonia in older people can be broadly classified into factors that alter host defenses and factors that increase exposure to bacteria. Aspiration of oropharyngeal secretions that are colonized by pathogenic bacteria and/or regurgitated gastric contents is one of the common causes of CAP. Several studies indicate that 5% of cases of CAP are aspiration pneumonia (2,3). The incidence of aspiration pneumonia increases to 18% in nursing home-acquired pneumonia (NHAP) (2). Aspiration pneumonia with Mendelson's syndrome or the acute aspiration of gastric content is called chemical pneumonitis and is less common. Aspiration pneumonia is also used to describe the bacterial infection of the lung that results from aspiration of bacteria contained in oropharyngeal or gastric secretions. Such silent aspiration frequently occurs and is a more important cause of pneumonia than acute aspiration of gastric content in older people (2). The lack of specific and sensitive markers of aspiration complicates the epidemiologic study of aspiration pneumonia. A witnessed aspiration event was defined as a history of choking after emesis or eating. An unwitnessed aspiration event was defined as the development of at least one of the following within 24 hr of a witnessed episode of emesis, coughing while eating, or the presence of vomitus on a pillow or clothing: a new infiltrate on chest radiograph, a chest radiograph with an infiltrate consistent with aspiration (lower lobe infiltrate), new tachypnea (respiratory rate >18 breaths/min), new fever ($\geq 37.8°C$), or a change in mental status not explained by another cause (3). However, when the term aspiration pneumonia is used, it refers to the development of a pneumonia in the setting of patients with risk factors for increased oropharyngeal aspiration (4). Kikuchi et al. (5) evaluated the occurrence of silent aspiration in otherwise healthy elderly patients with CAP and age-matched control subjects using[111]indium chloride scanning. Silent aspiration was demonstrated in 71% of patients with CAP compared with 10% in control subjects during a single examination night. Approximately half of all healthy adults aspirate small amounts of oropharyngeal secretions during sleep. The incidence of silent aspiration was increased to 94% in patients in nursing homes (6). If the mechanical, humoral, or cellular host defense mechanisms are impaired, or if the aspirated innoculum is large enough, pneumonia may follow. A large number of cases of aspiration pneumonia in the elderly are CAP; however, only 5% of CAP has been attributed to aspiration pneumonia. The latter low incidence may be related to varying definitions of aspiration pneumonia and/or the infrequent direct witnessing of aspiration or its associated symptoms (emesis, coughing while eating).

3. CLINICAL MANIFESTATIONS AND DIAGNOSTIC PROCEDURES OF PNEUMONIA IN OLDER PEOPLE

Cough, sputum, chills, and pleural pain are less frequent in NHAP than in CAP. In contrast, in older patients, altered mental status including delirium is more often reported in NHAP than in CAP. Fever is frequently absent in older patients with pneumonia (7). In contrast, tachypnea (respiratory rate >20/min) and tachycardia (>100/min) were seen in two-thirds of older patients with pneumonia (7).

Plain chest radiographs are important for confirming the clinical suspicion of pneumonia in older patients with pneumonia. Computed tomography scans are helpful when diagnosing aspiration pneumonia occurring in the posterior portion of the lower lobe or airway obstruction by a proximal tumor. Leukocytosis and an increase in band forms develop less frequently in older people and are thus less sensitive in the detection of pneumonia. In contrast, C-reactive protein (CRP) is highly sensitive for the detection of pneumonia in older patients (7). To initiate pathogen-directed therapy, bacterial isolation from sputum is desirable. However, older patients are often too weak to provide an adequate sputum specimen, and the diagnostic yield of sputum is relatively low (7). Bronchoscopy appears to be well tolerated even in older patients.

Bronchoscopy is recommended when pneumonia responds poorly to treatment, or in immunocompromised patients, and may facilitate a diagnosis of unsuspected mycobacterial disease or unusual organisms (7). A search for urinary *Streptococcus pneumoniae* capsular antigen is useful in the diagnosis of pneumococcal pneumonia. Blood cultures and urinary legionella antigen tests are recommended in older patients with CAP and NHAP (7). A fourfold or greater rise of paired sera for respiratory viral causes should be obtained during the influenza season. *Legionella pneumophila* infection should be considered with a fourfold rise in titers to 1:128 or higher, or a single titer of 1:256 or higher with legionella immunofluorescent antibody tests. *Mycoplasma pneumoniae* infection may be the etiology in the presence of a fourfold rise in titers to 1:64 or higher, or a single titer of 1:256 or higher, in the mycoplasma-specific IgG immunofluorescent antibody test. For a diagnosis of *Chlamydia pneumoniae* infection there should be a fourfold rise in titers to 1:16 or higher, or a single titer of 1:128 or higher, in complement-fixing tests. For most of these serological tests, a fourfold rise or drop in antibody titers is also considered a positive response (7,8). All blood culture isolates, with the exception of *Staphylococcus epidermidis* and *Corynebacterium* species, should be considered to be etiologic agents of CAP.

4. MICROBIAL CAUSES OF PNEUMONIA IN OLDER PEOPLE

Despite extensive investigations, the diagnosis of the bacterial cause of CAP is made in no more than 50% of CAP overall, and this is particularly so in the elderly. The elderly have increased oropharyngeal colonization with pathogens such as *S. pneumoniae, Haemophilus influenzae, Staphylococcus aureus*, and aerobic gram-negative bacilli including *Klebsiella pneumoniae* and *Escherichia coli*. Among them *S. pneumoniae* remains the single most common implicated pathogen isolated from older patients with CAP and NHAP. Oropharyngeal colonization with these pathogens with subsequent aspiration presumably accounts for the greater prevalence of these pathogens in elderly patients with CAP. The most frequent pathogens in severe CAP in a critical care setting were *S. pneumoniae* (45%), *H. influenzae*, and gram-negative bacilli (4,7,8). These bacteria and *S. aureus* are also more frequently isolated in patients with mild to moderate HAP (4). *S. pneumoniae, H. influenzae, S. aureus*, or gram-negative bacilli should be considered to be the cause of the pneumonia if it is isolated in pure culture from expectorated sputum and if morphologic correlates of the bacterium predominated on the Gram stain. *S. aureus*, particularly species resistant to methicillin (MRSA), are increasingly recognized in the nursing home population (8). There is an increased likelihood of infection with resistant gram-negative organisms, including *Pseudomonas aeruginosa, Enterobacter* spp., and *Acinetobacter* spp., in patients with HAP after a prolonged hospital stay or after the use of antibiotics (4). The frequency of gram-negative bacteria pneumonia also increases in nursing home patients and in patients with decreased functional status. Isolation of the anaerobes including *Prevotella* and *Fusobacterium* species increases in elderly patients with pneumonia with aspiration (4,7).

5. CHOICE OF ANTIBIOTICS FOR PNEUMONIA IN OLDER PEOPLE

Table 1 shows the common pathogens and pathogen-directed antimicrobial therapy for pneumonia in older people (8). When the etiologic agent is established or strongly suspected, pathogen-directed therapy is recommended. In this therapy, antibiotics are decided according to the microbial pathogens. In contrast, in the absence of an etiologic diagnosis, empirical antibiotic therapy is initiated. The selection of antibiotics is based on many factors, including severity of the illness, the patient's age, antimicrobial intolerance or side effects, clinical features, and concomitant medications (8). In general, the empirical antimicrobial agents preferred for most patients, in no special order, are a macrolide, doxycycline, or a fluoroquinolone (8). The initial empirical therapeutic strategy for severe CAP is recommended to be high-dose ampicillin and erythromycin intravenously (2,7). Because there are no specific clinical studies on the use of antibiotics in HAP in older people, recommendations for management of HAP in older people are similar to those for HAP in younger adults (7).

In pathogen-directed therapy, preferred antibiotics are penicillin G and amoxicillin for penicillin-susceptible *S. pneumoniae* (8) (Table 1). Older people have a high incidence of multidrug-resistant *S. pneumoniae* infection (≈20%). Therefore, another alternative in the initial management of severe CAP with *S. pneumoniae*, β-lactamase-producing *H. influenzae*, and atypical pathogens could be the use of high-dose third-generation cephalosporins plus a macrolide agent (2). Use of cefotaxime and ceftriaxone, fluoroquinolone, and vancomycin are also recommended for penicillin-resistant *S. pneumoniae* based on in vitro susceptibility test (8). Cephalosporin (second or third generation), doxycycline, β-lactam/β-lactamase inhibitor, or azithromycin are used for the treatment of *H. influenzae*. For the treatment of methicillin-susceptible *S. aureus* (MSSA), nafcillin and oxacillin with or without the combination of rifampin or gentamicin are recommended (8). Vancomycin is recommended for the treatment of methicillin-resistant *S. aureus* (MRSA) (8). For the treatment of aerobic gram-negative bacilli including *K. pneumoniae* and *E. coli*, the use of third-generation cephalosporins with or without aminoglycoside, or a carbapenem are recommended (4,8). Furthermore, in severe hospital-acquired pneumonia, highly resistant gram-negative organisms including *P. aeruginosa* and *Acinetobacter* are likely to be involved (4). The antimicrobial agents recommended for the treatment of *P. aeruginosa* are an aminoglycoside plus antipseudomonal β-lactam (4,8) or an antipseudomonal β-lactam plus antipseudomonal quinolone (4). For the treatment of *M. pneumoniae* and *Chlamydia pneumoniae*, use of doxycycline and macrolide is recommended (8). For the anaerobes including *Prevotella* and *Fusobacterium* species isolated in elderly patients with aspiration pneumonia (4,8), use of β-lactam/β-lactamase inhibitor and clindamycin is recommended (8) (Table 1).

6. CHANGES IN PHARMACOKINETICS AND PHARMACODYNAMICS OF ANTIBIOTICS WITH AGING

Decline of renal function is a major contributor to drug toxicity in older people. The most important renal function to monitor with aging is the creatinine clearance. Due to the age-dependent decline of renal function, the pharmacokinetics of many drugs is altered in older adults (9). The therapeutic/toxic ratio of β-lactam compounds is much higher than that of aminoglycosides (9). Because aminoglycosides and vancomycin are more nephrotoxic agents, dosage intervals are recommended to be

Table 1 Common Pathogens and Pathogen-Directed Antimicrobial Therapy for Pneumonia in Older Adults

Organisms	Preferred antimicrobial agent	Alternative antimicrobial agent
Streptococcus pneumoniae		
Penicillin susceptible	Penicillin G, amoxicillin	Cephalosporins, imipenem or meropenem,
Penicillin resistant	Cefotaxime and ceftriaxone, fluoroquinolone, vancomycin	macrolides clindamycin, fluoroquinolone, deoxycycline
H. influenzae	Cephalosporin (second or third generation), doxycycline	Fluoroquinolone, clarithromycin
	β-lactam/β-lactamase inhibitor, azithromycin	
Anaerobe	β-lactam/β-lactamase inhibitor, clindamycin	Imipenem
Staphylococcus aureus		
Methicillin susceptible	Nafcillin/oxacillin ± rifampin or gentamicin	Cefazolin or cefuroxime, vancomycin, clindamycin
Methicillin resistant	Vancomycin ± rifampin or gentamicin	Quinapristin + dalfopristin, linezolid
Enterobacteriaceae[a]	Cephalosporin (third generation) + aminoglycoside, carbapenem	Aztreonam, β-lactam/β-lactamase inhibitor, fluoroquinolone
Pseudomonas aeruginosa	Aminoglycoside + antipseudomonal β-lactam	Aminoglycoside + ciprofloxacin, ciprofloxacin + antipseudomonal β-lactam
Legionella	Marcolide + rifampin, fluoroquinolone	Doxycycline ± rifampin
Mycoplasma pneumoniae	Doxycycline, macrolide	Fluoroquinolone
Chlamydia pneumoniae	Doxycycline, macrolide	Fluoroquinolone

[a]*E. coli, Klebsiella, Proteus,* and *Enterobacter.*

increased in the elderly with reduced renal function (9). However, the major route of elimination of macrolide antibiotics is the liver. Nevertheless, the pharmacokinetics of macrolides is also modified in elderly patients. Furthermore, reduction of orally administered doses of ciprofloxacin is proposed in older patients, because the bioavailability of ciprofloxacin increases after oral doses through facilitated absorption and/or reduced elimination. Thus, older adults have altered pharmacokinetics of antibiotics, including a difference in absorption, distribution, and elimination compared with healthy younger adults. Therapeutic drug monitoring may be needed more frequently (9).

7. PHARMACOLOGICAL TREATMENT OF PNEUMONIA OTHER THAN ANTIBIOTICS IN OLDER PEOPLE

The oral cavity, the skin, and the intestinal tract are the major reservoir and sites for bacteria, and miscellaneous microorganisms are normally swallowed without any consequences. Older people are less likely to cough these microorganisms from the respiratory tract because their coughing reflex is diminished. Coughing may also be associated with an abnormal swallowing reflex. The pathophysiology in the deterioration of both swallowing and cough reflexes is a decrease of substance P, which is created in the cervical ganglion of the sensory branches of the vagus or pharyngeal nerves (1). The reduction of substance P occurs when the production of dopamine by the nigrostriata deteriorates as a result of cerebral vascular diseases in the deep cortex (1). Because the amount of dopamine is decreased in patients with cerebral infarction, amantadine, which promotes dopamine synthesis, was administered for 3 years to a group of patients with cerebral infarction. The incidence of pneumonia was reduced to one-fifth of that of the control group (1).

An angiotensin-converting enzyme (ACE) inhibitor inhibits an enzyme to metabolize substance P. By administering an ACE inhibitor, the small amount of substance P in the pharynx or trachea will remain there and not be metabolized. The concentration of substance P increases with time, and this will, in turn, return the swallowing/coughing reflex to normal. With an ACE inhibitor, the side effect of coughing is three times more likely to happen in women than in men. When the ACE inhibitor imidapril was administered for 2 years, the incidence of pneumonia was reduced to one-third, compared with a group to which no imidapril was administered (1). The high risk factor of silent aspiration for CAP is confirmed by the fact that interventions to prevent silent aspiration decrease the incidence of CAP in older people.

While treating pneumonia with antibiotics in older people, recurrent or continued silent aspiration prolongs pneumonia and may lead to superinfection with resistant pathogens. Kanda et al. (10) studied the combination treatment of amantadine and/or ACE inhibitors with antibiotics for patients aged $\geq$65 years, who had a previous history of stroke and were admitted with CAP. The patients in the intervention group had a significantly shorter duration of using antibiotics (approximately half), and hospitalization (approximately two-thirds), and lower medical costs (approximately two-thirds), than their counterparts. Infections with MRSA and hospital deaths were significantly lower in the intervention group compared with the control group (Table 2). Reducing the duration of antimicrobial treatment by these pharmacological treatments is a potentially important strategy for preventing antimicrobial resistance.

In patients with stroke, the prevalence of swallowing dysfunction ranges from 40% to 70% (1). Nakagawa et al. (6) showed that the risk of pneumonia was

Table 2 Characteristics of Patients

Characteristics	Control group (n = 35)	Intervention group (n = 33)	p-value
Age, mean + SD	78 ± 8	78 + 7	0.83[a]
Sex, male/female	7/28	10/24	0.53[a]
Barthel index, mean ± SD	34 ± 15	35 ± 16	0.70[b]
Duration (days) of antibiotics, mean ± SD	39 ± 22	17 ± 12	<0.01[a]
Duration (days) of hospitalization use, mean ± SD	51 ± 36	37 ± 22	0.04[a]
Medical cost (US$/person), mean ± SD	15,114 ± 1,086	10,766 + 6,148	<0.05[a]
Infection of MRSA, n	16	4	<0.01[b]
Hospital death, n	15	5	0.03[b]

[a] Unpaired *t*-test.
[b] Chi-square test.

significantly higher in patients with basal ganglia infarcts than in patients with cerebral hemispheric strokes in other locations or without cerebral hemispheric strokes. At age ≥65 years, approximately half of older adults may have silent cerebrovascular accidents (CVA). In most cases, it lies in a deep cortex. Thirty percent of those who had a silent CVA in a deep cortex suffer from pneumonia for over 2 years (11). Therefore, the clinical problems of CVA and associated pneumonia are not restricted to only nursing home residents, the very frail, or those who are dying.

Preventing CVA may reduce the incidence of pneumonia among old people. A drug that appears to decrease the incidence of CVAs or cerebral infarction is cilostazol. It has an antithrombocyte action and an action of cerebral vasodilation. When cilostazol was administered for 3 years, it was possible to reduce the incidence of cerebral infarction by one-half, compared with a group that did not receive the drug. In addition, the incidence of pneumonia was also reduced by half (12) (Fig. 1).

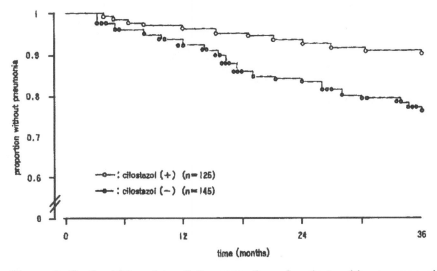

Figure 1 Kaplan-Meier plots of the proportion of patients without pneumonia using cliostazol (o) and not using cliostazol (•).

8. PREVENTION OF PNEUMONIA IN OLDER PEOPLE

There are a number of factors that increase risk of pneumonia in older people, which may also reduce the effectiveness of pneumonia. Homocystinuria gives rise to myocardial infarction and arteriosclerosis among small children. In the case of old people who have slight homocystinuria, the higher the value of homocysteine, the more likely a cerebral infarction (13). A high value of homocysteine among old people is, in part, due to genetic polymorphism. Those who have an inadequate intake of vitamin B12 and folic acid are prone to arteriosclerosis because the metabolism of homocysteine deteriorates. Folic acid is present in vegetables, and fish are rich in vitamin B12. Thus, vegetables and fish are important in the diet and potentially reduce the incidence of CVAs and hence, secondary pneumonia. Folate deficiency is common among the elderly, especially those who are institutionalized. High levels of homocysteine suggest that the levels of vitamin B12 or folic acid are low. Low levels of vitamin B12 or folic acid also suggest impaired dopamine metabolism in the central nervous system and may adversely impact brain function. Supplementing vitamin B12 or folic acid to older patients may improve their swallowing reflex and perhaps reduce the occurrence of pneumonia. A substance called capsaicin is thought to strongly promote the release of substance P. When capsaicin, the main substance of cayenne pepper and red peppers, is placed in the mouth, the swallowing reflex instantaneously improves (1). Oral health status has a positive influence on nutritional health status. Taking care of the oral cavity or giving mechanical stimulus to the gums gives rise to substance P, which, in turn, improves the swallowing reflex (14) (Fig. 2). A 2-year study was conducted with a group of older adults who preferred oral care and another group that did not. The incidence of pneumonia was reduced to 40% in the oral care group. Furthermore, particularly noteworthy is the fact that the study group consisted of older people living in a nursing home and once they developed pneumonia, 80% died of the disease regardless of therapy. However, when the oral cavity care and hygiene were provided, the rate of mortality from pneumonia was reduced by 50% compared with the nonoral care patients. Thus, good oral cavity care is effective in reducing mortality from pneumonia in older people (15).

Gastroesophageal reflux occurs in critically ill patients even in the absence of nasogastric tubes and enteral feedings; up to 30% of patients who are kept in a supine position are estimated to have gastroesophageal reflux. When gastric juice is aspirated, pneumonia becomes more serious. Older people who sit for ≈2 hr after a meal minimize gastroesophageal reflux, resulting in the reduction of the number of febrile days due to respiratory infection to one-third (16). In patients with swallowing dysfunction, a soft diet should be introduced, and the patients should be taught compensatory feeding strategies (e.g., reducing the bite size, keeping the chin tucked and the head turned while eating, and swallowing repeatedly).

Approximately half of all healthy elderly aspirate a small amount of oropharyngeal secretions during sleep (2,3). The swallowing reflex is normally not reduced during sleep at night. However, in those with a CVA in the cerebral basal nucleus the swallowing reflex sharply decreases during the day. When these people sleep at night, they do not cough at all. Their sleep was observed for 2 weeks. It was found that they slept unexpectedly well for 9.5 hr a day. They slept for 6 hr at night and as long as 3.5 hr during the day. However, patients asked for a sleeping pill because they felt they were not able to sleep at night. While taking a benzodiazepine sedative, their swallowing reflex did not decrease, but when taking

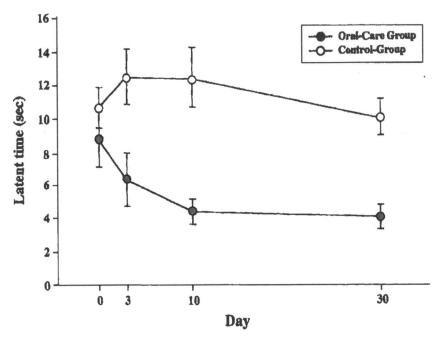

Figure 2 Daily oral care group (•) was associated with a significant decrease in latency time of the swallowing reflex at 3, 10, and 30 days compared with the control group (○) ($p < 0.001$).

neuroleptics, which are dopamine inhibitors, their swallowing reflex clearly was reduced. Those who were administered a psychotropic drug were threefold more prone to pneumonia (17). Effective intervention in sleep patterns using daytime physical activity, improvement in the night-time environment and nonpharmacologic sleep protocol provides an alternative to sedative–hypnotic drug use to promote sleep in older hospitalized patients.

Vaccines against influenza and pneumococcal diseases are effective means of preventing illness and death from both diseases. In 1999, 67% and 54% of older persons reported receiving influenza and pneumococcal vaccines, respectively. These rates are in contrast to the Healthy People 2010 goals for both immunization of 90% each among older people (18). Annual influenza vaccinations for all older adults aged ≥65 years are recommended (19). Pneumococcal vaccine should be administered to those aged ≥65 years.

9. CONCLUSION

Pneumonia in older people comes not only from a discrete infection to the lung but also from accumulated impairments in multiple systems, and develops when the accumulated effects of these impairments in multiple domains compromise compensatory mechanisms. Pneumonia in older people should be managed as a geriatric syndrome with adequate antimicrobial agents and pharmacological agents to prevent silent aspiration.

REFERENCES

1. Mylotte JM, Goodnough S, Naughton BJ. Pneumonia versus aspiration pneumonitis in nursing home residents: diagnosis and management. J Am Geriatr Soc 2003; 51:17–23.
2. American Thoracic Society. Hospital-acquired pneumonia in adults: diagnosis, assessment of severity, initial antimicrobial therapy, and preventive strategies. Am J Respir Crit Care Med 1996; 153:1711–1725.
3. Kikuchi R, Watanabe N, Konno T, Mishina N, Sekizawa K, Sasaki H. High incidence of silent aspiration in elderly patients with community-acquired pneumonia. Am J Respir Crit Care Med 1994; 150:251–253.
4. Nakagawa T, Sekizawa K, Arai H, Kikuchi R, Manabe K, Sasaki H. High incidence of pneumonia in elderly patients with basal ganglia infarction. Arch Intern Med 1997; 157:321–324.
5. Bartlett JG, Dowell SF, Mandell LA, File TM Jr, Musher DM, Fine MJ. Practice guidelines for the management of community-acquired pneumonia in adults. Clin Infect Dis 2000; 31:347–382.
6. Meyers BR, Wilkinson P. Clinical pharmacokinetics of antibacterial drugs in the elderly. Implications for selection and dosage. Clin Pharmacokinet 1989; 17:385–395.
7. Kanda A, Ebihara S, Yasuda H, Sasaki T, Sasaki H. A combinatorial therapy for pneumonia in elderly people. J Am Geriatr Soc 2004; 52:846–847.
8. Nakagawa T, Sekizawa K, Nakajo K, Tanji H, Arai H, Sasaki H. Silent cerebral infraction: a potential risk for pneumonia in the elderly. J Intern Med 2000; 247:255–259.
9. Yamaya M, Yanai M, Ohrui T, Arai H, Sekizawa K, Sasaki H. Anthithrombotic therapy for prevention of pneumonia. J Am Geriatr Soc 2001; 49:687–688.
10. Matsui T, Arai H, Yuzuriha T, Yano H, Miura M, Hashimoto S, Higuchi S, Matsushita S, Morikawa M, Kato A, Sasaki H. Elevated plasma homocysteine levels and risk of silent brain infarction in elderly people. Stroke 2001; 32:1116–1119.
11. Yoshino A, Ebihara T, Ebihara S, Fujii H, Sasaki H. Daily oral care and risk factors for pneumonia among elderly nursing home patients. J Am Med Assoc 2001; 286:2235–2236.
12. Yoneyama T, Yoshida M, Ohrui T, Mukaiyama H, Okamoto H, Hoshiba K, Ihara S, Yanagisawa S, Ariumi S, Morita T, Mizuno Y, Ohsawa T, Akagawa Y, Hashimoto K, Sasaki H. Oral care reduces pneumonia in older patients in nursing homes. J Am Geriatr Soc 2002; 50:430–433.
13. Matsui T, Yamaya M, Ohrui T, Arai H, Sasaki H. Sitting position to prevent aspiration in bed-bound patients. Gerontology 2002; 48:194–195.
14. Wada H, Nakajo K, Satoh-Nakagawa T, Suzuki T, Ohrui T, Arai H, Sasaki H. Risk factors of aspiration pneumonia in Alzheimer's disease patients. Gerontology 2001; 47: 271–276.
15. Santibanez TA, Nowalk MP, Zimmerman RK, Jewell IK, Bardella IJ, Wilson SA, Terry MA. Knowledge and beliefs about influenza, pneumococal disease, and immunizations among older people. J Am Geriatr Soc 2002; 50:1711–1716.
16. Fukushima T, Nakayama K, Monma M, Sekizawa K, Sasaki H. Benefits of influenza vaccination for bedridden patients. Arch Intern Med 1999; 159:1258.

SUGGESTED READING

Janssens JP, Krause KH. Pneumonia in the very old. Lancet Infect Dis 2004; 4:112–124.
Marik PE. Aspiration pneumonitis and aspiration pneumonia. N Eng J Med 2001; 344: 665–671.
Yamaya M, Yanai M, Ohrui T, Arai H, Sasaki H. Interventions to prevent pneumonia among older adults. J Am Geriatr Soc 2001; 49:85–90.

31
Tuberculosis

Shobita Rajagopalan
Department of Internal Medicine, Division of Infectious Diseases, Charles R. Drew University of Medicine and Science, Martin Luther King, Jr.–Charles R. Drew Medical Center, Los Angeles, California, U.S.A.

Key Points:

- Tuberculosis (TB) is a significant infectious disease in the elderly resulting in increased morbidity and mortality.
- Age-related decline in adaptive immune responses in addition to underlying comorbid illnesses (diabetes, cancer, immunosuppression) may enhance susceptibility to TB.
- Frail older persons may not exhibit the classical symptoms and signs of TB, i.e., fever, night sweats, weight loss, cough, and hemoptysis. TB must be treated as the "great masquerader" and considered in the differential diagnosis of unexplained malaise, anorexia, and low-grade fevers and nonspecific clinical manifestations of illness.
- Screening for TB, utilizing the two-step tuberculin skin testing, is routinely recommended in the initial assessment of elderly patients admitted to long-term care facilities (the utility of the QuantiFERON test as an alternative for latent TB diagnosis in this setting needs to be further evaluated). Increased efficiency of transmission of TB between elderly residents of such facilities has been reported.
- Diagnosis and management of TB in the geriatric population is similar to younger patients; close monitoring for adverse reactions to drug therapy is important particularly in patients taking multiple medications.

1. BACKGROUND AND EPIDEMIOLOGY

Tuberculosis (TB) continues to pose a significant global challenge to healthcare in the 21st century accounting for approximately 2 million deaths and 8 million infections each year (1). Complex social structures, overcrowding and homelessness, international migration, emergence of multidrug-resistant (MDR) strains of *Mycobacterium tuberculosis* (*Mtb*), the human immunodeficiency virus (HIV) acquired immunodeficiency syndrome (AIDS) epidemic, and the public health infrastructure burden for TB control have contributed to this difficult dilemma. Between 1993 and 2003, the overall trend in TB incidence in the United States has fortunately declined by 45% from the peak (2). However, foreign-born persons from high-burden countries for TB continue to contribute to the disproportionate and relative rise in TB cases in the

435

United States (3). Globally, it has been projected that between 2002 and 2020, ≈100 million new TB infections (TB infection or latent TB refers to infection with the tubercle bacillus which has been contained by the host immune response without overt clinical manifestations of illness), more than 150 million cases of TB disease (TB disease refers to symptomatic TB associated with clinical illness), and 36 million TB deaths will occur if TB control is not significantly enhanced (4).

Individuals aged 65 years and older constitute a large repository of *Mtb* infection in the United States. TB case rates are relatively higher for this age group across both genders and all races compared with younger age groups; likely risk factors include biological (compromised nutrition and immune status, underlying disease, medications, and possible racial susceptibility to *Mtb*) and socioeconomic factors (poverty, living conditions, and access to health care) (5). Although in 1987 the geriatric population represented ≈12% of the U.S. population, 6150 TB cases were reported in persons 65 years of age and older, accounting for 27% of the total U.S. TB morbidity (6). Centers for Disease Control and Prevention (CDC) surveillance data indicate that similar to younger age groups, 84% of older TB patients have pulmonary disease. Because more than half of these patients have sputum smears positive for acid-fast bacilli, they are potentially capable of transmitting the infection to other persons (7). In addition, based on data from CDC's National Center for Health Statistics, ≈5% of all elderly persons live in nursing homes (8). The potential efficiency for the transmission of TB in elderly residents of nursing homes is likely to be significantly higher than for the community-dwelling elders (9). In 1984–1985, a CDC-sponsored study of 15,379 routinely reported TB cases from 29 states indicated that the incidence of TB among nursing home residents was 39.2 cases per 100,000 persons. In comparison, the incidence of TB in community-dwelling elderly was 21.5 cases per 100,000 persons (7).

It is thus clearly important that clinicians caring for the elderly maintain a high index of suspicion for TB in this vulnerable age group. Many older individuals who are frail and debilitated may not present with classical symptoms and signs of TB disease and may manifest low-grade fevers, anorexia, weight loss, and unexplained weakness. The control and prevention of TB among the elderly must be strongly addressed to achieve the Institute of Medicine's goal of eliminating TB in the United States by 2010 (4). This chapter will further review the pathogenesis and immunologic aspects, unique clinical characteristics, and the current diagnosis and management of TB as it pertains to the aging population. The pharmacotherapy of TB will be reviewed in detail elsewhere in this chapter.

2. PATHOGENESIS AND IMMUNOLOGIC ASPECTS

TB is an airborne, highly communicable disease transmitted primarily via droplet nuclei that are expelled by coughing or sneezing from an actively infected individual (10,11). Infectious particles containing a relatively low inoculum of one to three viable tubercle bacilli are able to reach the alveolar spaces by inhalation. An estimated 5–200 inhaled bacilli are needed to initiate TB infection. Nonspecifically activated macrophages ingest the tubercle bacilli and transport them to the regional lymph nodes (most often hilar and mediastinal). The bacilli multiply or are inhibited or destroyed, based on the organisms' virulence and the macrophages' intrinsic killing ability. Infected macrophages release chemotactic factors such as complement component C5a, which attract additional macrophages and circulating monocytes to the infected area; monocytes transform into macrophages at the tissue level. Macrophages containing multiplying bacilli may die, releasing more bacilli and cellular debris that also attract monocytes. The balance between microbial virulence and host defense results in macrophages, still not specifically activated, that harbor multiplying organisms. Consequently, the number of organisms increases steadily. Monocytes continue to migrate to the site of infection during this stage. After about 3 weeks, the onset of cell-mediated immunity (CMI) and delayed-type hypersensitivity (DTH) responses set in resulting in a positive dermal reactivity to standard-dose tuberculin. Lymphokine-activated alveolar macrophages have an enhanced ability to destroy intracellular tubercle bacilli. The characteristic tubercle granuloma, or the Ghon complex, is formed consisting of organized collections of epithelioid cells, lymphocytes, and capillaries; caseous necrosis may result with eventual healing. Reactivation of a dormant focus occurs as a result of hydrolytic enzymes that liquefy the caseum, enabling the released bacilli to multiply freely in the extracellular environment, with cavity formation due to continued DTH responses. Tubercle bacilli then disseminate via the blood stream to distant sites. The tubercle bacilli can remain at a steady state of dormancy indefinitely as long as the host immune integrity remains intact. About 10% of infected persons may develop TB disease at some time in their lives, but the risk is considerably higher in persons who are immunosuppressed, especially those with HIV infection, those who use illicit drugs, or persons who are aging. Other factors, e.g., poor nutrition, homelessness, imprisonment, or alcoholism, also increase susceptibility to TB disease.

Although it is likely that the increased frequency of TB in the elderly could partly be due to CMI that is impaired by senescence, other concomitant age-related diseases (diabetes mellitus, malignancy), chronic kidney disease, malnutrition, and immunosuppressive agents may also contribute to this increase. In the elderly, ≈90% of TB disease cases are due to reactivation of primary infection (5). Persistent infection without disease may result in 30–50% of persons. Some elderly persons previously infected with *Mtb* may eventually eliminate the viable tubercle bacilli and revert to a negative tuberculin reactor state. These individuals are thus at risk for new infection (reinfection) with *Mtb*. Older persons can therefore develop disease in three possible ways: as primary TB disease, as persistent and latent primary infection that may reactivate, or as a new infection or reinfection.

3. UNIQUE CLINICAL CHARACTERISTICS

A major concern with TB disease in the elderly is the ability to recognize or diagnose the disease. TB disease in the elderly may not exhibit the classic features of TB, i.e., cough, bloody sputum, fever, chills, night sweats, and weight loss. Clinical presentations in this population may include loss of appetite, chronic malaise, cognitive impairment, unexplained prolonged low-grade fever, or changes in functional capacity (e.g., activities of daily living).

3.1. Pulmonary TB

The majority of older patients (75%) with *Mtb* infection manifest active disease in their lungs (12). Because of the propensity for minimal pulmonary symptoms associated with aging, a high index of suspicion for TB disease in the presence of unexplained constitutional symptoms, as mentioned in the previous paragraph, should be maintained. The chest radiographic characteristics of pulmonary TB in the elderly are discussed in the diagnosis section of this chapter.

3.2. Miliary TB

As seen with other forms of disseminated TB, miliary TB in the elderly is relatively common and occasionally an autopsy finding (5,13). One form of miliary TB seen in the elderly consists of repeated episodes of low-grade *Mtb* bacteremia and a protracted illness, associated with fever without localizing symptoms or signs, and with radiographic evidence of miliary mottling. A nonreactive form of miliary TB has also been described in older and immunosuppressed patients; this is an overwhelming tuberculous infection consisting of numerous small caseous lesions with large numbers of replicating bacilli, minimal neutrophilic infiltrate, and little or no granulomatous reaction. Clinical presentation includes fever, weight loss, and hepatosplenomegaly; older patients may occasionally present as a "fever of unknown origin."

3.3. Tuberculous Meningitis

Aging adults may develop TB meningitis due to reactivation of a latent primary focus or from miliary seeding of the meninges in primary, disseminated TB (14). This form of TB is associated with significant mortality and severe neurological sequelae in survivors. Elderly persons may present with unexplained encephalopathy and dementia, or as in younger individuals with this form of TB, with fever, headache, altered sensorium, and weakness.

3.4. Bone and Joint TB

Bone and joint TB most commonly involves the thoracic and lumbar spines (15,16). Paravertebral (cold) abscesses are classically described with spinal infection. TB of the spine is a common extrapulmonary form of this disease in the elderly, particularly in the United States and Europe. Presenting manifestations consist of pain over the involved spine, fever, weight loss, and constitutional symptoms and, in advanced cases, neurological deficits or sinus tract formation. Involvement of larger weight-bearing joints such as the hips may occur with TB infection. Older persons can sometimes present with *Mtb* involvement of other peripheral joints such as the knees, ankles, wrists, and metatarsophalangeal joints. Involvement of these smaller joints may be overlooked due to preexisting and concomitant degenerative joint disease in these patients.

3.5. Genitourinary TB

This relatively common form of TB in older adults may involve any part of the genitourinary (GU) tract (17). The kidney is one of the major sites of involvement in GU TB. Although localizing symptoms such as flank pain, dysuria, or hematuria may occur, $\approx$20–33% of patients remain asymptomatic. Sterile (no bacteria) pyuria has been described. Genital structures may be involved with scrotal or pelvic masses or draining sinuses and, occasionally, the absence of symptoms.

3.6. TB at Other Sites

Extrapulmonary TB at any age can involve virtually any organ in the body and must be kept in the differential of unexplained febrile illnesses and is hence referred to as "the great masquerader." Infection of lymph nodes, pleura, pericardium, peritoneum, gall bladder, small and large bowel, the middle ear, and carpal tunnel have been described.

4. DIAGNOSIS

TB in the elderly is commonly overlooked. A high index of suspicion for this fully treatable infectious disease is crucial for the diagnosis and management of these patients.

4.1. Tuberculin Skin Testing

The Mantoux method of tuberculin skin testing using the purified protein derivative (PPD) antigen still remains one of the diagnostic modalities of choice for TB infection, despite its potential for false-negative results (18). In the elderly, because of the increase in anergy to dermal antigens, the two-step tuberculin test is suggested as part of the initial geriatric assessment to avoid overlooking potentially false-negative reactions (19). The American Geriatrics Society routinely recommends two-step tuberculin testing as part of the baseline evaluation of all institutionalized elderly. The two-step tuberculin skin test involves initial intradermal placement of five tuberculin units of PPD, and the results are read at 48–72 hr. Patients are retested within 2 weeks after a negative response (induration of less than 10 mm). A positive "booster effect," and therefore a positive tuberculin skin test reaction, is a skin test of 10 mm or more and an increase of 6 mm or more over the first skin test reaction. The booster phenomenon must be differentiated from a true tuberculin conversion. The booster effect occurs in a person previously infected with *Mtb* but who has a false-negative skin test; repeat skin test elicits a truly positive test. Conversion occurs in persons previously uninfected with *Mtb* and who had a true negative tuberculin skin test but who become infected within 2 years as demonstrated by a repeat skin test induration that is positive and 10 mm or more during this period. Several factors influence the results and interpretation of the PPD skin test. Decreased skin test reactivity is associated with waning DTH with time, disseminated TB, other chronic and debilitating diseases such as cancer, immunosuppressive drug therapy, as well as the elimination of TB infection. False-positive PPD results occur with cross-reactions with nontuberculous mycobacteria and in persons receiving the Bacillus Calmette–Guerin (BCG) vaccine; the latter has an unpredictable effect on the PPD skin test reactivity and is presumed to wane after 10 years. The utility of anergy testing has been debated because of lack of a standardized protocol for selection of the number and type of antigens to be used, the criteria for defining positive and negative reactions, and administration and interpretation techniques (20).

Table 1 outlines the revised criteria for positive tuberculin skin test reactivity by size of induration necessitating drug treatment (21).

Table 1 Skin Test Criteria for Positive Tuberculin Reaction (mm Induration)

≥5 mm
  HIV-positive persons
  Recent contacts of person(s) with infectious tuberculosis
  Persons with chest radiographs consistent with tuberculosis (e.g., fibrotic changes)
  Patients with organ transplants and other immunosuppressed hosts receiving the
    equivalent of >15 mg/day prednisone for >1 month
≥10 mm
  Recent arrivals (<5 years) from high-prevalence countries
  Injection drug users
  Residents and employees of high-risk congregate settings: prisons, jails, nursing homes,
    other health care facilities, residential facilities for AIDS patients, and homeless shelters
  Mycobacteriology laboratory personnel
  High-risk clinical conditions: silicosis; gastrectomy; jejunoileal bypass; ≥10% below ideal
    body weight; chronic renal failure; diabetes mellitus; hematological malignancies
    (e.g., lymphomas, leukemias); other specific malignancies (carcinoma of the head or
    neck, and lung) (alcoholics are also considered high risk)
≥15 mm
  Persons with no risk factors for TB

Note: Chemoprophylaxis is recommended for all high-risk persons regardless of age.
Persons otherwise low-risk tested at entry into employment; ≥15 mm induration is positive.
Abbreviations: HIV, human immunodeficiency virus; AIDS, acquired immunodeficiency syndrome.
Source: Adapted from Ref. 21.

4.2. QuantiFERON-TB Testing

In 2001, the QuantiFERON-TB test was approved by the Food and Drug Administration (FDA) to aid in the detection of latent TB infection. This in vitro test measures
by an enzyme-linked immunosorbent assay (ELISA) the concentration of interferon-
gamma (IFN-γ) released from tuberculin PPD-sensitized lymphocytes in heparinized
whole blood incubated for 16–24 hr. Interpretation of QFT results is stratified by
estimated risk for *Mtb* infection in a manner similar to the tuberculin skin test testing
using different induration cutoff values as shown in Tables 2 and 3 (22). The role
for QFT in targeted testing has not yet been clearly defined and may be a useful
alternative to tuberculin skin testing in the future.

4.3. Chest Radiography

Chest radiography is indicated in all individuals with suspected TB infection, regardless of the primary site of infection. In the elderly, 75% of all TB disease occurs in the
respiratory tract and largely represents reactivation disease; 10–20% of cases may be
as a result of primary infection (23). Although reactivation TB disease typically
involves the apical and posterior segments of the upper lung lobes, studies have
shown that many elderly patients manifest their pulmonary infection variably in
either the middle or lower lobes or the pleura, as well as present with interstitial,
patchy, or cavitary infiltrates that may be bilateral. Primary TB can involve any lung
segment but more often tends to involve the middle or lower lobes as well as
mediastinal or hilar lymph nodes. Thus, radiographic diagnosis of pulmonary TB
in the elderly must be made with caution because of the atypical location of the
infection in the lung fields.

Table 2 Interim Recommendations for Applying and Interpreting QFT-TB

Reason for testing	Population	Initial screening	Positive results	Evaluation
Tuberculosis (TB suspect)	Persons with symptoms of active TB	Tuberculin skin testing (TST) might be useful; QFT not recommended	Induration ≥5 mm	Chest radiograph, smears, and cultures, regardless of test results
Increased risk of progression to active TB, if infected	Persons with recent contact with TB, changes on chest radiograph consistent with prior TB, organ transplants, or human immunodeficiency virus infection, and those receiving immunosuppressing drugs equivalent of ≥15 mg/day of prednisone for ≥1 month[a]	TST; QFT not recommended	Induration ≥5 mm	Chest radiograph if TST is positive; treat for latent TB infection (LTBI) after active TB disease is ruled out
	Persons with diabetes, silicosis, chronic renal failure, leukemia, lymphoma, carcinoma of the head, neck, or lung, and persons with weight loss of ≥10% of ideal body weight, gastrectomy, or jejunoileal bypass[a]	TST; QFT not recommended	Induration ≥10 mm	

(Continued)

Table 2 Interim Recommendations for Applying and Interpreting QFT-TB (*Continued*)

Reason for testing	Population	Initial screening	Positive results	Evaluation
Increased risk for LTBI	Recent immigrants, injection-drug users, and residents and employees of high-risk congregate settings (e.g., prisons, jails, homeless shelters, and certain health-care facilities)[a,b]	TST or QFT	Induration ≥10 mm; percentage tuberculin response ≥15%	Chest radiograph if either test is positive; confirmatory TST is optional if QFT is positive; treat for LTBI after active TB disease is ruled out; LTBI treatment when only QFT is positive should be based on clinical judgment and estimated risk
Other reasons for testing among persons at low risk for LTBI	Military personnel, hospital staff, and health-care workers whose risk of prior exposure to TB patients is low, and U.S.-born students at certain colleges and universities	TST or QFT	Induration ≥15 mm; percentage tuberculin response ≥30%	Chest radiograph if either test is positive; confirmatory TST if QFT is positive; treatment for LTBI (if QFT and TST are positive and after active TB disease is ruled out) on the basis of assessment of risk for drug toxicity, TB transmission, and patient preference

[a]QFT has not been adequately evaluated among persons with these conditions; it is recommended for such populations.
[b]QFT has not been adequately evaluated among persons aged <17 years, or among pregnant women; it is not recommended for such populations.
[c]The following additional conditions are required for QFT to indicate *Mycobacterium tuberculosis* infection: (1) mitogen—nil and tuberculin—nil are both >1.5 IU and (2) percentage avian difference is ≤10.
Source: Adapted from Ref. 22.

Table 3 QuantiFERON-TB Testing: Results and Interpretation

M − N[a] (IU/ mL)	T − N[b]+ (IU mL)	Avian difference (%)	Tuberculin response (%)[c]	Report and interpretation	Interpretation
≤1.5	All other response profiles	All other response profiles	All other response profiles	INY-γ response to mitogen is inadequate	Indeterminate
≥1.5	All other response profiles	All other response profiles	≤15	Percentage tuberculin response is <15 or not significant	Negative: *Mycobacterium tuberculosis* infection unlikely
≥1.5	≥1.5	≤10	≥15 but <30	Percentage tuberculin response is 15–30	Conditionally positive: *M. tuberculosis* infection likely if risk is identified, but unlikely for persons who are at low risk
≥1.5	≥1.5	≤10	≥30	Percentage tuberculin response is ≥30	Positive: *M. tuberculosis* infection likely

[a]M − N is the IFN-γ responses to mitogen minus the IFN-γ responses to nil antigen.
[b]T − N is the IFN-γ responses to purified protein derivative from *M. tuberculosis* infection. If T − N is <1.5 IU mL, the persons are deemed negative for *M. tuberculosis* infection, regardless of their percentage tuberculin response and percentage avian difference results.
[c]A percentage tuberculin response cutoff of 15% is used for persons with identified risk for tuberculosis infection, whereas a cutoff of 30% is used for persons with no identified risk factors.
Source: Adapted from Ref. 22.

4.4. Laboratory Diagnosis

Sputum samples must be collected from all patients, regardless of age, with pulmonary symptoms or chest radiographic changes compatible with TB disease and who have not been previously treated with antituberculous agents. In elderly patients unable to expectorate sputum, other diagnostic techniques such as sputum induction or bronchoscopy may be considered; in the frail and very old patients, the risk of such bronchoscopic procedures must be weighed against the benefits of potentially making a definite diagnosis of TB (24). In the case of pulmonary and GU TB, three consecutive early morning sputum or urine samples, respectively, are recommended for routine mycobacteriologic studies. Sputum samples are examined initially by smear and then cultured for *Mtb*. Because routine mycobacterial culture methods may require up to 6 weeks for growth of *Mtb*, many laboratories now use radiometric procedures for the isolation and susceptibility testing of this organism (25). Radiometric systems using ^{14}C-labeled liquid substrate medium may identify the organisms as early as after 8 days. Sterile body fluids and tissues can be inoculated into liquid media, which also allow the growth and detection of *Mtb* 7–10 days earlier than the solid media techniques. Histological examination of tissue from various sites such as the liver, lymph nodes, bone marrow, pleura may show the characteristic tissue reaction (caseous necrosis with granuloma formation) with or without AFB, which would also strongly support the diagnosis of TB disease.

Other diagnostic methods for TB that have been clinically evaluated include serology (e.g., ELISA, radioimmunoassay, latex particle agglutination assay) and gas chromatography assay for tuberculostearic acid (21). However, when applied to serum samples alone, these tests have not been considered sensitive and specific enough to be used as the sole diagnostic procedure for TB. Nucleic acid amplification (NAA) tests such as polymerase chain reaction and other methods for amplifying DNA and RNA may facilitate rapid detection of *Mtb* from respiratory specimens; the interpretation and use of the NAA test results has been recently updated by the CDC (26). Similar techniques that utilize DNA probes can be used to track the spread of the organism in epidemiologic studies and may be used to predict drug resistance prior to the availability of standard results; such methods are presently being used in some laboratories. Rapid diagnosis of TB is important in elderly patients, patients with immunocompromised states and with MDR TB.

5. MANAGEMENT

5.1. Pharmacotherapy

The drug treatment of TB including monitoring for adverse reactions is provided in detail in a separate chapter (see chapter "Antituberculous Drugs").

Because of the rise of MDR-TB cases, the TB treatment algorithm and recommendations have been accordingly modified (Fig. 1 and Table 4) (27). Clinicians must be aware of the potential for drug toxicity in the older patient population already burdened with polypharmacy. A shorter course and more intensive regimens, particularly when administered by directly observed therapy (DOT), are increasingly preferred to avoid the emergence of drug resistance resulting from poor compliance with antituberculous drug regimens.

Treatment of MDR-TB is complex and often needs to be individualized, requiring the addition of a minimum of two more antituberculous agents to which the organism is presumably susceptible. Consultation with a TB expert who is familiar with *Mtb* drug resistance is generally recommended. Alternative drugs may have to be used for treatment in such cases (27).

5.2. Treatment of Latent TB Infection

The drug treatment of latent TB infection is reviewed in detail in the chapter "Antituberculous Drugs." The recently modified therapy guidelines for latent TB infection (LTBI) in adults including the elderly is shown in Table 5 (28,29). Despite the fact that these new recommendations do not specifically address aging adults, one has to apply the concept of targeted skin testing and LTBI treatment of high-risk populations to include the elderly.

6. INFECTION CONTROL ISSUES

The primary goal of a TB infection control program is to detect TB disease early and to isolate and promptly treat persons with infectious TB. Prevention of transmission

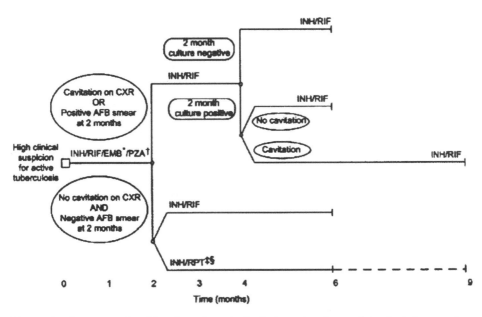

Figure 1 Treatment algorithm for tuberculosis. Patients in whom tuberculosis is proved or strongly suspected should have treatment initiated with isoniazid, rifampin, pyrazinamide, and ethambutol for the initial 2 months. A repeat smear and culture should be performed when 2 months of treatment has been completed. If cavities were seen on the initial chest radiograph or the acid-fast smear is positive at completion of 2 months of treatment, the continuation phase of treatment should consist of isoniazid and rifampin daily or twice weekly for 4 months to complete a total of 6 months of treatment. If cavitation was present on the initial chest radiograph and the culture at the time of completion of 2 months of therapy is positive, the continuation phase should be lengthened to 7 months (total of 9 months of treatment). If the patient has HIV infection and the CD4+ cell count is <100/μL, the continuation phase should consist of daily or three times weekly isoniazid and rifampin. In HIV-uninfected patients having no cavitation on chest radiograph and negative acid-fast smears at completion of 2 months of treatment, the continuation phase may consist of either once weekly isoniazid and rifapentine or daily or twice weekly isoniazid and rifampin, to complete a total of 6 months (bottom). Patients receiving isoniazid and rifapentine, and whose 2-month cultures are positive, should have treatment extended by an additional 3 months (total of 9 months). *EMB EMB may be discontinued when results of drug susceptibility testing indicate no drug resistance. †PZA may be discontinued after it has been taken for 2 months (56 doses). ‡RPT should not be used in HIV-infected patients with tuberculosis or in patients with extrapulmonary tuberculosis. §Therapy should be extended to 9 months if 2-month culture is positive. CXR, chest radiograph; EMB, ethambutol; INH, isoniazid; PZA, pyrazinamide; RIF, rifampin; RPT, rifapentine. *Source*: Adapted from Ref. 27.

of TB in any health care environment is of utmost importance both for patients and health care workers. Enhanced awareness of drug-resistant TB has prompted public health agencies to institute strict TB identification, isolation, treatment, and prevention guidelines. The TB infection control program in most acute care as well as long-term care facilities should consist of three types of control measures: administrative actions (i.e., prompt detection of suspected cases, isolation of infectious patients, and rapid institution of appropriate treatment), engineering control (negative-pressure ventilation rooms, high-efficiency particulate air filtration, and ultraviolet germicidal irradiation), and personal respiratory protection requirements (masks).

Table 4 Recommended Drug Regimens for Treatment of TB Disease in Adults (Including the Elderly)

| | Initial phase | | | Continuation phase | | | | Rating[c] (evidence)[d] | |
	Regimen	Drugs	Intervals and doses[a] (minimal duration)	Regimen	Drugs	Interval and doses[a,b] (minimal duration)	Range of total doses (minimal duration)	HIV−	HIV+
1		INH, RIF, PZA, EMB	Seven days per week for 56 doses (8 weeks) or day/week for 40 doses (8 weeks)	1a	INH/RIF	Seven days per week for 126 doses (18 weeks) or 5 days per weeks for 90 doses (18 weeks)[e]	182–130 (26 weeks)	A(I)	A(II)
				1b	INH/RIF	Twice weekly for 36 doses (18 weeks)	92–76 (26 weeks)	A(I)	A(II)[f]
				1c[g]	INH/RPT	Once weekly for 18 doses (18 weeks)	44–58 (26 weeks)	B(I)	E(I)
2		INH, RIF, PZA, EMB	Seven days per week for 14 doses (2 weeks), then twice weekly for 12 doses (6 weeks) or 5 days/week for 10 doses (2 weeks) then twice weekly for 12 doses (6 weeks)	2a	INH/RIF	Twice weekly for 36 doses (18 weeks)	62–58 (26 weeks)	A(II)	B(II)[f]

Initial phase	Drugs	Interval and doses[a]	Continuation phase	Drugs	Interval and doses[a,b]	Range of total doses (minimal duration)	Rating[c,d] HIV−	Rating[c,d] HIV+
			2b[g]	INH/RPT	Once weekly for 18 doses (18 weeks)	44–40 (26 weeks)	B(I)	E(I)
3	INH, RIF, PZA, EMB	Three times weekly for 24 doses (8 weeks)	3a	INH/RIF	Three times weekly for 54 doses (18 weeks)	78 (26 weeks)	B(I)	B(I)
4	INH, RIF, EMB	Seven days per week for 56 doses (8 weeks) or 5 days/week for 40 doses (8 weeks)	4a	INH/RIF	Seven days per week for 217 doses (31 weeks) or 5 days/week for 155 doses (31 weeks)[e]	273–195 (39 weeks)	C(I)	C(I)
			4b	INH/RIF	Twice weekly for 62 doses (31 weeks)	118–102 (39 weeks)	C(I)	C(II)

[a] When DOT is used, drugs may be given 5 days/week and the necessary number of doses adjusted accordingly. Although there are no studies that compare five with seven daily doses, extensive experience indicates this would be an effective practice.

[b] Patients with cavitation on initial chest radiograph and positive cultures at completion of 2 months of therapy should receive a 7-month [31 weeks; either 217 doses (daily) or 62 doses (twice weekly)] continuation phase.

[c] Definitions of evidence ratings: A, preferred; B, acceptable alternative; C, when A and B cannot be given; E, should never be given.

[d] Definitions of evidence ratings: I, randomized clinical trial; II, data from clinical trials that were not randomized or were conducted in other populations; III, expert opinion.

[e] Five-day-a-week administration is always given by DOT. Rating for 5 days/week regimens is AIII.

[f] Not recommended for HIV-infected patients with CD4 cell counts <100 cells/μL.

[g] Options 1c and 2b should be used only in HIV-negative patients who have negative sputum smears at the time of completion of 2 months of therapy and who do not have cavitation on initial chest radiograph (see text). For patients started on this regimen and found to have a positive culture from the 2-month specimen, treatment should be extended an extra 3 months.

Abbreviations: EMB, ethambutol; INH, isoniazid; PZA, pyrazinamide; RIF, rifampin; RPT, rifapentine.

Table 5 Revised Drug Regimens for Treatment of Latent TB Infection in Adults (Including the Elderly)

Drug	Interval and duration	Comments	Ratings (evidence) HIV negative	HIV infected
Isoniazid	Daily for 9 months	In HIV-infected persons, isoniazid may be administered concurrently with nucleoside reverse transcriptase inhibitors (NRTIs), protease inhibitors, or nonnucleoside reverse transcriptase inhibitors (NNRTIs)	A(II)	A(II)
	Twice weekly for 9 months	DOT must be used with twice-weekly dosing	B(II)	B(II)
Isoniazid	Daily for 6 months	Not indicated for HIV-infected persons, those with fibrotic lesions on chest radiographs, or children	B(I)	C(I)
	Twice weekly for 6 months	DOT must be used with twice-weekly dosing	B(II)	C(I)
Rifampin	Daily for 4 months	Used for persons who are contacts of patients with isoniazid-resistant, rifampin-susceptible TB In HIV-infected persons, most protease inhibitors or delavirdine should not be administered concurrently with rifampin. Rifabutin	B(II)	B(III)

Rifampin plus pyrazinamiade (RZ)	Daily for 2 months	with appropriate dose adjustments can be used with protease inhibitors (saquinavir should be augmented with ritonavir) and NNRTIs (except delavirdine). Clinicians should consult web-based updates for the latest specific recommendations	D(II)	D(II)
	Twice weekly for 2–3 months	RZ generally should not be offered for treatment of LTBI for HIV-infected or HIV-negative persons	D(III)	D(III)

Notes: Strength of the recommendation: (A) Both strong evidence of efficacy and substantial clinical benefit support recommendation for use. Should always be offered. (B) Moderate evidence for efficacy or strong evidence for efficacy but only limited clinical benefit supports recommendation for use. Should generally be offered. (C) Evidence for efficacy is insufficient to support a recommendation for or against use, or evidence for efficacy might not outweigh adverse consequences (e.g., drug toxicity, drug interactions) or cost of the treatment or alternative approaches. Optional. (D) Moderate evidence for lack of efficacy or for adverse outcome supports a recommendation against use: should generally not be offered. (E) Good evidence for lack of efficacy or for adverse outcome support a recommendation against use. Should never be offered. Quality of evidence supporting the recommendation: (I) Evidence from at least one properly randomized controlled trial. (II) Evidence from at least one well-designed clinical trial without randomization for cohort or case-controlled analytic studies (preferably from more that one center), from multiple time-series studies, or from dramatic results form uncontrolled experiments. (III) Evidence from opinions of respected authorities based on clinical experience, descriptive studies, or reports of expert committees. The substitution of rifapentine for rifampin is not recommended because rifapentine's safety and effectiveness have not been established for patients with LTBI.

Source: Adapted from Refs. 28, 29.

The Advisory Committee for the Elimination of Tuberculosis of the CDC has established recommendations for surveillance, containment, assessment, and reporting of TB infection and disease in long-term care facilities; health care professionals, administrators, and staff of such extended care programs must be alerted to these recommendations (30).

REFERENCES

1. World Health Organization. The World Health Report. Making a difference. World Health Organization 1999; 3:310–320.
2. Centers for Disease Control: http://www.cdc.gov/nchstp/tb/surv/surv2003/PDF/T1.pdf.
3. Zuber PLF, McKenna MT, Binkin NJ, Onorato IM, Castro KG. Long-term risk of tuberculosis among foreign-born persons in the United States. J Am Med Assoc 1997; 278:304–307.
4. Geiter L, ed. Institute of Medicine. Ending Neglect: The Elimination of Tuberculosis in the United States. Washington, DC: National Academy Press, 2000:1–269.
5. Yoshikawa TT. Tuberculosis in aging adults. J Am Geriatr Soc 1992; 40:178.
6. Centers for Disease Control and Prevention. Tuberculosis Statistics in the United States, 1987. Atlanta, GA: HHS Publication No. (CDC) 89–832, 1989.
7. Centers for Disease Control and Prevention. Fact Sheets. www.cdc.gov.
8. National Center for Health Statistics, Hing E. Use of Nursing Homes by the Elderly: Preliminary Data from the 1985 National Nursing Home Survey. Hyattsville, MD: National Center for Health Statistics. Vital and Health Statistics: Advance Data from Vital and Health Statistics, No. 135. DHHS Publication No. (PHS) 87–1250, 1987.
9. Ijaz K, Dillara JA, Yang Z, Cave MD, Bates JH. Unrecognized tuberculosis in a nursing home causing death with spread of tuberculosis to the community. J Am Geriatr Soc 2002; 50:1213–1217.
10. Adler JJ, Rose DM. Transmission and pathogenesis of tuberculosis. In: Rom WN, Garay SM, eds. Tuberculosis. 1st ed. New York: Little, Brown and Company, Inc., 1996.
11. Dannenberg AM. Pathogenesis of tuberculosis: native and acquired resistance in animals and humans. In: Leive L, Schlessinger D, eds. Microbiology. Washington, DC: American Society for Microbiology, 1984:344–354.
12. Perez-Guzman C, Vargas MH, Torres-Cruz A, Villareal-Velarde H. Does aging modify pulmonary tuberculosis? A meta analytical review. Chest 1999; 116:961–967.
13. Mert A, Bilir M, Tabak F. Miliary tuberculosis: clinical manifestations, diagnosis and outcome in 38 adults. Respirology 2001; 6:217–224.
14. Kalita J, Misra UK. Tuberculous meningitis with pulmonary miliary tuberculosis: a clinicoradiological study. Neurol India 2004; 52:194–196.
15. Shah AH, Joshi SV, Dhar HL. Tuberculosis of bones and joints. Antiseptic 2001; 98:385–387.
16. Malaviya A. Arthritis associated with tuberculosis. Best Pract Res Clin Rheumatol 2003; 17:319–343.
17. Lenk S, Schroeder J. Genitourinary tuberculosis. Curr Opin Urol 2001; 11(1):93–98.
18. Markowitz N, Hansen NI, Wilcosky TC, Hopewell PC, Glassroth J, Kvale PA, Mangura BT, Osmond D, Wallace JM, Rosen MJ, Reichman LB. Tuberculin and anergy testing in HIV-seropositive and HIV-seronegative persons. Ann Intern Med 1993; 119(3):185–193.
19. Tort J, Pina JM, Martin-Ramos A, Espaulella J, Armengol J. Booster effect in elderly patients living in geriatric institutions. Med Clin Barc 1995; 105:41–44.
20. Slovis BS, Plitman JD, Haas DW. The case against anergy testing as a routine adjunct to tuberculin skin testing. J Am Med Assoc 2000; 283:2003–2007.

21. American Thoracic Society. Diagnostic Standards and Classification of Tuberculosis in Adults and Children. Am J Resp Crit Care Med 2000; 161:1376–1395.
22. Centers for Disease Control Guidelines for using the QuantiFERON-TB test for diagnosing latent *Mycobacterium tuberculosis* infection. MMWR 2003; 52(RR02):15–18.
23. Woodring JH, Vandiviere HM, Fried AM, Dillon M, William T, Melvin I. Update: the radiographic features of pulmonary tuberculosis. Am J Roentgenol 1986; 146(3): 497–506.
24. Patel YR, Mehta JB, Harvill L, Gatekey K. Flexible bronchoscopy as a diagnostic tool in the evaluation of pulmonary tuberculosis in an elderly population. J Am Geriatr Soc 1993; 41:629–632.
25. Hanna BA. Diagnosis of tuberculosis by microbiologic techniques. In: Rom WN, Garay SM, eds. Tuberculosis. 1st ed. New York: Little, Brown and Company, Inc., 1996:153.
26. Centers for Disease Control and Prevention. Nucleic acid amplification tests for tuberculosis. MMWR 2000; 49:593–594.
27. Centers for Disease Control and Prevention, American Thoracic Society & Infectious Disease Society of America. Treatment of tuberculosis. MMWR 2003; 52(RR11):1–77.
28. American Thoracic Society. Targeted skin testing and treatment of latent tuberculosis infection. Am J Resp Crit Care Med 2000; 161:S221–S247.
29. MMWR Update. Fatal and severe liver injuries associated with rifampin and pyrazinamide for latent tuberculosis infection, and revisions in American Thoracic Society/Centers for Disease Control and Prevention—Recommendations—United States, 2001; 50(34): 733–735.
30. Centers for Disease Control and Prevention. Control of tuberculosis in facilities providing long-term care to the elderly: recommendations of the Advisory Committee for the Elimination of Tuberculosis. MMWR 1990; 39(RR10):7.

SUGGESTED READING

American Thoracic Society. Targeted skin testing and treatment of latent tuberculosis infection. Am J Resp Crit Care Med 2000; 161:S221–S247.

Centers for Disease Control, American Thoracic Society & Infectious Disease Society of America. Treatment of tuberculosis. MMWR 2003; 52(RR11):1–77.

MMWR Update. Fatal and severe liver injuries associated with rifampin and pyrazinamide for latent tuberculosis infection, and revisions in American Thoracic Society/Centers for Disease Control and Prevention—Recommendations—United States, 2001; 50(34): 733–735.

Rom WN, Garay SM, eds. Tuberculosis. 1st ed. New York: Little, Brown and Company, Inc., 1996.

32

Medical and Surgical Treatment of Intra-abdominal Infections

John G. Carson, Ryan W. Patterson, and Samuel Eric Wilson
Department of Surgery, University of California, Irvine, California, U.S.A.

Key Points:

- Intra-abdominal infections are associated with increased morbidity and mortality in elderly individuals.
- Atypical manifestations of such infections often lead to delay in the diagnosis; furthermore, underlying comorbid illnesses may complicate the overall clinical presentation.
- Prompt initiation of antibiotic therapy and supportive care is essential once the diagnosis is made.
- Appendicitis in the elderly frequently presents atypically at advanced stages leading to perforation, peritonitis and higher mortality.
- Diverticulitis is common in the elderly with higher incidence of diverticular perforation.
- Cholecystitis has a misleading benign course in the elderly; presentation in advanced stages is relatively common in the elderly.
- Choledocholithiasis is the most common cause of cholangitis in aging adults; endoscopic drainage is the preferred initial treatment.

1. INTRODUCTION

An aging population increases the need for healthcare services and the growing elderly are an expanding part of surgical workloads. The National Hospital Discharge Survey (NHDS) reported that in 1999, patients aged 65 years or older constituted 12% of the population, but constituted 40% of hospital discharges and 48% of days of inpatient care (1). Older patients who account for a considerable share of cases of intra-abdominal infections frequently present atypically, which can lead to misdiagnosis (2,3). Symptoms are not as clear-cut in the older patient. For example, Cooper et al. (4) found that elderly patients present with nausea, vomiting, and fever approximately one-half as often as do younger patients. Elderly patients who have intra-abdominal infection tend to have a lower mean core body temperature than the young and polymorphonuclear lymphocyte counts occasionally in the normal range. The etiologies of intra-abdominal sepsis in the elderly are different from the population less than 65 years of age (Fig. 1A and B).

(A) Etiologies of intra-abdominal sepsis of patients ≥65 years

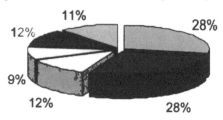

(B) Etiologies of intra-abdominal sepsis of patients <65 years

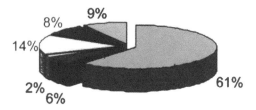

- ■ Appendicitis
- ■ Diverticulitis
- □ Cholecystitis
- □ Intra-abdominal abscess
- ■ Cholangitis
- ■ Colon cancer, sigmoid volvulus and mesenteric ischemia

Figure 1 Etiologies of intra-abdominal sepsis of patients: **(A)** ≥65 years; **(B)** <65 years. *Source*: Adapted from Ref. 4.

2. PHYSIOLOGIC CHANGES IN THE ELDERLY

Intra-abdominal sepsis affects all ages; however, in the elderly loss of physiologic reserve, combined with concomitant systemic illness, may result in a much worse outcome. As one ages, vital functions, such as wound healing, oxygen delivery to tissues, immunosurveillance, and depleted cardiopulmonary reserves blunt the response to peritonitis while they inhibit the ability to localize, combat, and eradicate infection. The nutritional status of the elderly may be deficient secondary to difficulty in mastication, decreased appetite, and lack of an appropriate diet. The aging skin loses elasticity and blood supply, rendering it fragile and more susceptible to injury and infection (5). Cardiovascular physiology deteriorates through arterial wall thickening (intimal hyperplasia) and resultant decrease in compliance. Cardiac output decreases with aging, resulting in an overall decrease in cardiac reserve. Increased rigidity of the chest wall and a decrease in respiratory muscle strength result in an increased closing capacity and a decreased forced expiratory volume in one second (FEV1) (6). The elderly have a diminished ventilatory response to hypercapnia and hypoxia. Chest wall stiffness increases, thus decreasing compliance and expiratory flow rates. These factors contribute to the increased risk for pulmonary complications.

Renal physiology is also affected with age. Starting at the age of 50, the kidney begins to decrease in weight from cortical loss. Glomerulosclerosis in turn leads to a decrease in the glomerular filtration rate (GFR). After the age of 40 years, the GFR decreases ≈ 1 mL/min/year (7) so that reduced renal reserves are common. This has major importance in dosing of certain antimicrobials, which may have nephrotoxicity as a side effect. In the event of surgery, the fluid, acid/base balance, and the serum electrolyte concentrations must be closely monitored, and dehydration or fluid overload avoided. Overall, the changes occurring in each organ system during aging lead to a depletion of physiologic reserve, which, in turn, complicates presentation as well as pre- and postoperative care.

Etiologies of intra-abdominal sepsis are age-dependent (Fig. 1A and B). Among patients 65 years and older, the leading causes of intra-abdominal infection include appendicitis (28%); diverticulitis (28%); cholecystitis (12%); cholangitis (12%); intra-abdominal abscess (9%); and colon cancer, sigmoid volvulus, and mesenteric ischemia ($\approx 11\%$ combined) (4). In contrast, the most common sources of intraperitoneal sepsis in patients younger than 65 years of age are appendicitis (61%); intra-abdominal abscess (14%); cholangitis (8%); diverticulitis (6%); cholecystitis (2%); and colon cancer, sigmoid volvulus, and mesenteric ischemia ($\approx 9\%$ collectively). Biliary and pancreatic foci of infection were nearly three times as common in geriatric patients compared with their younger cohort.

This chapter reviews the pathophysiology and clinical presentation of intra-abdominal sepsis in the group aged 65 and older and pre-, intra-, and postoperative management, including antimicrobial treatment. Specific sources of intra-abdominal sepsis are discussed along with potential complications and prognosis.

3. INTRA-ABDOMINAL SEPSIS/ACUTE SECONDARY PERITONITIS

Peritonitis is an inflammatory response of the peritoneal lining to direct irritation, which can occur after infectious, inflammatory, perforating, or ischemic injuries to the gastrointestinal or genitourinary system. Secondary peritonitis is caused by bacterial contamination originating from within the viscera or external to the abdomen. Localized infection can be eradicated by host defenses; however, untreated generalized peritonitis leads to septicemia with multiple organ failure. The severity of peritonitis is influenced by several factors including the amount of inoculum, type of bacterial or fungal infection, nature and duration of injury, and the host's immune and nutritional status (8). Minimal or well-localized (e.g., appendicitis) contamination progress to fulminant bacterial peritonitis relatively slowly (e.g., 12–24 hr). Conversely, infection associated with distal gut and biliary tract perforations as well as postoperative anastomotic leakage tend to progress rapidly. In the immunocompromised host, generalized peritonitis and sepsis advance even more quickly. Pathogens causing peritonitis include endogenous organisms of the gastrointestinal tract. The predominant Enterobacteriaccae include *Escherichia coli*, *Klebsiella*, and *Enterobacter*; other pathogens include *Enterococcus* and *Pseudomonas* species. In addition, anaerobes such as the *Bacteroides fragilis* group and streptococci are common (9).

Intra-abdominal infections present differently in the elderly, compared with younger patients (4). In geriatric patients symptoms are less acute or delayed. Comorbid illnesses, which include cardiac disease, peripheral vascular disease, hypertension, cerebrovascular disease, renal insufficiency, pulmonary disease, and malignancy, are common (10). Geriatric patients are less likely to develop nausea, vomiting, diarrhea, and fever (4). Also, in older patients the duration of symptoms to presentation is almost twice as long as in younger patients. The presenting diagnosis is more likely to be unknown or extraperitoneal in the elderly vs. younger patients. A higher percentage of elderly patients (14% vs. 3%) are hypothermic (temperature <36°C) with a lower average temperature (37.5°C vs. 38.2°C) compared with younger patients. Length of hospital stay and the number of days until normothermia is restored are significantly longer among the elderly treated for intra-abdominal sepsis. Except for an inappropriately low polymorpholeukocyte count of <2000 lymphocytes/mm^3, which occurs occasionally among geriatric patients, hematologic factors are comparable. On physical examination, peritoneal signs (abdominal pain and tenderness, guarding and rigidity, distention, free peritoneal air, diminished bowel sounds) and lethargy are similar (4). Other systemic findings include chills, tachypnea, dehydration, oliguria, tachycardia, sweating, disorientation, and ultimately refractory shock if disease is unchecked.

Laboratory tests include complete blood count, arterial blood gas, electrolytes, cross matching, and a blood clotting profile, as well as liver and renal function tests. Gram stain of infected material should be done for nosocomial infections to identify potential gram-positive organisms. An appropriate amount of intravenous fluids and colloid must be administered to replace the substantial transfer of protein-rich fluid to the peritoneal cavity. In the elderly or frail patient, central venous pressure or pulmonary artery wedge pressure as well as hourly urine output should be accurately charted. Adequate volumes of lactated Ringer's or balanced electrolyte solution must be infused rapidly to correct hypovolemia and restore blood pressure and urine output to acceptable levels. Potassium should be withheld until tissue and renal perfusion are sufficient as measured by urine output.

Infections involving the stomach, duodenum, biliary system, and proximal small bowel may be caused by gram-positive and gram-negative aerobic and facultative organisms. Distal small bowel perforations may lead to infections by gram-negative facultative and aerobic organisms, which, untreated, usually form abscesses progressing to bacteremia. *B. fragilis* is the predominant anaerobe in intra-abdominal infection. *E. coli* is the most common gram-negative facultative organism in intra-abdominal infections arising from colonic perforation or ischemia. Streptococci and enterococci are also commonly present.

Guidelines for antibiotic therapy are based on many well-studied single- and multi-drug therapies summarized by the Infectious Diseases Society of America (IDSA Guidelines for Intra-abdominal Infections, Table 1) (11). For patients with community-acquired intra-abdominal infections of mild to moderate severity, recommended antimicrobials include β-lactam/β-lactamase inhibitor combinations, ertapenem, cefazolin or cefuroxime plus metronidazole, and quinolones plus metronidazole. These antimicrobials are preferable to agents that have broader activity against resistant gram-negative organisms and/or greater toxicity. Recommended regimens for more severe infections include piperacillin/tazobactam, imipenem/cilastatin, meropenem, third-/fourth-generation cephalosporin (cefotaxime, ceftriaxone, ceftizoxime, ceftazidime, cefepime) in combination with metronidazole, ciprofloxacin with metronidazole, and aztreonam plus metronidazole. Depending on the patient's renal function as well as the excretion and toxicity of the antimicrobial agent, decreased dosing may be required (Table 2). Nosocomial (postoperative) infections are caused by more resistant flora, which include *Pseudomonas aeruginosa*, *Enterobacter* species, *Proteus* species, methicillin-resistant *Staphylococcus aureus* (MRSA), enterococci, and *Candida* species. Complex multidrug regimens are

Table 1 Recommended Treatment of Community Acquired Intra-abdominal Infections (Infectious Diseases Society of America Guidelines)

Antimicrobial drug	Mild–moderate infections	High severity infections
Single agent		
β-Lactam/β-Lactamase inhibitor	Ticarcillin/clavulanic acid	Piperacillin/tazobactam
Carbapenems	Ertapenem	Imipenem/cilastatin, meropenem
Combination regimens		
Cephalosporin + metronidazole	Cefazolin or cefuroxime + metronidazole	Third-/fourth-generation cephalosporin (cefotaxime, ceftriaxone, ceftizoxime, ceftazidime, cefepime) + metronidazole
Fluoroquinolone + metronidazole	Ciprofloxacin, levofloxacin, moxifloxacin, or gatifloxacin, each in combination with metronidazole[a]	Ciprofloxacin + metronidazole
Monobactam		Aztreonam + metronidazole

[a]Increasing resistance of *Bacteroides fragilis* group to available quinolones has been reported; these agents should be used in combination with metronidazole.
Source: Adapted from Ref. 11.

required for these infections and selection should be based on culture and susceptibility reports. Local nosocomial resistance patterns should dictate empirical treatment, and therapy should be changed according to results from the microbiology laboratory.

Once the diagnosis of intra-abdominal infection is suspected, appropriate antibiotic treatment should be initiated along with fluid resuscitation so that enough visceral perfusion has been restored to improve drug distribution. Completion of antibiotic courses with oral forms of a quinolone plus metronidazole or with oral amoxicillin/clavulanic acid is satisfactory for patients able to tolerate an oral diet. Prolonged preoperative length of stay and prolonged (>3 days) preoperative antimicrobial therapy are predictors of antibiotic failure and recurrent infections (12). Such patients should be treated as nosocomial infection. Antimicrobial therapy should be continued until resolution of clinical signs of infection occurs [normal temperature and white blood cell (WBC) count as well as bowel function]. Patients with persistent clinical evidence of intra-abdominal infection after 5–7 days of therapy should be reevaluated for persistent or recurrent infection using computed tomography (CT). *Candida albicans* or other fungi are isolated in about 20% of acute perforations. Antifungal agents are not necessary unless the patient is immunocompromised or has recurrent infection. If *C. albicans* is isolated as a pathogen, fluconazole is commonly used unless there is resistance, in which case caspofungin and voriconazole are less toxic choices than amphoterin B (13).

The objective of surgery for peritonitis is to remove all infected material, correct the underlying cause, and prevent late complications. Operative management

Table 2 Renal Dosing Adjustments for Selected Antimicrobials

Antimicrobial drug	Renal dosing
Ticarcillin/clavulanic acid	CrCl > 60: 3.1 g q4–6 hr; 30–60: q8–12 hr; 10–30: q12–24 hr or 2 g ivpb q8 hr; <10: 2 g q12 hr or 3.1 g q24–48 hr; <10+ hepatic dysfcn: 2 g q24 hr; PD: 3.1 g q12 hr; HD: 2 g q12 hr+ 3.1 g AD
Ertapenem	CrCl < 30: 500 mg qd
Cefazolin	CrCl 10–30: q12 hr; <10: q24 hr
Cefuroxime	CrCl 10–20: q12 hr; <10: q24 hr
Metronidazole	CrCl < 10: 500 mg ivpb q12 hr
Ciprofloxacin	CrCl 10–50: 50–75% of usual dose q12 hr; <10/50% of usual dose q12. Alternatives: (200 mg ivpb or 250 mg po q12 hr) or (400 mg ivpb or 500 mg po q24 hr); HD/PD: 250–500 mg po or 200–400 mg ivpb q24 hr AD or 200 mg ivpb or 250 mg po q12 hr
Levofloxacin	CrCl > 50/no change; 20–49: 500 mg × 1 then 250 mg q24 hr; <19/HD/PD: 500 mg × 1 then 250 mg q48 hr
Gatifloxacin	CrCl < 40, HD, CAPD: 400 mg PO/IV × 1 then 200 mg PO/IV qd
Piperacillin/tazobactam	CrCl 20–40: 2.25 g q6 hr; <20: 2.25 g q8 hr; HD: Max 2.25 g q8 hr 0.75 g AD; PD: 2.25 g q8 hr
Imipenem/cilastatin	CrCl 31–70: 500 mg q6–8 hr; 21–30: 500 mg q8–12 hr max; 0–20: 250–500 mg q12 hr max; HD: 250 mg AD + q12 hr; PD: max dose = 1 g/day, i.e., 500 mg ivpb q12 hr
Meropenem	CrCl 26–50: q12 hr; 10–25: 500 mg q12 hr; <10: 500 mg q24 hr; HD: suppl. dose w/HD
Cefotaxime	CrCl < 20: reduce dose 50%
Ceftriaxone	PD: 750 mg ivpb q12 hr
Ceftazidime	CrCl 30–50: q12 hr; 10–30: q24 hr; <10: q48 hr
Cefepime	CrCl 30–60: 0.5–2 g q24 hr; 11–29: 0.5–1 g q24 hr; <10:250–500 mg q24 hr or 0.5–2 g q48 hr; HD: 1g AD; PD: 1–2 g q48 hr
Aztreonam	CrCl 10–30: 50% of usual dose q6–8 hr; <10: 25% of usual dose q6–8 hr; HD/PD: see <10 guidelines (HD: 500 mg AD). Give loading dose of 1–2 g before starting above regimens

Abbreviations: CrCl, creatinine clearance; IVPB, intravenous piggyback; dysfcn, dysfunction; PD, peritoneal dialysis; HD, hemodialysis; AD, after dialysis; CAPD, chronic ambulatory peritoneal dialysis; po, oral; max, maximum; suppl, supplemental.
Source: Adapted from University of Pennsylvania Medical Center Guidelines for Antibiotic Use: http://www.uphs.upenn.edu/bugdrug/antibiotic_manual/renal.htm & www.epocrates.com.

includes control of the perforation, peritoneal lavage, peritoneal drainage, and management of abdominal distention secondary to ileus. A midline incision offers the best exposure except in localized disease (e.g., appendicitis). An aspiration (usually 5 mL) of purulent peritoneal fluid is sent for aerobic and anaerobic cultures immediately after the peritoneal cavity is entered. Contaminated and necrotic material is removed after a thorough exploration. The primary disease is then treated by repair (e.g., perforated ulcer), drainage (e.g., acute pancreatitis), or resection (e.g., ruptured appendix or necrotic gallbladder). Colonic reanastomosis in the presence of ischemia or extensive contamination increases the likelihood of leakage; thus, a temporary stoma is safer and can be closed several weeks later. Surgical wounds are often left open in grossly soiled cases and delayed primary closure may be performed in those with less contamination on the third or fourth postoperative day.

Diffuse peritonitis requires lavage with abundant amounts (>2 L) of warm isotonic crystalloid solution to remove blood and fibrin clots, and to dilute remaining bacteria. Use of antiseptics or antibiotics (e.g., povidone-iodine or tetracycline) are of little proven value and may increase the likelihood of forming adhesions. Lavage with aminoglycosides, which may induce respiratory depression via neuromuscular blockade, is avoided. Aspiration of all fluid should follow as it may hinder defense mechanisms by diluting opsonins and removing phagocytes. Pulsatile lavage may be used for gentle debridement of peritoneal surfaces.

Peritoneal drainage is useful when there is residual focal infection or continued contamination. For large volumes of fluid, a soft sump drain with continuous suction is effective. Smaller volumes are best evacuated by closed drain systems (e.g., Jackson–Pratt). Several large Penrose drains should be placed for large cavities with thick walls. In severe peritonitis, re-exploration of the abdomen after 1–3 days may be required; however, planned re-exploration should be restricted to patients with long-standing (>72 hr) extensive intra-abdominal sepsis who are predicted to develop recurrent abscess. Otherwise, relaparotomy is based on objective findings on CT examination, which are often confirmed by needle aspiration before percutaneous drainage or re-exploration.

Abdominal distention caused by ileus is common in patients who have peritonitis. Decompression of the intestine by nasogastric suction is often ineffective. Temporary closure of the abdomen with prosthesis avoids abdominal compartment syndrome (increased intra-abdominal pressure) in patients who have massive intestinal edema due to aggressive fluid replacement along with the inflammatory response to peritonitis. In the elderly, a gastrostomy may prevent aspiration, sinusitis, and nasopharyngeal erosion when prolonged nasogastric decompression is expected.

Postoperative intensive care monitoring and ventilatory support are often needed in unstable and frail patients. Besides fluids and blood products, inotropic agents may be required to achieve hemodynamic stability. Antibiotics are given for 7 days or longer depending on the resolution of peritonitis. Antimicrobial therapy is adjunctive to a definitive operation in management of peritonitis. The tripartite role of antibiotics is: first, to control preoperative sepsis; second, to combat bacteremia caused by intraoperative manipulation; and third, to speed resolution of peritoneal cellulitis. Source control is best achieved by operation or percutaneous drainage. Evidence of a favorable clinical response in the elderly includes reduction in fever and leukocytosis; resolution of ileus; satisfactory urine output; and return of sense of well-being, cognition, and basic functions. The risk of secondary infection is reduced by removal of all nonessential catheters as well as drains once drainage diminishes or becomes more serous. Early feeding and discontinuation of antibiotics are vital in controlling proximal gut colonization with candida, *Enterococcus faecium*, pseudomonas, MRSA, and coagulase-negative staphylococci, which cause secondary nosocomial infection with subsequent multiple organ failure.

Complications are frequent and may be considered as local or systemic. By the end of first postoperative week, residual abscesses, deep wound infections, anastomotic breakdown, and fistula formation may complicate recovery. General failure to improve despite appropriate treatment, persistent high or spiking fever, generalized edema with high fluid requirements, increased abdominal distention, inability to wean the patient from inotropes, and continued mental confusion point to residual intra-abdominal sepsis.

Geriatric patients are particularly susceptible to tertiary peritonitis, which is defined as the persistence or recurrence of intra-abdominal infection after appropriate management. This occurs most commonly in severe pancreatitis, after resection of necrotic bowel, and anastomotic breakdown, but may also follow complicated appendicitis, perforated ulcers, and diverticulitis. The most common organisms include *Enterococcus* species, *Candida* species, *Staphylococcus epidermidis*, *E. coli*, *Enterobacter* species, *B. fragilis*, and *Pseudomonas* species (14). Tertiary peritonitis has a poor outcome, as a consequence of patient risk and the severity of the pathologic process (15). Koperna et al. reported that relaparotomy within 48 hr after initial successful eradication significantly improves outcomes for elderly patients with tertiary peritonitis (16). Intra-abdominal abscesses, responsible for 50% of the nosocomial intra-abdominal infections among geriatric patients, may be more safely managed by image-guided percutaneous drainage.

A thorough physical examination and abdominal CT should be obtained when the resolution of peritonitis is slow. Open re-exploration or percutaneous catheter drainage of localized abscesses should be undertaken as needed. Supportive measures for uncontrolled sepsis with multiorgan failure include antibiotics, mechanical ventilation, total parenteral nutrition (TPN), hemodialysis, and trans fusions, which are ineffective unless combined with intervention to achieve source control.

Prognosis depends on the etiology and duration of intra-abdominal infection as well as the age and general health of the patient (Table 3). Mortality rates are below 10% for patients with appendicitis or perforated peptic ulcer, for those who have minimal bacterial contamination, and especially if diagnosis and operation are early. More often, geriatric patients are more likely to have coexisting illnesses, greater bacterial contamination, a delay in diagnosis and treatment, and greater risk for respiratory and renal failure. Distal small bowel and colonic perforation or postoperative sepsis are accompanied by mortality rates approaching 50%. Intra-abdominal infections with resistant gram-positive cocci on culture, while not an independent predictor of mortality, result in prolonged hospitalizations (17). Patients with tertiary peritonitis may have mortality as high as 63% (14). High-risk patients may be identified by noticeably poor physiologic indices (i.e., APACHE II or Mannheim Peritonitis Index), low preoperative serum albumin levels, and reduced cardiac status (18).

Table 3 Stratification of Outcomes of Peritonitis According to Etiology

Severity	Cause	Mortality rate (%)
Mild	Appendicitis Perforated peptic ulcer Acute salpingitis	<10%
Moderate	Diverticulitis (localized perforation) Nonvascular small bowel perforation Gangrenous cholecystitis Multiple trauma	<20%
Severe	Large bowel perforation Ischemic small bowel Acute necrotizing pancreatitis Postoperative complications	20–80%

Source: Adapted from Ref. 42.

3.1. Acute Appendicitis

Appendicitis is an urgent surgical illness with variable manifestations that causes significant morbidity when accompanied by the diagnostic delay common in the older patient. In patients 65 years and older, appendicitis is responsible for 28% of significant intra-abdominal infections. The surgeon's goals are to evaluate patients referred for suspected appendicitis and to minimize the negative appendectomy rate without increasing the incidence of perforation. Obstruction of the appendiceal lumen by fibrosis, lymphoid hyperplasia, fecaliths, calculi, neoplasms, or parasites is the primary cause of appendicitis. Ineffective lymphatic and venous drainage allows bacterial invasion of the appendiceal wall progressing to necrosis and, in advanced cases, perforation and spillage of purulence into the peritoneal cavity. With aging, changes occur in the appendix such as atrophy of the intraluminal lymphoid tissue causing thinning of the appendiceal wall, which increase its susceptibility to inflammation. Atherosclerosis decreases blood supply, the lumen becomes narrowed, and the muscularis, fibrotic. Therefore, small changes in intraluminal pressure can produce rapid ischemia, gangrene, and perforation more rapidly in the elderly (19). Summed up, the course of appendicitis in the elderly often leads to secondary complications before diagnosis is established.

Acute appendicitis in the elderly usually presents in a more advanced stage and may have an atypical presentation leading to delayed diagnosis and increased rate of perforation, generalized peritonitis, and death (20). Appendicitis does not present classically (e.g., anorexia, abdominal pain with shift to the right lower quadrant, and nausea/vomiting) in the elderly. Typical symptoms includes decreased incidence of nausea, vomiting, anorexia, periumbilical pain, and migration in pain [e.g., periumbilical to right lower quadrant (RLQ)]. In contrast, older patients have an increased rate of constipation and diffuse and more severe abdominal pain. On physical examination, there are often signs of established, generalized peritonitis, probably reflecting the higher perforation rate. Abdominal distention, generalized tenderness, guarding, rebound tenderness, and palpable abdominal mass are significantly increased; however, tenderness is less localized to the RLQ. McBurney's sign (RLQ pain on palpation), obturator sign (pain with internal rotation of flexed right thigh), psoas sign (pain with right thigh extension), and Rovsing's sign (RLQ pain on left lower quadrant rebound test) may also be present depending on the degree of peritoneal irritation. Fever and leukocytosis is common in the majority of elderly patients with appendicitis.

Spiral CT of the abdomen is of great value in geriatric patients with atypical clinical symptoms and signs. An enlarged appendix with periappendiceal fat stranding is found in 90% of patients with appendicitis. Plain films of the abdomen show a fecalith in about 20% of patients with early appendicitis, and may also be useful in determining the presence of free air in perforation as well as assessing the degree of ileus (20).

Complications include perforation, peritonitis, and appendiceal abscess. Perforation by the time of appendectomy occurs in nearly 50% of patients aged over 50 years resulting in generalized peritonitis to microabscesses (21). Appendiceal abscess develops when localized perforation and periappendiceal infection are walled off by the omentum, mesentery, and viscera. Patients present with clinical appendicitis and RLQ mass. An ultrasound and CT should be performed, and if an abscess is found, percutaneous image-guided drainage may be considered. Operation for appendectomy and abscess drainage may be done if the abscess is known with certainty to be caused by appendicitis. Pylephlebitis is suppurative thrombophlebitis of the portal venous system, which characteristically presents with fever, chills, low-grade jaundice, and eventually hepatic abscesses; however, this presentation is encountered rarely today. CT scan is the best method for detecting thrombosis and gas in portal venous system.

Treatment is appendectomy (open or laparoscopic), with few exceptions such as the unstable patient with severe comorbid conditions. The laparoscopic approach may be useful if the diagnosis is uncertain. Antibiotics (see Table 1), fluids, and electrolytes are given preoperatively.

In the elderly, the mortality rate for appendicitis is 2–14% (19). Mortality rates for elderly patients with ruptured appendix approach 10%.

3.2. Diverticulitis

Diverticula of the sigmoid colon, common in older patients in Western countries, are outpouchings or pseudodiverticulae formed by herniation of the colonic mucosa through the weak areas in muscularis created by penetration of the vasa recta. Diverticulosis is reported in up to one-third of the population less than 45 years of age and up to two-thirds of those greater than 85 years. Diverticulitis, which is inflammation caused by fecalith impaction of these outpouchings, results in the classic presentation of constipation, left lower quadrant pain/tenderness (93–100%), fever (57–100%), and leukocytosis (69–83%). Patients with acute uncomplicated diverticulitis may be treated by conservative measures with appropriate antibiotic therapy (see Table 1) for enteric organisms and bowel rest. Nasogastric suction may be employed to relieve vomiting or ileus. CT scan is recommended to exclude perforation or abscess formation. If a pericolonic abscess is found, CT-guided drainage with a staged primary resection is appropriate treatment. Failure to show improvement within 72–96 hr should lead to consideration of surgical intervention, such as resection of sigmoid and/or left colon. Diverticulitis may be complicated by pericolic or intermesenteric abscess, perforation, intestinal obstruction, and fistula formation. Colovesical fistulas are the most common. Free perforation is an uncommon complication of diverticulitis; however, it may carry a 6–35% mortality rate (22). Older patients are more likely than younger patients to have diverticular perforations that result in generalized, rather than localized, peritonitis (23). A single-stage resection can be performed in ≈70% of patients in stable condition avoiding colostomy and a secondary operation for closure (24).

3.3. Cholecystitis

Acute cholecystitis results from obstruction of the cystic duct, which causes gallbladder distention and inflammation, abdominal pain, and tenderness. Etiologies include cholelithiasis (≈90% of cases), ischemic damage in critically ill patients (acalculous cholecystitis), infection (cytomegalovirus in acquired immune deficiency syndrome) strictures of the common bile duct, and neoplasms. Even though most gallstones are asymptomatic, nearly 20% have serious complications (9). The most common organisms that colonize the gallbladder and biliary tree in the elderly are *E. coli*, *Klebsiella*, and *B. fragilis*. Cholecystectomy for symptomatic cholelithiasis is one of the most commonly performed procedures in older patients.

Geriatric patients present with a deceptively benign course of illness that does not correspond to the severity of the disease. Advanced pathology is the rule among older patients; for example, in one report, 40% of cases had empyema of the gallbladder, gangrenous cholecystitis, or free perforation, and 15% had subphrenic abscesses or liver involvement (25). Furthermore, gangrenous gallbladder disease may also be present with mild leukocytosis and no peritoneal signs (26). Symptoms initially consist of right upper quadrant (RUQ) pain with occasional referred pain to the right scapula, with progression to abdominal tenderness. Other symptoms include nausea and vomiting in about half of patients and mild icterus in 10% of cases. Fever may also accompany these symptoms (33% of cases). Onset of RUQ pain is often preceded by a history of ingestion of fatty meals or biliary colic. RUQ tenderness is present on physical examination and in about one-third of patients the gallbladder is palpable. Murphy's sign may be elicited as the patient breathes deeply, and inspiration ceases as tenderness is accentuated with palpation of the right subcostal region.

Laboratory findings usually include leukocytosis (12,000–15,000 WBC/mm^3), although normal counts are not uncommon. Elevated serum alkaline phosphatase, alanine transaminase, aspartate transaminase, and bilirubin are not unexpected. Bilirubin greater than 4 mg/dL suggests choledocholithiasis. Elevated serum amylase may be present, but pancreatitis should be considered if the value is greater than 500 IU/L.

Ultrasound will demonstrate calculi, sludge, and thickening of the gallbladder wall. If ultrasound in negative or equivocal, a radionucleotide scan [hepatobiliary iminodiacetic acid (HIDA) scan] should be performed. HIDA scans have a sensitivity and specificity greater than 90% for acute cholecystitis, and if the gallbladder is observed on HIDA scan, acute cholecystitis is excluded. In acute acalculous cholecystitis stones are not detectable, but the gallbladder wall is thickened. HIDA scans are unreliable if bilirubin is greater than 5 mg/dL.

The major complications of acute cholecystitis are empyema, gangrene, and perforation. Empyema (suppurative cholecystitis) is characterized by purulence in the gallbladder and presentation of spiking fevers, chills, and leukocytosis >15,000 WBC/mm^3. Parenteral antibiotics (see Table 1) should be given and cholecystectomy performed or in exceptionally high-risk cases, percutaneous cholecystostomy should be performed.

Perforation may result in pericholecystic abscess, free perforation, and cholecystenteric fistula. Pericholecystic abscess should be suspected when symptoms and signs progress with the appearance of a palpable mass. Cholecystectomy and drainage should be performed in the stable patient, but percutaneous cholecystostomy is favored in the unstable patient. Localized pain, sudden spread of pain, and tenderness to other areas of the abdomen suggests free perforation. When free perforation is suspected, emergency laparotomy must be performed with cholecystectomy. Cholecystenteric fistula decompresses the gallbladder and resolves acute disease after the inflamed gallbladder adheres to adjacent stomach, duodenum (most common), or colon; necrosis develops; and perforation may occur into lumen of the gut. If the gallstones are large enough and discharge into the gut lumen, they may cause gallstone ileus (obstruction of the small intestine). Symptomatic cholecystenteric fistulas should be treated with cholecystectomy, closure of the fistula, and removal of the stone that is lodged in the distal small bowel.

For uncomplicated acute cholecystitis, initial treatment includes intravenous hydration, analgesia, intravenous antibiotics, bowel rest, and, if indicated, insertion of a nasogastric tube. For acute cholecystitis of mild severity, a parenteral first-generation cephalosporin (e.g., cefazolin) may be given. For severe cases of acute cholecystitis, gentamicin with clindamycin or metronidazole, piperacillin-tazobactam, or third-generation cephalosporin with an antianaerobic agent provides adequate coverage. Laparoscopic cholecystectomy, if technically feasible, is the treatment of choice as it is associated with fewer complications and earlier discharge compared with the open approach. Intraoperative cholangiography should be performed in patients with bilirubin over 3 mg/dL who have not had preoperative endoscopic retrograde cholangiopancreatography (ERCP) and the common bile duct explored if indicated (e.g., choledocholithiasis). Elderly men require almost twice as much emergency treatment as elderly women (59% vs. 32%). Patients requiring emergency treatment are at a fivefold increased risk of necrotizing, suppurative, or hemorrhagic cholecystitis and a 50% increase in complications (27). Emergent situations include clinical signs that suggest progression (fever >39°C, marked leukocytosis >15,000, or chills), emphysematous cholecystitis, sudden onset of generalized abdominal pain indicating free perforation, and appearance of a mass suggesting local perforation or abscess, as well as acalculous acute cholecystitis. In the unusual circumstance when patient's health status is very poor, percutaneous cholecystostomy should be performed to decompress the gallbladder. Pre- and postoperative ERCP with sphincterotomy and stone extraction may be performed in conjunction with laparoscopic cholecystectomy for patients with choledocholithiasis.

The overall mortality for cholecystectomy for all ages is 0.5–1.8%. In the elderly, it increases to 0.8–4.4%. In the emergent setting, the mortality rate for cholecystectomy is 10–19% (28). In older patients, secondary cardiovascular and pulmonary complications contribute significantly to morbidity and mortality.

3.4. Cholangitis

The most serious biliary tract emergencies are acute cholecystitis, ascending cholangitis, and acute pancreatitis. These conditions usually result from obstruction of the common bile duct caused by calculi or less frequently by benign or malignant strictures of the biliary tree, biliary tree manipulation, or biliary sludge. Despite therapeutic advances, these conditions still cause significant morbidity and mortality in the elderly (29). The most common cause of cholangitis in the United States is choledocholithiasis secondary to cholelithiasis.

Acute cholangitis occurs as a result of bacterial infection superimposed on obstruction of the biliary tree. Of the complications of gallstones, cholangitis is the most rapidly lethal entity; thus, making an accurate diagnosis and initiating early treatment are imperative (30). For patients who fail initial conservative therapy and do not have drainage, mortality approaches nearly 100%. Normally bile is sterile, but once the bile duct is obstructed colonization by bacteria leads to ascending infection, which may spread to the lymphatics and bloodstream. Partial obstruction is associated with a higher rate of infection than complete obstruction and obstruction from calculi has a higher rate of cholangitis than neoplastic obstruction (31). After biliary enteric bypass, obstruction of the anastomosis is associated with a high risk of cholangitis. Organisms most commonly found in cholangitis are *Enterococcus*, *Klebsiella*, and *Enterobacter*. Anaerobes are found in up to 15%, most commonly in the elderly.

Clinical presentation of cholangitis classically presents with fever and chills, RUQ pain, and jaundice, which is known as Charcot's Triad. About 10–20% of the patients present with altered mental status and hypotension and with these two additional features the syndrome is termed Reynold's pentad. RUQ tenderness is present in two-thirds and severe cholangitis may be associated with small or microhepatic abscesses that carry a poor prognosis. Ultrasound or CT is the most commonly used first-line imaging modality. ERCP should be considered early in the course of presentation.

Treatment includes correction of fluid and electrolyte abnormalities. Patients should have blood cultures drawn to assist refining of antibiotic therapy. Almost all patients with ascending cholangitis require biliary drainage. Endoscopic drainage is the preferred initial treatment in most patients for decompressing the biliary system in acute cholangitis (32). ERCP has also been shown to have lower morbidity rates, shorter length of hospitalization, and a higher definitive success rate than percutaneous drainage. In the case where endoscopic drainage is unsuccessful, operation and common bile duct exploration may be required. In summary, acute cholangitis, cholecystitis, and gallstone pancreatitis are urgent biliary infections usually caused by biliary calculi with morbidity and mortality in the elderly higher than in the general population.

3.5. Colon Cancer Perforation

Approximately 140,000 Americans are diagnosed with colon cancer each year with the majority of patients aged 60 and over. In advanced tumors, perforation may cause peritonitis with an incidence of 2.6–10% (33). Elderly patients disproportionately suffer perforations at a site proximal to the obstructing lesion. Perforation is the most lethal complication of colon cancer (34).

Common symptoms and signs upon presentation of colon cancer preceding perforation are abdominal pain (100%), weight loss (71%), anemia (57%), and melena (46%) (33). After perforation, signs of peritoneal inflammation are present along with the development of leukocytosis and fever.

Decreased survival in the elderly results from poorer nutritional status, more advanced local disease, peritoneal seeding of the cancer, and the emergent nature of the operation (35).

Perforation of the large bowel secondary to colon cancer requires aggressive surgical treatment. The abdomen should be explored for multiple primary carcinomas of the colon, distant metastases, and associated abdominal disease. Surgery includes wide resection of the tumor and its lymphatic drainage. Anastomosis is usually delayed in perforation with the proximal colonic end exteriorized. Secondary anastomosis is performed after inflammation subsides.

The operative mortality of perforation from colon cancer is 33% among older patients (34). Perforation proximal to a cancer is associated with a higher perioperative mortality and worse long-term outcome when compared with acute perforations at the site of the tumor. Perforation of the sigmoid colon is associated with a mortality rate of 16–38%. Furthermore, the 5-year survival rate significantly decreases after perforation in colon cancer patients.

3.6. Acute Necrotizing Pancreatitis

Acute necrotizing pancreatitis (ANP) is the most severe manifestation of a spectrum of inflammation associated with pancreatitis. Severe pancreatic inflammation causes necrosis, which is likely to become infected. The amount of devitalized tissue is the strongest predictor of mortality in ANP. In severe pancreatitis, three potential outcomes exist: resolution, pseudocyst, and abscess. The incidence of pancreatitis is ≈185,000 cases per year. ANP is reported to occur in ≈5–10% of all episodes of pancreatitis. Although sterile necrosis may occur, a variable percentage of patients develop infection of the necrotic tissue. Organisms causing infection in ANP include predominantly gut-derived flora such as *E. coli*, *Pseudomonas*, *Klebsiella*, and *Enterococcus* species. Approximately 75% of infections are monomicrobial. Fungal and gram-positive infections are uncommon, but occur more frequently during antibiotic treatment. The mortality rate is 30% for infected necrosis or abscess even with appropriate surgical intervention and drainage (36).

Patients with pancreatitis who have more than four of Ranson's criteria, an unexpectedly prolonged course, hemodynamic instability, fever, and failure of medical therapy should have a contrast-enhanced CT scan. We routinely obtain a CT scan on all hospitalized pancreatitis patients for its prognostic value. On physical examination, epigastric abdominal pain and tenderness with a mass on palpation are sought. Grey–Turner sign (discoloration of flanks) or Cullen sign (periumbilical discoloration) are characteristic of retroperitoneal bleeding but rarely noted. Other findings include vital signs consistent with sepsis, abdominal guarding, rebound tenderness, vomiting, jaundice, fever, and leukocytosis. Serum amylase is elevated but <1000 IU/L. A serum albumin <2.5 g/dL and elevated alkaline phosphatase are characteristic of pancreatic abscess. Contrast-enhanced CT scans are examined for nonenhancing areas, which indicates loss of vascularity, necrosis, or, in the case of abscess, a fluid collection. Percutaneous needle aspiration of these areas may detect bacteria with Gram stain and culture.

For patients with APN involving a significant proportion of the pancreas (e.g., >30%), antimicrobial therapy may be initiated with imipenem or meropenem for at least 1 week (37). If the patient becomes unstable at any time or when conservative measures fail (e.g., malaise, inability to tolerate diet, or persistent pain), a necrosectomy should be performed to remove necrotic debris. Percutaneous CT-guided aspiration should be undertaken if there is no clinical improvement after 1 week of antibiotics (38). If bacterial infection is noted, necrosectomy should be considered. However, if the aspirate is sterile, conservative treatment should be continued for 4–6 weeks. During surgery, all peripancreatic spaces are opened and any necrotic tissue is removed by gentle blunt dissection. If bile duct obstruction is known, a T-tube may be inserted and cholecystectomy may be performed in the presence of gallbladder disease. Two large drains are placed within the debrided spaces and are sometimes used for postoperative lavage.

In the case of a defined pancreatic abscess, percutaneous drainage is the initial step but may not be definitive as the abscess often contains particulate necrotic debris, which cannot pass through the drainage tube. Necrosectomy followed by administration of postoperative broad-spectrum antibiotics and external drainage is often necessary. The mortality rate for APN ranges from 20% to 40%.

3.7. Perforated Gastroduodenal Ulcer

Peptic ulcer disease (PUD), a common disorder that affects millions of individuals in the United States each year, is caused by the corrosive effects of gastric acid on vulnerable epithelium usually colonized by *Helicobacter pylori* or weakened by nonsteroidal anti-inflammatory drugs. Over the last few decades, the incidence of ulcer perforation has been decreasing in the young and men, but increasing in the elderly and women (39). Perforation complicates nearly 10% of patients with PUD. Most perforated ulcers are located anteriorly, and unusually may be complicated by an acute hemorrhage secondary to a posterior "kissing ulcer" eroding into the gastroduodenal artery in less than 10% of patients. Perforations may be sealed by omentum or liver, with the subsequent development of subhepatic and subdiaphragmatic abscesses. Immediately after perforation, gastroduodenal secretions may flood the peritoneal cavity causing a chemical peritonitis. After 12–24 hr, bacterial peritonitis evolves, greatly increasing the mortality.

Sharp, severe, sudden-onset epigastric pain suggests perforation, which may or may not have been preceded by PUD symptoms. Shoulder pain reflects diaphragmatic irritation. Nausea may occur but vomiting and back pain are usually absent. A relative relief of symptoms has been described after the initial chemical peritonitis as the irritants are diluted with exudate from the peritoneal reaction. A typical patient presents in serious distress, lying quietly with knees drawn up and breathing shallowly. Abdominal rigidity, epigastric tenderness, tympany to percussion due to escaped air, and reduced/absent bowel sounds are also characteristic. The abdomen is "rigid as a board, silent as a grave." Patients are initially afebrile. If treatment is delayed, continued escape of enteric gas results in abdominal distention. Older patients may present less acutely without classical findings. Many of these atypical perforations occur in patients already hospitalized for other conditions, and the addition of new-onset abdominal pain is not appreciated. Serial abdominal x-rays should be obtained in this situation. Leak from a small duodenal ulcer may trace down the right lateral paracolic gutter and produce pain and rigidity in the RLQ (Valentino's sign) thereby confusing the diagnosis with acute appendicitis.

A mild leukocytosis (12,000 WBCs/mm^3) is common early, but after 12–24 hr white cell counts of 20,000 cells/mm^3 are noted. A mild rise in serum amylase may be expected due to absorption from the peritoneal cavity. Chest or abdominal roenterograms reveal free subdiaphragmatic air in 85% of cases. The left lateral decubitus position, which displaces air over the right lobe of the liver, may be more practical in the uncomfortable patient. If no free air is demonstrated, and the clinical findings are consistent perforated ulcer, an upper gastrointestinal series with gastrograffin contrast should be performed.

Severity of illness and mortality rate correlate directly with the time interval between perforation and surgical repair. The first step is to pass a nasogastric tube to reduce further contamination of the peritoneal cavity. Laboratory tests and x-rays should be obtained, and intravenous (IV) antibiotics (see Table 1) and IV fluids given. Operation and suture closure of perforation reinforced with omentum is a time tried and proven repair. Laparoscopic methods are reported to have less postoperative pain, fewer chest infections, and shorter hospital stay than in open repair, although most reports are testimonial, with one exception (40). All fluid should then be aspirated from the peritoneal cavity. In the case of bleeding "kissing ulcers," vagotomy and gastroenterostomy or pyloroplasty should be performed. Perforated anastomotic ulcers require vagotomy or partial gastrectomy (antrectomy).

There is a 15% overall mortality rate with perforated peptic ulcer, higher with increased age, female sex, and gastric perforations. Indeed, among patients 70 years and older the postoperative death rate may be as high as 41% (40). Delay in treatment, advanced age, and associated systemic diseases are consistent predictors of poor outcome.

3.8. Abdominal Trauma

Serious trauma refers to life-threatening injuries that require specialized surgical care for the patient to survive without disability. Patients aged 65 and older account for about 28% of all fatal injuries, even though they constitute only 12% of the population. Deaths from abdominal trauma are predominantly from postinjury hemorrhage and sepsis.

The principles for management of abdominal trauma change little with age; however, older patients are more intolerant of both shock and exploratory laparotomy. Penetrating abdominal injuries may cause sepsis if they perforate a hollow viscus, and therefore violating the peritoneal cavity; this results in increasing abdominal tenderness or hypovolemia, which demand surgical exploration. When the depth of injury is in question, local exploration assist in determining the presence of peritoneal penetration. All gunshot wounds should be explored as the incidence of intra-abdominal injuries exceeds 90% (41). Blunt trauma results from rapid deceleration, and fixed, noncompressive organs such as the liver, spleen, pancreas, and kidneys are at greatest risk of injury. Occasionally, hollow organs may be injured and lead to sepsis.

Diagnostic modalities include the "focused assessment with sonography for trauma" (FAST) scan, CT, diagnostic laparoscopy, diagnostic peritoneal lavage (DPL), and exploratory laparotomy. FAST scan is rapid, repeatable, and accurate for detecting intra-abdominal fluid or blood (42,43). CT is noninvasive, qualitative, and accurate for the diagnosis of intra-abdominal injury. In the stable patient who suffered a penetrating wound, diagnostic laparoscopy can repair certain injuries as well as quickly establish whether peritoneal penetration has occurred and thus lowering the number of negative laparotomies. The use of DPL has declined since the advent of FAST; however, it is very sensitive and specific for detecting intra-peritoneal blood and signs of perforation. The main indications for exploratory laparotomy are signs of peritonitis and unexplained hypovolemia.

Colon injuries are often associated with postoperative infection so the surgeon should attempt to divert the fecal stream or exteriorize the injury in major trauma. Wounds that involve less than one-half the bowel should be repaired primarily if vascular supply remains intact. Primary repair is contraindicated in patients who are in shock or require multiple transfusions. A delay of more than 6 hr between injury and operation or an extensive wound is relative contraindications to primary repair. Small, clean rectal wounds can be closed primarily. Larger rectal injuries should be treated with proximal diversion and presacral drains. Irrigation of the peritoneal cavity should also be performed. The internist or geriatrician is likely to become involved in consultation for postoperative sepsis. The CT is most useful to detect postoperative abscess or leak from visceral repair. Advice on antimicrobials is based on the expectation of polymicrobial, mixed aerobic, and anaerobic flora. If the patient has been in the ICU for more than 72 hr receiving broad-spectrum antibiotics, organisms may be typical of tertiary peritonitis and include *Enterococcus*, *Staphylococcus*, *Pseudomonas*, and other resistant gram-negative bacteria. In this setting culture and susceptibility results are paramount in antimicrobial selection. The death rate from visceral injuries in the elderly may be up to 80% depending on the severity of injury (41).

REFERENCES

1. Etzioni DA, Liu JH, O'Connell JB, Maggard MA, Ko CY. Elderly patients in surgical workloads: a population-based analysis. Am Surg 2003; 69:916–965.
2. Fenyo G. Acute abdominal disease in the elderly: experience from two series in Stockholm. Am J Surg 1982; 143:751–754.

3. Adelman RD, Berger JT, Macina LO. Critical care for the geriatric patient. Clin Geriatr Med 1994; 10:19–30.

4. Cooper G. Intra-abdominal infection: differences in presentation and outcome between younger patients and the elderly. Clin Infect Dis 1994; 19:146–148.

5. Freeman A, Gordon M. Dermatologic diseases and problems. In: Cassel CK, Leipzig RM, Cohen HJ, Carson EB, Meier DE, eds. Geriatric Medicine. An Evidence-Based Approach. 4th ed. New York: Springer-Verlag, 2003:869–881.

6. Knudson RJ, Lebowitz MD, Holberg CJ, Burrows B. Changes in the normal maximal expiratory flow-volume curve with growth and aging. Am Rev Respir Dis 1983; 127: 725–734.

7. Brenner BM, Meyer TW, Hostetter TH. Dietary protein intake and the progressive nature of kidney disease: the role of hemodynamically mediated glomerular injury in the pathogenesis of progressive glomerular sclerosis in aging, renal ablation and intrinsic renal disease. N Engl J Med 1982; 307:652–659.

8. Farthmann EH, Schoffel U. Epidemiology and pathophysiology of intraabdominal infections (IAI). Infection 1998; 26:329–334.

9. Margiotta SJ Jr, Horwitz JR, Willis IH, Wallack MK. Cholecystecomy in the elderly. Am J Surg 1988; 156:509–512.

10. Raymond DP, Pelletier SJ, Crabtree TD, Schulman AM, Pruett TL, Sawyer RG. Surgical infection and the aging population. Am Surg 2001; 67:827–832 (discussion 832–833).

11. Solomkin JS, Mazuski JE, Baron EJ, Sawyer RG, Nathens AB, DiPiro JT, Buchman T, Dellinger EP, Jernigan J, Gorbach S, Chow AW, Bartlett J. Infectious Diseases Society of America. Guidelines for the selection of anti-infective agents for complicated intra-abdominal infections. Clin Infect Dis 2003; 37:997–1005.

12. Solomkin JS, Wilson SE, Christou NV, Rotsetin OD, Dellinger EP, Bennison RS, Pak R, Tack K. Results of a clinical trial of clinafloxacin versus imipenem/cilastatin for intra-abdominal infections. Ann Surg 2001; 233:79–87.

13. Calandra T, Billie J, Schneider R, Mosimann F, Francioli P. Clinical significance of candida isolated from peritoneum in surgical patients. Lancet 1989; 2:1437–1440.

14. Nathens AB, Rotstein OD, Marshall JC. Tertiary peritonitis: clinical features of a complex nosocomial infection. World J Surg 1998; 22:158–163.

15. Evans HL, Raymond DP, Pelletier SJ, Crabtree TD, Pruett TL, Sawyer RG. Tertiary peritonitis (recurrent diffuse or localized disease) is not an independent predictor of mortality in surgical patients with intraabdominal infection. Surg Infect (Larchmt) 2001; 2:255–263 (discussion 264–265).

16. Koperna T, Schulz F. Relaparotomy in peritonitis: prognosis and treatment of patients with persisting intraadominal infection. World J Surg 2000; 24:32–37.

17. Pelletier SJ, Raymond DP, Crabtree TD, Gleason TG, Pruett TL, Sawyer RG. Outcome analysis of intraabdominal infection with resistant gram-positive organisms. Surg Infect (Larchmt) 2002; 3:11–19.

18. Christou NV, Barie PS, Dellinger EP, Waymack JP, Stone HH. Surgical infection. Society intra-abdominal infection study. Prospective evaluation of management techniques and outcome. Arch Surg 1993; 128:193–198 (discussion 198–199).

19. Lau WY, Fan ST, Yiu TF, Chu KW, Lee JM. Acute appendicitis in the elderly. Surg Gynecol Obstet 1985; 161:157–160.

20. Kraemer M, Franke C, Ohmann C, Yang Q. Acute Abdominal Pain Study Group. Acute appendicitis in late adulthood: incidence, presentation, and outcome. Results of a prospective multicenter acute abdominal pain study and a review of the literature. Langenbecks Arch Surg 2000; 385:470–481.

21. Frymark WB Jr, Jonasson O. Acute appendicitis in the elderly. IMJ III Med J 1986; 169:158–161.

22. Beart R. Diverticular disease of the colon. In: Cameron JL, ed. Current Surgical Therapy. 7th ed. St Louis: Mosby, 2001:179–180.

23. Watters JM, Blakslee JM, March RJ, Redmond ML. The influence of age on the severity of peritonitis. Can J Surg 1996; 39:142–143.
24. Podnos YD, Jiminez JC, Wilson SE. Intra-abdominal sepsis in the elderly persons. Clin Infect Dis 2002; 35(1):62–68.
25. Morrow DJ, Thompson J, Wilson SE. Acute cholecystitis in the elderly: a surgical emergency. Arch Surg 1978; 113:1149–1152.
26. Glenn F, McSherry CK. Calculous biliary tract disease. Curr Probl Surg 1975; June:1–38.
27. Strohl EL, Diffenbaugh WG, Baker JH. Gangrene and perforation of the gallbladder. Surg Gynecol Obstet 1962; 114:1–7.
28. Houghton PW, Jenkinson LR, Donaldson LA. Cholecystectomy in the elderly: a prospective study. Br J Surg 1985; 72:220–222.
29. Lillemoe KD. Surgical treatment of biliary tract infections. Am Surg 2000; 66:138–144.
30. Horton J, Bilhartz L. Gallstone disease and its complications. In: Feldman M, Friedman L, Sleisenger M, eds. Fortran's Gastrointestinal and Liver Disease: Pathophysiology, Diagnosis, Management. Philadelphia: WB Saunders, 2002:1065–1095.
31. Hanau LH, Steigbigel NH. Acute (ascending) cholangitis. Infect Dis North Am 2000; 14:521–546.
32. Leung JW, Chung SC, Sung JJ, Banez VP, Li AK. Urgent endoscopic drainage for acute suppurative cholangitis. Lancet 1989; 1:1307–1309.
33. Crowder VH Jr, Cohn I Jr. Perforation in cancer of the colon and rectum. Dis Colon Rectum 1967; 10:415–420.
34. Kelley WE Jr, Brown PW, Lawrence W Jr, Terz JJ. Penetrating, obstructing, and performing carcinomas of the colon and rectum. Arch Surg 1981; 116:381–384.
35. Chen HS, Sheen-Chen SM. Obstruction and perforation in colorectal adenocarcinoma: an analysis of prognosis and current trends. Surgery 2000; 127:370–376.
36. Nieuwenhuijs VB, Besselink MG, van Minnen LP, Gooszen HG. Surgical management of acute necrotizing pancreatitis: a 13-year experience and a systematic review. Scand J Gastroenterol Suppl 2003:111–116.
37. Clancey TE, Ashley SW. Current management of necrotizing pancreatitis. Adv Surg 2002; 36:103–121.
38. Freeny PC, Hauptmann E, Althaus SJ, Traverso LW, Sinanan M. Percutaneous CT-guided catheter drainage of infected acute necrotizing pancreatitis: techniques and results. AJR Am J Roentgenol 1998; 170:969–975.
39. Svanes C. Trends in perforated peptic ulcer: incidence, etiology, treatment, and prognosis. World J Surg 2000; 24:277–283.
40. Siu WT, Leong HT, Law BK, Chau CH, Li AC, Fung KH, Tai YP, Li MK. Laparoscopic repair for perforated peptic ulcer: a randomized controlled trial. Ann Surg 2002; 235:313–319.
41. Uccheddu A, Floris G, Atlanta ML, Pisanu A, Cois A, Farci SL. Surgery for perforated peptic ulcer in the elderly. Evaluation of factors influencing prognosis. Hepatogastroenterology 2003; 50:1956–1958.
42. Macho JR, Krupski WC, Lewis FR. Management of the injured patient. In: Way LW, Doherty G, eds. Current Surgical Diagnosis and Treatment. 11th ed. New York: Lange Medical Books/McGraw-Hill, 2003:230–266.
43. Udobi KF, Rodriguez A, Chiu WC, Scalea TM. Role of ultrasonography in penetrating abdominal trauma: a prospective clinical study. J Trauma 2001; 50:475–479.

SUGGESTED READING

Cooper G. Intra-abdominal infection: differences in presentation and outcome between younger patients and the elderly. Clin Infect Dis 1994; 19:146–148.

Farthmann EH, Schoffel U. Epidemiology and pathophysiology of intraabdominal infections (IAI). Infection 1998; 26:329–334.

Podnos YD, Jiminez JC, Wilson SE. Intra-abdominal sepsis in the elderly persons. Clin Infect Dis 2002; 35(1):62–68.

Raymond DP, Pelletier SJ, Crabtree TD, Schulman AM, Pruett TL, Sawyer RG. Surgical infection and the aging population. Am Surg 2001; 67:827–832 (discussion 832–833).

Solomkin JS, Mazuski JE, Baron EJ, Sawyer RG, Nathens AB, DiPiro JT, Buchman T, Dellinger EP, Jernigan J, Gorbach S, Chow AW, Bartlett J. Infectious Diseases Society of America. Guidelines for the selection of anti-infective agents for complicated intra-abdominal infections. Clin Infect Dis 2003; 37:997–1005.

Watters JM, Blakslee JM, March RJ, Redmond ML. The influence of age on the severity of peritonitis. Can J Surg 1996; 39:142–143.

33
Viral Hepatitis

Abbasi J. Akhtar and Made Sutjita
Department of Internal Medicine, Division of Infectious Diseases, Charles R. Drew University of Medicine and Science, Martin Luther King, Jr.–Charles R. Drew Medical Center, Los Angeles, California, U.S.A.

Key Points:

- Viral hepatitis may be an underdiagnosed condition in the elderly because high-risk behavior, a significant risk factor for this disease, is considered less likely in this age group.
- Decreased regenerative capacity of the aging liver may contribute to higher mortality due to viral hepatitis.
- The decline in cell-mediated immune response seen with aging may be associated with a higher propensity for the hepatitis B career state.
- Effective antiviral agents such as interferon, lamivudine, and adefovir are available for the treatment of infection with the hepatitis B virus.
- Pegylated interferons and ribavirin combination therapy is the mainstay therapy in hepatitis C virus infection.

1. INTRODUCTION

It is predicted that by the year 2050 approximately 78 million Americans will be aged ≥ 65 years and 18 million ≥ 85 years (1). Hence, caring for the elderly will require increasing awareness of certain diseases and disabilities in this population. There is a relative unawareness among the primary care healthcare providers about the significance of viral hepatitis in the elderly population. Viral hepatitis is a worldwide disease, caused mainly by hepatotropic viruses, including A, B, C, D, and E, or less commonly by nonhepatotropic viruses such as the herpes group of viruses. Although there is a plethora of published information about this subject, the data are scant about viral hepatitis in the elderly population. There is a high threshold for the screening and treatment of viral hepatitis in the elderly with a presumption that this age group has negligible, if any, high-risk behavior and/or exposure for viral hepatitis compared with younger individuals. Consequently, elderly patients with viral hepatitis may remain undiagnosed until they present with more severe disease such as fulminant liver failure or the complications of cirrhosis, such as gastrointestinal bleeding, encephalopathy, and hepatocellular carcinoma.

Table 1 Characteristics of Viral Hepatitides

	HAV	HBV	HCV	HDV	HEV
Transmission (usual mode)	Enteral	Parenteral	Parenteral	Parenteral	Enteral
Incubation period (days)	15–50	30–180	15–180	30–180	15–70
Diagnosis	IgM anti-HAV	IgM anti-HBc HBsAg, HBV-DNA	anti-HCV HCV-RNA	IgM anti-HDV	IgM anti-HEV HEV-RNA
Chronic liver disease	No	Yes	Yes	Yes	No
Association with HCC	No	Yes	Yes	Yes	No
Specific treatment	—	Interferon, lamivudine, adefovir	Interferon, ribavirin	—	—
Vaccine availability	Yes	Yes	—	—	—

Abbreviations: HAV, hepatitis A virus; HBV, hepatitis B virus; HCV, hepatitis C virus; HDV, hepatitis D virus; HEV, hepatitis E virus; HCC, hepatocellular carcinoma.

The aging liver maintains its anatomical integrity and physiological capacity reasonably well. However, decreased regenerative capacity of the aging liver (2) may contribute to increased mortality following a microbial or toxic injury. This review will elaborate contemporary management of viral hepatitis in the population in general and highlight unique aspects of such antiviral treatment in the elderly.

Common clinical varieties of viral hepatitis include hepatitis A, B, C, D, and E (Table 1). Both hepatitis A and hepatitis E are often self-limiting diseases, acquired by fecal–oral transmission, and hence require no specific therapy. Hepatitis B and hepatitis D are transmitted parenterally and have a tendency for chronicity. Hepatitis C spreads by parenteral routes and is associated with the highest chronicity rate among the viral hepatitides. Various forms of viral hepatitides cannot be distinguished from each other clinically or by biochemical tests, and hepatitis serology is necessary for accurate diagnosis. Currently available antiviral therapies for hepatitis B and hepatitis C show promising results; however, novel treatments for these infections continue to evolve. Vaccination against hepatitis A and hepatitis B are available. Although the overall incidence of hepatitis A and hepatitis B may be less in the elderly in comparison to younger individuals, older individuals suffer from higher morbidity and mortality from these illnesses.

2. HEPATITIS A

Hepatitis A is generally a benign and self-limited condition. However, it may be associated with increased morbidity and mortality in elderly patients. Forbes et al. in their study (3) found that the mortality rate of patients with hepatitis A over a period of 6 years was 0.03–0.06% in the group aged 25–35 years. The mortality rate increased 100-fold to 3–6% for patients >55 years old and close to 15% in patients >75 years of age.

2.1. Epidemiology and Clinical Relevance

Hepatitis A virus (HAV) is single-stranded RNA virus belonging to the family Picornaviridae. Fecal–oral transmission is the predominant mode of HAV transmission; however, by virtue of initial viremia, parenteral transmission of HAV is possible (4,5). Therefore, prevalence of HAV antibody is inversely proportional to the sanitary conditions. The incidence of hepatitis A is decreasing globally with improvement in the standards of hygiene and socioeconomic development. Outbreaks of new cases of hepatitis A are reported from otherwise low-prevalence areas because of decrease in immunity (6–8). HAV is reported to be the cause of fever in 1–2% of nonimmunized travelers returning from high-risk areas, after a stay of a month or more (9).

2.2. Clinical Features

The incubation period of HAV infection is about 30 days, with a range of 15–50 days. Many cases remain clinically undiagnosed. Symptoms, when present, may include flu-like illness, fever, anorexia, nausea, vomiting, diarrhea, abdominal pain, and fatigue. Physical signs when present are also nonspecific including mild jaundice, mild to moderate tenderness in the right upper quadrant of the abdomen, and dark urine. Fulminant hepatic failure (FHF) because of massive hepatocyte necrosis may occasionally occur. FHF is associated with a high mortality (>80%) unless timely liver transplantation is available. Those at high risk of FHF due to HAV include persons having hepatitis B, hepatitis C, alcoholic liver disease, chronic liver disease due to other causes, and the elderly. However, those who survive from FHF, regain normal liver function; there is no carrier state. Hepatitis A does not cause chronic liver disease or cirrhosis.

2.3. Diagnosis

History, physical findings, and routine laboratory tests including elevated liver enzymes are of only suggestive value, and a definitive diagnosis of acute hepatitis A is based on the presence of IgM anti-HAV antibody in the serum. IgG anti-HAV is more of an epidemiological importance, as it does not distinguish between current and past infection.

2.4. Management

No specific antiviral therapy is available for HAV. Most mild to moderate cases may be managed as outpatients. Patients should be advised to take adequate rest, generous fluid intake, and a healthy appetizing diet and to avoid alcohol and hepatotoxic medications. Frail elderly patients with moderate disease and patients with more severe illness should be hospitalized, and clinicians must be vigilant of early signs of hepatic decompensation and impending FHF such as encephalopathy. FHF should be managed in the intensive care unit setting and a liver transplant center should be consulted early, rather than as a last resort, for patients who can tolerate this procedure. It is unclear what an appropriate age cutoff is for eligibility for a liver transplant.

2.5. Prevention

Principles of basic sanitation should be observed, including enteric precautions, good hand washing by healthcare providers and household (10) after contact with patient, and safe sex. Immunoglobulin containing HAV antibodies may provide short-term protection to susceptible individuals against HAV and may also be helpful in postexposure prophylaxis in household or sexual contacts of the patient with HAV infection (11). Long-term protection can be acquired by HAV vaccination with a high success rate. Currently available HAV vaccines, including HAVRIX (SmithKline Beecham) and VAQTA (Merck), have high immunogenicity and excellent safety profiles (12). Ideally, HAV vaccine should be included in universal vaccination regimen to all susceptible individuals including children and newborn babies. HAV vaccination must be offered to all high-risk groups for HAV infection, including children in areas where HAV is endemic, travelers (including nonimmune elderly) (13) to areas where HAV is common, men who have sex with men (MSM), household or sexual contacts of an infected person, and users of illicit drugs. Elderly persons, hepatitis B virus (HBV) carriers, and individuals with chronic liver disease due to HBV, hepatitis C virus (HCV), or other causes, are more prone to severe complications of HAV and should be vaccinated if susceptible to HAV (14,15).

3. HEPATITIS B

3.1. Epidemiology and Clinical Relevance

HBV is an important cause of acute and chronic liver disease affecting more than 350 million people worldwide. Prevalence of HBV is higher in Africa, Southeast Asia, China, and the Mediterranean countries. In the United States 250,000 cases of acute viral hepatitis are reported annually due to HBV, about half of these remain asymptomatic, and 5% develop chronic disease. HBV belongs to the Hepadnaviridae family of hepatotropic viruses. Prior to current blood screening strategies, at least 10% of HBV infection was blood transfusion related. Currently, intravenous drug abuse, homosexuality, and high-risk sexual practices are the common modes of transmission of HBV. Such practices are relatively uncommon in the elderly as compared with their younger counterparts. However, hepatitis B transmission has been demonstrated in nursing homes for the elderly. Therefore, susceptible nursing home residents should be considered for vaccination (16). Definite source of infection may not be identified in up to 50% cases of HBV. Some intravenous drug users may have dual infection with both hepatitis B and hepatitis C viruses. Hepatitis B infection may also coexist with human immunodeficiency virus (HIV) infection. The prevalence of serological markers of HBV in alcoholics is significantly higher than in the general population (17). The combined impact of HBV infection and alcohol results in enhanced liver injury and a significantly higher incidence of cirrhosis and hepatocellular carcinoma (18).

3.2. Clinical Features

The incubation period of HBV infection is longer than HAV, ranging from several weeks to 6 months. During this period the patient may transmit infection and yet remain asymptomatic. Clinical spectrum of HBV infection varies from subclinical stage, acute hepatitis without presence of jaundice, to chronic hepatitis or asymptomatic carrier. Elderly patients have been reported to have a higher tendency of becoming HBV carriers after acute HBV infection, perhaps due to age-related decline in immune competence (19). Fifty percent of all patients who develop HBV infection, remain asymptomatic throughout the period of their illness. Approximately one-third of patients infected with HBV develop acute hepatitis, which is clinically indistinguishable from other viral hepatitides. Mortality rate is reported to be higher in elderly patients 3–6%, as compared to 0.1–1.0% in the younger persons.

FHF is the main cause of death in acute HBV infection, whereas complications of cirrhosis such as gastrointestinal bleeding and hepatocellular carcinoma are the main causes of long-term mortality. Although HBV is a hepatotropic virus, hepatic injury is probably immune mediated and not due to direct HBV toxicity (20). Extrahepatic manifestation such as serum sickness-like syndrome presenting as urticaria, arthritis, and fever, may precede hepatitis in some patients. Other extrahepatic manifestations include polyarteritis nodosa (21), glomerulonephritis (22), essential mixed cryoglobulinemia (23), and aplastic anemia (24). Extrahepatic manifestations may be caused by direct pathogenic effect of HBV or via immune complexes (25).

3.3. Diagnosis

Like other viral hepatitides, diagnosis of HBV infection is based on the presence of its serological markers. Hepatitis B surface antigen (HBsAg) appears within 6 weeks after infection and is usually cleared by 3 months. Hepatitis e antigen (HBeAg) appearing soon after HBsAg indicates active viral replication. Antibody to hepatitis B core antigen (anti-HBc) appears in acute phase. High titers of IgM anti-HBc indicate acute HBV infection whereas lower titers of IgG anti-HBc along with antibody to hepatitis B surface antigen (anti-HBsAg) indicate past infection and immunity. Hepatitis B viral DNA (HBV DNA) level in serum is the most precise marker of active viral replication.

3.4. Management

Management of acute HBV infection is supportive and most often can be carried out at the patient's home or nursing home. Symptomatic supportive measures including maintenance of adequate hydration and nutrition and avoiding hepatotoxic medications including alcohol may suffice. The aim of antiviral therapy in chronic HBV infection is to stop HBV replication and eradicate it if possible, in order to prevent the progression of liver disease and its complication such as cirrhosis and hepatocellular carcinoma (HCC). Loss of HBeAg in serum and sustained suppression of serum HBV DNA to undetectable levels, normalization of liver chemistry, and improvement in liver histology are the key indicators of successful therapy (26,27).

Interferon alpha (INF-α) (subcutaneous injections, 5 million units daily or 10 million units three times weekly) for at least 16 weeks and antiviral agent, lamivudine 100 mg orally for 52 weeks, are approved by the Food and Drug Administration for treatment for chronic HBV, and are indicated in patients with elevated serum aminotransferases and HBV DNA levels $>10^5$ copies/mL. The exact mechanism of action of interferon is not clear; it may be a combination of antiviral and immunomodulatory effects. The latter effect of interferon is manifested by increase in transaminases just before clearance of HBeAg. Therefore, interferon treatment is contraindicated in HBV patients with advanced liver disease at the risk of precipitating liver failure. Side effects of interferon therapy include flu-like syndrome, leucopenia, thrombocytopenia, and depression and many patients, especially the elderly, cannot tolerate interferon therapy. In the management of chronic HBV infection in the elderly, particular attention should be given to the screening of hepatocellular carcinoma and the presence of serious comorbidities. Not all elderly patients with HBV infection require antiviral therapy. Risk and benefits of treatment, current state of health, severity of liver disease, and HBV DNA level should be considered in making treatment decisions. Lamivudine may be the preferred therapy due to its better tolerability. Dose adjustment of lamivudine may only be necessary in the presence of renal insufficiency (27). Successful vaccination of the elderly against HBV is feasible and should be recommended to all susceptible patients in general and to high-risk nursing home patients in particular.

Seroconversion from HBeAg to anti-HBeAb along with biochemical improvement is noticed only in 30% of patients (28). However, a reduction in the risk of HCC is reported following successful therapy with interferon (29). Serum alanine aminotransferase (ALT) levels before starting treatment is a reliable predictor of response. Higher pretreatment ALT levels are associated with a better response, whereas normal ALT levels predict poor response. No correlation has been demonstrated between pretreatment serum HBV DNA levels or histological activity index with HBeAg seroconversion (30).

The advantages of lamivudine, a nucleoside analog, are that it is administered orally, inhibits HBV replication, is effective in clearance of HBV DNA from serum, and has fewer side effects as compared with INF-α. However, recurrence of viremia and development of YMDD mutant lamivudine-resistant HBV strains are the major shortcomings of therapy. Combination therapy with INF-α and lamivudine has not shown to be more effective against HBV infection than monotherapy with either of these two drugs. A novel therapeutic agent, adefovir dipivoxil (10 mg orally daily), appears to be safe, effective, and well tolerated; other agents being studied for more effective and safer therapy of HBV infection include tenofovir, emtricitabine, famciclovir, and entecavir (31) (see also chapter "Antiviral Drugs").

3.5. Prevention

Currently available recombinant hepatitis B vaccines include Energix-B and Recombivax HB. More recently, Twinrix, a combined HAV and HBV vaccine, has also become available (32). Three doses of vaccines are administered intramuscularly into deltoid muscle over a 6-month period. Antibodies are produced against HBsAg, and anti-HBs titers of 10 mIU/mL or higher are considered protective for a period of 15–20 years or more. Elderly patients and immunocompromised patients may have suboptimal response to vaccination and a second vaccination series may be helpful (33). Hepatitis B immunoglobulin (HBIG) 0.04–0.07 mL/kg should be given along with the first dose of vaccine in cases of postexposure prophylaxis (34).

4. HEPATITIS C

4.1. Epidemiology and Clinical Relevance

Approximately 170 million people, i.e., 3% of the world's population, are infected with HCV. In the United States, about 4 million people are infected with HCV and of these, approximately 2.7 million have ongoing infection. Although during recent years the incidence of HCV infection in developed countries has fallen, its prevalence remains high. Prior to modern screening measures HCV was the most common cause of post-transfusion hepatitis. At present, sharing the needles among illicit drug users is the main mode of transmission of HCV. Other less efficient modes of transmission of HCV include sexual activity, perinatal contact, and accidental exposure as in healthcare workers. The source of exposure remains undetermined in some patients. Hepatitis C is the most frequent cause of viral hepatitis in older adults.

HCV is an RNA virus belonging to *Hepacivirus* genus of the Flaviviridae family. HCV genotypes 1a and 1b account for 75% of HCV infections in the United States. More genotypes and quasispecies are being recognized (35). The exact role of ethnicity in the prevalence of disease progression of HCV is unclear but appears to be substantial. Serum iron, ALT levels, histological disease activity index, and response to treatment were significantly lower in African–American as compared with Caucasian patients (36). In the United States HCV-associated cirrhosis is an important cause of hepatocellular carcinoma and is the most common reason for liver transplantation; HCV accounts for approximately 12,000 deaths every year. Approximately three-fourths of infected persons will develop chronic infection with approximately one-quarter going on to cirrhosis. As the population ages, it is anticipated that there will be an increasing number of individuals with chronic hepatitis C infection.

4.2. Clinical Features

The incubation period of HCV ranges between 2 and 26 weeks (average 6 weeks). Heterogeneity of HCV helps it escape detection by the host immune system for a long time. Consequently, acute HCV may be an unnoticed benign event. Patients may remain asymptomatic and unaware of infection and being potentially infectious, while disease progresses. Symptoms are present only in one-third of the patients and jaundice is noticed in only 20% patients. Up to 70% of patients infected with HCV proceed to chronicity, 85% having persistent infection and at high risk of developing cirrhosis and HCC. The spectrum of extrahepatic manifestations is wider than in other viral hepatitides. Extrahepatic manifestation similar to those observed in HBV infection can also occur in HCV infection (37). In addition, pulmonary fibrosis (38), type 2 diabetes mellitus (39), dermatological manifestations (40), corneal ulceration (41), pancreatitis (42), etc., have been reported.

4.3. Diagnosis

Enzyme immunoassay anti-HCV antibody (EIA) is an initial screening test, the latest version being EIA-3, which is simple to perform and is widely available. Recombinant immunoblot assay (RIBA-3) is a more specific anti-HCV antibody test used to eliminate the false-positive EIA test. However, when treatment is planned the standard test of choice is measurement of viral load by quantitative HCV-RNA by polymerase chain reaction (PCR) or signal amplification methods. This test serves as a reliable guide for the beginning, monitoring, completing, and success or failure of therapy.

4.4. Management

The aim of antiviral therapy is to eliminate the HCV from blood and achieve sustained viral remission, whereas the long-term goal is to prevent or halt the progression of liver disease and prevent its complication such as cirrhosis and hepatocellular carcinoma. Although all HCV-infected patients should be considered for therapy, not everybody will be eligible for it. The decision of intent to treat will have to be individualized. The treatment of acute hepatitis C has not been well studied because of its declining incidence and the difficulty in recognizing it during the acute stage. Choices include immediate therapy (43) with INF-α 2b for 24 weeks or wait and watch for spontaneous recovery (44). Patient motivation, prescription drug coverage, and financial factors, absence of significant comorbidity, uncontrolled psychiatric illness or thyroid disease, and pancytopenia are important considerations for initiating treatment. The patient's full understanding and cooperation are of paramount importance in the management of HCV. Therefore, patients should receive optimal information in the form of brochures, videos, and health personnel counseling. In particular, information should be provided about the risks of consuming excess alcohol substance abuse and intravenous drug abuse. Younger patients should be warned about the risk of serious consequences of pregnancy during therapy or shortly thereafter. Experience in treating older hepatitis patients with interferon is limited. Age, independent of physiological function or comorbidities, does not appear to affect response rates. The most important factors to determine whether older patients may be considered for interferon therapy will be motivation, comorbidities, presence of psychiatric disorders, and cognitive capacity. Viral genotype and HCV-RNA level should be obtained before starting therapy. Liver biopsy is useful and informative but not mandatory in all patients. Baseline liver chemistries and complete blood count should be obtained and used as a reference for subsequent visits to monitor response and potential toxicity of the therapy. Two formulations of pegylated interferon are currently licensed in the United States: IFN-α-2b 1.5 μg/kg body weight or IFN-α-2a 180 μg subcutaneously once a week along with oral ribavirin 13–15 mg/kg daily. Neutrophil count, platelet count, and hemoglobin should be checked at 2 and 4 weeks after the start of therapy and throughout the duration of therapy for necessary modification of therapy. Patients in whom the HCV-RNA level fails to drop by 1–2 logs during the first 12 weeks of combined therapy are unlikely to respond and continuation of therapy any longer may be futile. A virologic response is determined by the absence of detectable HCV-RNA by PCR after the first 6 months of therapy. Sustained virologic response is indicated by the absence of HCV-RNA 6 months after the completion of the therapy. Viral relapse has been reported in 50–75% of patients treated with IFN monotherapy, 30–45% of patients treated with nonpegylated combination therapy, and 15% of patients treated with pegylated combination therapy. Re-treating with the same agent is not indicated. However, re-treating the nonresponders to monotherapy with combination therapy using pegylated IFN may be successful (45). New developments in treatment are awaited (46). Response to conventional therapy in African–Americans (47) and the elderly is less favorable as compared with younger patients. The associated comorbidities adversely affect the prognostic outcome and preclude use of more effective combination therapy with ribavirin. Safer and more effective therapies are needed in this group of the fastest growing population (48,49) (see also chapter "Antiviral Drugs").

4.5. Prevention

Immunoglobulin, given previously, has not shown any reliable evidence of protection after exposure to HCV. Attempts to develop a vaccine against HCV have been futile and yet no vaccine is available. However, patients infected with HCV should be offered vaccination against hepatitis A and B if found susceptible. Healthcare counseling regarding standard hygienic precautions should be offered to the patients and to those at high risk of infection.

5. HEPATITIS D

Hepatitis delta virus (HDV) infection is present globally. The presence of HBsAg in blood is required for HDV to cause infection as it is a defective RNA-virus (50). Consequently, the incidence of HDV infection is directly proportional to the prevalence of HBV prevalence in any community. Infection with HDV can be acquired simultaneously along with HBV or may occur later as superinfection. HDV infection increases the severity of liver disease due to HBV and hastens the development of cirrhosis. Prevalence data are not available on HDV infection in the elderly or in nursing home residents. The diagnosis of HDV infection is based on detection of anti-HDV antibody in serum or hepatitis D antigen in liver. The treatment with INF-α is effective in a minority of patients. Liver transplantation if feasible is a valid option for advanced HDV infection. Prevention of HBV prevents HDV as well (51).

6. HEPATITIS E

Hepatitis E virus (HEV) is a RNA virus usually transmitted by fecal–oral route (52). Therefore, it is more prevalent in areas of poor sanitation and contaminated water supply. Parenteral transmission is rare. In the United States HEV infection is mainly diagnosed in returning travelers. However, HEV is the most common cause of enterically transmitted non-A hepatitis in the developing countries. The diagnosis of HEV infection is made by finding anti-HEV antibodies in serum. The incubation period ranges from 2 to 10 weeks. Clinical and biochemical features of HEV infection mimic other forms of viral hepatitides. Fulminant hepatitis is rare except in pregnant women, particularly in the third trimester, in whom the mortality may be as high as 25%. Chronic HEV infection has not been reported. There is no specific therapy for HEV infection nor is any vaccine available yet. Reports on HEV infection in the elderly are lacking or inadequate to make any conclusions about their role in this population.

7. NOVEL AND PRESUMED HEPATOTROPIC VIRUSES

Non-A through E viral hepatitis has been an enigma until recent years, when newer viral agents including the hepatitis G virus (53), virus GB agent (54), TT virus (55), and SEN virus (56) are being recognized. However, their natural history, epidemiology, and exact clinical relevance have yet to be determined. There are no standard diagnostic tests or specific treatment available at present, and their role in infection and morbidity in the elderly are unknown.

REFERENCES

1. Schneider EL. Aging in the third millennium. Science 1999; 283:796–797.
2. Sanz N, Diez-Fernandez C, Alvarez AM, Fernandez-Simon L, Cascales M. Age-related changes on parameters of experimentally-induced liver injury and regeneration. Toxicol Appl Pharmacol 1999; 154:40–49.
3. Forbes A, Williams R. Increasing age—an important adverse prognostic factor in hepatitis A virus infection. J R Coll Physicians Lond 1988; 4:237–239.
4. Grinde B, Stene-Johansen K, Sharma B, Hoel T, Jensenius M, Skaug K. Characterization of an epidemic of hepatitis A virus involving intravenous drug abusers: infection by needle sharing? J Med Virol 1997; 53:69–75.
5. Bell BP, Shapiro CN, Alter MJ, Moyer LA, Judson FN, Mottram K, Fleenor M, Ryder PL, Margolis HS. The diverse pattern of hepatitis A epidemiology in the United States-implication for vaccination strategies. J Infect Dis 1998; 178:1579–1584.
6. Cuthbert JA. Hepatitis A: old and new. Clin Microbiol Rev 2001; 14:38–58.
7. Brown GR, Persley K. Hepatitis A epidemic in the elderly. South Med J 2002; 95: 826–833.
8. Willner IR, Howard SC, Williams EQ, Riely CA, Waters B. Serious hepatitis A: an analysis of patients hospitalized during an urban epidemic in the United States. Ann Intern Med 1998; 128:111–114.
9. Steffen R. Risk of hepatitis A in travelers: the European experience. J Infect Dis 1995; 171:S24–S28.
10. Floreani A, Chiaramonte M. Hepatitis in nursing homes. Incidence and management strategies. Drugs Aging 1994; 5:96–101.
11. Center for Disease Control and Prevention. Prevention of hepatitis A through active or passive immunization: recommendations of the Advisory Committee on Immunization Practices. MMWR 1999; 48(RR12):1–37.

12. Ashur Y, Adler R, Rowe M, Shouval D. Comparison of immunogenicity of two hepatitis A vaccines VAQTA and HAVRIX in young adults. Vaccine 1999; 17:2290–2296.

13. Leder K, Weller PF, Wilson ME. Travel vaccines and elderly persons: review of vaccines available in the United States. Clin Infect Dis 2001; 33:1553–1566.

14. Kemmer NM, Miskovsky EP. Hepatitis A. Infect Dis Clin North Am 2000; 14:605–615.

15. Pramoolsinsap C, Poorvorawan Y, Hirsch P, Busagorn N, Attamasirikul K. Acute, hepatitis-A super-infection in HBV carriers, or chronic liver disease related to HBV or HCV. Ann Trop Med Parasitol 1999; 93:745–751.

16. Sugauchi F, Mizokami M, Orito E, Ohno T, Kato H, Maki M, Suzuki H, Ojika K, Ueda R. Hepatitis B virus infection among residents of a nursing home for the elderly: seroepidemiological study and molecular evolutionary analysis. J Med Virol 2000; 62:456–462.

17. Laskus T, Radkowski M, Lupa E, Horban A, Cianciara J, Slusarczyk J. Prevalence of markers of hepatitis viruses in out-patient alcoholics. J Hepatol 1992; 15:174–178.

18. Shiomi S, Kuroki T, Minamitani S, Ueda T, Nishiguchi S, Nakajima S, Seki S, Kobayashi K, Harihara S. Effect of drinking on the outcome of cirrhosis inpatients with hepatitis B or C. J Gastroenterol Hepatol 1992; 7:274–276.

19. Kondo Y, Tsukada K, Takeuchi T, Mitsui T, Iwano K, Masuko K, Itoh T, Tokita H, Okamoto H, Tsuda F. High carrier rate after hepatitis B virus infection in the elderly. Hepatology 1993; 18:768–774.

20. Chisari FV, Ferrari C. Hepatitis B virus immunopathogenesis. Annu Rev Immunol 1995; 13:29–60.

21. Guillevin L, Lhote F, Cohen P, Sauvaget F, Jarrousse B, Lortholary O, Noel LH, Trepo C. Polyarteritis nodosa related to hepatitis B virus. A prospective study with long-term observation of 41 patients. Medicine 1995; 74:238–253.

22. Conjeevaram HS, Hoofnagle JH, Austin HA, Park Y, Fried MW, Di Bisceglie AM. Long-term outcome of hepatitis B virus-related glomerulonephritis after therapy with interferon alfa. Gastroenterology 1995; 109:540–546.

23. Cesur S, Akin K, Kurt H. The significance of cryoglobulinemia in patients with chronic hepatitis B and C virus infection. Hepatogastroenterology 2003; 50:1487–1489.

24. Brown KE, Tisdale J, Barrett J, Dunbar CE, Young NS. Hepatitis-associated aplastic anemia. N Engl J Med 1997; 336:1059–1064.

25. Trepo C, Guillevin L. Polyarteritis nodosa and extrahepatic manifestations of HBV infection: the case against autoimmune intervention in pathogenesis. J Autoimmun 2001; 16:269–274.

26. Lok AS, Heathcote EJ, Hoofnagle JH. Management of hepatitis B 2000—summary of a workshop. Gastroenterology 2001; 120:1828–1953.

27. Merle P, Trepo C, Zoulim F. Current management strategies for hepatitis B in the elderly. Drugs Aging 2001; 18:725–735.

28. Wong DK, Cheung A, O'Rourke K, Naylor CD, Detsky AS, Heathcote J. Effect of alpha-interferon in patients with hepatitis B e antigen-positive chronic hepatitis B: a meta-analysis. Ann Intern Med 1993; 119:312–323.

29. Ikeda K, Saitoh S, Suzuki Y, Kobayashi M, Tsubota A, Fukuda M, Koida I, Arase Y, Chayama K, Murashima N, Kumada H. Interferon decreases hepatocellular carcinogenesis in patients with cirrhosis caused by hepatitis B virus: a pilot study. Cancer 1998; 82:827–835.

30. Chien RN, Liaw YF, Atkins M. Pretherapy alanine transaminase level as a determinant for hepatitis B e antigen seroconversion during lamivudine therapy in patients with chronic hepatitis B. Asian Hepatitis Lamivudine Trial Group. Hepatology 1999; 30:770–774.

31. Ganem D, Prince AM. Hepatitis B virus infection—natural history and clinical consequences. N Engl J Med 2004; 350:1118–1129.

32. Van Damme P, Van Herck K, Van der Wielen M. Combined hepatitis A and B vaccine in elderly. Vaccine 2004; 22:303–304.

33. Jadoul M, Goubau P. Is anti-hepatitis B virus (HBV) immunization successful in elderly hemodialysis (HD) patients? Clin Nephrol 2002; 58:301–304.

34. Zuckerman JN, Zuckerman AJ. Current topics in hepatitis B. J Infect 2000; 41:130–136.

35. Bukh J, Miller RH, Purcell RH. Genetic heterogeneity of hepatitis C virus: quasispecies and genotypes. Semin Liver Dis 1995; 15:41–63.
36. Howell C, Jeffers L, Hoofnagle JH. Hepatitis C in African Americans: summary of a workshop. Gastroenterology 2000; 119:1385–1396.
37. Mayo MJ. Extrahepatic manifestations of hepatitis C infection. Am J Med Sci 2002; 325:135–148.
38. Ueda T, Ohta K, Suzuki N, Yamaguchi M, Hirai K, Horiuchi T, Watanabe J, Miyamoto T, Ito K. Idiopathic pulmonary fibrosis and high prevalence of serum antibodies to hepatitis C virus. Am Rev Respir Dis 1992; 146:266–268.
39. Mason A, Nair S. Is type II diabetes another extrahepatic manifestation of HCV infection? Am J Gastroenterol 2003; 98:243–246.
40. Schwaber MJ, Zlotogorski A. Dermatologic manifestations of hepatitis C infection. Int J Dermatol 1997; 36:251–254.
41. Wilson SE, Lee WM, Murakami C, Weng J, Moninger GA. Mooren-type hepatitis C virus-associated corneal ulceration. Ophthalmology 1994; 101:736–745.
42. Alvares-Da-Silva MR, Francisconi CF, Waechter FL. Acute hepatitis C complicated by pancreatitis: another extrahepatic manifestation of hepatitis C virus? J Viral Hepatitis 2000; 7:84–86.
43. Jaeckel E, Cornberg M, Wedemeyer H, Santantonio T, Mayer J, Zankel M, Pastore G, Dietrich M, Trautwein C, Manns MP and German Acute Hepatitis C Therapy Group. Treatment of acute hepatitis C with interferon alfa-2b. N Engl J Med 2001; 345: 1452–1457.
44. Hoofnagle JH. Therapy for acute hepatitis C. N Engl J Med 2001; 345:1495–1497.
45. Seeff LB, Hoofnagle JH. National Institute of Health Consensus Development Conference: management of hepatitis C: 2002. Hepatology 2002; 36:S1–S2.
46. Rossi SJ, Wright TL. New developments in the treatment of hepatitis C. Gut 2003; 52:756–757.
47. Theodore D, Shiffman ML, Sterling RK, Bruno CJ, Weinstein J, Crippin JS, Garcia G, Wright TL, Conjeevaram H, Reddy RK, Nolte FS, Fried MW. Intensive interferon therapy does not increase virological response rate in African Americans with chronic hepatitis C. Dig Dis Sci 2003; 48:140–145.
48. Brind AM, Watson JP, James OF, Bassendine MF. Hepatitis C virus infection in the elderly. QJM 1996; 89:291–296.
49. Hayashi J, Kashiwagi S. Hepatitis C virus infection in the elderly. Epidemiology, prophylaxis and optimal treatment. Drugs Aging 1997; 11:296–308.
50. Bean P. Latest discoveries on the infection and coinfection with hepatitis D virus. Am Clin Lab 2002; 21:25–27.
51. Taylor JM. Therapy of HDV. Hepatology 2003; 38:1581–1582.
52. Hyams KC. New perspectives on hepatitis E. Curr Gastroenterol Rep 2002; 4:302–307.
53. Alter MJ, Gallagher M, Morris TT, Moyer LA, Meeks EL, Krawczynski K, Kim JP, Margolis HS. Acute non-A-E hepatitis in the United States the role of hepatitis G virus infection. N Engl J Med 1997; 336:741–746.
54. Simons JN, Desai SM, Mushahwar IK. The GB viruses. Curr Top Microbiol Immunol 2000; 242:341–375.
55. Bendinelli M, Pistello M, Maggi F, Fornai C, Freer G, Vatteroni ML. Molecular properties, biology, and clinical implications of TT virus, a recently identified widespread infectious agent of humans. Clin Microbiol Rev 2001; 14:98–113.
56. Umemura T, Yeo AE, Sottini A, Moratto D, Tanaka Y, Wang RY, Shih JW, Donahue P, Primi D, Alter HJ. SEN virus infection and its relationship to transfusion-associated hepatitis. Hepatology 2001; 33:1303–1311.

SUGGESTED READING

Brown GR, Persley K. Hepatitis A epidemic in the elderly. South Med J 2002; 95:826–833.

Center for Disease Control and Prevention. Prevention of hepatitis A through active or passive immunization: recommendations of the Advisory Committee on Immunization Practices. MMWR 1999; 48(RR12):1–37.

Keeffe EB, Dieterich DT, Han SH, Jacobson IM, Martin P, Schiff ER, Tobias H, Wright TL. A treatment algorithm for the management of chronic hepatitis B virus infection in the United States. Clin Gastroenterol Hepatol 2004; 2:87–106.

Seeff LB, Hoofnagle JH. National Institute of Health Consensus Development Conference: management of hepatitis C: 2002. Hepatology 2002; 36:S1–S2.

Van Damme P, Van Herck K, Van der Wielen M. Combined hepatitis A and B vaccine in elderly. Vaccine 2004; 22:303–304.

34
Urinary Tract Infection

L. E. Nicolle
Departments of Internal Medicine and Medical Microbiology, University of Manitoba, Health Sciences Centre, Winnipeg, Manitoba, Canada

Key Points:

- The clinical diagnosis of urinary tract infection in cognitively and functionally impaired elderly patients is often not straightforward.
- Factors to consider in antimicrobial selection include efficacy of the agent for urinary infection, patient tolerance, patient renal function, and the potential for an antimicrobial resistant organism.
- An appropriately collected urine specimen should be obtained for culture prior to initiation of antimicrobial therapy for the treatment of urinary infection.
- Asymptomatic bacteriuria is common in elderly populations and should not be screened for or treated except prior to a genitourinary intervention with a high likelihood of mucosal trauma and bleeding.
- Pyuria accompanies most urinary tract infections, but does not differentiate symptomatic from asymptomatic infection for treatment in the absence of acute symptoms attributable to urinary infection.

1. EPIDEMIOLOGY AND CLINICAL RELEVANCE

Urinary tract infection is the most common bacterial infection that occurs in elderly populations. It is considered acute uncomplicated urinary infection when it presents as acute cystitis in women with a normal genitourinary tract (1). These women also experience acute nonobstructive, or uncomplicated, pyelonephritis. Complicated urinary infection occurs in individuals with functional or structural abnormalities of the genitourinary tract (1). Asymptomatic bacteriuria is isolation of microorganisms in a urine specimen with quantitative counts consistent with infection in the absence of acute signs or symptoms attributable to urinary infection. A characteristic of elderly individuals with urinary infection is the high frequency of recurrence. Recurrent infection is considered a reinfection if the infecting organism originates outside the urinary tract, and relapse if the infection recurs with an organism that has persisted within the urinary tract.

Urinary infection in elderly populations is generally considered to be complicated urinary tract infection. For older men, infection is most frequently attributable to benign prostatic hypertrophy with urethral obstruction and turbulent urine flow, and chronic bacterial prostatitis. For women, abnormalities such as increased postvoid residual urine volume, cystoceles, and bladder diverticuli all contribute. Women with a genetic predisposition for acute uncomplicated cystitis, which manifests with infection at younger ages, remain at increased risk of infection in the postmenopausal period (2). Thus, urinary infection occurring in elderly female populations reflects both a genetic propensity, and increased frequency of genitourinary abnormalities in postmenopausal women. Urinary infection is a common problem in residents of nursing homes (3). Associated comorbidities, especially chronic neurologic illnesses that lead to impaired voiding, are likely the major determinants of urinary infection in this setting. The use of indwelling catheters and, for men, condom drainage, is an additional important contributor to infection (4).

Urinary infection is an important cause of morbidity in elderly populations. While acute cystitis is less frequent in older women than in young sexually active women, hospitalization rates for urinary infection are higher in older women (5). For men, urinary infection is rare prior to 60 years of age, but after age 60 there is a substantial morbidity, including hospitalization, attributable to urinary infection. In the relatively well elderly resident in the community, even mild symptomatic episodes interfere with social function. New or increased incontinence associated with urinary infection may be particularly troubling for patients and their families. In long-term care facilities, symptomatic urinary infection is second only to respiratory infections as a site of infection (3). Urinary infection is the most common cause of bacteremia in elderly populations presenting to acute care emergency departments or who are resident in long-term care facilities, but is an infrequent cause of mortality. While symptomatic urinary infection does cause morbidity in elderly populations, most urinary infection is asymptomatic. Asymptomatic bacteriuria is not associated with excess morbidity or mortality (6).

Geriatric populations exhibit a wide range of health status including chronic medical illnesses and functional impairment. The spectrum extends from the healthy elderly individual resident in the community to the fully dependent bed-bound resident in a nursing home. The risks of developing infection and the relative impacts of infection vary depending on comorbidities and functional status. This discussion of urinary infection is presented in the context of the elderly population living in the community, representing the relatively well elderly, and the population in the nursing home, representing the frail and impaired elderly. However, there are substantial variations among individuals in both these groups, and unique characteristics of the individual must always be considered, regardless of the residential location.

2. ETIOLOGIC PATHOGENS

The most important uropathogen in elderly populations is *Escherichia coli*. However, a wide range of other organisms may also be isolated, consistent with the spectrum of infecting organisms in other populations with complicated urinary infection (Table 1). The infecting organism is influenced by prior antimicrobial therapy, noso-comial exposure, and the presence of indwelling catheters. Enterobacteriaceae other than *E. coli*, such as *Klebsiella* spp., *Citrobacter* spp., and *Enterobacter* spp. are frequent. Urease producing organisms including *Proteus mirabilis*, *Morganella morganii*, and *Providencia stuartii* are also common. These organisms may be associated with renal and bladder stone formation, but despite a very high

Table 1 The Relative Frequency of Isolation of Bacterial Species in Elderly Subjects with Urinary Infection According to Residence Status

| | Percentage of infections with organism isolated | | | | |
| | Community | | Long-term care facility | | |
Organism	Women	Men	Women	Men	CIC
Escherichia coli	75	44	54	25	10–37
Klebsiella spp.	5.3	6.3	11	8.3	3–21
Citrobacter spp.			3.6		
Enterobacter spp.	3.5	13	1.8	2.7	
Proteus mirabilis	11	19	25	67	9–36
Providencia spp.				28	5–61
M. morganii				2.7	5–19
P. aeruginosa	2	19	3.6	33	5–30
Other gram-negative bacteria					7–16
Enterococcus spp.			1.8	5.6	7–28
Coagulase-negative staphylococci				2.7	1–9
Other gram-positive bacteria					5–20

Abbreviation: CIC, chronic indwelling catheter.

prevalence of *P. mirabilis* infection in male nursing home patients, urolithiasis has not been identified as a significant problem in these populations. *Pseudomonas aeruginosa* and other nonfermenting gram-negative species are also isolated. Gram-positive organisms are common, including enterococci species, coagulase-negative staphylococci, and group B streptococci. *Staphylococcus aureus* and other streptococcal species are less frequent. Yeast species are occasionally isolated, usually from patients characterized by risk factors including diabetes mellitus, presence of chronic indwelling catheters, and exposure to broad-spectrum antibiotics. *Candida albicans* is most common, but other species such as *C. tropicalis*, *C. glabrata*, *C. parapsilosis*, and *C. kreusii* also occur.

Specific organism virulence factors in elderly populations are likely similar to younger populations. Bacteremic *E. coli* strains from elderly subjects without urinary obstruction express the pap G adhesin and other potential virulence factors such as hemolysin or aerobactin (7). The prevalence of virulence factors is much lower in *E. coli* strains isolated from persons with structural abnormalities, consistent with complicated urinary infection. There is relatively little information describing potential virulence factors in infecting organisms other than *E. coli*.

About 5–10% of elderly nursing home patients have voiding managed by chronic indwelling catheters (4). These catheters, and other indwelling urinary devices such as ureteric stents or nephrostomy tubes, are exposed continuously to the urinary stream and become coated with a biofilm within a few days of insertion. The biofilm is a complex organic material that includes microorganisms, extracellular substances produced by these microorganisms, and urinary components such as calcium, magnesium, and Tamm–Horsfall protein. There are usually at least three to five organisms growing in the biofilm. Urease-producing organisms are common, and struvite formation associated with these organisms may lead to catheter obstruction. Microorganisms in the biofilm live in a relatively protected environment. Antimicrobials in the urine and the host immune and inflammatory response have limited efficacy in eradicating these organisms. Thus, organisms persist in the biofilm despite antimicrobial therapy, facilitate emergence of antimicrobial resistant organisms, and are a source for relapse of both symptomatic and asymptomatic urinary infection (8).

3. CLINICAL MANIFESTATIONS

The clinical manifestations of symptomatic urinary infection in elderly individuals are often consistent with those recognized in younger populations. Cystitis, or bladder infection, is characterized by lower tract irritative symptoms including frequency, dysuria, urgency, and suprapubic pain. An additional common symptom in elderly individuals, particularly women, is new or worsening incontinence. Patients with pyelonephritis, or kidney infection, present with costovertebral angle pain or tenderness with or without fever or associated lower tract irritative symptoms. While older populations have an attenuated febrile response compared with younger patients, the majority of elderly individuals with significant infection, including severe pyelonephritis, will have fever (9).

The symptoms of urinary infection differ for residents with chronic indwelling catheters. While these patients may present with costovertebral angle pain or tenderness, consistent with pyelonephritis, fever without localizing genitourinary symptoms is a more common presentation of urinary infection. A resident with a chronic indwelling catheter and fever without localizing findings will have a urinary source in 30–50% of sporadic episodes (10). Urinary infection presenting with fever alone in subjects with chronic indwelling catheters likely reflects mucosal trauma from the catheter, or the large bioburden of organisms in the associated biofilm.

4. DIAGNOSIS

4.1. Clinical Manifestations

The presence of characteristic upper or lower urinary tract symptoms may be reliable indicators for the clinical diagnosis of urinary infection. However, for the functionally impaired elderly, including many nursing home residents, the diagnosis may be problematic (3). Characterization of symptoms is impaired by limitations in communication due to hearing loss, aphasia, or cognitive impairment. Evaluation is also hampered by chronic symptoms accompanying chronic illness, such as chronic incontinence, frequency, or nocturia. In the nursing home population, over 50% of men or women with incontinence and cognitive impairment have asymptomatic bacteriuria at any time. The most highly functionally impaired elderly are most likely to have both chronic genitourinary symptoms and asymptomatic bacteriuria. Because these patients usually have a positive urine culture at any time, any change in clinical status, regardless of whether localizing genitourinary signs or symptoms are present, is frequently diagnosed as acute urinary infection. However, in the absence of acute genitourinary symptoms, fever without localizing symptoms or signs in bacteriuric noncatheterized residents is attributable to urinary infection in only 10% of episodes (10). Unfortunately, there are no clinical variables other than presence of an indwelling catheter that are useful to identify the episodes likely attributable to urinary infection. Thus, in the absence of localizing genitourinary symptoms, the diagnosis of symptomatic urinary infection should be made cautiously in functionally impaired nursing home residents.

An additional problem in the management of residents of long-term care facilities is a complaint of cloudy or foul smelling urine, especially in incontinent residents. Pyuria accompanies bacteriuria in most long-term care residents (6). Cloudy urine may be attributable to pyuria, but other potential causes, such as urinary phosphate crystals, may be an explanation. While bacteriuria may be associated with an unpleasant odor through production of volatile amines by bacteria in the urine, the odor is neither sensitive nor specific to identify bacteriuria. Subjective urine characteristics such as cloudiness or foul smell, in the absence of other symptoms, are not indications for antimicrobial therapy irrespective of whether bacteriuria is present. One potential approach to management, when possible, is to increase fluid intake to dilute the urine.

4.2. Urine Culture

A urine specimen for culture should be obtained prior to institution of antimicrobial therapy in any elderly individual where a clinical diagnosis of urinary infection is entertained. A positive urine culture not only confirms the clinical diagnosis but also identifies the specific infecting organism with antimicrobial susceptibility to assist in therapeutic decisions.

The microbiologic diagnosis of urinary infection is based on the quantitative count of organisms isolated from the urine specimen. Specimens must be collected in a manner to minimize contamination by periurethral or, in women, vaginal secretions, and be forwarded expeditiously to the laboratory for processing. A clean-catch specimen obtained with voiding is adequate for most women. A voided specimen is not feasible for some women, especially with significant functional impairment. In-and-out catheterization should be performed to collect a specimen from these women when there is a clinical indication. Urine specimens obtained from bedpans or diapers are subject to considerable contamination, and are not appropriate. For men, a clean-catch midstream specimen can usually be obtained. When voiding is managed using a condom catheter, a clean catheter and leg bag should be applied and the urine specimen collected immediately after voiding. For subjects with indwelling urethral catheters, the urine specimen should be obtained by aspiration through the sampling port or tubing, and not from the drainage bag.

For voided urine specimens in men or women, $\geq 10^5$ colony-forming units (cfu)/mL is the appropriate quantitative count of organisms to identify symptomatic urinary infection. Lower quantitative counts of $\geq 10^3$ cfu/mL have been suggested to be appropriate for voided specimens from ambulatory men, but this criterion has not been validated for elderly populations. If the specimen is collected by condom drainage, $\geq 10^5$ cfu/mL is as the appropriate quantitative criterion (3). Quantitative counts of $\geq 10^2$ cfu/mL are consistent with acute uncomplicated cystitis in premenopausal women, but have not been evaluated in elderly women. As the majority of elderly subjects are considered to have complicated urinary infection, the criterion of $\geq 10^5$ cfu/mL seems most appropriate, pending further evaluation of quantitative urine cultures in well-characterized older populations. Lower quantitative counts may occur in patients experiencing diuresis due to renal failure, diuretic therapy, or hydration. In clinical situations where symptomatic urinary infection is a diagnostic consideration and lower quantitative counts of potential uropathogens are isolated, the relevance of the urine specimen results should be interpreted critically in the context of the clinical presentation. In most cases, lower quantitative counts will likely represent contamination.

When urine specimens are obtained by either indwelling or in-and-out urethral catheterization, any quantitative bacterial growth is considered significant. A urine specimen collected through a chronic indwelling catheter reflects the microbiology of the biofilm as well as the urine. Where symptomatic urinary infection is diagnosed, the chronic catheter should be replaced immediately prior to the initiation of antimicrobial therapy. A urine specimen obtained from the freshly placed catheter will reflect the microbiology of bladder urine rather than the biofilm, and is more relevant for treatment decisions (8).

4.3. Other Diagnostics Tests

Pyuria uniformly accompanies symptomatic urinary infection. In elderly populations, pyuria is also present in at least 90% of nursing home patients with asymptomatic bacteriuria (6). The presence or degree of pyuria in a subject with asymptomatic bacteriuria has no prognostic significance. In particular, it does not predict subsequent development of symptomatic infection, or adverse long-term outcomes such as renal failure or mortality. Thus, the presence or absence of pyuria does not differentiate symptomatic and asymptomatic infection and is not, by itself, an indication for antimicrobial treatment.

Additional diagnostic tests may be indicated in subjects presenting with more severe clinical findings, including sepsis syndrome. Appropriate investigations may include blood cultures, peripheral leukocyte count, and an assessment of renal function including blood urea nitrogen and serum creatinine. If urinary obstruction or other abnormalities are present or suspected, further investigations to identify obstruction or abscess, including a renal or pelvic ultrasound or other diagnostic imaging, should be considered. These investigations are indicated not only to characterize abnormalities that increase the likelihood of infection, but also may direct therapeutic interventions such as drainage, where necessary.

5. ANTIBIOTIC TREATMENT

5.1. Asymptomatic Bacteriuria

Asymptomatic bacteriuria should not be treated in elderly individuals. Prospective, randomized comparative trials have consistently failed to document benefits with treatment of asymptomatic bacteriuria in these populations (6). Antimicrobial treatment does not decrease the frequency of symptomatic urinary infection, including episodes of fever without localizing signs or symptoms. Chronic genitourinary symptoms, particularly chronic incontinence, are not improved with antimicrobial therapy. There is no improved survival with antimicrobial treatment. There are, however, negative clinical outcomes reported with antimicrobial treatment of asymptomatic bacteriuria. These include an increased frequency of adverse antimicrobial effects, increased likelihood of reinfection with more resistant bacteria, and increased costs. Recurrence of bacteriuria following treatment is expected. At least 50% of elderly nursing home residents will be bacteriuric again by 4 weeks after discontinuation of therapy (3,11). Thus, maintaining sterile urine through treatment of asymptomatic bacteriuria is not a realistic therapeutic goal. Treatment of asymptomatic bacteriuria in nursing home residents is unnecessary and increases the intensity of antimicrobial exposure contributing to the high prevalence of resistant organisms in some nursing homes.

Pyuria accompanies asymptomatic bacteriuria for at least 90% of nursing home subjects. The pyuria persists as long as bacteriuria is present. About 30% of nursing home residents without bacteriuria also have pyuria. The presence or absence of pyuria, or the degree of pyuria, has not been shown to have any prognostic significance. Thus, for elderly subjects with asymptomatic bacteriuria, the presence of pyuria in a urine specimen is not an indication for antimicrobial therapy.

The exceptional situation, when asymptomatic bacteriuria should be treated, is in elderly subjects who undergo invasive genitourinary manipulations with a high risk of mucosal trauma and bleeding. Following procedures such as transurethral resection of the prostate, about 60–70% of bacteriuric men have bacteremia, and 6–15% may have sepsis syndrome. In fact, antimicrobial therapy in this situation should be considered prophylactic therapy to prevent bacteremia and sepsis, rather than treatment of bacteriuria. A urine specimen for culture should be obtained within 1 week prior to the procedure. Antimicrobial selection should be directed by the organisms isolated, and initiated only shortly before the procedure—within 12 hr. In the absence of an indwelling catheter, antimicrobial therapy does not need to be continued beyond the procedure. When an indwelling catheter remains in place, therapy is usually continued until the catheter is removed. Prophylactic antimicrobial therapy is not indicated for all invasive procedures. It should be considered only for procedures with a high likelihood for mucosal trauma with bleeding. For instance, antimicrobial therapy is not required prior to replacement of a chronic indwelling catheter, as bacteremia is uncommon with this manipulation (3).

5.2. Symptomatic Infection

The optimal treatment of symptomatic infection in elderly populations is based upon a precise knowledge of the microbiology obtained from the urine or blood culture, which identifies the specific infecting organism and susceptibilities. When symptoms are mild, antimicrobial therapy should be withheld until urine culture results are available. For patients with moderate or severe symptoms, empirical therapy is initiated but should be reassessed at 48–72 hr, when culture results are available. Parenteral therapy is indicated for individuals with severe systemic manifestations including high fever, hemodynamic instability, nausea or vomiting, where gastrointestinal absorption is problematic, or where the infecting organism is resistant to available oral antimicrobials. Other considerations relevant to initiating therapy include known or anticipated antimicrobial resistance, and patient tolerance. For all patients, renal function, prior history of adverse reactions, and potential interactions with other medications must be evaluated. If underlying genitourinary abnormalities are present or suspected, they should be fully characterized by appropriate diagnostic or functional studies. The presence of abnormalities may influence the effectiveness of therapy. For patients with chronic indwelling catheters, the catheter should be replaced immediately prior to institution of antimicrobial therapy. Apart from allowing more appropriate specimen collection, catheter replacement removes much of the biofilm, and decreases the likelihood of early symptomatic relapse following therapy (10).

5.3. Comparative Clinical Trials in Elderly Populations

Comparative clinical trials of antimicrobial treatment for symptomatic urinary infection in elderly patients are summarized in Table 2. Given the magnitude of the problem of urinary infection in elderly populations and the large number of potentially affected individuals, there is remarkably little systematic evaluation of the relative efficacy and safety of different antimicrobial regimens. Most of these few studies are compromised by small study numbers, failure to fully characterize the study population, and, for some, enrollment of both asymptomatic and symptomatic patients. One notable study is that by Gomolin et al. (18). This nonblinded study was adequately powered and enrolled a diverse population of elderly women with symptomatic urinary infection. It reported improved clinical and bacteriologic

Table 2 Comparative Clinical Trials of Antimicrobial Therapy for Treatment of Urinary Infection in Elderly Populations

Population (Ref.)	Antibiotic regimens, days	No. of subjects	Short-term cure number (%)
Not stated (12), symptoms not stated	Norfloxacin 400 mg bid, 7	20	19 (95)
	Amoxicillin 250 mg tid, 7	20	15 (75)
Ambulatory (13), symptoms not stated	Norfloxacin 400 mg bid, 10	17	15 (88)
	Amoxicillin 250 mg tid, 10	18	11 (61)
"Geriatric patients" (14)	Ciprofloxacin 100 mg bid, 5	16	16 (100)
	Trimethoprim 200 mg bid, 5	16	12 (75)
Hospitalized (15), 10% asymptomatic	Norfloxacin 400 mg bid, 3	49	42 (86)[a]
	Trimethoprim 300 mg qd, 3	51	35 (69)[a]
"Geriatric patients" (16)	Cefetamet 2 g qd, 10	18	16 (89)
	Cefadroxil 2 g qd, 10	21	14 (67)
Nursing home (17)	Ofloxacin 200 mg qd or bid, 10	12 ⎫	
	Ciprofloxacin 500 mg bid, 10	13 ⎬	24 (96)
Community and nursing home, women (18)	Ciprofloxacin 250 bid, 10	129	108 (96)[a]
	TMP–SMX 160/800 bid, 10	132	95 (87)[a]

[a] $p < 0.05$.
Abbreviations: TMP-SMX, trimethoprim–sulfamethoxazole; bid, two times a day; tid, three times a day; qd, daily.

outcomes with ciprofloxacin compared with trimethoprim/sulfamethoxazole, with part of this improved efficacy attributable to an increased frequency of trimethoprim–sulfamethoxazole-resistant isolates.

A few other comparative studies have analyzed urinary infection outcomes stratified by age. For women presenting with acute cystitis, 3-day therapy with a β-lactam antimicrobial cured 74% of women over 50 years compared with 94% under 30 years (19). In another study, outcomes with either lomefloxacin or trimethoprim–sulfamethoxazole for 14 days in ambulant men or women with complicated urinary infection were similar for subjects greater or less than 60 years (20).

Clinical trials of treatment of urinary infection, including those performed for licensure of new antimicrobials, frequently restrict enrollment to individuals <65 years of age. This further compromises our knowledge of optimal therapeutic regimens for elderly populations. Effectively, this means that antimicrobials are marketed, and frequently intensely used, for treatment of urinary infection without prior evaluation in elderly populations. Overall, the knowledge base on which to develop specific recommendations for treatment of symptomatic urinary infection in elderly patients is limited, and is required further investigation.

5.4. Antimicrobial Agents

Agents for treatment of urinary infection are listed in Table 3. Antimicrobial selection or dose is not influenced by age itself. There is a consistent decline in renal function with aging, but this is highly variable among individuals, and dose modification is based on individual renal function rather than age. Preferred antimicrobials are those with renal excretion that achieve high urinary levels, have limited toxicity, and a narrow bacterial spectrum. Substantial prior experience with the antimicrobial in treatment of urinary infection is preferred.

First-line oral agents, depending on organism susceptibility and patient tolerance, include trimethoprim–sulfamethoxazole, trimethoprim by itself, amoxicillin, nitrofurantoin and fluoroquinolones such as norfloxacin and ciprofloxacin (1) Cephalosporins are not generally recommended for first-line therapy because of their broad-spectrum activity, but are effective for susceptible organisms and may be appropriate depending on patient tolerance. More recently introduced fluoroquinolones such as levofloxacin or gatifloxacin are effective for urinary infection, but there is relatively limited experience with these agents, and they do not appear to provide a therapeutic advantage for treatment of urinary infection over earlier fluoroquinolones. Concerns about QT prolongation on electrocardiogram and hypoglycemia in patients on oral hypoglycemic therapy are also a consideration with these agents. Nitrofurantoin has been used for many years as an effective agent for treating lower urinary infections. Although other antibiotics have become first-line treatment for urinary infections in recent times, nitrofurantoin may be prescribed in older adults with lower urinary infections that fail to respond to other antibiotics. However, patients with renal impairment (creatinine clearance $< 60 \, mL/min$) should not be prescribed nitrofurantoin (see also chapter "Nitrofurans").

First-line empirical parenteral therapy remains an aminoglycoside–gentamicin or tobramycin together with ampicillin if enterococcus is of concern. Following initiation of parenteral therapy, a clinical response will generally be observed within 48–72 hr, when urine culture results are usually available. If the clinical status has stabilized, a change to oral therapy with an antimicrobial selected based on known

Table 3 Antimicrobials for Treatment of Urinary Infection in Subjects with Normal Renal Function

Agent	Dose	
	Oral	Parenteral
First line		
Amoxicillin/ampicillin	500 mg tid	1 g q4–6 hr
Nitrofurantoin	50–100 mg qid	
Macrocrystals/monohydrate	100 mg bid	
Trimethoprim–sulfamethoxazole	160–800 mg bid	160–800 mg bid
Trimethoprim	100 mg bid	
Gentamicin		1–1.5 mg/kg q8 hr or 4–5 mg/kg q24 hr
Tobramycin		1–1.5 mg/kg q8 hr or 4–5 mg/kg q24 hr
Other		
Amikacin		5 mg/kg q8 hr or 15 mg/kg q24 hr
Amoxicillin–clavulanic acid	500 mg tid	
Aztreonam		1–2 g q6 hr
Cefaclor	500 mg qid	
Cefadroxil	1 g qd or bid	
Cefepime		2 g q12 hr
Cefixime	400 mg qd	
Cefotaxime		1–2 g q8 hr
Cefpodoxime proxetil	100–400 mg bid	
Ceftriaxone		1–2 g q24 hr
Ceftazidime		0.5–2 g q8 hr
Cefuroxime axetil	250 mg bid	
Cephalexin/cefazolin	500 mg qid	1–2 g q8 hr
Ciprofloxacin	250–500 mg bid	200–400 mg q12 hr
Gatifloxacin	400 mg qd	
Imipenem-cilastatin		500 mg q6 hr
Lomefloxacin	400 mg qd	400 mg qd
Norfloxacin	400 mg bid	
Ofloxacin	200–400 mg bid	400 mg bid
Piperacillin		3 g q4 hr
Piperacillin–tazobactam		4 g/500 mg q8 hr
Vancomycin		500 mg q6 hr or 1 g q12 hr

Abbreviations: qd, daily; bid, two times a day; tid, three times a day.

susceptibilities is usually possible. Short-term empirical therapy, with early review of clinical status and culture results to reassess whether continued parenteral therapy with an aminoglycoside is appropriate, will limit ototoxicity or nephrotoxicity with aminoglycoside use. Additional practical benefits of aminoglycosides are once daily dosing and intramuscularly administration. This facilitates use in many nursing homes, where establishing and maintaining intravenous lines may be problematic. Other empirical parenteral options include extended-spectrum cephalosporins, such as ceftriaxone and ceftazidime, extended-spectrum penicillins, such as piperacillin, or fluoroquinolones.

5.5. Duration of Therapy

The optimal duration of therapy for symptomatic urinary infection is also not well studied for elderly populations. For women who present with acute cystitis, there are concerns that a short course of therapy is less effective in older than in younger women, and 5–7 days of therapy is suggested. However, a recent prospective, randomized trial of 3 or 7 days' ciprofloxacin reported similar cure rates for both treatment durations, and decreased adverse effects for 3-day therapy (21). This study enrolled women of mean age 78.7 years, with the exclusion of patients with any complicating factors. For men, 7-day therapy for cystitis is recommended. For pyelonephritis, 10–14 days of therapy is recommended for both women and men.

The duration of therapy for treatment of febrile urinary infection in subjects with chronic indwelling catheters has not been adequately studied. It is recommended that as short a course of therapy as possible, usually 7 days, be given if the catheter must remain in place. The continuing presence of the catheter means there is a substantial continuing risk of superinfection. The more prolonged the duration of antimicrobial therapy, the greater the likelihood of resistant organisms emerging, which may complicate further management.

Many antimicrobials diffuse poorly into the prostate. In addition, prostate stones are common in older men and provide a protected nidus for bacteria, which may cause relapsing cystitis. Studies have reported improved outcomes for men with relapsing urinary infection of prostatic origin when retreatment for 6 or 12 weeks is given for recurrence, rather than 7–10 days. More prolonged therapy is assumed to be more effective because the longer antimicrobial course is more likely to eradicate prostatic bacterial foci. However, men enrolled in these studies had asymptomatic bacteriuria, and the relevance of more prolonged therapy for symptomatic infection is not clear. Currently, a man presenting with urinary infection should receive initial therapy for 7–10 days. If a symptomatic relapse with the same organism occurs within 4 weeks following discontinuation of therapy, consideration may be given to a more prolonged course of therapy.

5.6. Follow-Up After Therapy

The anticipated microbiologic outcome for an individual with complicated urinary infection is relapse in over 50% of individuals by 6 weeks. The majority of these individuals will not be symptomatic. Posttreatment urine cultures are not indicated unless the patient has recurrent or persistent symptoms. The goal of therapy is to ameliorate symptoms, not to sterilize the urine.

5.7. Guidelines

Confirming a diagnosis of symptomatic urinary infection in a functionally impaired bacteriuric nursing home resident is frequently, as previously discussed, imprecise. Thus, deciding whether or not to initiate antimicrobial therapy may be problematic. Consensus guidelines have been published with recommendations for minimum clinical criteria to be met prior to initiating empirical antimicrobial therapy in these settings (22). For suspected urinary infection in residents without a chronic indwelling catheter, fever over 38.5°C or an acute confusional state together with any acute localizing genitourinary symptoms are indications for initiation of antimicrobial therapy. Empirical therapy is also appropriate for women with acute, severe dysuria without fever. For residents with indwelling catheters, fever or confusion without localizing genitourinary symptoms or signs is sufficient to initiate antimicrobial therapy. In all cases, a urine culture should be obtained prior to initiating the antimicrobial.

There are few guidelines that address antimicrobial treatment of urinary infection in elderly populations. The Society of Health Care Epidemiology of America Long Term Care Committee position paper on use of antimicrobials in nursing homes makes some recommendations for treatment of urinary infection (11). This paper recommends empiric therapy with trimethoprim–sulfamethoxazole while awaiting urine culture results, and avoidance of broader-spectrum agents such a fluoroquinolones or amoxicillin/clavulanic acid unless there is known or anticipated antimicrobial resistance. Aminoglycosides are recommended for empiric treatment of patients who are ill enough to require parenteral therapy. A treatment duration of 3–7 days for women with cystitis, and 10–14 days for pyelonephritis is recommended. The paper also notes, however, the limited evidence base for development of guidelines, and that specific recommendations are based largely on expert opinion.

6. PREVENTION

6.1. General Approaches

Urinary infection in elderly men and women is usually secondary to voiding abnormalities accompanying chronic comorbid illnesses, prior genitourinary interventions, and, in men, prostatic hypertrophy. The extent to which urinary infection can realistically be prevented given the inability to alter underlying factors that promote infection is questionable. A reasonable goal seems to be to focus prevention on more severe manifestations of infections, such as bacteremia and invasive infection. Early identification and management of obstruction could certainly prevent some serious complications. This is particularly an issue for men, where prostate obstruction is always a consideration. Appropriate use and care of indwelling and condom catheters will prevent some infections. Attention to sterilization and disinfection of equipment and fluids for any urologic procedures is also important.

Some elderly nursing home residents with impaired voiding have bladder emptying managed by intermittent catheterization. A prospective, randomized comparative trial reported that symptomatic urinary infection was similar for nursing home residents managed with intermittent catheterization regardless of whether a clean or sterile catheterization procedure was followed (23). While this is a negative study with respect to prevention of infection, it enlarges our understanding of appropriate catheter management in the long-term care facility. Clean intermittent catheterization is more efficient and cheaper, so should be recommended.

6.2. Nonantimicrobial Interventions

Cranberry juice contains hippuric acid, which is bacteriostatic, and other molecules which have been shown to interfere with adherence of organisms to the bladder wall, at least in vitro. Clinical trials in young women with frequent recurrent acute cystitis have suggested a modest benefit of daily cranberry juice intake in preventing recurrent infection (24). Studies in elderly populations are limited and, to date, do not show a convincing benefit. One study in a nursing home population reported that daily cranberry juice decreased the frequency of bacteriuria associated with pyuria, but not overall prevalence of bacteriuria or episodes of symptomatic infection (25). The interpretation of observations of this study is further limited because subjects randomized to the placebo arm had a greater frequency of urinary infection prior to enrollment, introducing a bias in the comparative groups. Thus, a benefit of cranberry juice in elderly populations remains unproven.

In postmenopausal women, topical vaginal estriol cream in a group of women of mean age 65 years (26) and an estradiol-releasing vaginal ring in women with a mean age of 67 years (27) had significantly decreased episodes of recurrent symptomatic infection in postmenopausal women. Prospective and case–control studies that have evaluated the efficacy of systemic estrogens have consistently reported no decrease in urinary infections with estrogen use. In fact, several studies report increased rates of infection with estrogen use, possibly explained by an increase in sexual activity in women who use systemic estrogens. A prospective, randomized trial of estriol pessaries compared with prophylaxis with nitrofurantoin reported a much greater benefit with nitrofurantoin and no apparent efficacy of the pessary (28). Thus, the use of topical estrogen to prevent urinary infection in elderly women remains controversial. It is likely premature to recommend vaginal estrogen therapy solely for an indication of prevention of urinary infection.

6.3. Antimicrobial Therapy

Prophylactic antimicrobial therapy is effective for the prevention of recurrent acute cystitis in elderly women. Women with recurrent episodes of acute uncomplicated cystitis who receive long-term low-dose prophylactic antimicrobial therapy have a 90–95% decrease in recurrences (27). Only nitrofurantoin has been evaluated specifically in elderly women (27), but it is likely that agents shown to be as effective as nitrofurantoin in younger women are also effective in older women. Trimethoprim–sulfamethoxazole and trimethoprim are, with nitrofurantoin, first-line prophylactic therapy. Norfloxacin or ciprofloxacin may be considered second-line agents for women who cannot be managed with one of the three first-line agents. Long-term low-dose prophylactic antimicrobial is appropriate for women with frequent recurrent infections who are distressed by the symptoms. The role of postcoital prophylaxis in postmenopausal women has not been well studied. Most of these women are less sexually active then younger women, so the role for postcoital prophylaxis needs to be evaluated specifically in this population.

Another use of antimicrobials for "prevention" is in suppressive therapy. This is given not to prevent infection, but to prevent recurrent symptomatic episodes in a clinical setting where cure of the underlying infection may not be achieved. This approach is appropriate for only highly selected patients with persistent genitourinary abnormalities that prevent eradication of infecting bacteria, and who are experiencing frequent and severe symptomatic episodes. Examples include men with recurrent cystitis with bacteria from a prostatic source, or individuals with renal failure. Generally, suppressive therapy is initiated at a full antimicrobial dose. If the patient has a satisfactory clinical response after several weeks, the dose may be decreased to about one-half the daily full therapeutic dose. The duration of therapy is determined by characteristics of the individual patient, and therapy may need to be continued indefinitely. The indication for continuing suppressive therapy should, however, be periodically reevaluated in each patient.

REFERENCES

1. Rubin RH, Shapiro ED, Andriole VT, Davis RJ, Stamm WE. Evaluation of new anti-infective drugs for the treatment of urinary tract infection. Clin Infect Dis 1992; 15(suppl 1):S216–S227.

2. Raz R, Gennesin Y, Wasser J, Stoler Z, Rosenfeld S, Rottensterichh E, Stamm WE. Recurrent urinary tract infections in postmenopausal women. Clin Infect Dis 2000; 30:152–156.

3. Nicolle LE. SHEA Long Term Care Committee—Urinary tract infections in long-term care facilities. Infect Control Hosp Epidemiol 2001; 22:167–175.

4. Nicolle LE. The chronic indwelling catheter and urinary infection in long-term care facility residents. Infect Control Hosp Epidemiol 2001; 22:316–321.

5. Nicolle LE, Friesen D, Harding GKM, Ross LL. Hospitalization for acute pyelonephritis in Manitoba, Canada during the period from 1989 to 1992. Impact of diabetes, pregnancy, and aboriginal origin. Clin Infect Dis 1996; 22:1051–1056.

6. Nicolle LE. Asymptomatic bacteriuria in the elderly. Infect Dis Clin North Am 1997; 11:647–662.

7. Nicolle LE. Urinary tract pathogens in complicated urinary infection and in the elderly. J Infect Dis 2001; 183(suppl 1):S5–S8.

8. Raz R, Schiller D, Nicolle LE. Chronic indwelling catheter replacement prior to antimicrobial therapy for symptomatic urinary infection. J Urol 2000; 164:1254–1258.

9. Bentley DW, Bradley S, High K, Schoenbaum S, Taler G, Yoshikawa TT. Practice guideline for evaluation of fever and infection in long-term care facilities. Clin Infect Dis 2000; 31:640–653.

10. Orr P, Nicolle LE, Duckworth H, Brunka J, Kennedy J, Murray D, Harding GKM. Febrile urinary infection in the institutionalized elderly. Am J Med 1996; 100:71–77.

11. Nicolle LE, Bentley DW, Garibaldi R, Neuhaus EG, Smith PW, the SHEA Long-term Care Committee. Antimicrobial use in long term care facilities. Infect Control Hosp Epidemiol 2000; 21:537–545.

12. Leigh DA, Smith EC, Marriner J. Comparative study using norfloxacin and amoxycillin in the treatment of complicated urinary tract infections in geriatric patients. J Antimicrob Chemother 1984; 13(suppl B):79–83.

13. Hill S, Yeates M, Pathz J, Morgan JR. A controlled trial of norfloxacin and amoxycillin in the treatment of uncomplicated urinary tract infection in the elderly. J Antimicrob Chemother 1985; 15:505–506.

14. Newson SWB, Murphy P, Matthews J. A comparative study of ciprofloxacin and trimethoprim in the treatment of urinary tract infections in geriatric patients. J Antimicrob Chemother 1986; 18(suppl D):111–115.

15. Ewer TC, Barley RR, Gilchrist NL, Aitken JM, Sainsbury R. Comparative study of norfloxacin and trimethoprim for the treatment of elderly patients with urinary tract infection. NZ Med J 1988; 101:537–539.

16. Sourander L, Becq-Giraudon B, Bernstein-Hahn L, Germano G, Kissling M. Cefetamet pivoxil in geriatric patients with complicated urinary tract infection. Drug Invest 1989; 1:34–39.

17. McCue JD, Gaziano P, Orders D. A randomized controlled trial of ofloxacin 200 mg 4 times daily or twice daily vs ciprofloxacin 500 mg twice daily in elderly nursing home patients with complicated UTI. Drugs 1995; 49:368–373.

18. Gomolin IH, Siami PF, Reuning-Scherer J, Haverstock DC, Heyd A. Efficacy and safety of ciprofloxacin oral suspension versus trimethoprim-sulfamethoxazole oral suspension for treatment of older women with acute urinary tract infection. J Am Geriatr Soc 2001; 49:1606–1613.

19. Nicolle LE, Hoepelman AIM, Floor M, Verhoef J, Norgard K. Comparison of three days therapy with cefcanel or amoxicillin for the treatment of acute uncomplicated urinary tract infection. Scand J Infect Dis 1993; 25:631–637.

20. Nicolle LE, Louie TJ, Dubois J, Martel A, Harding GKM, Sinave CP. Treatment of complicated urinary tract infection with lomefloxacin compared with trimethoprim-sulfamethoxazole. Antimicrob Agents Chemother 1994; 38:1368–1373.

21. Vogel T, Verreault R, Gourdeau M, Morin M, Grenier-Gosselin L, Rochette L. Optimal duration of antibiotic therapy for uncomplicated urinary tract infection in older women: a double-blind randomized controlled trial. Can Med Assoc J 2004; 170:469–473.

22. Loeb M, Bentley DW, Bradley S, Crossley K, Gantz N, Garibaldi R, McGeer A, Muder R, Mylotte J, Nicolle LE, Nurse B, Paton S, Simor AE, Smith P, Strausbaugh L. Development of minimum criteria for the initiation of antibiotics in residents of long-term care facilities: results of a consensus conference. Infect Control Hosp Epidemiol 2001; 22:120–124.

23. Duffy LM, Cleary J, Ahern S, Kuskowski MA, West M, Wheeler L, Mortimer JA. Clean intermittent catheterization: safe, cost-effective bladder management for male residents of VA nursing homes. J Am Geriatr Soc 1995; 43:865–870.

24. Raz R, Chazan B, Dan M. Cranberry juice and urinary tract infection. Clin Infect Dis 2004; 38:1413–1419.

25. Avorn J, Monane M, Gurwitz HH, Glynn RJ, Choodnovskiy I, Lipsitz LA. Reduction of bacteriuria and pyuria after ingestion of cranberry juice. J Am Med Assoc 1994; 9:751–754.

26. Raz R, Stamm WE. A controlled trial of intravaginal estriol in postmenopausal women with recurrent urinary tract infections. New Engl J Med 1993; 329:753–756.

27. Eriksen B. A randomized, open, parallel group study on the preventive effect of an estradiol-releasing vaginal ring on recurrent urinary tract infections in postmenopausal women. Am J Obstet Gynecol 1999; 180:1077–1079.

28. Raz R, Colodner R, Rohana Y, Bathino S, Rottensterich E, Wasser I, Stamm W. Effectiveness of estriol-containing vaginal pessaries and nitrofurantoin macrocrystal therapy in the prevention of recurrent urinary tract infection in postmenopausal women. Clin Infect Dis 2003; 36:1362–1368.

SUGGESTED READING

Loeb M, Bentley DW, Bradley S, Crossley K, Gantz N, Garibaldi R, McGeer A, Muder R, Mylotte J, Nicolle LE, Nurse B, Paton S, Simor AE, Smith P, Strausbaugh L. Development of minimum criteria for the initiation of antibiotics in residents of long-term care facilities: results of a consensus conference. Infect Control Hosp Epidemiol 2001; 22:120–124.

Nicolle LE. Asymptomatic bacteriuria in the elderly. Infect Dis Clin North Am 1997; 11:647–662.

Nicolle LE. SHEA Long Term Care Committee. Urinary tract infections in long-term care facilities. Infect Control Hosp Epidemiol 2001; 22:167–175.

Stamm WE, Raz R. Factors contributing to susceptibility of postmenopausal women to recurrent urinary tract infections. Clin Infect Dis 1999; 28:723–725.

Yoshikawa T, Norman D, Nicolle LE. Management of complicated urinary tract infections in elderly patients. J Am Geriatr Soc 1996; 44:1235–1241.

35
Skin and Soft Tissue Infections

Made Sutjita
Department of Internal Medicine, Division of Infectious Disease, Charles R. Drew University of Medicine and Science, Martin Luther King, Jr.–Charles R. Drew Medical Center, Los Angeles, California, U.S.A.

Key Points:

- Skin and soft tissue infections occur commonly in elderly patients.
- The aging skin has increased susceptibility to infections due to physiological changes and associated pathological conditions, i.e., vascular insufficiency and/or lymphedema.
- Because of age-related decline in immune function associated with underlying comorbid conditions, elderly patients may present with more severe forms of soft tissue infection such as cellulitis, necrotizing fasciitis, diabetic foot infection, or infected pressure ulcers with recurrent sepsis.
- Dose adjustment is needed for various antimicrobial agents with renal clearance mechanisms because of age-associated decline in kidney function.
- Immobility, malnutrition, underlying metabolic disease, and vascular insufficiency that occur in debilitated and frail older patients may delay the healing process.

Skin and soft tissue infections are frequently encountered in the elderly. The skin and soft tissue is the third most common site of infection after the urinary and respiratory tracts, respectively, as a recognizable focus for sepsis in the elderly (1). The aging skin is more fragile and susceptible to infection as a consequence of intrinsic physiological changes, the effects of chronic sun exposure, and a variety of common eczematous skin problems which include atopic, seborrheic, contact, and asteatotic eczema. Declining age-related immune function may result in common skin infections such as cellulitis, which present with varying degrees of severity, such as toxic forms of erysipelas or a toxic necrotizing fasciitis, diabetic foot infection, infected pressure ulcers with recurrent sepsis, or herpes zoster infections associated with severe postherpetic neuralgia (PHN) (see also "Herpes Zoster"). Skin and soft tissue infections unique to the elderly will be reviewed in this chapter.

1. GENERAL APPROACH TO SKIN AND SOFT TISSUE INFECTIONS

Physicians examining a discrete skin lesion should determine if the lesion is a localized skin infection or a manifestation of more serious systemic diseases such as bacteremia, fungemia, or seeded septic emboli. Patients should be assessed immediately to ascertain if they are toxic or ill. Toxic appearance is commonly associated with more serious illnesses such as sepsis. Diffuse or rapidly spreading skin lesions are usually manifestations of life-threatening infection and warrant hospital admission, prompt diagnosis, and aggressive medical and surgical management. Frail elderly patients with immune compromised states such as those with poorly controlled diabetes mellitus, chronic liver diseases, malignancy, and acquired immunodeficiency syndrome (AIDS) are prone to severe skin and soft tissue infections compared with younger or immune-competent persons. Immobility commonly results in frail elders in the community or long-term care facilities acquiring pressure ulcers with superimposed infection of the surrounding soft tissue and skin.

2. PRESSURE ULCERS AND INFECTION

2.1. Epidemiology, Risk Factors, and Clinical Criteria

Pressure ulcers, also referred to as decubitus ulcers or pressure sores, are destructive lesions of the skin and subcutaneous tissues with varying degree and depth of involvement of the integument as a result of pressure. Generally, the term pressure sores or pressure ulcers are preferred over decubitus ulcers, due to the variety of locations in which pressure ulcers develop and the multiple precipitating circumstances that cause them. Pressure ulcers frequently occur among elderly patients who are bedridden or unable to reposition themselves. The skin in frail and debilitated elderly patients is thin and friable and associated with less fat and muscle with which to dissipate pressure. Vitamin C deficiency in the elderly may contribute to the fragility of blood vessels and connective tissue and lower the threshold of pressure-induced injury. An age-related decrease in the number of dermal blood vessels may also place an elderly person at risk of ischemic injury caused by pressure and shearing forces. The most common locations for pressure ulcers to develop are the sacrum, ischial tuberosities, greater trochanters, heels, and lateral malleoli (2). The incidence of pressure ulcers among patients in acute care hospitals ranges from 1% to 5% and prevalence rate ranges from 3% to 14%. The prevalence rate of pressure ulcers among patients admitted to skilled nursing facilities ranges between 5% and 25% (3).

Pressure ulcers are the result of soft tissue compression between bony prominences and external surfaces over a period of time causing localized tissue necrosis. Many local and systemic risk factors may contribute to the development of pressure ulcers (4). Local risk factors include: (1) direct pressure to skin and subcutaneous tissue (the greater the pressure, the less the time required for tissue necrosis due to impaired capillary perfusion); (2) shearing forces: when skin and subcutaneous tissue adhere to the linen, movement of the patients either by nursing staff or patient themselves, may shear the underlying blood vessel causing microhemorrhage and tissue necrosis; (3) moisture and increase in skin temperature: mattresses retain heat causing increased skin temperature and moisture, which increase tissue metabolic rate and accelerate the effects of ischemia causing breaks in the skin. Systemic risk factors which play a role in pressure ulcer development include: (1) aging of the skin, which can lead to reduced elasticity and thinning, as well as loss of water and fat content; (2) immobility and inactivity, which may render elderly patients prone to pressure ulcers; (3) malnutrition, which causes delay in wound healing; (4) peripheral vascular disease, which impairs adequate oxygenation of tissue; and (5) sensory loss, (e.g., stroke patients), which may cause patients to be less aware of pain and damage due to continued pressure.

Pressure ulcers are classified or graded using a standardized system. The most common staging system used is based on the recommendation by the Agency for Health Care Policy and Research (now called Agency for Healthcare Research and Quality) (5).

Stage I: Nonblanching erythema of intact skin, the heralding lesion of skin ulceration. In individuals with darker skin, discoloration of the skin, warmth, edema, induration, or hardness may also be indicators.

Stage II: Partial-thickness skin loss involving epidermis, dermis, or both. The ulcer is superficial and presents clinically as an abrasion, blister, or shallow crater.

Stage III: Full-thickness skin loss involving necrosis of subcutaneous tissue that may extend down to (but not through) underlying fascia. The ulcer presents clinically as a deep crater with or without undermining the adjacent tissue.

Stage IV: Full-thickness skin loss with extensive destruction; tissue necrosis, or damage to muscle, bone, or supporting structures (i.e., tendon, joint capsule).

Pressure ulcers can cause pain and discomfort in people with intact sensory mechanisms (6); patients with spinal cord injuries may not present with pain. Because of the loss of the normal protective layers of the skin which are broken down with pressure ulcer development, superimposed infections such as cellulitis, fasciitis, and osteomyelitis with associated bacteremia are common (5). Although superficial infections may be caused by common skin organisms such as *Staphylococcus aureus* and streptococci, deeper ulcers generally over the sacrum and coccyx are colonized with enteric gram-negative and anaerobic organisms, which can invade the ulcers and result in polymicrobial infections. Elderly residents of long-term care facilities may present with such infected pressure ulcers secondary to resistant microflora, which can pose a treatment challenge.

2.2. General Management

A thorough examination of the skin surfaces is necessary in evaluating patients with pressure ulcers. All necrotic tissue should be debrided prior to the staging of the ulcers. Once appropriate debridement is completed, a detailed examination of the area should be performed to establish staging. Included in the documentation is the length, width, and depth of the wound, and presence or absence of sinus tracts, undermining, exudates, and granulation tissue (5). Instant photography can be utilized for patient's chart documentation, which can be compared with subsequent assessments of the progression or improvement of the pressure ulcers. General examination should also include the overall evaluation of strength, muscle tone, spasticity, and range of motion of the patient's extremities. The other comorbid conditions, nutritional status, pain scale, and mental health should be assessed. Once a patient develops a pressure ulcer, the ulcer should be examined on a regular basis to monitor progression or improvement. The presence of bacterial infection, underlying osteomyelitis, related abscess, or sinus tract should be determined, and managed appropriately. Plain films, computerized tomography, bone scan, or magnetic resonance imaging (MRI) are useful in assessing the underlying tissue and bone involvement.

The principles of treatment are focused on medical or surgical management while addressing the factors that led to ulcer formation. In general, the management of pressure ulcers includes: (1) debriding of necrotic tissue, (2) cleaning the wound with normal saline initially and with each dressing change, (3) preventing infection and treating infection if present, and (4) dressing of ulcers to keep them moist and the surrounding tissue dry (6).

Patients must be positioned to keep pressure off the ulcer area. Patient's position should be changed on a regular basis or at least every 2 hr to keep the ulcer area pressure free. Underlying diseases such as diabetes mellitus and depression should be managed properly. If malnutrition is an issue, it should be corrected by aggressive nutritional supplements. Vitamin C and zinc should be prescribed if deficiencies are detected. Pain status should also be assessed and treated appropriately.

2.3. Antibiotic Treatment for Infected Pressure Ulcers

The presence of infection in chronic wounds is based on clinical signs of surrounding erythema, edema, ulcer odor, purulent exudates, and fever. A foul odor is an important clinical sign and may signify the presence of anaerobic organisms (7). Occasionally, wounds with a reported foul odor are not always infected. If the pressure ulcers are infected, systemic antibiotics are required. Reduction of colony-forming units (CFUs) of organisms has been used as the end point in evaluating antimicrobial efficacy in acute wounds. Topical antimicrobial agents have not been shown to be effective. However, several topical antibiotic agents may reduce CFUs without damaging the wound. These include silver sulfadiazine 1% cream, combination antibiotic ointments, and propylene glycol (8). Topical gentamicin and silver sulfadiazine have been used for treatment of infected pressure ulcers and shown to improve the clinical appearance of the ulcers (9,10). Infections with anaerobes may respond to topical metronidazole. Systemic antibiotics should be administered if the clinical condition suggests accompanying cellulitis or spread of the infection to bone or to the bloodstream.

As in diabetic ulcers, most pressure ulcers in the elderly yield multiple organisms when cultured. Making an accurate bacteriologic diagnosis is difficult. *Pseudomonas aeruginosa* and *Providencia* spp. colonies were significantly increased in worsening pressure ulcers compared with stationary or rapidly healing ulcers. Peptococci, *Bacteroides* species, or *Clostridium* were also found in more than half of worsening or stationary ulcers but were absent in healing pressure ulcers. Therefore, *P. aeruginosa* and *Providencia* species should not be regarded as simple colonization (11,12).

In addition to debridement, systemic antibiotics are indicated in the presence of systemic signs of infection or underlying osteomyelitis. A variety of empirical antibiotic regimens have been suggested for patients with pressure ulcer-associated cellulitis, osteomyelitis, or bacteremia. Bacteremia in this situation is usually caused by *Pseudomonas mirabilis*, *S. aureus*, or *Bacteroides fragilis* (12). Any antibiotic that is active against the majority of organisms that are causing pressure ulcer infection is appropriate. In the absence of osteomyelitis, a 10–14-day course of antibiotic treatment is commonly administered, but no studies have carefully defined the duration of therapy. If osteomyelitis is present, it requires a more extended (6 weeks or longer) course of therapy. Frequently, bone debridement is also necessary for optimal healing. In older patients or the presence of renal failure, the dose of antibiotics that are excreted in the kidney should be adjusted appropriately.

Surgical options are available to close stage III and IV pressure ulcers that do not heal by conservative treatment modalities. Possible surgical interventions include direct closure, split- or full-thickness skin grafts, skin flaps, musculocuta-neous flaps, and free flaps. The decision for surgical intervention depends on the location of the ulcer, the primary diagnosis, comorbid conditions, and the goal of the treatment (5).

2.4. Complication of Pressure Ulcers

Serious complications may occur in pressure ulcers that are not optimally treated. These include cellulitis, fistula formation, sinus tract and abscess, osteomyelitis, septic arthritis, bacteremia, infective endocarditis, and meningitis (6). Diagnosis and management of such complications can be found in other sections of this textbook, and thus will not be discussed here.

3. CELLULITIS

Cellulitis is an acute spreading infection of the skin and subcutaneous tissue characterized by localized pain, erythema, swelling, and heat. Cellulitis can affect virtually any part of the body, but commonly affects the lower and upper extremities.

The primary portal of entry of pathogens is nonintact integument or cracked skin, for example, due to skin dryness, intertrigo, tinea pedis, or athlete's foot (14,15). In a study conducted in elderly patients with cellulitis of the feet and legs, 83% had tinea pedis (16). Cellulitis resulting from gluteal fold intertrigo associated with hip replacement therapy has also been reported (17). Previous trauma such as lacerations, puncture wounds, insect bites, surgical incision sites, illicit substance injection sites, liposuction sites, or pressure ulcers can be associated with spreading cellulitis (18–20). In nursing home residents, a common portal of entry of bacteria causing local cellulitis is the site of gastrostomy tube insertion (21). Additional risk factors for cellulitis include conditions that disrupt the lymphatic and venous flow. These include obesity, history of deep venous thrombosis, breast cancer with axillary node dissection, cancer of the cervix, cancer of the uterus, radical pelvic surgery, nephritic syndrome, right-sided congestive heart failure, previous saphenous vein harvesting (during coronary artery bypass surgery), and hip replacement surgery (21–24). Other predisposing factors include a previous history of cellulitis, peripheral vascular disease, alcoholism, immunosuppressive drugs such as corticosteroid, and any underlying chronic disease (18,21,25).

The most common microorganisms involved in cellulitis are group A *Streptococcus* and *S. aureus* (26). Other organisms such as groups B, C, G streptococci and others are occasionally implicated. Group B streptococcal (*Streptococcus agalactiae*) infection can cause cellulitis in adults, particularly those with diabetes mellitus, underlying malignancies, and AIDS (27). From the portal of entry or primary site, the organisms spread locally and cause an inflammatory reaction. The involved area is red, hot, and swollen. The border of lesion is not well demarcated and elevated. Bullous lesions may be found in severe forms of cellulitis due to streptococci and some gram-negative organisms such as *Aeromonas hydrophila*, *Vibrio vulnificus*, and *Escherichia coli*. *A. hydrophila* infection is acquired through a laceration after contact or swimming in freshwater (28,29). Regional lymphadenitis is common and bacteremia may occur.

The diagnosis of cellulitis is made based on clinical evaluation. Patients may complain of fever, chills, and malaise. Culture of the skin aspirate is rarely positive.

Blood cultures drawn during spikes of temperature prior to initiating antibiotics may be useful to guide therapy.

3.1. Antibiotic Therapy

Nafcillin (a penicillinase-resistant penicillin) or cefazolin (a first-generation cephalosporin) are drugs-of-choice for simple cellulitis. Both antibiotics are excellent for streptococci and susceptible *S. aureus*. Unfortunately, skin and soft tissue infection due to methicillin-resistant *S. aureus* (MRSA) is increasing in the community (30). It is probably wise to include broad-spectrum antibiotics effective against both MRSA as well as sensitive streptococci such as vancomycin, doxycycline, or trimethoprim-sulfamethoxazole (TMP-SMZ). For patients allergic to penicillin, doxycycline, clindamycin, vancomycin, quinupristin–dalfopristin, linezolid, or daptomycin are appropriate alternatives. Antibiotics dosing should be appropriately adjusted in elderly patients with renal failure.

3.2. Erysipelas

Erysipelas is a variant of cellulitis with prominent lymphatic involvement. Erysipelas involves the superficial layers of the skin and cutaneous lymphatics compared with cellulitis, which extends more deeply into the layers of the skin (19). Erysipelas involves the skin of the face and extremities and is characterized by painful, bright red, edematous, indurated lesions. The lesions have raised borders that are sharply demarcated from the adjacent normal skin (Fig. 1). Erysipelas has been reported in all age groups,

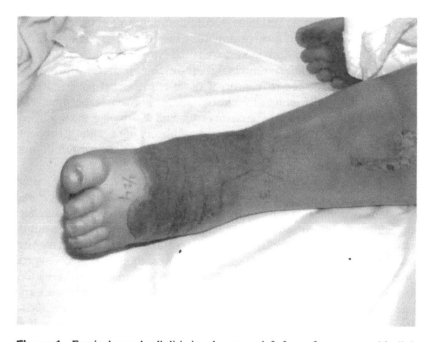

Figure 1 Erysipelas and cellulitis in edematous left foot of a woman with diabetes mellitus and renal failure. The lesion on the foot has a raised border that sharply demarcated from the adjacent skin. Further proximal the lesion margin is blurry, which is more consistent with cellulitis.

but elderly patients are the most commonly affected. Peak incidence has been reported to be in patients aged 60–80 years, particularly in individuals with high risk of and those with lymphatic drainage disruption (e.g., after mastectomy, pelvic surgery, bypass grafting) (31). The most common microorganism responsible in erysipelas is group A *Streptococcus* (32). The treatment of choice is penicillin or penicillinase-resistant penicillin or first-generation cephalosporins. For patients allergic to penicillin, clindamycin or erythromycin are acceptable alternatives.

3.3. Cellulitis Due to *Vibrio vulnificus*

V. vulnificus is a gram-negative bacillus usually found in warm, shallow, coastal salt waters in temperate climates. It causes infection by two mechanisms. First, infection occurs by ingestion of contaminated seafood such as raw oysters. Second, infection occurs through an open wound exposed to contaminated seawater. Infection with *V. vulnificus* has been reported in adults; in a case series in Taiwan the ages of patients ranged from 19 to 76 years; the ratio of male to female patients was 2:1 (33). Patients with chronic liver diseases and other immunocompromised states are prone to have severe infection including life-threatening septic shock and blistering skin lesions (34). Most patients infected with *V. vulnificus* have bullous skin lesions, which are found on the trunk and lower extremities. These hemorrhagic bullae can progress to necrotic ulcerations or to necrotizing fasciitis. In such a case surgical debridement in addition to systemic antibiotic is needed. The effective antibiotics include tetracycline, third-generation cephalosporins, and fluoroquinolones; an aminoglycoside may be needed in seriously ill patients. This infection is associated with high morbidity and mortality.

4. FURUNCLES AND CARBUNCLES

Furuncles (boils) are inflammatory skin nodules or abscesses that usually develop from preexisting folliculitis. It is a deeper infection of the hair follicle than folliculitis and consists of an inflammatory nodule with a pustular center through which hair emerges (26). Furuncles occur in skin area that contain hair follicles and are subject to friction and perspiration such as in the face, neck, axilla, and buttocks (34). Furuncles begin as tender, red skin nodules that soon become fluctuant often with spontaneous drainage of pus with subsiding of the lesion.

Carbuncles involve several adjacent hair follicles, creating an inflammatory mass with pus discharging from several follicular orifices. Carbuncles commonly occur on the face, neck, upper extremities, and buttocks. Compared with furuncles, carbuncles are frequently accompanied by constitutional symptoms (26). Both furuncles and carbuncles drain to the skin surface along the hair follicles. Carbuncles are often associated with diabetes mellitus. The most common etiologic agent is *S. aureus*. Both strains of *S. aureus*, methicillin-sensitive *S. aureus* (MSSA), and MRSA can cause furuncles and carbuncles. The community-acquired furuncle is usually caused by MSSA. However, recent increase in community-acquired MRSA infection has been observed (35). If MRSA infection is suspected or confirmed by culture, the antibiotic regimen should include antibiotics that are effective against MRSA. Involvement of the skin of the perineal region is likely to be caused by either coliform or anaerobic organisms.

Elderly patients with cutaneous abscesses should be carefully assessed for the presence of fever, chills, sweats, and other constitutional symptoms, keeping in mind that frail older patients may not have classical manifestations of infection. Blood cultures should ideally be drawn prior to the initiation of antibiotics. Fluctuant abscesses can be aspirated and aspirates sent for Gram stain and culture for aerobic and anaerobic organisms. Patients with abscesses should also be assessed for the presence of systemic diseases such as diabetes mellitus, valvular heart disease, and immunologic abnormalities. The medical management of these conditions is usually more complicated than in normal persons. Most skin abscesses will require incision and drainage unless drainage occurs spontaneously. Incision and drainage or manipulation should be avoided for lesions on the lips and nose. Manipulation of lesions on these sites may allow the organism to spread through the facial and emissary veins and lead to cavernous sinus thrombophlebitis or brain abscess.

A simple drained furuncle may not require systemic antibiotic therapy. In cases where an abscess occurred with extension of infection to adjacent tissues such as cellulitis, osteomyelitis, and blood stream invasion, and/or coexisting diabetes mellitus and immune compromised states should be treated with systemic antibiotics. Patients with abscesses and underlying cardiac valve diseases should be given prophylactic antibiotics prior to incision and drainage.

4.1. Antibiotic Therapy

Acutely ill patients may benefit from parenteral antibiotic therapy. Intravenous nafcillin or cefazolin, which have activity against MSSA and other gram-positive cocci, are preferred choices. Otherwise, if MRSA is suspected the patients may need vancomycin, quinupristin–dalfopristin, linezolid, or daptomycin or other effective antibiotics against MRSA. For less ill patients, oral antibiotics such as dicloxacillin or cephalexin are reasonable choices. Clindamycin, quinupristin–dalfpopristin, linezolid, and daptomycin are alternatives for patients allergic to penicillin. Quinupristin–dalfopristin, linezolid, and daptomycin are effective against both MSSA and MRSA. Depending on the severity of infection, a 10–14-day course of antibiotics is usually sufficient to treat the infection.

In patients with perianal abscesses, empirical antibiotic regimens which cover aerobic gram-negative and anaerobic organisms must be used. Commonly recommended regimens include a β-lactam–β-lactamase inhibitor combination agent and an aminoglycoside or a fluoroquinolone and metronidazole.

5. PARONYCHIA

Paronychia is a superficial infection of epithelium lateral to the nail plate. This acute painful purulent infection is most frequently caused by *S. aureus* and *Streptococcus* species. Occasionally, *P. aeruginosa* may play a role in the pathogenesis, particularly if green discoloration is found (29). A mixed infection is not uncommon in patients with diabetes mellitus. If the infection is chronic, fungal etiology should be considered. Infection usually starts in the lateral nail fold. Occasionally, it may spread to the complete margin of skin around the nail plate. Early in the course of the disease, cellulitis is usually observed and subsequently may progress to abscess. A simple drainage procedure to this abscess would generally improve the patient's condition and discomfort.

The treatment of choice for a paronychia is incision and drainage. Warm compresses or soaks with half-strength hydrogen peroxide can be provided. The presence of a subungual abscess requires nail plate removal. The degree of debridement depends on the degree of nail bed infection. Antibiotics are not necessary if the incision successfully achieves adequate drainage. If cellulitis is present, antibiotics are indicated. Cephalexin, which has activity against both *S. aureus* and streptococci, is a reasonable choice. If the infection is caused by MRSA, the antibiotic prescribed should include antibiotic that is active against MRSA as mentioned earlier.

6. PUNCTURE WOUNDS

Wound infection after a puncture wound occurs because of dirt pushed deep into the skin by the object (typically a nail) puncturing the tissue. Complications of puncture wounds can be serious. These include local soft tissue infection, cellulitis, osteomyelitis, and tetanus. *P. aeruginosa* is one of the common microorganisms isolated from the infected puncture wound ("sweaty tennis shoe syndrome") (36). The management of puncture wounds includes cleaning of the wound with a detergent or iodophor, surgical debridement of necrotic tissue, removal of residual foreign bodies, tetanus prophylaxis, and prophylactic antibiotics. Generally, prophylactic antibiotics are not routinely indicated unless the wound has gone unattended for more than 6 hr or unless adjacent soft tissue infection has already occurred. If local soft tissue infection or cellulitis results from a puncture wound, it should be treated with systemic antibiotic. The antibiotics regimen should cover *S. aureus*, and streptococci as mentioned in the cellulitis section. If *P. aeruginosa* infection is suspected, as in the case of penetrating puncture wound in a person wearing a sweaty tennis shoe, adding ciprofloxacin for a 14-day course of therapy is reasonable (37). Abscess resulting from puncture wounds should be surgically drained.

7. BITE WOUNDS

Bite wounds range from minimal scratches, punctures, lacerations, to evulsions. Bite wounds can be due to dog, cat, other animals, or occasionally human. The origin of the infecting microorganism can be from the normal oral flora of the biter, the environment, or the victim's skin flora (38)

7.1. Dog Bites

Dogs are responsible for almost 80% of animal bite wounds. The common organisms isolated from dog bite wounds are alpha-hemolytic streptococci, *Pasteurella multocida* (20–30%), and *S. aureus* (20–30%) (38). Other pathogens include *Eikenella corrodens*, *Capnocytophaga canimorsus*, and other anaerobic microorganisms.

The management of bite wounds includes irrigation of the wound with normal saline. Depending on the severity of tissue injury, debridement and surgical repair may be needed. Infected wounds and those that are seen more than 24 hr after the bite occurs should be left open. Approximately 20% of the dog bites become infected (Fig. 2). Therefore, it may be prudent to treat patients with a 5–7-day course of antibiotics after most of the dog bites. For severe infected wounds, ampicillin–sulbactam is the drug-of-choice. Amoxillin–clavulanate is recommended for outpatient antibiotic therapy. For those who are allergic to penicillin, a combination of clindamycin and a fluoroquinolone such as levafloxacin is recommended. Patients should be assessed for the need of tetanus vaccine and rabies postexposure prophylaxis.

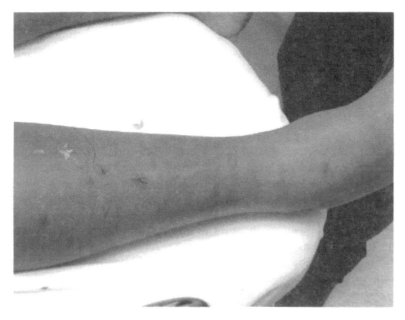

Figure 2 Cellulitis after a dog bite. Dark crusted puncture wounds can be seen surrounded by spreading erythema, swelling of the skin, and subcutaneous tissue.

7.2. Cat Bites

The incidence of infection after a cat bite is >50% (26). The most frequent organism isolated is *P. multocida*. Otherwise the spectrum of pathogens is similar to those of dog bites. Infection by *Bartonella henselae*, the cause of cat-scratch disease, may occur after a cat bite. The management step is similar to dog bite wounds including the need of tetanus toxoid and risk assessment for rabies postexposure prophylaxis.

8. NECROTIZING SOFT TISSUE INFECTION OR NECROTIZING FASCIITIS

8.1. Clinical Features

Clinicians need to be familiar to the symptoms and signs of necrotizing fasciitis. Necrotizing soft tissue infection has a high morbidity and mortality rate. Necrotizing fasciitis is characterized by rapidly progressing inflammation and necrosis of the skin, subcutaneous connective tissue, fascia, and sometimes muscle. Infection spreads through the fascial plane, causing rapid destruction of flesh. The terminology of "flesh-eating bacteria" refers to the destructive nature of bacteria causing necrotizing fasciitis. The organism most closely linked to necrotizing fasciitis is beta hemolytic group A *Streptococcus*, although the majority of cases may be caused by the other organisms. Necrotizing fasciitis is classified into three types (39). Type I is polymicrobial in etiology; at least one anaerobic species is isolated in combination with one or more facultative anaerobic species such as streptococci (other than group A) and other members of the Enterobacteriaceae (40). Type I necrotizing fasciitis usually occurs after trauma or surgery. It may initially be mistaken for a simple wound cellulitis. Type II is caused by group A *Streptococcus* either alone or in combination with other species such as *S. aureus*. It is commonly referred to as "flesh-eating bacterial infection." Type III is also referred to as gas gangrene or clostridial myonecrosis. This skeletal muscle infection may also be associated with recent surgery or trauma. Fournier gangrene is a variant of necrotizing soft tissue infections involving the genitalia and usually results from polymicrobial infection. It may occur as a result of trauma, extension of a urinary tract infection, perianal, or retropenitoneal infection (41).

There are many underlying conditions that can predispose patients to develop necrotizing fasciitis. Immunocompromised states such as in patients with diabetes mellitus, AIDS, and malignancy are predisposing factors (42). The other predisposing factors for development of streptococcal necrotizing fasciitis include varicella, penetrating injuries, minor cuts, burns, splinters, surgical procedures, blunt trauma, and muscle strains (43). The organism may enter the subcutaneous tissue through nonintact integument and spread along the superficial and deep fascial planes. Rapid spread of infection is facilitated by bacterial toxins and enzymes such as hyaluronidase, collagenase, streptokinase, and lipase. The progression of bacterial penetration results in tissue necrosis and thrombosis of the vasculature. Initially, patients often present with clinical manifestation similar to cellulitis (44). One important clue is the degree of pain which is typically disproportionate to the severity of the findings on physical examination (i.e., erythema, swelling, and tenderness). Anesthesia may develop later after necrosis of the peripheral nerve due to the thrombosis of vasa nervorum. Infection progresses in 2–3 days, causing the redness of the skin to turn purple or purple-black (45). Clear or hemmorhagic bullae may develop. When bullae rupture, a dry, black eschar may develop at the site of rupture. During progression of disease, patients may have high fever, chills, a toxic appearance, hypotension, shock, multiorgan failure, and death.

Early diagnosis and prompt intervention is critical to reduce the mortality rate. The clinician should have a high index of suspicion based on clinical findings, such as appearance of the skin and extreme pain out of proportion to the clinical examination. The presence of fever and toxic appearance should raise suspicion for necrotizing fasciitis. In addition to routine laboratory test, radiologic imaging, aspirate Gram stain and culture, and blood culture should be performed. Immediate surgical consultation is needed for all patients with necrotizing soft tissue infection.

8.2. Treatment

The most effective management found to decrease mortality is early diagnosis and prompt surgical debridement (44). Intensive care unit admission is needed in most patients with necrotizing fasciitis. A combination of intravenous antibiotics such as penicillin, an aminoglycoside or third-generation cephalosporin, and clindamycin or metronidazole, is typically administered to provide broad bacterial coverage (42). The antibiotic regimen can be modified later, once the Gram stain, culture, and sensitivity results are obtained.

REFERENCES

1. Chassagne P, Perol MB, Doucet J, Trivalle C, Menard JF, Manchon ND, Moynot Y, Humbert G, Bourreille J, Bercoff E. Is presentation of bacteremia in the elderly the same as in younger patients? Am J Med 1996; 100:65–70.
2. Agris J, Spira M. Pressure ulcers: prevention and treatment. Clin Symp 1979; 31:1–32.
3. The National Pressure Ulcer Advisory Panel. Pressure ulcers prevalence, cost and risk assessment: consensus development conference statement. Decubitus 1989; 2:4–8.

4. Fisher AR, Wells G, Harrison MB. Factors associated with pressure ulcers in adults in acute care hospitals. Adv Skin Wound Care 2004; 17:80–90.

5. Bergstrom N, Allman RM, Alvarez OM, Bennett MA, Carlson CE, Frantz RA, Garber SL, Jackson BS, Kaminski MV, Kemp MG, Krouskop TA, Lewis VL, Maklebust J, Margolis DJ, Marvel EM, Reger SI, Rodeheaver GT, Salcido R, Xakellis GC, Yarkony GM. Pressure Ulcer Treatment. Clinical Practice Guideline No. 15. Rockville, MD: U.S. Department of Health and Human Services, Public Health Service, Agency for Health Care Policy and Research. AHCPR Publication No. 95–0652, 1994.

6. Rehm CR, Siebens H. Pressure ulcers. In: Fontera W, Silver J, eds. Essentials of Physical Medicine and Rehabilitation. Philadelphia, PA: Hanley and Belfus, 2002:699–704.

7. Sapico FL, Ginunas VJ, Thornhill-Joynes M, Canawati HN, Capen DA, Klein NE, Khawam S, Montgomerie JZ. Quantitative microbiology of pressure sores in different stages of healing. Diagn Microbiol Infect Dis 1986; 5:31–38.

8. Bolton L, Oleniacz W, Constantine B. Repair and antibacterial effects of topical antiseptic agents in vivo. Models Dermatol 1985; 2:145–158.

9. Bendy RH Jr, Nuccio PA, Wolfe E. Relationship of quantitative wound bacterial counts to healing of decubiti: effect of topical gentamicin. Antimicrob Agents Chemother 1964; 4:147–155.

10. Kucan JO, Robson MC, Heggers JP, Ko F. Comparison of silver sulfadiazine, povidone-iodine and physiologic saline in the treatment of chronic pressure ulcers. J Am Geriatr Soc 1981; 29:232–235.

11. Daltrey DC, Rhodes B, Chattwood JG. Investigation into the microbial flora of healing and non-healing decubitus ulcers. J Clin Pathol 1981; 34:701–705.

12. Seiler WO, Stahelin HB, Sonnabend W. Effect of aerobic and anaerobic germs on the healing of decubitus ulcers. Schweiz Med Wochenschr 1979; 109:1594–1599.

13. Bryan CS, Dew CE, Reynolds KL. Bacteremia associated with decubitus ulcers. Arch Intern Med 1983; 143:2093–2095.

14. Day MR, Day RD, Harkless LB. Cellulitis secondary to web space dermatophytosis. Clin Podiatr Med Surg 1996; 13:759–766.

15. Robbins JM. Recognizing, treating, and preventing common foot problems. Cleveland Clin J Med 2000; 67:45–56.

16. Semel JD, Goldin H. Association of athlete's foot with cellulitis of the lower extremities: diagnostic value of bacterial cultures of ipsilateral interdigital space samples. Clin Infect Dis 1996; 23:1162–1164.

17. Studer-Sachsenberg EM, Ruffieux P, Saurat JH. Cellulitis after hip surgery: long term follow-up of seven cases. Dermatology 1997; 137:133–136.

18. Ginsberg MD. Cellulitis: analysis of 101 cases and review of literature. South Med J 1981; 74:350–533.

19. Bisno AL, Stevens DL. Streptococcal infections of skin and soft tissues. N Engl J Med 1996; 334:240–245.

20. Swartz MN. Cellulitis. N Engl J Med 2004; 350:904–912.

21. Schamader K, Twersky J. Herpes zoster, cellulitis, and scabies. In: Yoshikawa TT, Ouslander JG, eds. Infection Management for Geriatrics in Long-Term Care Facilities. New York: Marcel Dekker, Inc., 2002:283–303.

22. Baddour LM, Bisno AL. Recurrent cellulitis after coronary bypass surgery. Association with superficial fungal infection in saphenous venectomy limbs. J Am Med Assoc 1984; 251:1049–1052.

23. Dupuy A, Benchikhi H, Roujeau JC, Bernard P, Vaillant L, Chosidow O, Sassolas B, Guillaume JC, Grob JJ, Bastuji-Garin S. Risk factors for erysipelas of the leg (cellulitis): case–control study. Br Med J 1999; 318:1591–1594.

24. Studer-Sachsenberg EM, Ruffieux P, Saurat JH. Cellulitis after hip surgery: long-term follow-up of seven cases. Br J Dermatol 1997; 137:133–136.

25. Parada JP, Maslow JN. Clinical syndromes associated with adult pneumococcal cellulitis. Scand J Infect Dis 2000; 32:133–136.

26. Magnussen RC. Skin and soft tissue infections. In: Reese RE, Betts RF, eds. A Practical Approach to Infectious Diseases. Boston: Little, Brown and Company, 1996:109–114.

27. Farley MM, Harvey C, Stull T, Smith JD, Schuchat A, Wenger JD, Stephens DS. A population based assessment of invasive disease due to group B streptococci in non pregnant adults. N Engl J Med 1995; 328:1807–1811.

28. Heckerling PS, Stine TM, Pottage JC, Levin S, Harris AA. *Aeromonas hydrophilia* myonecrosis and gas gangrene in a nonimmunocompromised host. Arch Intern Med 1983; 143:2005–2007.

29. Hall JH, Callaway JL, Tindall JP, Smith JG Jr. *Pseudomonas aeruginosa* in dermatology. Arch Dermatol 1968; 97:312–324.

30. Iyer S, Jones DH. Community-acquired methicillin-resistant *Staphylococcus aureus* skin infection: a retrospective analysis of clinical presentation and treatment of a local outbreak. J Am Acad Dermatol 2004; 50(6):854–858.

31. Davis L, Benbeniskty K. Erysipelas, 2003. http://www.emedicine.com/derm/topic 129.htm.

32. Bernard P, Bedame C, Mounier M, Denis F, Catanzano G, Bonnetblanc JM. Streptococcal cause of erysipelas and cellulitis in adults. Arch Dermatol 1989; 125:779–782.

33. Chuang YC, Yuan CY, Liu CY, Lan CK, Huang AH. Vibrio vulnificus infection in Taiwan: report of 28 cases and review of clinical manifestations and treatment. Clin Infect Dis 1992; 15:271–276.

34. Jagar C. Vibrio vulnificus infections, 2003. www.emedicine.com/DERM/topic847.htm.

35. Okuma K, Iwakawa K, Turnidge JD, Grubb WB, Bell JM, O'Brien FG, Coombs GW, Pearman JW, Tenover FC, Kapi M, Tiensasitorn C, Ito T, Hiramatsu K. Dissemination of new methicillin-resistant Staphylococcus aureus clones in the community. J Clin Microbiol 2002; 40:4289–4294.

36. Fitzgerald RH Jr, Cowan JD. Puncture wounds of the foot. Orthop Clin North Am 1975; 6:965–972.

37. Raz R, Miron D. Oral ciprofloxacin for treatment of infection following nail puncture wounds of the foot. Clin Infect Dis 1995; 21:194–195.

38. Goldstein EJ. Bite wounds and infection. Clin Infect Dis 1992; 14:633–638.

39. Schwartz RA. Necrotizing fasciitis, 2004. www.emedicine.com/derm/topic743.htm.

40. Swartz MN. Skin and soft tissue infections. In: Mandell GL, Bennett JE, Dolin R, eds. Principles and Practice of Infectious Diseases. Vol. 1. 5th ed. Philadelphia, PA: Churchill Livingstone, 2000:1037–1066.

41. Kilic A, Aksoy Y, Kilic L. Fournier's gangrene: etiology, treatment, and complications. Ann Plast Surg 2001; 47:523–527.

42. Trent JT, Kirsner RS. Necrotizing fasciitis. Wounds 2002; 14:284–292.

43. Stevens DL. Invasive group A streptococcus infections. Clin Infect Dis 1992; 14:2–11.

44. Childers BJ, Potyondy LD, Nachreiner R, Rogers FR, Childers ER, Oberg KC, Hendricks DL, Hardesty RA. Necrotising fasciitis: a fourteen-year retrospective study of 163 consecutive patients. Am Surg 2002; 68:109–116.

45. Jarrett P, Rademaker M, Duffill M. The clinical spectrum of necrotizing fasciitis. A review of 15 cases. Aust NZ J Med 1997; 27:29–34.

SUGGESTED READING

Childers BJ, Potyondy LD, Nachreiner R, Rogers FR, Childers ER, Oberg KC, Hendricks DL, Hardesty RA. Necrotising fasciitis: a fourteen-year retrospective study of 163 consecutive patients. Am Surg 2002; 68:109–116.

Fisher AR, Wells G, Harrison MB. Factors associated with pressure ulcers in adults in acute care hospitals. Adv Skin Wound Care 2004; 17:80–90.

Kilic A, Aksoy Y, Kilic L. Fournier's gangrene: etiology, treatment, and complications. Ann Plast Surg 2001; 47:523–527.

Swartz MN. Cellulitis. N Engl J Med 2004; 350:904–912.

36
Herpes Zoster

Kenneth E. Schmader
*Center for the Study of Aging and Human Development, Duke University and
Durham Veterans Affairs Medical Centers, Durham, North Carolina, U.S.A.*

Key Points:

- Acyclovir, valacyclovir (a prodrug of acyclovir), and famciclovir (a prodrug of penciclovir) are deoxyguanosine analogs converted by viral thymidine kinase and then cellular kinases to a triphosphate form that stops varicella-zoster virus (VZV) replication by inhibiting VZV DNA polymerase and by acting as a chain terminator by incorporation into the VZV DNA chain.
- Although all three agents are renally eliminated and have similar plasma half-lives (2–3 hr), the oral bioavailability of valacyclovir (54%) and famciclovir (77%) is much greater than that of acyclovir (10–20%).
- Oral acyclovir (800 mg every 4 hr, i.e., five times daily), valacyclovir (1 g every 8 hr, i.e., three times daily), and famciclovir (500 mg every 8 hr, i.e., three times daily) accelerated cutaneous healing, reduced acute herpes zoster (HZ) and the duration of chronic pain and were well tolerated in randomized controlled trials in immunocompetent older patients where all patients received the drug within 72 hr of rash onset; all three drugs are recommended for treatment of HZ in older adults with cost and dosing schedule determining the choice of agent.
- The disadvantages of antiviral therapy for HZ older adults include nausea/vomiting, headache, and, rarely, confusion; many treated patients still develop chronic pain (e.g., 25–35% of antiviral-treated patients have pain 3 months from rash onset); and the effectiveness of antiviral agents is uncertain if the patient presents more than 72 hr since rash onset, except perhaps for patients who have ophthalmic HZ or continue to have new vesicle formation.
- Corticosteroids are not recommended for routine use for HZ older adults because they do not prevent postherpetic neuralgia or reduce the duration of chronic pain and have significant adverse effects.

1. EPIDEMIOLOGY AND CLINICAL RELEVANCE

Herpes zoster (HZ) is a neurocutaneous disease that is caused by the reactivation of varicella-zoster virus (VZV) from a latent infection of dorsal sensory or cranial nerve ganglia. HZ may cause sensory disturbances, visual impairment, motor neuropathy, and other central nervous system (CNS) inflammatory conditions, but pain is the most clinically significant problem associated with HZ in older persons.

The likelihood of developing HZ increases sharply with aging. In a seminal study in England, Hope–Simpson detected the incidence of HZ to be 2.5 per 1000 person-years in adults aged 20–50 years and 7.8 per 1000 person-years in those aged >60 years (1). The increased risk of HZ with aging was confirmed in Boston where investigators reported an incidence of 1.9, 2.3, 3.1, 5.7, and 11.8 per 1000 person-years for the age groups 25–34, 35–44, 45–54, 55–64, and 65–75+ years, respectively (2). In the Duke Established Populations for Epidemiological Studies of the Elderly (EPESE), the lifetime risk of HZ increased significantly with age even among elderly individuals [odds ratio, 1.20 for every 5-year interval >65 years, 95% confidence interval (CI), 1.10–1.31] (3). Second attacks of HZ occur in 4–5% of individuals. The lifetime incidence of HZ is estimated to be 10–20% in the general population and as high as 50% of a cohort surviving to age 85 years. Although precise figures are not available, epidemiological data suggest that there are several hundred thousand cases of HZ in the United States each year.

Defective cell-mediated immunity is the other major predictor of HZ (4). Individuals with human immunodeficiency syndrome (HIV) infection, hematological malignancies, bone marrow and solid organ transplantation, systemic lupus erythematosus, and immunosuppressive therapy experience HZ at rates 20–100 times greater than that of immunocompetent individuals. For example, the incidence of HZ ranges from 29 to 51 per 1000 person-years in HIV-infected individuals. Among cancer patients, one study reported a cumulative 5-year incidence rate of HZ to be 62.5 per 1000 person-years, with the highest incidence in patients with Hodgkin's disease. Among bone marrow transplant recipients, 13–55% of patients develop HZ within 1 year of transplantation.

White race, psychological stress, and physical trauma also appear to be risk factors for HZ. Factors that do not affect the risk of HZ include sex, marital status, educational level, geographic location, season, or urban vs. rural residence.

Patients with HZ may transmit VZV via direct contact, airborne, or droplet nuclei to nonimmune individuals during the vesicular stage of the rash and cause varicella. There is no danger of transmission if the rash is only maculopapular or crusted. The incubation period of varicella is usually between 14 and 16 days with a range of 8–21 days. Important groups at risk for varicella include children who have not received the varicella vaccine or who have had an insufficient response to the vaccine, and susceptible healthcare workers and staff particularly if they are pregnant or immunocompromised. As most adults are latently infected with VZV, and therefore immune, they are not at risk for varicella. In addition, the exposure of a latently infected individual to HZ does not cause HZ or varicella.

2. ETIOLOGIC PATHOGEN

VZV is a double-stranded DNA human herpesvirus (4). The DNA genome is surrounded by an icosahedral protein capsid. The nucleocapsid in turn is surrounded by a protein layer called the tegument and a lipoprotein envelope studded with glycoproteins. The intact spherical virion is about 150–200 nm in diameter. The virus is infectious only if enveloped and is therefore quite labile as many physical forces (i.e., enzymes, heat, detergents, etc.) damage the envelope.

The VZV genome contains approximately 125,000 nucleotide base pairs and encodes about 70 gene products. These products include immediate early gene proteins which regulate early and late gene expression; early gene proteins such as the enzymes thymidine kinase and viral DNA polymerase; and late gene structural proteins, such as nucleocapsid and membrane proteins. Viral thymidine kinase catalyzes the transformation of nucleoside analogs such as acyclovir and penciclovir to the triphosphate form that inhibits VZV DNA polymerase and viral replication. Membrane glycoproteins in the viral envelope bind to host cell receptors, initiate cellular infection, and stimulate the host immune response.

VZV latently infects sensory ganglia at the time of primary infection and persists for life in neurons and/or satellite cells in the ganglia. A few latency-associated transcripts and proteins have been detected and are thought to maintain latency and the ability to reactivate. Periodic productive infection occurs throughout life but the host cellular immune response usually contains full reactivation to HZ. However, with the age-related decline in cellular immunity to VZV, reactivated VZV may not be contained and HZ results, partially explaining the increased risk of HZ in older persons.

3. CLINICAL MANIFESTATIONS

HZ begins when VZV spreads in the affected sensory ganglion and peripheral sensory nerve as well as the corresponding dorsal root and adjacent spinal cord. These events cause intense neuronal inflammation, hemorrhage, and destruction. Before the virus reaches the skin, the patient experiences a prodrome of pain or discomfort in the affected dermatome. Prodromal sensations include aching, burning, or lancinating pain as well as itching or tingling. This troublesome prologue confuses patients and physicians and imitates many other painful conditions in older persons, such as migraine headaches, trigeminal neuralgia, myocardial infarction, cholecystitis, biliary or renal colic, appendicitis, lumbosacral strain, "pulled" muscles, or herniated lumbar intervertebral disks. Very sensitive skin in the affected dermatome before the rash breaks out is one clue to incipient HZ. The prodrome usually lasts a few days, although there are case reports of it lasting weeks to months. In some patients, VZV never reaches the skin so they experience neuralgia without ever developing a rash. This phenomenon is known as zoster sine herpete.

In most cases, VZV reaches the skin and produces the characteristic rash (Fig. 1). A typical rash is unilateral and located in a dermatome, most commonly involving the Tl–L3 and VI dermatomes. It begins as a red, maculopapular eruption, usually develops vesicles within hours to days, starts crusting over in a week to 10 days, and heals within 2–4 weeks. The rash may involve adjacent dermatomes and a few vesicles distant from the primary dermatome due to hematogenous spread. Atypical rashes are not uncommon in older persons and immunocompetent individuals. The rash may be limited to a small patch located within a dermatome or may remain maculopapular without ever developing vesicles. Conversely, vesicles may form for several days and involve several dermatomes or disseminate widely, resembling varicella.

Most patients experience dermatomal pain or discomfort due to acute neuritis at the onset of the rash. A small percentage of patients never develop pain while others may experience the delayed onset of pain days or weeks after rash onset. The neuritis is usually described as burning, deep aching, tingling, itching, or

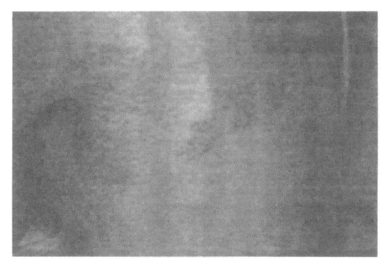

Figure 1 Herpes zoster. Involvement of a thoracic dermatome with erythema, maculopapular, and vesicular lesions within the dermatome.

stabbing. A subset of patients, especially those with trigeminal nerve involvement, may develop severe or even excruciating pain acutely. This pain has a profound negative impact on the functional status and quality of life and usually results in substantial health service utilization, including hospitalization.

The most common and feared complication of HZ is postherpetic neuralgia (PHN) (5). PHN is defined as pain 90–120 days after rash onset. The pathogenesis of PHN includes ectopic discharge from damaged peripheral, primary afferent nerves; decreased inhibition of neuronal activity in central structures; and central sensitization such that normal sensory input is amplified and perceived as painful. Older age is the most powerful predictor of PHN but greater acute pain severity, prodromal pain, and greater rash severity are also important risk factors. The patient with PHN may suffer from non-stimulus-evoked constant burning or aching pain, non-stimulus-evoked intermittent stabbing or shooting pain, and/or stimulus-evoked pain, the worst of which is allodynia. Allodynia is pain after a nonnoxious stimulus such that severe pain may be induced by the lightest touch of clothing or the wind. These subtypes of pain may produce disordered sleep, depression, anorexia, weight loss, chronic fatigue, and social isolation. Furthermore, PHN can impair basic and instrumental activities of daily living, depending on the severity and location of the pain.

Other neurological complications of HZ include cranial polyneuropathy, motor paralysis, meningoencephalitis, transverse myelitis, and stroke after ophthalmic HZ due to VZV-induced granulomatous angiitis of the nearby internal carotid artery(6). Cranial nerve (CN) symptoms include facial weakness with involvement of CN V or VII; hearing loss, imbalance, hyperacusis, and tinnitus with CN VIII; dysgeusia and mouth lesions with CN V, mandibular branch, and CN IX; and pharyngitis and laryngitis with CN IX, X. Ramsay–Hunt syndrome refers to

VZV-induced facial palsy and otic vesicles, often in association with CN VIII and/or other CN symptoms. Up to 5% of HZ patients develop focal motor pareses involving muscle groups innervated by ventral horn neurons in proximity to dorsal horn neurons of the affected dermatome. The most commonly affected muscles are those of the extremities and the face. These deficits usually occur at the time of or within a few weeks after the onset of the rash. Full or partial recovery of motor function occurs in 65–85% of patients within months of the onset of weakness but VZV-induced facial palsy has a much lower rate of recovery (30–40%).

HZ occurs in the ophthalmic division of the trigeminal nerve in 10–15% of patients and may cause ocular complications. The likelihood of inflammation of the eye appears to be higher when the rash is on the tip of the nose (nasociliary branch involvement) but in general the appearance and location of the facial rash does not predict the presence or extent of eye involvement. VZV-induced damage to the cornea and uvea and other eye structures can cause corneal anesthesia and ulceration, glaucoma, optic neuritis, eyelid scarring and retraction, visual impairment, and blindness in patients who did not receive antiviral therapy.

4. DIAGNOSIS

4.1. Clinical Diagnosis

HZ is easy to identify when the characteristic unilateral, dermatomal rash and pain syndrome described in the previous section presents in an older patient (7). Herpes simplex virus (HSV) infection is important to differentiate from HZ. Features that may distinguish HSV from HZ include multiple recurrences, especially around the genitals or mouth, and the absence of chronic pain. However, it may be impossible to distinguish the two conditions on clinical grounds because HSV presents with a unilateral, red, maculopapular, vesicular rash and acute pain similar to HZ. The differential diagnosis also includes contact dermatitis, burns, and vesicular lesions associated with fungal infections but the history and examination usually make the distinction clear.

4.2. Laboratory Diagnosis

Laboratory diagnostic testing is useful for differentiating herpes HZ from HSV, for suspected organ involvement, and for atypical presentations. The best specimen is vesicle fluid which contains abundant VZV. Tzanck smears may suggest VZV infection if multinucleated giant cells and intranuclear inclusions are demonstrated in stained vesicle scrapings but the technique cannot differentiate VZV from HSV infections. Available diagnostic tests include immunofluorescence antigen (IFA) or enzyme immunoassay (EIA) antigen detection, viral culture, polymerase chain reaction (PCR), and serology. IFA or EIA detection of VZV antigens in vesicle scrapings, crusts, tissue biopsy, or cerebrospinal fluid (CSF) is rapid (hours), specific, and sensitive (about 90%) when performed by technicians experienced laboratory. VZV culture from vesicle fluid, blood, CSF, or infected tissue specimens (but not crusts) is slower and less sensitive ($\approx$40%) than IFA. However, culture is the standard for the definitive diagnosis and the only method that yields infectious VZV for further analysis, such as determination of resistance to antiviral drugs. VZV DNA detection using the PCR of vesicle fluid, cells scraped or swabbed from skin lesions, crusts, respiratory secretions, CSF, or tissue obtained by biopsy is very sensitive (nearly 100%) and specific. IFA and/or culture are the primary diagnostic tests because they are more available and less expensive than PCR. However, PCR is extremely valuable in diagnosing VZV infections, particularly in unusual specimens or when the clinician suspects that IFA or culture has yielded false-negative test results. Serology can be used to diagnose zoster sine herpete or HZ retrospectively using acute and convalescent VZV IgG titers. Enzyme-linked immunosorbent assay (ELISA) is commonly used to measure antibodies to VZV because it is simple to perform and available commercially. However, commercial ELISA assays may lack sensitivity and specificity. Experts often recommend more sensitive and specific tests such as an immunofluorescence assay for antibody to VZV-induced membrane antigens (FAMA) or a VZV latex agglutination test.

5. TREATMENT

5.1. Antiviral Agents—Pharmacology

Acyclovir, valacyclovir, and famciclovir are currently available anti-VZV drugs for routine use (7) (see also chapter "Antiviral Drugs"). These drugs are deoxyguanosine analogs that are converted first by viral thymidine kinase and then cellular kinases to the nucleoside triphosphate form. The conversion by viral thymidine kinase allows for the accumulation of the drugs in infected cells but not in uninfected cells so the drug acts only in target cells. The triphosphate form stops VZV from replicating by inhibiting VZV DNA polymerase and by acting as a chain terminator by incorporation into the VZV DNA chain.

Acyclovir has poor gastrointestinal (GI) absorption with a bioavailability of 10–20%. It is extensively distributed throughout the body including CSF. The major route of elimination is the kidney via glomerular filtration and tubular secretion. The elimination half-life is 2–3 hr in patients with normal renal function.

Valacyclovir is a valine ester prodrug of acyclovir that is well absorbed in the GI tract and metabolized in the intestine and the liver to acyclovir, thereby bypassing the poor GI absorption of acyclovir. This formulation yields a higher oral bioavailability of acyclovir of about 54%. The route of elimination and half-life are the same as for acyclovir.

Famciclovir is a diacetyl 6-deoxy prodrug that is well absorbed in the GI tract and metabolized in the liver to penciclovir. Penciclovir has a chemical structure and mechanism of action that is very similar to that of acyclovir. The major route of elimination is the kidney via glomerular filtration and tubular secretion. The elimination half-life is 2–3 hr in patients with normal renal function, although the intracellular half-life of about 7 hr is much longer than that of acyclovir triphosphate. Valacyclovir and famciclovir achieve plasma levels of antiviral activity similar to that of intravenously administered acyclovir.

Foscarnet is an analog of inorganic pyrophosphate that inhibits VZV DNA polymerase at the pyrophosphate-binding site. It is structurally unrelated to acyclovir or penciclovir and does not require viral thymidine kinase for activity. Therefore, it is useful for treatment of HZ due to thymidine kinase-negative, acyclovir/penciclovir-resistant VZV. Thus far, acyclovir-resistant VZV has only been reported in patients

Table 1 Pharmacology of Anti-Varicella Zoster Virus Medications

Parameter	Acyclovir (Zovirax®)	Valacyclovir (Valtrex®)	Famciclovir (Famvir®)
Structure	Deoxyguanosine analog	Valine ester of acyclovir	Diacetyl 6-deoxy analog of penciclovir, a deoxyguanosine analog
Active agent	Acyclovir triphosphate	Acyclovir triphosphate	Penciclovir triphosphate
Conversion to active drug	None	First-pass intestinal and/or hepatic metabolism to acyclovir	Hepatic metabolism to penciclovir
Mechanism of action	Competitive inhibition VZV DNA polymerase	Competitive inhibition VZV DNA polymerase	Competitive inhibition VZV DNA polymerase
Oral bioavailability	10–20%	54%	77%
Elimination, plasma half-life	Renal, 2–3 hr	Renal, 2–3 hr	Renal, 2–3 hr

with advanced acquired immunodeficiency syndrome. Foscarnet is only given intravenously, 40 mg every 8 hr, and is eliminated via the kidney (Table 1).

5.2. Antiviral Agents—Pharmacotherapy

The principal goal of the treatment of HZ in older patients is the reduction of acute and chronic pain. Other important goals are to accelerate rash healing, prevent ocular damage in patients with ophthalmic HZ, and prevent disease spread and visceral and central nervous system complications in older patients with deficiencies in cell-mediated immunity (i.e., hematological malignancies). Antiviral therapy is useful in meeting these goals (Table 2).

5.2.1. Acyclovir

Oral acyclovir significantly reduced the time to rash healing by 1–2 days and acute pain in randomized controlled trials in patients >50 years old who were treated within 72 hr of rash onset (8,11). The trials demonstrated conflicting results regarding the efficacy of preventing PHN but meta-analyses of the individual acyclovir trials indicated a reduction in the duration of chronic pain (8,11). In a meta-analysis of three acyclovir trials, the adjusted hazard ratio (acyclovir vs. placebo) for the time to complete cessation of pain in patients $\geq$50 years of age was 2.13 (95% CI = 1.42–3.19) (8). This meta-analysis excluded an acyclovir trial that demonstrated no difference in pain outcomes between acyclovir vs. placebo because data were not available on time to complete cessation of pain, although these data were available on time to first cessation of pain. Including all four studies, the hazard ratio for time to first pain-free period was 1.31 (95% CI = 1.08–1.60) (8). Intravenous acyclovir is effective in limiting disease and treating visceral and CNS complications in immunocompromised individuals (12).

Table 2 Oral Antiviral Treatment of Herpes Zoster in Older Adults

Feature	Acyclovir	Valacyclovir	Famciclovir
Regimen	800 mg every 4 hr (five times a day) for 7 days	1 g every 8 hr (three times a day) for 7 days	500 mg every 8 hr (three times a day) for 7 days
Benefit: pain median days to resolution, drug vs. control (8–10)	41 vs. 101 (placebo)	38 vs. 51 (acyclovir)	63 vs. 163 (placebo)
Risks: adverse events common (>5%)	Nausea/vomiting, headache, diarrhea	Nausea/vomiting, headache, diarrhea	Nausea/vomiting, headache, diarrhea
Uncommon	Confusion, hallucinations TTP/HUS	Confusion, hallucinations TTP/HUS	Confusion, hallucinations
Precautions	Renal insufficiency	Renal insufficiency	Renal insufficiency
Drug interactions	Reduces phenytoin levels Probenecid impairs clearance	Reduces phenytoin levels Probenecid impairs clearance	Increases digoxin levels Probenecid impairs clearance
Renal dosing	CrCl ≥25 mL/min, no adjustment CrCl 10–24 mL/min: 800 mg every 8 hr CrCl <10 mL/min: 800 mg every 12 hr	CrCl ≥50 mL/min: no dosage adjustment CrCl 30–49 mL/min: 1 g every 12 hr CrCl 10–29 mL/min: 1 g every 24 hr CrCl <10 mL/min: 500 mg every 24 hr	CrCl ≥60 mL/min: no dosage adjustment CrCl 40–59 mL/min: 500 mg every 12 hr CrCl 20–39 mL/min: 500 mg every 24 hr CrCl <20 mL/min: 250 mg every 24 hr
How supplied	200 mg capsules; 200, 400, 800 mg tablets; 200 mg/5 mL solution	500 mg, 1 g tablets	125, 250, and 500 mg tablets

Abbreviation: TTP/HUS, thrombotic thrombocytopenic purpura/hemolytic-uremic syndrome.

The most common adverse effects of acyclovir are nausea/vomiting, headache, and diarrhea. It may cause renal insufficiency via precipitation in renal tubules, especially when given intravenously to patients with dehydration or preexisting renal insufficiency. The dose of oral acyclovir in patients with normal renal function is 800 mg every 4 hr (five times daily) for 7 days. Dose adjustments are necessary for renal insufficiency (Table 2). For older patients who cannot swallow tablets or capsules, acyclovir comes in an oral solution (unlike valacyclovir or famciclovir) at 200 mg/5 mL. The dose of intravenous acyclovir in patients with normal renal function is 10 mg/kg every 8 hr for 7 days.

5.2.2. Valacyclovir

Valacyclovir was compared to acyclovir in patients ≥50 years of age and older in a randomized, controlled trial (9). Median time to cessation of new lesion formation or healed rash was equivalent in the two groups. The hazard ratio (valacyclovir vs. acyclovir) for the time to complete cessation of pain was 1.34 [95% CI = 1.12–1.60] and the median days to resolution of pain was 38 days vs. 51 days, $p = 0.001$. There was no benefit in lengthening the duration of valacyclovir treatment from 7 to 14 days. The adverse effect profile of valacyclovir is the same as for acyclovir. The dose of oral valacyclovir in patients with normal renal function is 1 g every 8 hr (three times daily) for 7 days. Dose adjustments are necessary for renal insufficiency (Table 2).

5.2.3. Famciclovir

Famciclovir (500 and 750 mg doses) was compared to placebo in patients ≥18 years of age. A subgroup analysis was performed on patients ≥50 years of age (10). The median time to resolution of crusts (skin healing) was 2 days shorter in the 500 mg group vs. placebo (19 vs. 21 days). The proportion of patients who had pain at the time of rash healing was the same in all groups. In the subgroup analysis of older patients who had pain at rash healing, the median duration of pain was shorter in the treated group vs. placebo (63 vs. 163 days, $p = 0.004$). Randomized controlled trials comparing acyclovir to famciclovir and valacyclovir to famciclovir demonstrated equivalent results in rash healing, acute pain, and the duration of chronic pain (13,14).

All three drugs are recommended for the treatment of HZ in older adults with cost and dosing schedule determining the choice of agent. Antiviral therapy has helped with HZ pain but many treated patients still develop chronic pain. For example, 25–35% of antiviral-treated patients had pain 3 months from rash onset in the ideal setting of clinical trials (15). The effectiveness of antiviral agents is uncertain if the patient presents more than 72 hr since rash onset, except perhaps for patients who have ophthalmic HZ or continue to have new vesicle formation (7).

Ophthalmic HZ is an important form of HZ in older patients because of the risk of visual impairment or blindness in persons who may already have compromised vision from glaucoma, macular degeneration, cataracts, or diabetic neuropathy. Oral acyclovir was effective for the prevention of ocular complications of ophthalmic HZ in a randomized, controlled trial (16). Famciclovir and valacyclovir have comparable efficacy to acyclovir in the treatment of ophthalmic HZ (17,18). Ophthalmologist consultation is recommended in older patients with ophthalmic HZ to determine the presence and extent of ocular involvement and to determine the utility of local treatments such as mydriatics, glucocorticoids, or topical antivirals.

HZ in immunocompromised patients presents a special challenge because of the risk of VZV dissemination, visceral infection, and CNS involvement. Intravenous acyclovir significantly accelerated VZV shedding, hastened rash healing, reduced pain, and reduced the incidence of visceral and cutaneous dissemination progression, both in patients with localized disease and in those with cutaneous dissemination before treatment, in a randomized double-blind, placebo-controlled trial (10). In patients with mild immunocompromise and localized HZ, oral acyclovir, valacyclovir, or famciclovir will usually suffice. A randomized, controlled trial of oral famciclovir vs. oral acyclovir in localized HZ in immunocompromised patients following bone marrow or organ transplantation or oncology treatment found that the two treatments were equivalent in rash healing and loss of acute pain and that both were well tolerated (19). In patients with severe immune compromise or severe HZ, intravenous acyclovir is recommended. Patients with acyclovir-resistant VZV require intravenous foscarnet.

5.2.4. Corticosteroids

Corticosteroids have been advocated for decades in the treatment of HZ but the evidence indicates no efficacy in preventing PHN. In older patients, two randomized controlled trials that included data on corticosteroids vs. placebo showed equal rates of chronic pain in the two groups (20,21). In two randomized controlled clinical trials of acyclovir with or without corticosteroids, rates of chronic pain were not significantly different in those who did or did not receive corticosteroids (21,22). GI symptoms (dyspepsia, nausea, vomiting), edema, and granulocytosis were the most common adverse effects. Hence, corticosteroids are not recommended for routine use in elderly HZ patients. In the most recent trial of acyclovir and prednisone, time to uninterrupted sleep, return to daily activity, and cessation of analgesic therapy were significantly accelerated in patients who received corticosteroids. The patients in the trial had an average age of 60 years and no relative contraindications to corticosteroids such as hypertension, diabetes mellitus, or osteoporosis. Therefore, some experts advocate oral corticosteroids for otherwise healthy older adults with moderate to severe pain and no contraindications to corticosteroids. Corticosteroids may be useful for VZV-induced facial paralysis and cranial polyneuritis to improve motor outcomes and pain. Antiviral therapy should be used concomitantly in any patient receiving corticosteroids for HZ.

5.2.5. Analgesics

Acute HZ pain should be managed carefully just as any other pain syndrome. Clinicians should prescribe scheduled analgesics and use standardized pain measures, such as a 0–10 numerical rating scale, to determine pain severity and monitor therapy. Moderate to severe pain often necessitates scheduled opioid analgesia, which should be accompanied by scheduled laxatives. Regional or local anesthetic nerve blocks are useful if pain control from antiviral agents and analgesics is inadequate. The benefits of anticonvulsants or tricyclic antidepressants for acute HZ pain are unknown. Topical preparations such as the lidocaine patch or capsaicin have no role in treating acute HZ pain.

5.3. Postherpetic Neuralgia

Tricyclic antidepressants, gabapentin, pregabalin, opiates, and the topical lidocaine patch are effective in reducing PHN in a substantial number of older patients (5). The tricyclic antidepressants amitriptyline, desipramine, and nortriptyline produced moderate to good pain relief in 44–67% of elderly patients with PHN in several randomized, controlled trials. Nortriptyline and desipramine are preferred alternatives to amitriptyline because they cause less sedation, cognitive impairment, orthostatic hypotension, and constipation in older patients. In a comparative trial, amitriptyline and nortriptyline were equally effective in relieving pain but nortriptyline was better tolerated. Gabapentin and pregabalin significantly reduced average pain scores in patients with PHN in randomized, placebo controlled trials. The adverse effects of gabapentin and pregabalin included somnolence, dizziness and peripheral edema. Sustained-release oxycodone and morphine significantly reduced average pain ratings in older patients with PHN in two randomized, placebo-controlled crossover trials. The most frequently reported adverse effects were constipation, nausea, and sedation. Finally, the topical lidocaine patch and eutectic mixture of local anesthetics cream produced significant pain relief in patients with PHN in controlled clinical trials without systemic lidocaine toxicity. The patch may cause skin redness or rash.

6. PREVENTION

Interventions that prevent varicella and the establishment of latent VZV infection will prevent HZ in persons receiving the intervention. Varicella is effectively prevented by the live attenuated varicella vaccine. The vaccine is safe and well tolerated and induces protective antibodies and cellular immunity for many years in susceptible children and adults. In clinical practice, the vaccine is about 85% effective in protection against varicella (23). A small percentage of vaccines may not obtain an adequate immune response and develop "breakthrough" varicella but the resultant illness usually has less fever, constitutional symptoms, and cutaneous lesions than varicella due to wild-type VZV.

After Food and Drug Administration approval of the vaccine in 1995, the Centers for Disease Control and Prevention established a rigorous, active varicella surveillance program at sentinel sites in Antelope Valley, CA, West Philadelphia, PA, and Travis County, TX (24). From 1995 to 1999, varicella vaccination rates in children aged 12–23 months increased from <10% to ≈70% in 1999 at these sites. At the same time, varicella incidence declined by ≈80%, varicella seasonality was attenuated, and varicella-related hospitalizations declined markedly at all sites. The vaccine appears to be preventing most primary wild-type VZV infections in the United States, although clusters of breakthrough cases of varicella in vaccines have been reported in day care centers.

The Advisory Committee on Immunization Practices and American Academy of Pediatrics recommend the varicella vaccine for (1) routine childhood immunization, one dose at 12–18 months of age; (2) susceptible, immunocompetent older children, adolescents and adults, using two doses, 4–8 weeks apart for persons >13 years old; (3) individuals at high risk of exposure or transmission, including susceptible healthcare workers, the family of immunosuppressed individuals, teachers of children, day care workers, residents and staff in institutional settings, nonpregnant women of childbearing age, and college students; (4) postexposure prevention and outbreak control; and (5) day care and school entry.

The effect that prevention of primary wild-type VZV infection and varicella with the varicella vaccine will have on the incidence and natural history of HZ in the United States is unknown but will require careful study. As the children now receiving the vaccine become older adults, it is likely that there will be a decline in the incidence of wild-type VZV-related HZ and PHN. This result requires continued vaccination of high percentages of immune-naive individuals. The vaccine virus does establish a latent infection and can reactivate to cause HZ in vaccinated children and adults. However, thus far, vaccine virus-associated HZ appears to be less frequent and severe in older adults than natural HZ because the vaccine virus is highly attenuated. Conversely, the vaccine may affect the epidemiology of HZ in latently infected persons. A decline in the incidence of varicella will reduce the population's exposure to VZV and could prevent subsequent immune boosting to VZV. Reduced immune boosting to VZV could possibly increase the risk of VZV reactivation and HZ. Therefore, theoretically, the incidence of HZ in latently infected individuals could increase as varicella incidence declines.

A recent VA Cooperative Trial tested the hypothesis that vaccination against VZV would decrease the incidence, severity, or both of herpes zoster and postherpetic neuralgia among older adults (25). The study enrolled 38,546 adults 60 years of age or older in a randomized, double-blind, placebo-controlled trial of a more potent zoster vaccine than the currently licensed varicella vaccine. A total of 957 confirmed cases of herpes zoster (315 among vaccine recipients and 642 among placebo recipients) and 107 cases of postherpetic neuralgia (27 among vaccine recipients and 80 among placebo recipients) were included in the efficacy analysis. The zoster vaccine reduced the burden of illness due to herpes zoster by 61.1 percent ($P < 0.001$), reduced the incidence of postherpetic neuralgia by 66.5 percent ($P < 0.001$), and reduced the recidence of herpes zoster by 51.3 percent ($P < 0.001$). Reactions at the injection site were more frequent among vaccine recipients but were generally mild. This landmark study showed that the zoster vaccine markedly reduced morbidity from herpes zoster and postherpetic neuralgia among older adults.

Infection control measures are important for HZ patients during the vesicular phase of the rash with respect to preventing varicella in individuals at high risk for serious primary VZV infections. High-risk persons include immune-naive, susceptible patients with HIV disease, those undergoing immunosuppressive therapy, those with hematological malignancies, those with bone marrow transplantation, susceptible newborn infants, and even normal adults. Available approaches to prevent or modify varicella in these high-risk individuals include passive immunization with varicella-zoster immune globulin, active immunization with the varicella vaccine, chemoprophylaxis with acyclovir, and prevention of exposure via infection control practices. No preventive measures are recommended for a normal susceptible child because of the low likelihood of serious illness and the development of lifelong immunity and for latently infected, nonsusceptible persons.

ACKNOWLEDGMENTS

This work was supported by the Durham VA Medical Center Geriatric Research, Education and Clinical Center (GRECC) and K24-AI-51324-03 from the National Institute of Allergy and Infectious Diseases.

REFERENCES

1. Hope-Simpson RE. The nature of herpes zoster: a long-term study and new hypothesis. Proc R Soc Med (Lond) 1965; 58:9–20.

2. Donahue JG, Choo PW, Manson JE, Platt R. The incidence of herpes zoster. Arch Intern Med 1995; 155:1605–1609.
3. Schmader KE, George LK, Hamilton JD. Racial differences in the occurrence of herpes zoster. J Infect Dis 1995; 171:701–705.
4. Straus S, Schmader KE, Oxman MN. Varicella and herpes zoster. In: Freedberg I, Katz S, Wolff K, et al., eds. Fitzpatrick's Dermatology in General Medicine. 6th ed. New York: McGraw-Hill, 2003:2070–2086.
5. Dworkin RH, Schmader KE. The treatment and prevention of postherpetic neuralgia. Clin Infect Dis 2003; 36:877–882.
6. Gilden DH, Kleinschmidt-DeMasters BK, LaGuardia JJ, Mahalingam R, Cohrs RJ. Neurologic complications of the reactivation of varicella-zoster virus. N Engl J Med 2000; 342:635–645.
7. Gnaim JW, Whitley RJ. Herpes zoster. N Engl J Med 2002; 347:340–346.
8. Wood MJ, Kay R, Dworkin RH, Soong SJ, Whitley RJ. Oral acyclovir accelerates pain reduction in herpes zoster: a meta-analysis of placebo-controlled trials. Clin Infect Dis 1996; 22:341–347.
9. Beutner KR, Friedman DJ, Forszpaniak C, Andersen PL, Wood MJ. Valaciclovir compared with acyclovir for improved therapy for herpes zoster in immunocompetent adults. Antimicrob Agents Chemother 1995; 39:1546–1553.
10. Tyring S, Barbarash RA, Nahlik JE, Cunningham A, Marley J, Heng M, Jones T, Rea T, Boon R, Saltznan R. Famciclovir for the treatment of acute herpes zoster: effects on acute disease and postherpetic neuralgia: a randomized, double-blind, placebo-controlled trial. Ann Intern Med 1995; 123:89–96.
11. Jackson JL, Gibbons R, Meyer G, Inouye L. The effect of treating herpes zoster with oral acyclovir in preventing postherpetic neuralgia. Arch Intern Med 1997; 157: 909–912.
12. Balfour HH Jr, Bean B, Laskin OL, Ambinder RF, Meyers JD, Wade JC, Zaia JA, Aeppli D, Elirk LE, Segreti AC, Keeney RE. Acyclovir halts progression of herpes zoster in imm-unocornpromised patients. N Engl J Med 1983; 308:1448–1453.
13. deGreef H, Famciclovir Herpes Zoster Clinical Study Group. Famciclovir, a new oral antiherpes drug: results of the first controlled clinical study demonstrating its efficacy and safety in the treatment of uncomplicated herpes zoster in immunocompetent patients. Int J Antimicrob Agents 1995; 4:241–246.
14. Tyring SK, Beutner KR, Tucker BA, Anderson WC, Crooks RJ. Antiviral therapy for herpes zoster: randomized, controlled clinical trial of valacyclovir and famciclovir therapy in immunocompetent patients 50 years and older. Arch Fam Med 2000; 9: 863–869.
15. Dworkin RH, Schmader KE. The epidemiology and natural history of herpes zoster and postherpetic neuralgia. In: Watson CPN, ed. Herpes Zoster and Postherpetic Neuralgia. Amsterdam: Elsevier, 2001:39–65.
16. Cobo LM, Foulks GN, Liesegang T, Lass J, Sutphin IE, Wilhelmus K, Jones DB, Chapman S, Segreti AC, King DH. Oral acyclovir in the treatment of acute herpes zoster ophthalmicus. Ophthalmology 1986; 93:763–770.
17. Tyring S, Engst R, Corriveau C, Robillard N, Trottier S, Van Slycken S, Crann RA, Locke LA, Saltzman R, Palestine AG. Famciclovir for ophthalmic zoster: a randomized, aciclovir controlled study. Br J Ophmahnol 2001; 85:576–581.
18. Colin J, Prisant O, Cochener B, Lescale O, Rolland B, Hoang-Xuan T. Comparison of the efficacy and safety of valaciclovir and acyclovir for the treatment of herpes zoster ophthalmicus. Ophthalmology 2000; 107:1507–1511.
19. Tyring S, Belanger R, Bezwoda W, Ljungman P, Boon R, Saltzman RL. A randomized, double-blind trial of famciclovir versus acyclovir for the treatment of localized dermatomal herpes zoster in immunocompromised patients. Cancer Invest 2001; 19:13–22.

20. Esmann V, Geil JP, Kroon S, Fogh H, Peterslund NA, Petersen CS, Ronne-Rasmussen JO, Danielsen L. Prednisolone does not prevent postherpetic neuralgia. Lancet 1987; 2:126–129.

21. Whitley RJ, Weiss H, Gnann JW, Tyring S, Mertz GJ, Pappas PG, Schleupner CJ, Hayden F, Wolf J, Soong SJ. Acyclovir with and without prednisone for the treatment of herpes zoster: a randomized placebo-controlled trial. Ann Intern Med 1996; 125:376–383.

22. Wood MJ, Johnson RW, McKendrick MW, Taylor J, Mandal BK, Crooks J. A randomized trial of acyclovir for 7 days or 21 days with and without prednisolone for treatment of acute herpes zoster. N Engl J Med 1994; 330:896–900.

23. Vazquez M, LaRussa PS, Gershon AA, Niccolai LM, Muehlenbein CE, Steinberg SP, Shapiro ED. Effectiveness overtime of varicella vaccine. J Am Med Assoc 2004; 91:851–855.

24. Seward JF, Watson BM, Peterson CL, Mascola L, Pelosi JW, Zhang JX, Maupin TJ, Goldman GS, Tabony LJ, Brodovicz KG, Jumaan AO, Wharton M. Varicella disease after introduction of varicella vaccine in the United States, 1995–2000. J Am Med Assoc 2002; 287:606–611.

25. Oxman MN, Levin MJ, Johnson GR, Schmader KE, Straus SE, Gelb LD. et al. for the Shingles Prevention Study Group. A vaccine to prevent herpes zoster and postherpetic neuralgia in older adults. N Engl J Med 2005; 352:2271–2284.

SUGGESTED READING

Dworkin RH, Schmader KE. The treatment and prevention of postherpetic neuralgia. Clin Infect Dis 2003; 36:S77–S882.

Gnann JW, Whitley RJ. Herpes zoster. N Engl J Med 2002; 347:340–346.

37
Bacterial Meningitis

Chester Choi

Department of Medicine, St. Mary Medical Center, Long Beach, California, U.S.A. and David Geffen School of Medicine, University of California at Los Angeles, Los Angeles, California, U.S.A.

Key Points:

- The antibiotic treatment of bacterial meningitis in older adults is complicated by the greater range of etiologies and the increasing antibiotic resistance of some meningopathogens.
- The empirical treatment of bacterial meningitis in older adults should include ceftriaxone or cefotaxime plus ampicillin. Vancomycin should be added when *Streptococcus pneumoniae* resistant to third-generation cephalosporins is prevalent.
- Dexamethasone should be utilized for patients with known or suspected *S. pneumoniae* meningitis.
- Older adults with fever and altered mental status pose a particularly difficult clinical dilemma. Common infections such as pyelonephritis or pneumonia may lead to altered mental status in the absence of meningeal involvement or brain abscess. Most such patients will require a lumbar puncture and cerebrospinal fluid analysis to exclude bacterial meningitis.
- Pneumococcal vaccination is underutilized, yet may provide significant protection against meningitis caused by this organism.

1. EPIDEMIOLOGY AND CLINICAL RELEVANCE

The epidemiology of bacterial meningitis has changed markedly from a disease affecting mostly children to one increasingly of adults, especially older adults (1). In nationwide surveys from the 1970s to 1980s, an estimated 20,000 cases of bacterial meningitis occurred annually with 45% of the cases due to *Haemophilus influenzae* in children (2,3). Effective and universally applied vaccination for this organism has altered the epidemiology of bacterial meningitis such that the median age has changed from 15 months to 25 years and the number of cases due to *H. influenzae* has decreased by 94%. Current estimates are that about three cases of bacterial meningitis occur per 100,000 persons in the United States annually and that about 20% involve patients over 60 years of age. The latter percentage is a significant increase from an earlier survey where 8.6% involved older adults (4). The case fatality rate

Table 1 Surveillance Studies of Bacterial Meningitis in Older Adults (Age > 60 Years)

| | Studies | | | | | |
| | Wenger et al. | | Schlech et al. | | Schuchat et al. | |
Organisms	AR	CFR	AR	CFR	AR	CFR
S. pneumoniae	1.5	31	0.5	54	1.9	20
L. monocytogenes	0.5		0.1	41	0.6	
H. influenzae	0.2		0.09	24	0.07	
N. meningitidis	0.1		0.2	29	0.1	
Group B *Streptococcus*	0.2	51	0.02	23	0.1	18

Abbreviations: AR, attack rate per 100,000; CFR, case fatality rate (percent).
Source: From Wenger et al. (2)—incomplete data on CFRs for all organisms, Schlech et al. (3), and Schuchat et al. (4)—incomplete data on CFRs for all organisms.

in older adults is ≈20%, and Gorse and colleagues found that significant complications occurred in 85% of individuals over the age of 50 compared to 41% for a younger cohort in their retrospective comparison (5).

Epidemiological studies reveal that a broader array of organisms may cause meningitis in older adults, and that viral etiologies are distinctly less common (5,6). The bacterial etiologies include *S. pneumoniae*, *Listeria monocytogenes*, gram-negative bacilli such as *Escherichia coli* or *Klebsiella* species, *Streptococcus agalactiae*, and less commonly, *Neisseria meningitidis* and *H. influenzae*. Table 1 lists the attack rate and case fatality rates for some of these organisms in older adults.

The broader range of responsible organisms and increased incidence of bacterial meningitis in the elderly is multifactorial, including a higher likelihood of underlying chronic illnesses and the possible influence of immunosenescence, a decline in immune function related to aging. Many of the epidemiological studies link etiologies such as *S. pneumoniae*, *L. monocytogenes*, and *S. agalactiae* with underlying pneumonia, diabetes mellitus, renal or hepatic failure, or other chronic diseases with bacterial meningitis in older adults (5,6).

The development of most cases of meningitis is thought to involve (1) nasopharyngeal colonization, (2) access to and survival in the bloodstream, (3) traversal of the blood–brain barrier (BBB), and (4) replication in the subarachnoid space. Bacteria can replicate to numbers as high as 10^{10} in the cerebrospinal fluid (CSF) as host defenses are ineffective in that environment. Antibiotics or bacterial autolysins then cause the release of bacterial components which induce an inflammatory response in the CSF by activating mediator cytokines such as tumor necrosis factor and interleukins. These mediators, along with bacterial products, may result in alteration of the BBB and subsequent vasogenic cerebral edema, neuronal cell death, and cytotoxic edema, and reduction in cerebral blood flow and CSF outflow leading to interstitial edema (7,8).

2. ETIOLOGIC PATHOGENS

2.1. *Streptococcus pneumoniae*

This organism is the most frequent cause (70%) of bacterial meningitis in older adults and may be recognized as gram-positive diplococci with elongation or lancet-shaped morphology (4). Over 85 serotypes are identified with some known to more frequently cause severe disease due to capsular and other bacterial virulence factors. Treatment of this organism is complicated by penicillin and cephalosporin resistance mediated by alterations in penicillin-binding proteins. This resistance is particularly problematic in the treatment of meningitis since CSF levels of penicillins and cephalosporins adequate enough to overcome this resistance may be difficult to achieve.

Approximately 25–35% of isolates in the United States are nonsusceptible to penicillin (intermediate- or high-level resistance). Approximately 10–15% of isolates are multi-antibiotic resistant, including resistance to cephalosporins, trimethoprim-sulfamethoxazole (TMP–SMZ), erythromycin, azithromycin, clarithromycin, clindamycin, and chloramphenicol. All isolates remain susceptible to vancomycin (9,10).

The National Committee for Clinical Laboratory Standards changed the break point designations for nonmeningeal isolates of *S. pneumoniae* for ceftriaxone and cefotaxime (susceptible: $\geq 1\,\mu g/mL$, intermediate: $2\,\mu g/mL$, and resistant: $\geq 4\,\mu g/mL$) in 2002, but retained the previous values for meningeal isolates (susceptible: $\leq 0.5\,\mu g/mL$, intermediate: $1\,\mu g/mL$, and resistant: $\geq 2\,\mu g/mL$). The effect of this change is that fewer isolates overall are now deemed resistant to third-generation cephalosporins, so these antibiotics may be used more widely for nonmeningeal infections. However, the situation with meningeal pathogens remains the same, i.e., those with intermediate or resistant isolates are at risk of failure to treatment with third-generation cephalosporins alone. Clear communication between hospital laboratories and clinicians will be vital to avoid misidentifying a meningeal isolate as susceptible by mistakenly utilizing the nonmeningeal break points (11).

A recent development has been the recognition of meningitis caused by *S. pneumoniae* as a complication of implantation of cochlear devices to correct hearing loss. Most of these cases have been reported in children, but ≈13,000 of these devices have been implanted in older adults. This situation has been added as a new indication for the use of pneumococcal vaccine utilizing the preparation approved for that age range (conjugate vaccine, Prevnar®, in children and polysaccharide vaccine, Pneumovax®, in adults) (12).

2.2. *Listeria monocytogenes*

This gram-positive bacillus is found with increased frequency as a cause of meningitis in older adults (22%) as well as with immunocompromised individuals, particularly those with alterations in cell-mediated immunity (4). It is often a food-borne pathogen and has been identified as a contaminant of a variety of processed foods and food handling equipment, but this epidemiological feature is infrequently linked to adults with meningitis. Eleven serotypes are known, but most diseases are caused by types Ia, Ib, and IVb. A sometimes helpful property in identification of this organism is its "end-over-end" tumbling motility; this property, as well as its associated beta hemolysis, can be used to help differentiate it from other gram-positive bacilli such as *Corynebacteria* species which can sometimes contaminate CSF specimens (13).

2.3. Aerobic Gram-Negative Bacilli

Older adults are susceptible to meningitis caused by these agents through either bacteremic spread from distant foci such as urinary tract infections and intra-abdominal abscesses or direct extension to the meninges from traumatic or surgical causes. *Klebsiella* sp. and *E. coli* are the predominant organisms encountered; however, any of a number of gram-negative bacilli, including some that are multi-antibiotic resistant, have been implicated. Meningitis caused by these organisms results less often in a positive CSF Gram stain and may present with fewer neutrophils on CSF examination (14).

2.4. *Neisseria meningitidis*

On gram-stained smears, this organism appears as gram-negative, kidney-shaped diplococci with their concave surfaces opposite to each other. There are five main serotypes (A, B, C, Y, and W135) which cause disease in humans, but only about 5% of bacterial meningitis in older adults is due to this organism.

Complement deficiency, particularly of the late components (C5-9), has been strongly associated with severe or recurrent infections with this organism. The complement deficiency may be either congenital or acquired (15).

2.5. *Haemophilus influenzae*

This pleomorphic, gram-negative, and coccobacillary organism is a less common ($\approx$2.5%) cause of meningitis in older adults (4). Most invasive disease, including meningitis, is caused by encapsulated type B isolates. These organisms often produce a β-lactamase, which allows them to resist the effects of some penicillins including ampicillin or amoxicillin. Approximately 35–40% of isolates are β-lactamase positive (8).

2.6. *Streptococcus agalactiae*

The group B streptococci are increasingly being found as pathogens in community-acquired bacterial meningitis. Risk factors in addition to more advanced age include underlying diseases such as diabetes mellitus, renal insufficiency or failure, and advanced hepatic disease. The infection often results from bacteremic spread with blood cultures positive in almost 80% of patients in one series. A distant focus of infection, such as infective endocarditis, pneumonia, or female genital tract infection, was found in 40% of the patients (16).

3. CLINICAL MANIFESTATIONS

The presence of all three classical symptoms including fever, altered mentation, and neck stiffness may be present in less than half the adults with bacterial meningitis (1). However, in the elderly even the presence of all three symptoms is not sufficiently specific for diagnosis. The absence of all the three symptoms, though, does appear to be sufficient to exclude the diagnosis as determined in a comprehensive literature review (17).

Fever is less frequently found in older adults with a variety of infectious diseases, including meningitis (18). In older adults, neck stiffness may be found from prior neurological disease such as stroke or from cervical arthritis. Alteration in mental function may result from a number of causes in the elderly, including infectious diseases without direct central nervous system (CNS) involvement. In these latter situations, it is felt that cytokines may be responsible for the altered neurological function (19).

Thomas and colleagues found that physical examination findings, including neck stiffness, Kernig's sign, and Brudzinski's signs were not sensitive or specific enough to aid in the diagnosis of meningitis. Kernig's sign is sought by extending the knee to ascertain increased pain while the patient is in the supine position with the hip and knee flexed at 90°. Brudzinski's signs include the nape of the neck sign, whereby the examiner flexes the patient's neck (patient is in supine position) to determine if there is increased neck pain, resistance to this motion, and flexing of the hips or knees. Nuchal rigidity was found in 50% of those patients with moderate meningeal inflammation as classified by CSF white blood cell counts (WBCs) > 100 cells/mm^3. Thus, this study indicates that physical examination is insensitive and nonspecific in diagnosing meningitis, although no specific directions were given to the participating emergency medicine physicians regarding the proper technique or interpretation of these tests (20).

4. DIAGNOSIS

Since the clinical examination is not sufficiently specific, the diagnosis of bacterial meningitis rests on the results of lumbar puncture (LP) with CSF testing. In general, patients with bacterial meningitis will have WBCs in their CSF of >500–1000 cells/mm^3 with >85% of the cells being polymorphonuclear leukocytes. The CSF glucose is usually less than one-third of the simultaneous peripheral blood glucose, and the protein may be significantly elevated. The Gram stain is positive in ≈85% of cases in the absence of prior antibiotic therapy (21). Table 2 lists typical findings in bacterial and other types of meningitis.

The decisions regarding the performance of an LP and other neurological assessment of bacterial meningitis are complex and it is difficult to provide a rigid guideline. Older adults may have nonmeningeal infection as a cause of their altered mental function and fever; their altered mental function may be due to cytokines or other inflammatory responses to the infection or it may be due to a variety of other causes such as adverse drug reactions, dementia, or cerebral infarction (19). In a study of fever and altered mental status occurring in hospitalized patients who had not had neurosurgical procedures, LP did not reveal meningitis as a cause of these symptoms (22). However, the study was relatively small, making it difficult to draw firm conclusions. In deciding whether LP is indicated or not, one must consider the pretest probability of meningitis. Some patients with fever, acutely depressed mental function, and infection at a nonmeningeal site can be closely observed without an LP while their infection is treated. Most such patients, however, should undergo LP if it is safe to do so, particularly if their symptoms began before hospitalization (23).

LP is a procedure which raises concerns about possible serious complications such as cerebral herniation. In many urban centers, it has become routine to perform a computed tomography (CT) scan of the brain prior to performing an LP, but the test does not completely exclude the possibility of this complication and it may delay the appropriate antibiotic treatment of patients with bacterial meningitis. A careful neurological assessment, including a funduscopic examination, should be performed. In younger patients, if there is no evidence of papilledema, especially if venous pulsations are visualized and there are no findings of focal neurological deficit or rapid neurological progression, the risk of herniation from LP is considered negligible (24).

Table 2 CSF Findings in Meningitis

	Normal CSF	Acute bacterial	Viral	Tuberculous
Opening pressure	6–20 cm H$_2$O	Usually elevated	Moderately elevated	Usually elevated
CSF WBCs	0–5 (about 85% lymphs)	Usually several hundred to >60,000, PMNs predominate	Five to a few hundred but may be more than 1000; lymphocytes predominate but may be >80% PMNs in the first few days	Usually 25–100, rarely >500; lymphocytes predominate except in early stages where PMNs may account for >80% of cells
Protein	18–45 mg/dL	Usually 100–500, occasionally >1000	Frequently normal or slightly elevated (<100); may show greater elevation in severe cases	Nearly always elevated; usually 100–200 but may be much higher if dynamic block
Glucose	45–80 mg/dL, or 0.6 × serum glucose	Usually 5–40 mg/dL or <0.3 × serum glucose	Usually normal, but can be low with mumps, HSV2	Usually reduced; <45 in three-fourths of cases
Miscellaneous	For traumatic taps add 1 WBC and 1 mg/dL protein for each 1000 RBCs	Gram's stain+ in about 60–80%; Sp = gram-positive diplococci, Nm = gram-negative diplococci, Lm = gram-positive rods	Usually do not need to find specific causal virus	AFB+ stain in <25%, culture+ in >2/3 of cases (but may take 4–8 weeks for growth)

Abbreviations: Sp, *Streptococcus pneumoniae*; Nm, *Neisseria meningitidis*; Lm, *Listeria monocytogenes*; AFB, acid fast bacilli; HSV2, Herpes simplex type II; PMNs, polymorphonuclear neutrophils; WBC, white blood cell; RBCs, red blood cells.
Source: Adapted from Refs. 21,23,26.

Older adults may have brain pathology such as tumors, abscesses, infarcts, or hemorrhage that could lead to herniation if LP is performed. In addition, they may have ocular diseases that make visualization of the optic fundi for papilledema more difficult. In a recent retrospective study concerning this risk, the authors noted that the greatest identifiable risks of a subsequently abnormal CT scan were age >60 years, immunocompromised state, previous CNS disease, recent seizure, and focal abnormalities found on a bedside diagnostic neurological examination using the modified National Institutes of Health Stroke Scale. CT brain scans should generally be performed in older adults prior to LP (25).

Attempts to facilitate the diagnosis of bacterial meningitis have been sought. These include the use of bacterial antigen testing in CSF utilizing a variety of techniques such as latex agglutination or coagglutination to detect *S. pneumoniae*, *H. influenzae* type B, *N. meningitidis* (all five serotypes), *E. coli*, and *S. agalactiae*. However, these tests are relatively expensive and are not routinely necessary since Gram stains are frequently positive. Instead, the antigen testing should be reserved for situations where prior antibiotic therapy may have changed the yield of Gram stains or cultures or where bacterial meningitis seems very likely from the CSF results, but no organism has been identified on culture. In the latter situation, a stored tube of CSF may prove useful (26).

Other diagnostic tests under investigation include polymerase chain reaction (PCR) tests to detect specific bacteria and a broad-range bacterial PCR to diagnose bacterial meningitis in its early stages and differentiate it from other causes of meningitis (27). The latter test might obviate the need for further testing or for immediate antibiotic therapy if it is sufficiently sensitive to exclude the diagnosis of bacterial meningitis. Similarly, serum procalcitonin is being investigated to help diagnose or exclude bacterial meningitis. Magnetic resonance imaging may reveal enhancement of the meninges on gadolinium-enhanced T-1 weighted images (26).

5. ANTIBIOTIC TREATMENT

The treatment of bacterial meningitis is predicated on several key assumptions and principles. First, treatment must be instituted as soon as possible or patient outcomes will be adversely affected. Aronin and colleagues retrospectively reviewed almost 300 cases of bacterial meningitis in four hospitals in the northeastern United States. These authors examined a simple prognostic scoring model. By stratifying patients based on the presence of altered mentation, hypotension, and seizures, the authors were able to show that patients who progressed from two of these findings to all three prior to the institution of antibiotic therapy had significantly worse outcomes (28).

Second, bactericidal antibiotics should be chosen. This is based on earlier attempts at therapy with bacteriostatic antibiotics with seemingly worsened outcomes. Similarly, animal models of this disease do seem to provide evidence that bactericidal antibiotics are the preferred treatment. However, a possible dichotomy exists in the rationale. Bactericidal antibiotics would result in more rapid killing of bacteria, seemingly with a greater or more abrupt release of cytokines and bacterial products, which may portend increased inflammatory effect and, perhaps, worsened outcome. However, in an animal model of *E. coli* meningitis, bacterial killing resulted in lesser amounts of endotoxin release compared with untreated infection (29). In comparative studies of the treatment of *H. influenzae* meningitis in children, ceftriaxone

Table 3 Antibiotic Penetration of CSF

Excellent	Good (with inflammation)	Poor or negligible
Rifampin	Penicillins	Most first- and second-generation cephalosporins
TMP–SMZ	Third-generation cephalosporins	Aminoglycosides: tobramycin, and gentamicin
Chloramphenicol	Cefuroxime	
Metronidazole	Vancomycin (variable), erythromycin (variable), and tetracyclines (variable)	

Note: Excellent, >15–20% penetration; good, 5–20% penetration; poor or negligible, <1–5% penetration.
Abbreviations: TMP-SMZ, trimethoprim-sulfamethoxazole.
Source: Adapted from Refs. 23,26,29,31.

proved to be superior to cefuroxime due to the former drug's more rapid killing of bacteria and sterilization of the CSF (30). Thus, more rapid bactericidal activity seems to be beneficial, resulting in fewer serious sequelae.

Third, the ability of the chosen antibiotics to cross the BBB and achieve significant levels in the CSF is essential. This is the rationale for the utilization of high doses of antibiotics, particularly penicillins and cephalosporins, which cross the BBB only in the presence of inflammation and achieve levels ≈5–10% of serum concentrations. This phenomenon relates to the inability of these drugs to penetrate the tight junctions of meningeal lining cells or to be transported via pinocytosis at this barrier in the absence of inflammation. β-lactam antibiotics manifest time-dependent killing for most bacteria; thus, maintenance of adequate levels of these drugs in the CSF through either more frequent dosing or more prolonged duration of action would be optimal. Some other agents, such as TMP–SMZ, metronidazole, chloramphenicol, and rifampin, are able to penetrate this barrier well, due to their lipid solubility, and achieve CSF levels of 30–40% of serum concentrations even in the absence of inflammation (29). Table 3 lists antibiotics and their ability to penetrate the CSF.

In addition to the effects of inflammation and antibiotic lipid solubility, levels in the CSF are affected by an antibiotic's degree of ionization at physiologic pH, molecular size and shape, and degree of protein binding. Some antibiotic metabolites, e.g., desacetylcefotaxime, retain a significant degree of bactericidal activity while others, e.g., desacetylcephalothin, do not. Once antibiotics reach the CSF space, their efficacy is affected by protein binding since it is only the free or unbound drug which possesses antibacterial activity. Some antibiotics are associated with an inoculum effect such that the large organism burden seen in meningitis may require a higher level of such antibiotics than would be apparent from in vitro testing. Antibiotics may also vary in their CSF concentrations due to differences in their removal from the subarachnoid space. They are typically either resorbed from the CSF through the arachnoid villi or removed by a facilitated transport mechanism in the choroid plexus (31).

5.1. Empirical Antibiotic Therapy

A difficult dilemma for clinicians is the initiation of antibiotic therapy for suspected meningitis. In older adults, a broader range of organisms may be responsible for the

Table 4 Recommended Antibiotic Therapy for Bacterial Meningitis

Organism	Antibiotic	Total daily dose
Empirical treatment for bacterial meningitis[a]	Ceftriaxone plus Ampicillin[b]	4 g 12 g
S. pneumoniae (penicillin sensitive)	Penicillin G	20–24 million units
S. pneumoniae[c] (penicillin or cephlosporin resistant)	Vancomycin plus Ceftriaxone	2 g 4 g
L. monocytogenes	Ampicillin plus an aminoglycoside: gentamicin and tobramycin	12 g 3–6 mg/kg
N. meningitidis	Penicillin G or Ampicillin	20–24 million units 12 g
H. influenzae	Ceftriaxone	4 g
Enterobacteriaceae (gram-negative bacilli)	Ceftriaxone[d]	4 g
Staphylococcus aureus (methicillin sensitive)	Nafcillin or oxacillin	8–12 g
S. aureus (methicillin resistant)	Vancomycin	2 g

[a] Add vancomycin if highly penicillin-resistant S. pneumoniae suspected.
[b] If patient is penicillin allergic, consider use of vancomycin plus TMP–SMZ (15–20 mg/kg/day divided into doses every 6–8 hr) with or without aztreonam 8 g/day (divided into doses every 6 hr); add rifampin (600 mg/day) if dexamethasone utilized.
[c] Use vancomycin plus ceftriaxone plus rifampin (600 mg/day) if penicillin- or cephalosporin-resistant S. pneumoniae are identified and dexamethasone utilized.
[d] Ceftazidime (6 g/day) or cefepime (4 g/day) if P. aeruginosa is suspected or proven.
Source: Adapted from Refs (23,26,29).

illness and empirical antibiotic therapy must take into account this difference. Thus, recommendations for treatment have included ceftriaxone or cefotaxime for S. pneumoniae, N. meningitidis, H. influenzae, and some aerobic gram-negative rods and ampicillin for L. monocytogenes. In areas where S. pneumoniae is often highly resistant to penicillin and to third-generation cephalosporins, vancomycin should be added. The combination of vancomycin and ceftriaxone has been shown in vitro to provide synergistic killing of penicillin- and cephalosporin-resistant S. pneumoniae. In penicillin-allergic patients, empirical treatment for older adults is problematic as there are few efficacy studies, but such treatment recommendations could include vancomycin + TMP–SMZ ± aztreonam for aerobic gram-negative bacilli. Table 4 lists empirical and specific antibiotic regimens for bacterial meningitis in older adults.

There is an important multicenter trial from Europe utilizing dexamethasone as part of the initial therapy to reduce the effects of inflammatory cytokines with demonstrated improved outcomes, but the routine use of this agent may further complicate treatment decisions. High-dose dexamethasone (10 mg intravenously every 6 hr for 4 days) was beneficial in S. pneumoniae meningitis as shown by decreases in mortality and in other adverse complications such as seizures, impairment of consciousness, and cardiorespiratory failure. In this study, however, none of the patients had penicillin- or cephalosporin-resistant S. pneumoniae. Thus, the authors did not need to address the particularly problematic penetration of vancomycin into the CSF with the reduction of inflammation caused by the use of the steroid medication (32).

The accompanying editorial recommends the use of dexamethasone for known or suspected *S. pneumoniae* meningitis and its administration prior to or with the first dose of antibiotic. If the patient has a different etiologic organism, is in septic shock, or has already received antibiotic therapy, dexamethasone would not be recommended. However, the use of this agent and its effect of decreasing inflammation could decrease the levels of β-lactam antibiotics and especially vancomycin in the CSF. If penicillin- and cephalosporin-resistant *S. pneumoniae* is involved and dexamethasone is instituted, vancomycin should not be used as a single agent, but instead the combination of vancomycin plus ceftriaxone has been recommended and some experts would add rifampin to the combination. If the patient is intolerant of cephalosporins or has had a major reaction to penicillin (anaphylaxis or urticaria), vancomycin plus rifampin could be utilized, but a repeated LP should be performed to monitor the therapeutic effect. Patients with penicillin-resistant *S. pneumoniae* meningitis should have follow-up LPs at 24–48 hr to ensure appropriate response to therapy with a prompt increase in the CSF glucose and negative CSF cultures (33). Figure 1 depicts an algorithm for the management of bacterial meningitis in the elderly.

L. monocytogenes is best treated with a combination of intravenous ampicillin plus an aminoglycoside (gentamicin or tobramycin). Patients in whom aminoglycosides are contraindicated may be treated with ampicillin alone. Those who are penicillin allergic should receive TMP–SMZ. This organism may be susceptible to vancomycin in in vitro testing, but clinical failures have occurred when vancomycin has been utilized in *Listeria* meningitis and in other severe infections. Additionally, meropenem has in vitro activity against *L. monocytogenes*, but there is currently insufficient data to recommend its use and there may be allergic cross-reactivity for some patients with this agent and penicillin (28).

N. meningitidis should be treated with penicillin or ampicillin. Other agents such as third-generation cephalosporins may be equally effective, but there is less clinical experience with such treatment. Penicillin-allergic patients may be treated with chloramphenicol, although there are now reports of the emergence of chloramphenicol-resistant organisms in other countries (34).

The treatment of *H. influenzae* meningitis is complicated by antibiotic resistance also, with up to 35–40% of strains producing a β-lactamase rendering ampicillin or amoxicillin ineffective. These organisms generally respond to third-generation cephalosporins such as ceftriaxone or cefotaxime.

S. agalactiae is best treated with a combination of penicillin plus an aminoglycoside if the patient's renal function permits its use.

The duration of treatment for these pathogens has not been rigorously tested. In general, *S. pneumoniae* meningitis is treated for 10–14 days while *H. influenzae* and *N. meningitidis* require a shorter duration of about 7 days. *L. monocytogenes* and *S. agalactiae* are usually treated for 14–21 days and gram-negative bacilli require more prolonged therapy of about 21 days (29).

6. PREVENTION

The efficacy of the *H. influenzae* conjugate vaccine has been a major advance in health care, and there are attempts to duplicate its success with vaccines directed against

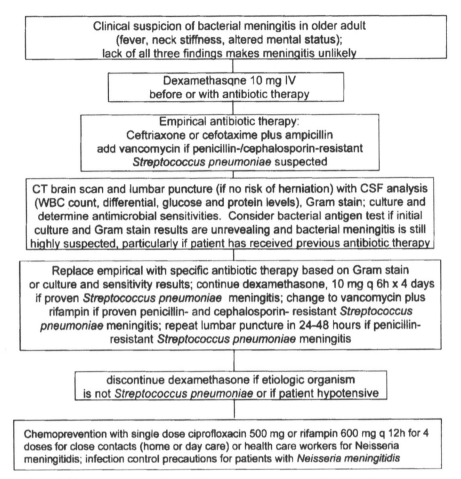

Clinical suspicion of bacterial meningitis in older adult
(fever, neck stiffness, altered mental status);
lack of all three findings makes meningitis unlikely

Dexamethasqne 10 mg IV
before or with antibiotic therapy

Empirical antibiotic therapy:
Ceftriaxone or cefotaxime plus ampicillin
add vancomycin if penicillin-/cephalosporin-resistant
Streptococcus pneumoniae suspected

CT brain scan and lumbar puncture (if no risk of herniation) with CSF analysis
(WBC count, differential, glucose and protein levels), Gram stain; culture and
determine antimicrobial sensitivities. Consider bacterial antigen test if initial
culture and Gram stain results are unrevealing and bacterial meningitis is still
highly suspected, particularly if patient has received previous antibiotic therapy

Replace empirical with specific antibiotic therapy based on Gram stain
or culture and sensitivity results; continue dexamethasone, 10 mg q 6h x 4 days
if proven *Streptococcus pneumoniae* meningitis; change to vancomycin plus
rifampin if proven penicillin- and cephalosporin- resistant *Streptococcus
pneumoniae* meningitis; repeat lumbar puncture in 24–48 hours if penicillin-
resistant *Streptococcus pneumoniae* meningitis

discontinue dexamethasone if etiologic organism
is not *Streptococcus pneumoniae* or if patient hypotensive

Chemoprevention with single dose ciprofloxacin 500 mg or rifampin 600 mg q 12h for 4
doses for close contacts (home or day care) or health care workers for Neisseria
meningitidis; infection control precautions for patients with *Neisseria meningitidis*

Key: CSF = cerebrospinal fluid; CT = computed tomography; IV = intravenous;
WBC = white blood cell;

Figure 1 Algorithm for the diagnosis and treatment of bacterial meningitis in older adults.

other meningopathogens. The 23-valent polysaccharide vaccine for *S. pneumoniae*,
Pneumovax, is an effective one, but the degree of efficacy is not definitively proven
(35). A recent study showed efficacy for bacteremic pneumococcal pneumonia, but
not for community-acquired pneumonia overall (36). Since bacteria or bloodstream
survival is presumed to be an important part of the pathogenesis of pneumococcal
meningitis, this polysaccharide vaccine may still provide significant protection for
this disease. The vaccine is significantly underutilized with less than one-third of
eligible candidates having received it in earlier surveys. The Centers for Disease
Control and Prevention have put forth targets of 60% vaccination rates for eligible
older adults and 90% for the institutionalized elderly (35).

The development of an improved vaccine is also a major goal, and a protein
conjugate vaccine has been developed for use in children and infants (Prevnar).
An interesting effect of the use of this vaccine, which also decreases colonization
rates of *S. pneumoniae*, is that adult infection rates, especially those in older adults,
were also decreased by the use of this vaccine in children. This may have a significant

beneficial effect on the rates of infection with antibiotic-resistant *S. pneumoniae* (37). *N. meningitidis* vaccine is a quadrivalent vaccine in the United States, containing antigenic material for serotypes A, C, Y, and W135. However, it is not of long-lasting efficacy and again research is under way to improve the duration of protection and to extend its efficacy to serotype B. Currently, indications for the use of this vaccine include prior severe meningococcal infection, asplenia, complement deficiency, and planned travel to areas with endemic meningococcal meningitis or planned residence in areas where the disease occurs more frequently. Individuals with close residential exposure to index cases of meningococcal meningitis should be treated with chemoprophylaxis (rifampin 600 mg twice a day for 2 days or a single dose of ciprofloxacin 500 mg) as should contacts, including healthcare workers, exposed to "mucosal splash" from an index case. Patients with this disease should be isolated with droplet-type precautions for the first 24 hr of treatment (15).

Efforts to prevent severe infections with *L. monocytogenes* have focused on food safety and awareness. A *S. agalactiae* vaccine is under development with the intent of preventing perinatal transmission of this organism and the resultant disease in the neonate. No trials involving older adults with underlying risk factors such as diabetes, renal or hepatic failure, or malignancy have been reported.

REFERENCES

1. van de Beek D, de Gans J, Spanjaard L, Weisfelt M, Reitsma JB, Vermueller M. Clinical features and prognostic factors in adults with bacterial meningitis. N Engl J Med 2004; 351:1849–1859.
2. Wenger JD, Hightower AW, Facklam RR, Gaventa S, Broome CV. Bacterial meningitis in the United States, 1986: report of a multistate surveillance study. J Infect Dis 1990; 162:1316–1323.
3. Schlech WF III, Ward JI, Band JD, Hightower A, Fraser DW, Broome CV, The Bacterial Meningitis Study Group. Bacterial meningitis in the United States, 1978 through 1981: the national bacterial meningitis surveillance study. J Am Med Assoc 1985; 253: 1749–1754.
4. Schuchat A, Robinson K, Wenger JD, Harrison JH, Farley M, Reingold AL, Lefkowitz L, Perkins BA. Bacterial meningitis in the United States in 1995. Active Surveillance Team. N Engl J Med 1997; 337:970–976.
5. Gorse GJ, Thrupp LD, Nudelman KL, Wyle FA, Hawkins B, Cesario TC. Bacterial meningitis in the elderly. Arch Intern Med 1984; 144:1603–1607.
6. Behrman RE, Meyers BR, Mendelson MH, Sacks HS, Hirschman SZ. Central nervous system infections in the elderly. Arch Intern Med 1989; 149:1596–1599.
7. Scheld WM, Koedel U, Nathan B, Pfister H. Pathophysiology of bacterial meningitis: mechanism(s) of neuronal injury. J Infect Dis 2002; 186(suppl 2):S25–S33.
8. Quagliarello V, Scheld WM. Bacterial meningitis: pathogenesis, pathophysiology, and progress. N Engl J Med 1992; 327:864–872.
9. Thornsberry C, Sahm DF, Kelly LJ, Critchley IA, Jones ME, Evangelista AT. Regional trends in antimicrobial resistance among clinical isolates of *Streptococcus pneumoniae*, *Haemophilus influenzae*, and *Moraxella catarrhalis* in the United States: results from the TRUST surveillance program, 1999–2000. Clin Infect Dis 2002; 34(suppl 1):S14–S16.
10. Whitney CG, Farley MM, Hadler J, Harrison LH, Lexau C, Reingold A, Lefkowitz L, Cieslak PR, Cetron M, Zell E, Jorgensen JH, Schuchat A. Active Bacterial Core Surveillance Program of the Emerging Infections Program Network. Increasing prevalence of multidrug-resistant Streptococcus pneumoniae in the United States. N Engl J Med 2000; 343:1917–1924.

11. Centers for Disease Control and Prevention. Effect of new susceptibility breakpoints on reporting of resistance in Streptococcus pneumoniae—United States 2003. MMWR 2004; 53:152–153.

12. Centers for Disease Control and Prevention. Pneumococcal vaccination for cochlear implant recipients. MMWR 2002; 51:931.

13. Nieman RE, Lorber B. Listeriosis in adults: a changing pattern. Report of eight cases and review of the literature, 1968–1978. Rev Infect Dis 1980; 2:207–227.

14. Berk Sl, McCabe WR. Meningitis caused by gram-negative bacilli. Ann Intern Med 1980; 93:253–260.

15. Rosenstein NE, Perkins BA, Stephens DS, Popovic T, Hughes JM. Meningococcal disease. N Engl J Med 2001; 344:1378–1388.

16. Domingo P, Barquet N, Alvarez M, Coll P, Marti-Vilatta JL. Group B streptococcal meningitis in adults: report of twelve cases and review. Clin Infect Dis 1997; 25: 1180–1187.

17. Attia J, Hatala R, Cook DJ, Wong JG. Does this adult patient have acute meningitis? J Am Med Assoc 1999; 282:175–181.

18. Norman DC. Fever in the elderly. Clin Infect Dis 2000; 31:148–151.

19. Flacker JM, Lipsitz LA. Neural mechanisms of delirium: current hypotheses and evolving concepts. J Gerontol A Biol Sci Med Sci 1999; 54A:B239–B246.

20. Thomas KE, Hasbun R, Jekel J, Quagliarello V. The diagnostic accuracy of Kernig's sign, Brudzinski's sign, and nuchal rigidity in adults with suspected meningitis. Clin Infect Dis 2002; 35:46–52.

21. Fishman RA. CSF findings in diseases of the nervous system. In: Fishman RA, ed. Cerebrospinal Fluid in Diseases of the Nervous System. 2nd ed. Philadelphia, PA: WB Saunders, 1992:253–343.

22. Metersky ML, Williams A, Rafanan AL. Retrospective analysis: are fever and altered mental status indications for lumbar puncture in a hospitalized patient who has not undergone neurosurgery? Clin Infect Dis 1997; 25:285–288.

23. Choi C. Bacterial meningitis in aging adults. Clin Infect Dis 2001; 33:1380–1385.

24. Tauber MG. Editorial response: to tap or not to tap? Clin Infect Dis 1997; 25:289–291.

25. Hasbun R, Abrahams J, Jekel J, Quagliarello V. Computed tomography of the head before lumbar puncture in adults with suspected meningitis. N Engl J Med 2001; 345:1727–1733.

26. Roos KL, Tunkel AR, Scheld WM. Acute bacterial meningitis in children and adults. In: Scheld WM, Whitley RJ, Durack DT, eds. Infections of the Central Nervous System. 2nd ed. Philadelphia, PA: Lippincott-Raven Publishers, 1997:335–402.

27. Saravolatz LD, Manzor O, VanderVelde N, Pawlak J, Belian B. Broad-range bacterial polymerase chain reaction for early detection of bacterial meningitis. Clin Infect Dis 2003; 36:40–45.

28. Aronin SI, Peduzzi P, Quagliarello VJ. Community-acquired bacterial meningitis: risk stratification for adverse clinical outcome and effect of antibiotic timing. Ann Intern Med 1998; 129:862–869.

29. Quagliarello VJ, Scheld WM. Treatment of bacterial meningitis. N Engl J Med 1997; 336:708–716.

30. Schaad U, Suter S, Gianella-Borradori A, Pfenninger J, Auckenthaler R, Bernath O, Cheseaux JJ, Wedgwood J. A comparison of ceftriaxone and cefuroxime for the treatment of bacterial meningitis in children. N Engl J Med 1990; 322:141–147.

31. Andes DR, Craig WA. Pharmacokinetics and pharmacodynamics of antibiotics in meningitis. Infect Dis Clin North Am 1999; 13:595–618.

32. de Gans J, van de Beek D. Dexamethasone in adults with bacterial meningitis. N Engl J Med 2002; 347:1549–1556.

33. Tunkel AR, Scheld WM. Corticosteroids for everyone with meningitis? N Engl J Med 2002; 347:1613–1614.

34. Antignac A, Ducos-Galand M, Guiyoule A, Pires R, Alonso J, Taha M. Neisseria meningitidis strains isolated from invasive infections in France (1999–2002): phenotypes and antibiotic susceptibility patterns. Clin Infect Dis 2003; 37:912–920.

35. Centers for Disease Control and Prevention. Prevention of pneumococcal disease; recommendations of the advisory committee on immunization practices (ACIP). MMWR 1997; 46(RR-8):1–24.

36. Jackson LA, Neuzil KM, Yu O, Benson P, Barlow WE, Adams AL, Hanson CA, Mahoney LD, Shay DK, Thompson WW, Vaccine Safety Datalink. Effectiveness of pneumococcal polysaccharide vaccine in older adults. N Engl J Med 2003; 348: 1747–1755.

37. Whitney CG, Farley MM, Hadler J, Harrison LH, Bennett NM, Lynfield R, Reingold A, Cieslak PR, Pilishvili T, Jackson D, Facklam RR, Jorgensen JH, Schuchat A, Active Bacterial Core Surveillance of the Emerging Infections Program Network. Decline in invasive pneumococcal disease after the introduction of protein–polysaccharide conjugate vaccine. N Engl J Med 2003; 348:1737–1746.

SUGGESTED READING

de Gans J, van de Beek D. Dexamethasone in adults with bacterial meningitis. N Engl J Med 2002; 347:1549–1556 and accompanying editorial Tunkel AR, Scheld WM. Corticosteroids for everyone with meningitis? N Engl J Med 2002; 347:1613–1614.

Quagliarello VJ, Scheld WM. Treatment of bacterial meningitis. N Engl J Med 1997; 336: 708–716.

Tunkel AR, Harman BJ, Kaplan SL, Kaufman BA, Roos KL, Scheld WM, Whitley RJ. Practice guidelines for the management of bacterial meningitis. Clin Infect Dis 2004; 39:1267–1284.

van de Beek D, de Gans J, Spanjaard L, Weisfelt M, Reitsma JB, Vermueller M. Clinical features and prognostic factors in adults with bacterial meningitis. N Engl J Med 2004; 351:1849–1859.

38
Infective Endocarditis

Vinod K. Dhawan
Charles R. Drew University of Medicine and Science, Martin Luther King, Jr.–Charles R. Drew Medical Center, UCLA School of Medicine, Los Angeles, California, U.S.A.

Key Points:

- Age has been shown to be an important risk factor for infective endocarditis (IE), with an incidence rate ratio of 8.8:1 for age ≥65 years vs. age <65 years.
- Degenerative valvular heart disease is being increasingly associated with endocarditis among the elderly. Degenerative valve lesions are present in 50% of patients aged >60 years who have IE. Common lesions include degenerative aortic valve disease, calcified mitral annulus, and calcific aortic stenosis.
- The presentations of IE in the elderly are often nonspecific and atypical, resulting in delayed diagnosis. Optimal diagnosis of IE in the elderly requires sound clinical judgment and a high index of suspicion.
- The predominant organisms, responsible for ≈80% cases of IE in the elderly are *Staphylococcus aureus*, *Streptococcus* spp., and Enterococci.
- Effective therapy of IE requires timely identification of the microbial etiology. Empirical intravenous antibiotic therapy should be initiated promptly after blood and other appropriate samples have been taken for culture. Bactericidal antibiotics are a cornerstone of therapy. Due to impaired renal clearance in the elderly, doses of antibiotics, including vancomycin, aminoglycosides, and β-lactams, should be adjusted appropriately.

1. EPIDEMIOLOGY AND CLINICAL RELEVANCE

Infective endocarditis (IE) is a serious endovascular infection with changing epidemiology. Developments in antibacterial therapy, clinical microbiology, cardiac imaging, and cardiac surgery have revolutionized its diagnosis and prognosis (1). The newer risk groups of elderly people, intravenous drug users, patients with prosthetic valves and pacemakers, and those on hemodialysis are increasingly represented among patients with IE. The overall incidence of IE ranges between 2 and 6 per 100,000 persons per year. The reported incidence of IE in the United States is ≈1 per 1000 hospital admissions (2). Age was an important risk factor for IE in a retrospective study in Olmsted County, MN, USA, with an incidence rate ratio of 8.8:1 for age ≥65 years vs. age <65 years (3). A more recent series of 108 patients with IE reported a mean age of 57 years (4). This is in sharp contrast to the reports in the early 1940s with the mean age of 35 years and only 10% of cases of IE occurring in patients >60 years (5). Several factors account for the increased incidence of IE in elderly patients: (a) decreased pool of patients with rheumatic heart disease, which predominantly affects the younger patients and predisposes to IE; (b) increased longevity of patients with underlying heart diseases through surgical interventions has expanded the pool of at-risk patients with older individuals; (c) the incidence of calcific/degenerative heart disease (typically seen in old age) and its related IE has increased commensurate with increased life expectation; (d) newer invasive therapeutic interventions, particularly intravenous catheters, pacemakers, and the dialysis shunts, to which the elderly are more likely to be subjected, have all increased the risk of bacteremia and subsequent IE among the elderly; and (e) more frequent prosthetic cardiac valve placement in recent years has added a unique category of patients at risk for IE, a larger proportion of which are elderly (6). The diagnosis and treatment of IE in the elderly are particularly challenging, requiring a high index of suspicion and careful monitoring for complications (7).

Infective endocarditis in older patients is somewhat more common in the males. Male to female ratio is 2 to 8:1 in patients >60 years of age (3,8). Mitral valve involvement is more frequent in the elderly with IE. In a series of 44 elderly patients with IE diagnosed by the Duke criteria, mitral valve was affected in 20 (45%), aortic valve in 14 (32%), and both the mitral and aortic valves were involved in two (5%) patients (9). Similarly, a retrospective review of IE (diagnosed by the Duke criteria) noted mitral valve involvement in 52% of the elderly, whereas the aortic valve was the site of involvement in 55% of younger patients (10).

Degenerative valvular heart disease is being increasingly associated with endocarditis among the elderly. It was noted to be the most common underlying factor in patients with native valve endocarditis in Israel (4). Degenerative valve lesions are present in 50% of patients aged >60 years who have IE (11). Common lesions include degenerative aortic valve disease (occurring on a previously normal valve or complicating a bicuspid aortic valve), calcified mitral annulus, and calcific aortic stenosis. Degenerative calcification of the normal aortic valve occurs with advancing age and causes functional stenosis due to the restricted mobility of its cusps. The resulting turbulence predisposes the elderly patient to IE. Autopsy findings have revealed calcification of congenitally bicuspid valve to be the most frequent cause of aortic stenosis between 60 and 75 years (12). Likewise, progressive calcification of mitral annulus occurs with advancing age, occurring in 3.2% of women before age 70 years, but in 44% of females aged >90 years (13). Patients with mitral valve prolapse and mitral regurgitation are more susceptible to IE, a risk particularly pronounced in men >45 years.

Due to the improved surgical techniques, a growing number of elderly patients receive bioprosthetic valves placing them at risk for subsequent IE. Prosthetic valve endocarditis accounts for 7–25% of cases of IE in most developed countries. The average incidence of prosthetic valve endocarditis is ≈1% at 12 months and 2–3% at 60 months. It has been noted that 42% of nursing home patients aged >60 have one or another underlying cardiac abnormality predisposing them to IE (14).

2. ETIOLOGIC PATHOGENS

Infective endocarditis pathogens have the ability to adhere to and colonize the damaged valves through several surface ligands. The predominant organisms, responsible for ≈80% cases of IE in the elderly, are *Staphylococcus aureus*, *Streptococcus* spp., and enterococci. Some studies have noted a higher prevalence of enterococci among the elderly with IE (15). Also, *S. bovis*, an organism associated with colonic malignancy, may be noted more commonly in the elderly with IE (16). HACEK group of organisms (*Haemophilus* spp., *Actinobacillus actinomycetemcomitans*, *Cardiobacterium hominis*, *Eikenella corrodens*, and *Kingella kingae*) may be occasionally responsible. *Staphylococcus lugdenesis*, a relatively virulent coagulase-negative staphylococcal species, may cause IE in older patients (17). It causes a rather acute disease with rapid valve destruction and paravalvular leak. Nosocomial endocarditis has emerged as a significant entity. In a recent study it accounted for 22% of 109 cases overall and 16% of cases excluding early prosthetic valve endocarditis in cardiac surgery patients (18). Nosocomial endocarditis is important because its case fatality rate is >50%. Intravascular and urinary catheters in the elderly may trigger bacteremia and IE. Staphylococci and enterococci are the most common organisms in nosocomial IE. In a recent report, up to 13% of nosocomial *S. aureus* bacteremia resulted in IE (19). Newly identified pathogens, which are difficult to cultivate, e.g., *Bartonella* spp. and *Tropheryma whipplei*, are present in selected individuals, and resistant organisms are challenging conventional antimicrobial therapy.

3. CLINICAL MANIFESTATIONS

Unlike the younger patients, elderly patients with IE often present with nonspecific and atypical findings, resulting in delayed diagnosis (20–26). Optimal diagnosis of IE in the elderly requires sound clinical judgment and a high index of suspicion. The older patients with IE may present with constitutional symptoms such as lethargy, fatigue, malaise, anorexia, backache, arthralgia, and weight loss, all of which may be attributed to aging and other disorders more likely among the elderly. IE may be complicated by congestive heart failure, paravalvular abscess formation, and embolic events, the most worrisome of which is a stroke. In addition, septic arthritis, vertebral osteomyelitis, pericarditis, metastatic abscesses, peripheral nervous system abnormalities, and an array of renal problems ranging from immune-complex glomerulonephritis to renal abscesses may be noted (20,27). The febrile response is often blunted in older patients. Some elderly patients manifest worsening of their congestive heart failure. New cardiac murmurs, due to progressive valvular damage damage and valvular incompetence, are highly indicative of IE. However, about one-third of patients with tricuspid valve disease , and those with only mural involvement, may not have a pathologic murmur on initial presentation. Additionally, heart murmurs in the elderly may be erroneously attributed to the underlying valvular calcification, and therefore neglected. In 1994, Durack et al. refined the existing clinical criteria for the diagnosis of IE through incorporation of echocardigraphic findings (28). Further modifications of the Duke criteria have been proposed more recently in an effort to improve the accuracy of clinical diagnosis of IE (29) (Table 1). Studies using the Duke criteria for diagnosis of IE have found no relevant differences in the frequency of fever, heart failure, embolic events, neurological symptoms, distribution of causative organisms, and cerebral deficit at the time of discharge as compared with their younger counterparts (9,10). On the contrary, renal insufficiency on admission and malignancy are significantly more common among elderly patients with IE (9,10). The elderly are particularly at risk of poor outcome in the absence of a timely and aggressive intervention. Age-dependent increase in mortality up to 32% has

Table 1 Modified Duke Criteria for Diagnosis of Infective Endocarditis

Major criteria
(1) Blood cultures positive for IE
   (a) Typical microorganism consistent with IE from two separate blood cultures as noted
     below
     (i) Viridans streptococci, *S. bovis, S. aureus* or HACEK group; or
     (ii) Community-acquired enterococci in the absence of a primary focus; or
   (b) Microorganisms consistent with IE from persistently positive blood cultures defined as
     (i) At least two positive cultures of blood samples drawn >12 hr apart; or
     (ii) All of three or a majority of four or more separate cultures of blood, the first and the
       last sample drawn >1 hr apart; or
   (c) Single positive blood culture for *Coxiella burnetti* or antiphase I IgG antibody titer
     >1:800
(2) Evidence of endocardial involvement
   (a) Positive echocardiogram for IE (TEE recommended for prosthetic valve, possible IE by
     clinical criteria, or complicated IE, i.e., paravalvular abscess) defined as
     (i) Oscillating intracardiac mass on valve or supporting structures in the path of
       regurgitant jets or on implanted material in the absence of an alternative anatomic
       explanation; or
     (ii) Abscess; or
     (iii) New partial dehiscence of valvular prosthesis; or
   (b) New valvular regurgitation (worsening or changing or preexisting murmur not
     sufficient)
Minor criteria
   (1) Predisposing heart disease or intravenous drug use
   (2) Fever >38°C
   (3) Vascular phenomenon: major arterial emboli, septic pulmonary infarcts, mycotic
     aneurysm, intracranial or conjunctival hemorrhage, Janeway's lesions
   (4) Immunologic phenomenon: glomerulonephritis, Osler's nodes, Roth's spots,
     rheumatoid factor
   (5) Microbiologic evidence: positive blood culture that does not meet a major criterion as
     noted above or serologic evidence of active infection with organism consistent with IE
Diagnosis
  Definite endocarditis
    (1) Histologic/microbiologic evidence of infection at surgery or autopsy; or
    (2) Two major criteria; or
    (3) One major and three minor criteria; or
    (4) Five minor criteria
  Possible endocarditis
    (1) One major and one minor criterion; or
    (2) Three minor criteria
  No endocarditis
    (1) Negative findings at surgery/autopsy, after antibiotic therapy for ≤4 days; or
    (2) Firm alternative diagnosis; or
    (3) Resolution of illness with antibiotic therapy for ≤4 days; or
    (4) Failure to meet criteria for possible endocarditis, as above

Abbreviations: HACEK, *Haemophilus* spp., *A. actinomycetemcomitans, C. hominis, E. corrodens,* and
K. kingae; TEE, transesophageal echocardiogram.
Source: Adapted from Refs. 28,29.

Table 2 Distinctive Features of Infective Endocarditis in Elderly Patients

Feature	Comments
Presentation	The febrile response is frequently blunted in the elderly patients
	Preexisting murmurs from degenerative valvular disease may confound cardiac auscultation
	Endocarditis-induced murmurs may not be easily appreciated on initial presentation due to emphysema and narrow intercostal spaces
Microbiology	Streptococci and staphylococci are the predominant organisms, recovered in ≈80% cases of IE
	Enterococci are somewhat more prevalent in the elderly with IE
	Streptococcus bovis may cause IE in association with colonic lesions
Underlying diseases	Degenerative valvular disease, mitral valve prolapse, and the presence of a prosthetic valve are important risk factors predisposing the elderly to infective endocarditis
Valvular involvement	Infective endocarditis in older patients is somewhat more frequent on the mitral valve as compared to the aortic valve
Sex distribution	Endocarditis in the elderly is somewhat more common in the males
Echocardiography	Presence of calcific valvular lesions and prosthetic valves make the echocardiographic findings difficult to interpret
	Transesophageal echocardiogram provides better diagnostic information in elderly patients with calcific valvular lesions and prosthetic valves
Diagnosis	Frequently delayed due to atypical presentations and difficulty in interpreting echocardiographic findings
Prognosis	Generally poor as compared to the nonelderly and is largely related to delayed diagnosis and therapy

been reported in patients >60 years (30). This may be largely due to the fact that atypical presentations of IE in the elderly result in its delayed recognition and therapy (31). Recent studies have noted that age itself is not an independent predictor of adverse outcome (10,32). Improved diagnostic modalities, particularly the early use of transesophageal echocardiographic examinations and equal therapeutic options, are responsible for this improved outcome (33). Unfavorable prognostic factors include the presence of neurologic sequelae, acute myocardial infarction, and infection with *S. aureus* and fungi. The distinctive features of IE in the elderly are listed in Table 2.

4. DIAGNOSIS

The diagnosis of IE in the elderly requires heightened suspicion and integration of clinical, laboratory, and echocardiographic data. Leukocytosis with left shift is common, while leukopenia and thrombocytopenia are noted rarely (34). Anemia may be present in the subacute disease. The erythrocyte sedimentation rate is elevated except in elderly patients with congestive heart failure. Microscopic hematuria, proteinuria, red blood cell casts, and bacteriuria may be noted on urine microscopy. Rheumatoid factor may be present, complement levels may decrease, and immune complexes may be noted.

The intravascular location of IE produces continuous high-grade bacteremia. The causative organism can be recovered in about 98% of patients by obtaining three sets of blood cultures. Prior antibiotic therapy may lower this yield. Identification of the pathogen in culture-negative disease depends on special procedures, which comprise inactivating antibiotics in the culture media, prolonging incubation (>2 weeks), and serology for select organism (agglutination, indirect fluorescence, enzyme-linked immunosorbent assay, complement fixation). More recently molecular approach of polymerase chain reaction amplification of specific gene targets and universal loci for bacteria (16S rRNA) and fungi (18S, 28S, and 5.8S rRNA) and subsequent sequencing has been used to identify the possible causal microbial agent in blood culture and heart valve material from patients with suspected IE (35,36). This approach is particularly helpful in patients with culture negative IE. However, microbial contamination of clinical samples may lead to false-positive results. It has been proposed that the Duke criteria be modified to include the positive identification of organisms consistent with IE by molecular methods (37).

The diagnosis of IE has been greatly enhanced by the advent of echocardiography (38). Transesophageal echocardiography (TEE) is more sensitive and specific than transthoracic echocardiogram (TTE). Elderly patients are more likely to have predisposing valvular conditions, e.g., degenerative and calcific lesions and prosthetic valves that decrease the sensitivity of TTE to 45% (15). Its sensitivity is also decreased among elderly patients in the presence of obesity, chest wall deformities, and chronic obstructive pulmonary disease (39). TEE has increased the diagnostic yield of IE in the elderly patients by 45% (15). TEE, with its overall sensitivity of 90%, is also superior to TTE in detecting smaller (5 mm) vegetations, diagnosing valvular perforation, demonstrating valvular regurgitation, and in delineating aneurysm and periannular abscess formation (40).

Radiographic examinations may be helpful in the evaluation of patients with IE. Chest X-rays of patients with right-sided IE may reveal multiple round densities, cavitary multilobar infiltrates, and pleural effusions due to septic emboli. Electrocardiogram may show conduction defects secondary to interventricular septal abscess formation (40). Computed tomographic (CT) scanning of the head of patients manifesting central nervous system abnormalities may reveal macroscopic abscess in 0.5% and diffuse cerebritis in 0.9–3.8% due to IE with highly virulent organisms (27,34). Arteriography is useful in outlining the mycotic aneurysms. The roles of imaging modalities including CT, magnetic resonance imaging, and nuclear imaging in the localization of endocardial lesions have yet to be fully evaluated.

5. ANTIBIOTIC TREATMENT

Rational therapy of IE requires timely identification of the microbial etiology. Empirical intravenous antibiotic therapy should be initiated promptly after blood and other appropriate samples have been taken for culture. Bactericidal antibiotics are a cornerstone of therapy. High concentrations of antibiotic in the serum are desirable to ensure diffusion into the vegetations. Long-term treatment is mandatory to kill dormant bacteria clustered in the infected foci. Therapeutic regimens recommended for the most commonly encountered pathogens in the elderly with IE are presented in Table 3. In the usual patient with a subacute presentation, therapy of

Table 3 Treatment of Elderly with Infective Endocarditis Due to Common Pathogens

Pathogen	Antibiotic regimen	Duration (weeks)
Native valve endocarditis		
Penicillin-susceptible (MIC ≤ 0.1 µg/mL) *viridans* streptococci and *S. bovis*	Aqueous penicillin G, 10–20 million U daily, divided q 6 hr, IV	4
	Aqueous penicillin G, 10–20 million U daily, divided q 6 hr, IV with gentamicin 3 mg/kg IV daily	2
	Ceftriaxone 2 g q 24 hr IV	4
	Ceftriaxone 2 g q 24 hr IV with gentamicin 3 mg/kg IV daily	2
	Vancomycin 15 mg/kg/day q 12–24 hr IV	4
Penicillin-resistant (MIC ≥ 1.0 µg/mL) streptococci and *Enterococcus* spp.	Aqueous penicillin G, 10–20 million U daily, divided q 6 hr, IV with gentamicin 3 mg/kg IV daily	4–6
	Ampicillin 2 g q 4 h IV with gentamicin 3 mg/kg IV daily	4–6
	Vancomycin 15 mg/kg/day q 12–24 hr IV with gentamicin 3 mg/kg IV daily	4–6
HACEK group organisms	Ceftriaxone 1–2 g q 24 hr IV	4
	Ampicillin 2 g q 4 hr IV with gentamicin 3 mg/kg IV daily	4
Methicillin-susceptible staphylococci	Oxacillin or nafcillin 2 g q 4 hr IV with (optional) gentamicin 3 mg/kg IV daily for 3–5 days	4–6
	Cefazolin 2 g q 8 hr IV (or cephalothin, 2 g IV q 4 hr) with (optional) gentamicin 3 mg/kg IV daily for first 3–5 days of therapy	4–6
	Vancomycin 15 mg/kg/day q 12–24 hr IV	4–6
Methicillin-resistant staphylococci	Vancomycin 15 mg/kg/day q 12–24 hr IV	4–6
Prosthetic valve endocarditis		
Methicillin-susceptible staphylococci	Oxacillin or nafcillin 2 g q 4 hr IV with gentamicin 3 mg/kg IV daily (for first 2 weeks of therapy) with rifampin 300 mg q 12 hr PO	6
Methicillin-resistant staphylococci	Vancomycin 15 mg/kg/day q 12–24 hr IV with gentamicin 3 mg/kg IV daily (for first 2 weeks of therapy) with rifampin 300 mg q 12 hr PO	6

Abbreviations: IV, intravenous; u, units; MIC, minimum inhibitory concentration; HACEK, *Haemophilus* spp., *A. actinomycetemcomitans*, *C. hominis*, *E. corrodens*, and *K. kingae*; PO, oral.

IE should be directed at streptococci with a combination of ampicillin (or penicillin) with an aminoglycoside, e.g., gentamicin. In the presence of an acute onset, where staphylococci are considered more likely, therapy should be initiated with semisynthetic penicillin such as nafcillin (or vancomycin, in the presence of penicillin allergy or suspected methicillin resistance) along with an aminoglycoside, e.g., gentamicin.

For prosthetic valve endocarditis, treatment should be empirically begun with vancomycin, gentamicin, and rifampin.

Once the etiologic agent of IE has been identified, antibiotic therapy should be re-evaluated and optimized. If penicillin-susceptible streptococci [minimum inhibitory concentration (MIC) $\leq 0.1\,\mu g/mL$] are implicated, treatment of IE may be continued for a period of 4 weeks with intravenous (IV) aqueous penicillin G (10–20 million U daily, divided every 6 hr), ceftriaxone (2 g every 24 hr), or, in the elderly with serious penicillin allergy, with vancomycin. Many experts use a 2-week regimen of penicillin along with gentamicin for penicillin-susceptible viridans streptococcal IE, but this regimen is frequently avoided in the elderly with fragile renal function. A randomized, multicenter, open-label study reported a 2-week regimen of 2 g ceftriaxone in combination with 3 mg/kg of gentamicin given once daily to be as effective as 2 g of ceftriaxone administered once daily for 4 weeks (41). The combination therapy group included 25 patients with ages ranging from 27 to 92 years (mean $\pm$ SD, 59.5 ± 15.5 years). Adverse effects were minimal in both groups. Treatment of IE due to enterococci or other penicillin-resistant streptococci (MIC $\geq 1.0\,\mu g/mL$) requires a combination of aqueous penicillin G, 20 million U daily, divided every 6 hr, IV, or ampicillin, 2 g every 4 hr IV with gentamicin. Therapy is continued for 4–6 weeks. Vancomycin is substituted for penicillin or ampicillin in the elderly patients allergic to β-lactams. A recent analysis of data from the national registry of Sweden suggested that a shortened aminoglycoside treatment of enterococcal endocarditis, i.e., for 2–3 weeks may be equally effective and potentially less nephrotoxic in the elderly (42).

Infective endocarditis due to methicillin-susceptible staphylococci can be treated with penicillinase-resistant penicillin (nafcillin or oxacillin, 2 g every 4 hr IV) or a cephalosporin [cephalothin, 2 g IV every 4 hr or cefazolin, 1–2 g IV or intramuscular (IM) every 8 hr]. The usual duration of therapy of IE is 4–6 weeks. An aminoglycoside, such as gentamicin, may be added during the first 3–5 days of therapy to achieve a rapid clearance of bacteremia, and a possible rapid decline in the number of bacteria in vegetations, while avoiding potential aminoglycoside nephrotoxicity (34). Experience with once daily aminoglycoside therapy in the treatment of staphylococcal IE is limited. Uncomplicated right-sided IE, with a susceptible strain of *S. aureus* can usually be cured with a 2-week combination of semisynthetic penicillin (e.g., nafcillin) and an aminoglycoside (43). However, this abbreviated treatment has not been studied in the elderly patients and should be avoided due to the potential of aminoglycoside toxicity. Vancomycin is less rapidly bactericidal than nafcillin in vitro against *S. aureus*, especially at high inocula, resulting in clinical failure rates of $\approx 40\%$ (44). Vancomycin therapy should be reserved for staphylococcal endocarditis in the presence of methicillin resistance or severe penicillin allergy. The role of newer antimicrobial agents, such as quinupristin–dalfopristin and linezolid, in the treatment of IE due to antibiotic-resistant gram-positive cocci in the elderly, has not been established. A recent report described the failure of linezolid therapy in two elderly patients who had IE due to methicillin-resistant *S. aureus* (45). Elderly patients with IE due to HACEK group of organisms may be treated with ceftriaxone, 2 g every 24 hr IV for 4 weeks. The alternative combination of ampicillin 2 g every 4 hr IV with gentamicin 3 mg/kg IV daily for the treatment of HACEK group endocarditis may cause nephrotocity in the elderly patients.

Treatment of other somewhat fastidious organisms, as noted in culture-negative endocarditis, may be challenging. Endocarditis caused by *Brucella* sp. responds to 3 months or more of treatment with doxycycline (100–200 mg every 12 hr) plus co-trimoxazole (960 mg every 12 hr) or rifampicin (300–600 mg daily) combined or not with streptomycin (16 mg/kg/day). Surgery might be needed. Disease associated with *Coxiella burnetii* is often treated with doxycycline combined with a fluoroquinolone. Surgery is necessary for cure as recurrences are common with medical therapy. Infective endocarditis caused by *Bartonella* sp. responds to β-lactams (amoxicillin or ceftriaxone) combined with aminoglycosides (e.g., gentamicin) for at least 2 weeks, or β-lactams combined with other drugs, e.g., doxycycline for 6 weeks or more. Combination with surgery is reported in at least 90% of cases. There is no effective medical therapy for IE caused by *Chlamydia* spp., *Mycoplasma* spp., and *Legionella* spp. Surgery is necessary for cure. However, since these organisms are highly susceptible to newer fluoroquinolones in vitro, this drug type should probably be part of the treatment. Infective endocarditis associated with *Tropheryma whipplei* is rare. In Whipple's disease not associated with IE, co-trimoxazole (960 mg every 12 hr) given for at least 1 year is recommended. Surgical valve-replacement may be necessary for successful therapy of endocarditis due to *T. whipplei*.

It is particularly important to consider the impact of aging on specific drug kinetics in order to optimize the dose. Due to impaired renal clearance in the elderly, doses of antibiotics, including vancomycin, aminoglycosides, and β-lactams, should be adjusted appropriately. Most elderly patients achieve therapeutic levels with vancomycin dose administered once a day. Serum concentration of vancomycin should be obtained for optimal dosing. Elderly patients are particularly prone to the nephrotoxicity and the ototoxicity of aminoglycosides. Careful attention to renal function and aminoglycoside serum concentration are particularly important in older patients to minimize toxicity. When synergy with another agent is demonstrated, serum level of aminoglycoside lower than generally considered "therapeutic" may be adequate. Dose adjustment is also necessary for many β-lactams excreted predominantly by the kidneys. Furthermore, many elderly patients are taking other medications for a variety of acute or chronic underlying diseases. As a consequence, it is important to consider potential drug interactions of these medications with antibiotics prescribed for IE.

Most patients with IE will experience defervesce of fever within a week of treatment. Those with persistent fever should be evaluated for the presence of a septic embolic focus (kidney, spleen, or liver), inadequate therapy, drug hypersensitivity, immune complex tissue injury, and valve ring abscess. Antibiotic therapy decreases the risk of first and recurrent embolization. With effective therapy the risk of embolization decreases from 17 events per 100 patient days in the first week to <5 events per 100 patient days during the second and third weeks (46). In general, elderly patients with IE generally have longer hospitalization as compared with the younger patients (42 vs. 32 days in one study) (9).

Surgical intervention is indicated in selected patients with IE. Several studies suggest that combined medical and surgical therapy of IE reduces mortality among patients with congestive heart failure, perivalvular invasive disease, or uncontrolled infection despite appropriate antimicrobial therapy. Patients with IE have been operated upon with acceptable morbidity and mortality due to the improved surgical techniques and the availability of longer lasting prosthetic valves. Results of studies on surgery for active IE indicate mortality rates of 8–16%, with actuarial survival at 5 years of 75–76%, and at 10 years of 61% (47). Accepted indications for surgery in the setting of IE are summarized in Table 4 and include: (a) failure of medical management and continuing bacteremia, unrelated to a metastatic abscess formation—such a patient is likely to have valve ring abscess; (b) acute left heart failure, unresponsive

Table 4 Indications for Surgery in Patients with Infective Endocarditis

Persistent sepsis caused by a surgically removable focus or a valvular ring or myocardial abscess
Acute left heart failure, unresponsive to medical therapy
Endocarditis due to organisms for which curative antimicrobial therapy is not available, e.g., fungi, rickettsiae, vancomycin-resistant enterococcus
Ruptured sinus of valsalva mycotic aneurysm
Prosthetic valve endocarditis with unstable prosthesis, progressive paravalular leak, or persistent infection after 7–10 days of appropriate antibiotic therapy
Persistent life-threatening embolization

to medical therapy; (c) IE due to organisms for which curative antimicrobial therapy is not available, e.g., fungi, rickettsiae, vancomycin-resistant enterococcus; (d) ruptured sinus of Valsalva mycotic aneurysm; (e) myocardial abscess as suggested by new conduction abnormalities or by echocardiography; (f) prosthetic valve endocarditis

Table 5 American Heart Association Recommendations for Endocarditis Prophylaxis

Oral cavity and upper respiratory tract procedures	
No allergy to penicillin	Amoxicillin 2 g po, 1 hr before procedure or ampicillin 2 g IM/ IV, 30 min before the procedure
Penicillin allergy present	Clindamycin 600 mg po, cephalexin/ cefadroxil 2 g po, azithromycin 500 mg po, or clarithromycin 500 mg po (all given as a single dose, 1 hr prior to procedure) Parenteral alternatives include clindamycin 600 mg IV or cefazolin 1 g IM/IV administered 30 min before the procedure
Gastrointestinal and genitourinary procedures	
No allergy to penicillin	Ampicillin 2 g IM/IV plus gentamicin 1.5 mg/kg, 30 min before procedure and followed by a dose of ampicillin 1 g IM/IV or amoxicillin 1 g po, 6 hr later
Penicillin allergy present	Vancomycin 1 g IV (1–2 hr infusion completed 30 min before procedure) plus gentamicin 1.5 mg/kg may be used 30 min before procedure
Low-risk patients	Amoxicillin 2 g, po, 1 hr before procedure or ampicillin 2 g IM/IV 30 min before procedure or vancomycin 1 g IV (1–2 hr infusion completed 30 min before procedure)

Abbreviations: po, oral; IV, intravenous; IM, intramuscular.
Source: Adapted from Ref. 50.

with unstable prosthesis, progressive paravalular leak, or persistent infection after 7–10 days of appropriate antibiotic therapy; and (g) persistent life-threatening embolization (48). While valve replacement is necessary for the left-sided IE, tricuspid valvulectomy or "vegetectomy" with valvuloplasty may be adequate for tricuspid valve disease. Elderly patients are at greater risk of postoperative complications, i.e., prosthetic dysfunction, pericardial tamponade, renal insufficiency, rhythm disturbances, and the necessity for a second intervention (10). Video-assisted cardioscopy avoids the need for extended cardiac incisions and has been recently used successfully for resection of endocardial vegetations (49).

6. PREVENTION

Preventive approached are important for diseases with serious consequences such as IE. Chemoprophylaxis should be considered for all elderly patients at risk for IE undergoing procedures that are likely to cause bacteremia. Such procedures include dental manipulations, instrumentation involving the respiratory, genitourinary, or gastrointestinal tract. For effective prophylaxis, it is necessary to have appropriate serum levels of antibiotic prior to a bacteremic episode. The American Heart Association has recently updated recommendations for prophylaxis of IE and these are summarized in Table 5 (50). There has been shift toward use of prophylaxis in fewer "high-risk" dental, genitourinary, or gastrointestinal tract procedures; fewer selected "high-risk" cardiac lesions; and a single-dose prophylaxis. Pre-existing cardiac conditions and the relative risk of IE are listed in Table 6. The prophylactic

Table 6 Cardiac Conditions Associated with Infective Endocarditis

---

Endocarditis prophylaxis recommended
High-risk category
  Prosthetic cardiac valves, including bioprosthetic and homograft valves
  Previous bacterial endocarditis
  Complex cyanotic congenital heart disease (e.g., single ventricle states, transposition of the great arteries, tetralogy of Fallot)
  Surgically constructed systemic pulmonary shunts or conduits
Moderate-risk category
  Most other congenital cardiac malformations (other than above and below)
  Acquired valvular dysfunction (e.g., rheumatic heart disease)
  Hypertrophic cardiomyopathy
  Mitral valve prolapse with valvular regurgitation and/or thickened leaflets
Endocarditis prophylaxis not recommended
Negligible-risk category (no greater risk than the general population)
  Isolated secundum atrial septal defect
  Surgical repair of atrial septal defect, ventricular septal defect, or patent ductus arteriosus (without residua beyond 6 months)
  Previous coronary artery bypass graft surgery
  Mitral valve prolapse without valvular regurgitation
  Physiologic, functional, or innocent heart murmurs
  Previous Kawasaki disease without valvular dysfunction
  Previous rheumatic fever without valvular dysfunction
  Cardiac pacemakers (intravascular and epicardial) and implanted defibrillators

---

Source: Adapted from Ref. 50.

regimen is directed at the putative organisms during the anticipated bacteremic episode. For dental, oral, respiratory, or esophageal procedures, antibiotic prophylaxis directed at viridans streptococci may be provided with oral amoxicillin 2 g, 1 hr before procedure or parenteral ampicillin 2 g, 30 min before the procedure. Alternative oral regimens for penicillin-allergic patients (given as a single dose, 1 hr prior to procedure) include oral clindamycin 600 mg, oral cephalexin/cefadroxil 2 g, oral azithromycin 500 mg, or oral clarithromycin 500 mg. Parenteral alternatives for penicillin-allergic patients include clindamycin 600 mg IV or cefazolin 1 g IM/IV administered 30 min before the procedure.

Prophylactic regimens for genitourinary and gastrointestinal (except esophageal) procedures target enterococci and take into account the risk of IE relative to the underlying cardiac conditions. Patients with high-risk conditions (prosthetic heart valve, prior endocarditis, complex cyanotic congenital heart disease, and surgically constructed systemic-pulmonary shunts) should receive ampicillin 2 g IM/IV plus gentamicin 1.5 mg/kg, 30 min before procedure and followed by a dose of ampicillin 1 g IM/IV or oral amoxicillin 1 g, 6 hr later. Alternatively, vancomycin 1 g IV (1–2 hr infusion completed 30 min before procedure) plus gentamicin 1.5 mg/kg may be used 30 min before procedure. Moderate risk of IE is posed by other underlying cardiac diseases such as unrepaired congenital cardiac malformations (except isolated secundum atrial septal defect), most acquired valve dysfunction, hypertrophic cardiomyopathy, and mitral valve prolapse with regurgitation (and/or thickened leaflets). Such patients may receive IE prophylaxis with oral amoxicillin 2 g, 1 hr before procedure or ampicillin 2 g IM/IV 30 min before procedure or vancomycin 1 g IV (1–2 hr infusion completed 30 min before procedure).

REFERENCES

1. Moreillon P, Que YA. Infective endocarditis. Lancet 2004; 363:1391–1349.
2. Hoesley CJ, Cobbs CG. Endocarditis at the millennium. J Infect Dis 1999; 179(suppl 2): S360–S365.
3. Steckelberg JM, Melton LJ III, Ilstrup DM, Rouse MS, Wilson WR. Influence of referral bias on the apparent clinical spectrum of infective endocarditis. Am J Med 1990; 88: 582–588.
4. Fefer P, Raveh D, Rudensky B, Schlesinger Y, Yinnon AM. Changing epidemiology of infective endocarditis: a retrospective survey of 108 cases, 1990–1999. Eur J Clin Microbiol Infect Dis 2002; 21:432–437.
5. Von Reyn CF, Levy BS, Arbeit RD, Friedland G, Crumpacker CS. Infective endocarditis: an analysis based on strict case definitions. Ann Intern Med 1981; 94:505–518.
6. Cabell CH, Heidenreich PA, Chu VH, Moore CM, Stryjewski ME, Corey GR, Fowler VG Jr. Increasing rates of cardiac device infections among Medicare beneficiaries: 1990–1999. Am Heart J 2004; 147:582–586.
7. Dhawan VK. Infective endocarditis in elderly patients. Clin Infect Dis 2002; 34: 806–812.
8. Cunha BA, Gill MV, Lazar JM. Acute infective endocarditis. Diagnostic and therapeutic approach. Infect Dis Clin North Am 1996; 10:811–834.
9. Gagliardi JP, Nettles RE, McCarty DE, Sanders LL, Corey GR, Sexton DJ. Native valve infective endocarditis in elderly and younger adult patients: comparison of clinical features and outcomes with use of the Duke criteria and the Duke Endocarditis Database. Clin Infect Dis 1998; 26:1165–1168.

10. Netzer RO, Zollinger E, Seiler C, Cerny A. Native valve infective endocarditis in elderly and younger adult patients: comparison of clinical features and outcomes with use of the Duke criteria. Clin Infect Dis 1999; 28:933–935.

11. McKinsey DS, Ratts TE, Bisno AL. Underlying cardiac lesions in adults with infective endocarditis. The changing spectrum. Am J Med 1987; 82:681–688.

12. Pomerance A. Pathogenesis of aortic stenosis and its relation to age. Br Heart J 1972; 34:569–574.

13. Pomerance A. Pathological and clinical study of calcification of the mitral valve ring. J Clin Pathol 1970; 23:354–361.

14. Felder RS, Nardone D, Palac R. Prevalence of predisposing factors for endocarditis among an elderly institutionalized population. Oral Surg Oral Med Oral Pathol 1992; 73:30–34.

15. Werner GS, Schulz R, Fuchs JB, Andreas S, Prange H, Ruschewski W, Kreuzer H. Infective endocarditis in the elderly in the era of transesophageal echocardiography: clinical features and prognosis compared with younger patients. Am J Med 1996; 100:90–97.

16. Leport C, Bure A, Leport J, Vilde JL. Incidence of colonic lesions in *Streptococcus bovis* and enterococcal endocarditis. Lancet 1987; 1:748.

17. Lessing MP, Crook DW, Bowler IC, Gribbin B. Native-valve endocarditis caused by *Staphylococcus lugdunensis*. QJM 1996; 89:855–858.

18. Bouza E, Menasalvas A, Munoz P, Vasallo FJ, del Mar Moreno M, Garcia Fernandez MA. Infective endocarditis—a prospective study at the end of the twentieth century: new predisposing conditions, new etiologic agents, and still a high mortality. Medicine (Baltimore) 2001; 80:298–307.

19. Fowler VG Jr, Sanders LL, Kong LK, McClelland RS, Gottlieb GS, Li J, Ryan T, Sexton DJ, Roussakis G, Harrell LJ, Corey GR. Infective endocarditis due to *Staphylococcus aureus*: 59 prospectively identified cases with follow-up. Clin Infect Dis 1999; 28:106–114.

20. Terpenning MS, Buggy BP, Kauffman CA. Infective endocarditis: clinical features in young and elderly patients. Am J Med 1987; 83:626–634.

21. Habte-Gabr E, January LE, Smith IM. Bacterial endocarditis: the need for early diagnosis. Geriatrics 1973; 28:164–170.

22. Applefeld MM, Hornick RB. Infective endocarditis in patients over age 60. Am Heart J 1974; 88:909–914.

23. Thell R, Martin FH, Edwards JE. Bacterial endocarditis in subjects 60 years of age and older. Circulation 1975; 51:174–182.

24. Tenenbaum MJ, Kaplan MH. Infective endocarditis in the elderly: an update. Geriatrics 1984; 39:121–123, 126–127.

25. Gantz NM. Geriatric endocarditis: avoiding the trend toward mismanagement. Geriatrics 1991; 46:66–68.

26. Selton-Suty C, Hoen B, Grentzinger A, Houplon P, Maignan M, Juilliere Y, Danchin N, Canton P, Cherrier F. Clinical and bacteriological characteristics of infective endocarditis in the elderly. Heart 1997; 77:260–263.

27. Cantrell M, Yoshikawa TT. Infective endocarditis in the aging patient. Gerontology 1984; 30:316–326.

28. Durack DT, Lukes AS, Bright DK. New criteria for diagnosis of infective endocarditis: utilization of specific echocardiographic findings. Duke Endocarditis Service. Am J Med 1994; 96:200–219.

29. Li JS, Sexton DJ, Mick N, Nettles R, Fowler VG Jr, Ryan T, Bashore T, Corey GR. Proposed modifications to the Duke criteria for the diagnosis of infective endocarditis. Clin Infect Dis 2000; 30:633–638.

30. Watanakunakorn C, Burkert T. Infective endocarditis at a large community teaching hospital, 1980–1990. A review of 210 episodes. Medicine (Baltimore) 1993; 72:90–102.

31. Wang JL, Hung CC, Hsieh SM, Chang SC. Clinical features and outcome analysis of infective endocarditis in elderly patients. J Formos Med Assoc 2004; 103:416–421.
32. Robbins N, De Maria A, Miller MH. Infective endocarditis in the elderly. South Med J 1980; 73:1335–1338.
33. Zamorano J, Sanz J, Moreno R, Almeria C, Rodrigo JL, de Marco E, Serra V, Samedi M, Sanchez-Harguindey L. Better prognosis of elderly patients with infectious endocarditis in the era of routine echocardiography and nonrestrictive indications for valve surgery. J Am Soc Echocardiogr 2002; 15:702–707.
34. Bayer AS. Infective endocarditis. Clin Infect Dis 1993; 17:313–320.
35. Lang S, Watkin RW, Lambert PA, Bonser RS, Littler WA, Elliott TS. Evaluation of PCR in the molecular diagnosis of endocarditis. J Infect 2004; 48:269–275.
36. Millar B, Moore J, Mallon P, Xu J, Crowe M, McClurg R, Raoult D, Earle J, Hone R, Murphy P. Molecular diagnosis of infective endocarditis—a new Duke's criterion. Scand J Infect Dis 2001; 33:673–680.
37. Lisby G, Gutschik E, Durack DT. Molecular methods for diagnosis of infective endocarditis. Infect Dis Clin North Am 2002; 16:393–412.
38. Evangelista A, Gonzalez-Alujas MT. Echocardiography in infective endocarditis. Heart 2004; 90:614–617.
39. Pedersen WR, Walker M, Olson JD, Gobel F, Lange HW, Daniel JA, Rogers J, Longe T, Kane M, Mooney MR, et al. Value of transesophageal echocardiography as an adjunct to transthoracic echocardiography in evaluation of native and prosthetic valve endocarditis. Chest 1991; 100:351–356.
40. Daniel WG, Mugge A, Martin RP, Lindert O, Hausmann D, Nonnast-Daniel B, Laas J, Lichtlen PR. Improvement in the diagnosis of abscesses associated with endocarditis by transesophageal echocardiography. N Engl J Med 1991; 324:795–800.
41. Sexton DJ, Tenenbaum MJ, Wilson WR, Steckelberg JM, Tice AD, Gilbert D, Dismukes W, Drew RH, Durack DT. Ceftriaxone once daily for four weeks compared with ceftriaxone plus gentamicin once daily for two weeks for treatment of endocarditis due to penicillin-susceptible streptococci. Endocarditis Treatment Consortium Group. Clin Infect Dis 1998; 27:1470–1474.
42. Olaison L, Schadewitz K. Enterococcal endocarditis in Sweden, 1995–1999: can shorter therapy with aminoglycosides by used? Clin Infect Dis 2002; 34:159–166.
43. DiNubile MJ. Abbreviated therapy for right-sided Staphylococcus aureus endocarditis in injecting drug users: the time has come? Eur J Clin Microbiol Infect Dis 1994; 13: 533–534.
44. Small PM, Chambers HF. Vancomycin for Staphylococcus aureus endocarditis in intravenous drug users. Antimicrob Agents Chemother 1990; 34:1227–1231.
45. Ruiz ME, Guerrero IC, Tuazon CU. Endocarditis caused by methicillin-resistant Staphylococcus aureus: treatment failure with linezolid. Clin Infect Dis 2002; 35: 1018–1020.
46. Steckelberg JM, Murphy JG, Ballard D, Bailey K, Tajik AJ, Taliercio CP, Giuliani ER, Wilson WR. Emboli in infective endocarditis: the prognostic value of echocardiography. Ann Intern Med 1991; 114:635–640.
47. Larbalestier RI, Kinchla NM, Aranki SF, Couper GS, Collins JJ Jr, Cohn LH. Acute bacterial endocarditis. Optimizing surgical results. Circulation 1992; 86:1168–1174.
48. Olaison L, Pettersson G. Current best practices and guidelines indications for surgical intervention in infective endocarditis. Infect Dis Clin North Am 2002; 16:453–475.
49. Miyaji K, Murakami A, Suematsu Y, Takamoto S. Video-assisted cardioscopy for infectious endocarditis. Pediatr Cardiol 2002; 23:562–563.
50. Dajani AS, Taubert KA, Wilson W, Bolger AF, Bayer A, Ferrieri P, Gewitz MH, Shulman ST, Nouri S, Newburger JW, Hutto C, Pallasch TJ, Gage TW, Levison ME, Peter G, Zuccaro G Jr. Prevention of bacterial endocarditis. Recommendations by the American Heart Association. Circulation 1997; 96:358–366.

SUGGESTED READING

Dhawan VK. Infective endocarditis in elderly patients. Clin Infect Dis 2002; 34:806–812.

Fefer P, Raveh D, Rudensky B Schlesinger, Yinnon AM. Changing epidemiology of infective endocarditis: a retrospective survey of 108 cases, 1990–1999. J Clin Microbiol Infect Dis 2002; 21:432–437.

Moreillon P, Que YA. Infective endocarditis. Lancet 2004; 363:139–149.

Steckelberg JM, Melton LJ III, Ilstrup DM, Rouse MS, Wilson WR. Influence of referral bias on the apparent clinical spectrum of infective endocarditis. Am J Med 1990; 88:582–588.

Zamorano J, Sanz J, Moreno R. Better prognosis of elderly patients with infectious endocarditis in the era of routine echocardiography and nonrestrictive indications for valve surgery. J Am Soc Endocardiogr 2002; 15:702–707.

39

Bone and Joint Infections

Parmis Pouya and Thomas T. Yoshikawa
*Department of Internal Medicine, Charles R. Drew University of Medicine and Science,
Martin Luther King, Jr.–Charles R. Drew Medical Center, Los Angeles,
California, U.S.A.*

Key Points:

- The elderly are at higher risk of developing septic arthritis and osteomyelitis. The morbidity and mortality associated with these infections are higher in the elderly.
- *Staphylococcus aureus* is still the most common bacterium infecting bones and joints in elderly and it is associated with worse outcomes.
- Early diagnosis and intervention can be challenging in the elderly population, secondary to the often more indolent, nonspecific, and at times asymptomatic course of these infections.
- Osteomylitis and septic arthritis are traditionally treated with weeks of parenteral antibiotics, requiring long periods of hospitalization, which can be particularly detrimental to the elderly.
- Drainage of infected joint fluid is important for relief of pressure and enhancing good outcome. Physical therapy, good nutrition, and managing the underlying diseases are essential to maintain good functional status.

1. EPIDEMIOLOGY AND CLINICAL RELEVANCE

In the elderly, many specific host factors influence the likelihood of acquiring bone and joint infections. Advanced age, prior illnesses, previous damage to bone and joints, nutritional status, coexisting illnesses, impaired immune system, and, perhaps, emotional well-being all have some impact on the risk of infection after exposure to a potential pathogen. The aging population in general requires more medical care, which in itself increases the risk of acquiring an infection, by way of frequent or extended hospitalization (nosocomial infection), increasing invasive investigations and interventions, introduction of implantable foreign devices, and administration of medications, such as corticosteroids and other immunosuppressants.

Septic arthritis is an infection of the joint, and the elderly are at higher risk of developing bacterial arthritis. In a prospective study, age >80 years was found to be an independent risk factor to joint infections (1). The reported incidence of septic arthritis is 2–5 per 100,000 per year in the general population. The older population accounts for ≈25% of these cases (2,3). There is a high prevalence of joint disease in

561

the elderly, and it is a well-known fact that diseased or damaged joints are more predisposed to infections. These arthropathies include rheumatoid arthritis, crystal arthropathies, prosthetic joints, osteoarthritis, and neuropathic joints (1,4). A prospective study of 154 patients with bacterial arthritis found that 40% had preexisting joint disease, mostly rheumatoid arthritis or degenerative arthritis (5). Also, the reported incidence of septic arthritis in patients with rheumatoid arthritis is as much as 10 times higher when compared with the general population (3). The pathogenesis of septic arthritis in the elderly may also be partly due to immunologic defects, since most of the other risk factors are associated with states of decreased immunity; for example, patients with diabetes mellitus or those on immunosuppressants are at risk of septic arthritis (3). Prosthetic joint placement also places the elderly at increased risk of septic arthritis, especially in those with rheumatoid arthritis (3,6).

The mortality associated with septic arthritis is higher in the elderly. Old age is associated with poor joint recovery, severe functional deterioration, and the poorest prognosis (3,5). Early recognition and institution of appropriate treatment is essential for a favorable outcome of this condition (4,5). The most common nonprosthetic joints involved are the knees and the hips. The shoulders, ankles, wrists, elbows, and interphalangeal joints are also commonly affected (3). In a retrospective study of 191 patients, the most frequent joints involved were also the knees (54%) and the hips (13%) (7).

Osteomyelitis is an infection of the bone and is second only to soft tissue infections, as the most common musculoskeletal infection in the elderly (6). It has a bimodal age distribution and overall is an uncommon but significant infection. Osteomyelitis results in bone necrosis, destruction of bone architect, and new bone formation; it can be acute, subacute, or chronic in nature. It is often difficult to diagnose in its early stages and requires long-term therapy that often fails. These conditions generate substantial health care costs, morbidity, and disability (8,9). Although most children diagnosed with osteomyelitis have no identifiable risk factors, the opposite is true for the elderly among whom the majority of cases occur in diabetics, and those with peripheral vascular diseases and other chronic illnesses. These conditions are both predisposing and complicating factors for osteomyelitis (10). The elderly population is also predisposed to developing both bone and joint infections secondary to frequently performed orthopedic or surgical procedures and interventions that can lead to bacteremia or a local infection. Furthermore, foreign prosthesis creates an ideal setting for these infections. The reported incidence of septic arthritis in patients with joint prosthesis is as much as 40–68 cases per 100,000 per year as compared with two to four cases per 100,000 per year in the general population (3).

Bone and joint infections, like other more prevalent musculoskeletal disorders, in the elderly cause pain, stiffness, imbalance, and weakness secondary to muscle disuse. These will inevitably make the older person more predisposed to falls and immobility. Such problems are more pronounced when the lower extremities are involved. In an elderly patient who may be already somewhat incapacitated by arthritis or any other comorbid condition, the further insult of a musculoskeletal infection may worsen the patient's mobility and tendency to fall. Prolonged bed rest results in imbalance, which together with the fear of falling is the major cause of immobilization. Thus, the vicious cycle of immobility, disability, and loss of independence may be perpetuated. Immobilization secondary to bed rest has its own consequences, some of which are very serious, i.e., thrombophlebitis, pulmonary embolism, and cardiac deconditioning, the last of which occurs at an accelerated rate in the elderly. Muscular atrophy, functional incontinence, and pressure ulcers may also occur, and thus these skeletal infections may ultimately manifest themselves as one of the geriatric syndromes. Also, the elderly are more likely to suffer from the side effects of the long-term antibiotic regimens used to treat these infections.

2. ETIOLOGIC PATHOGENS

Bacterial infections are the most common cause of septic arthritis and osteomyelitis at all ages. Rickettsia, viruses, and fungi are the other etiologic pathogens, but they are relatively infrequent causes of skeletal infection in the elderly (Tables 1 and 2).

The pathogenesis of septic arthritis and osteomyelitis is multifactorial. Virulence of the infecting organisms, host immune status, preexisting or underlying diseases, and presence of synthetic materials are some important factors which determine whether a local or a systemic infection is eliminated or develops into osteomyelitis or septic arthritis (1,11).

The specific organism(s) isolated in bacterial osteomyelitis and arthritis is/are often associated with the age of the patient or a common clinical scenario (i.e., source of bacteremia, trauma, or recent surgery). The routes and molecular mechanisms used by pathogens to colonize, invade, and infect bone and joints are diverse. The virulence of different pathogenic bacteria not only determines whether an infection develops but also influences the outcome of the infection. *Staphylococcus aureus* possesses various virulence factors such as surface-associated adhesion mechanisms that enable it to adhere tightly to cartilage and bone, thereby escaping host defenses as well as allowing it to express phenotypic changes, which makes it resistant to antimicrobial treatment. It produces numerous toxins including chondrocyte protease, which promotes chondrocyte-mediated breakdown of the articular cartilage. The bacterium can also persist within osteoblasts and can produce other toxins that subvert the immune system (10,11). These properties make *S. aureus* not only the most common bacterium infecting bones and joints via all routes and at all ages, but they are associated with worse outcomes when compared with less virulent organisms. In a study of patients with pneumococcal bacterial arthritis, for example, only 5% of adults did not return to baseline joint function. These results are in contrast to other studies of *S. aureus* bacterial arthritis that report 50% with poor joint outcomes following therapy (2).

All bacteria enter the bone and joint by three different mechanisms. These three pathogenic mechanisms in osteomyelitis were defined by Waldvogel et al. in the 1970s and for the most part, the first two mechanisms are responsible for the development of joint infections (12).

3. PATHOGENETIC MECHANISMS

3.1. Hematogenous Spread of Infection

This is the commonest route of joint infection at all ages. In a retrospective study of 191 patients, 72% of infections were from hematogenous spread (7). However, it only accounts for ≈20% of cases of osteomyelitis and mainly affects children, elderly, and intravenous (IV) drug users (13). Whenever this route of infection is suspected, especially with septic arthritis, one must seek a preceding or a current source of bacteremia (mainly monomicrobial), which is often a clue to the identity of the etiologic

Table 1 Osteomyelitis

Risk factors/clinical associations/routes	Predilection for sites	Etiologic pathogen(s)
Normal host, any age		*Staphylococcus aureus*
Elderly	Any, vertebral	*S. aureus* and gram-negative bacilli
IV drug user	Vertebrae	*Pseudomonas aeruginosa, Serratia marcescens*, and *S. aureus*
Diabetes mellitus	Feet	*S. aureus*, Group B streptococci, *Enterococcus* species, *Proteus mirabilis, P. aeruginosa*, and anaerobes
Sickle cell/hemoglobinopathies	Long bones	*Salmonella* species, *S. aureus*, and *Streptococcus pneumoniae*
Tuberculosis endemic area	Thoracic spine, ribs, sternum, hand, and feet Metaphysis of long bones	*Mycobacterium tuberculosis*
Postreduction and internal fixation of fracture		*E. coli, S. aureus*, and *P. aeruginosa*
Postoperative prosthetic joint osteomyelitis, infection post intra-articular injection		*S. epidermidis, S. aureus, P. aeruginosa*, and Enterobacteriaceae
Immunocompromised		Atypical mycobactera, fungi, and *Bartonella henselae*
UTI/instrumentation	Vertebrae	Gram-negative bacilli
Orthopedic devices/ foreign body		*S. epidermidis*, and *Propionibacterium* species
Nosocomial infections		Enterobacteriaceae and *P. aeruginosa*
Human bites		*Streptococcus* species and anaerobes
Human immunodeficiency virus		*B. henselae, Pasteurella multocida*, and *Eikenella corrodens*
Endemic, middle east (domestic animals)	Sacroiliac joint	*Brucella* species
Postcardiac surgery	Sternal osteomyelitis	*S. aureus, S. epidermidis*, gram-negative bacilli, atypical mycobacteria, and mycoplasma
Wounds, puncture wounds of feet	Foot	*P. aeruginosa*
Extremity decubitus ulcer, stage 4	Extremity	*S. aureus*
Sacral decubitus ulcer	Sacrum	*S. aureus*, gram-negative bacilli, and *Bacteroides fragilis*
Cat/dog bites		*P. multocida*
Poor dentition, periodontal disease	Mandibles	Oral anaerobes

Abbreviations: IV, intravenous; UTI, urinary tract infection.

Table 2 Septic Joint

Risk factors/clinical associations	Etiologic pathogen(s)
Normal host, any age	*Staphylococcus aureus* (most common bacterium), *Streptococcus* species, and *Neisseria gonorrhoeae*
Elderly	*S. aureus* and gram-negative bacilli
Sexually active, gonococcal infection, and urethritis	*N. gonorrhoeae*
Immunocompromised host	Gram-negative bacilli, mycobacteria, and fungi
Gastrointestinal infections	Gram-negative bacteria
Rheumatoid arthritis	*S. aureus*
Prosthetic joints/postarthroscopy	*Staphylococcus epidermidis*, *S. aureus*, *Pseudomonas aeruginosa*, and enterobacteriaceae
Skin breach/postsurgical procedure, penetrating injuries	*S. aureus*
Splenic dysfunction	*Streptococcus* species and *Salmonella* species
Tick exposure	*Borellia burgdorferi*
Human immunodeficiency virus	*S. aureus*, *Streptococcus pneumoniae*, *Salmonella*, *Hemophilus influenzae*, and mycobacteria
Endocarditis	*S. aureus*, enterococci, and *Streptococcus* species
Alcoholics/hemoglobinopathies	*Streptococcus pneumoniae*
Intravenous drug abuse	*Staphylococcus* species, *P. aeruginosa*, *Streptococcus* species, and other gram-negative bacilli

pathogen. For example, a joint infection following a urinary tract infection (UTI) may make one suspect gram-negative bacilli as a likely pathogen. UTIs, pneumonias, IV drug use, infected intravascular devices, soft tissue infections, dental procedures, and infective endocarditis are some of the notable sources of bacteremia and may lead to bone and joint infections by "seeding" (14).

Septic arthritis secondary to hematogenous spread occurs via synovial capillaries, which have no limiting basement membranes. Bacteria and inflammatory cells, leading to damage and destruction, quickly invade the cartilage. In osteomyelitis, the bacteria enter the metaphyseal vasculature and initiate an infection. In the older person, the most common sites of hematogenous-spread osteomyelitis are the thoracic and the lumbar vertebrae following bacteremia. Diabetes mellitus is also associated with an increased risk of vertebral osteomyelitis. This route of infection may be acquired in the presence of bone and joint trauma, ischemia, or foreign bodies. Elderly persons with joint replacements are at increased risk of infection (15). In the elderly population, especially in men, UTI is a common source of bacteremia. *S. aureus* causes the majority of the cases of hematogenous-spread osteomyelitis and septic arthritis in all adults >40 years of age. *Escherichiae coli* and other enteric bacilli account for a quarter of cases of vertebral osteomyelitis (13). *Neisseria gonorrhoeae* is a much less common cause of septic arthritis in the elderly. In a retrospective study of 191 patients with septic arthritis, the causative organisms included *S. aureus* (37%), *Streptococcus pyogenes* (16%), and *N. gonorrhoeae* (12%) (7).

3.2. Contiguous Focus of Infection

The second route implicated in the development of osteomyelitis and septic arthritis is infection from a contiguous focus. This is the most common route of infection leading to osteomyelitis in adults; however, it is a much less frequent cause of septic arthritis. Elderly frequently fall and may sustain open or closed fractures which may require orthopedic surgery, with or without foreign body placement. The infection may originate from penetrating traumatic injuries, surgical procedures involving bone and joints or from adjacent bones, joints, and soft tissues. In bedridden elderly, infected pressure ulcers may lead to osteomyelitis of the underlying bone. These infections are very often polymicrobial and are very difficult to treat.

3.3. Poor Vascular Supply

Osteomyelitis can also result from inadequate blood supplies to vulnerable tissues and almost always affects diabetics between 50 and 70 years of age, although it also occurs in patients with other causes of peripheral vascular disease. This variety of osteomyelitis tends to be polymicrobial (8). The organisms responsible for osteomyelitis and septic arthritis depend on the route and stage of infection as well as the age and comorbidities of the patient (Tables 1–3) (2,4,10,13,14).

4. CLINICAL MANIFESTATIONS

It is a well-known fact that clinical presentations of diseases are often atypical in the elderly population and classic symptoms may be "blunted" (see chapter "Clinical Manifestations of Infections"). Bone and joint infections are no exception. Osteomyelitis and septic arthritis in the older person may be asymptomatic and indolent in nature. Pain may be the only presenting feature without the usual signs of inflammation and infection (4). Geriatric syndromes such as acute confusion, depression, incontinence, and falls may be the presenting features. However, musculoskeletal complaints in the elderly are frequently secondary to pathology in other organ systems or of other etiology, such as endocrine, metabolic, neoplastic, and even psychological. These factors may make the diagnosis of skeletal infections more challenging in the elderly. The lack of symptomatology may further be complicated by the use of corticosteroids or immunosupressants or presence of comorbid conditions and

Table 3 Associated Clinical Scenarios and Sites of Infection

Intravenous drug abuse	Sternoclavicular joints, sternomanubrial joints, symphysis pubis joint, and sacroiliac joints.
Intra-abdominal abscesses	Hip joints
Femoral venipuncture	Hip joints
Ruptured colonic diverticuli	Hip joints
Subclavian vein catheterization	Sternoclavicular joints
Diabetes, hemodialysis	Vertebral osteomyelitis
Postincontinence surgery in females, athletes, and pelvic malignancy	Symphysis pubis

impaired immunity associated with diabetes mellitus, rheumatoid arthritis, hepatic, or renal dysfunction (4,13).

Septic arthritis in the elderly usually presents as monoarticular pain and tenderness in an already diseased joint. The knee is the joint most frequently involved (3,4). Polyarticular involvement usually occurs with rheumatoid arthritis, gonococcemia, rheumatic fever, acute hepatitis B, and overwhelming sepsis. Systemic infections in the frail elderly may not be accompanied by fever or leukocytosis. Elderly may have a normal white blood cell (WBC) count, may have no evidence of obvious inflammation, and may even be afebrile (4) (see chapter "Clinical Manifestations of Infections"). Nevertheless, most septic joints will manifest heat, swelling, effusion, erythema, and decreased range of motion; however, the elderly are less frequently completely immobilized by pain and less often experience associated muscle spasms (3). Fatigue and malaise may also be present as a part of the systemic manifestations of both osteomyelitis and septic arthritis. These patients may also present with associated symptoms and signs from the primary source or site of bacteremia, for example, pneumonia. It is important to note that septic arthritis in the elderly is more frequently associated with osteomyelitis (3).

Chronic osteomyelitis may present with symptoms and signs of its complications, such as pus drainage from a sinus tract, localized cellulitis, and abscess formation should a fistula become obstructed, pathologic fractures, and squamous cell carcinoma of the sinus tract (14). Subacute osteomyelitis in the elderly usually occurs in the vertebrae and may present with back pain at the site of the infection or as pain elsewhere, secondary to nerve root irritation. Paraspinal muscle spasm may exist and WBC count may be normal. A more indolent course is noted with tuberculous spinal osteomyelitis, which is also common in the elderly. However, it has a higher rate of abscess formation compared with pyogenic vertebral osteomyelitis (6). Radicular pain and eventual paralysis may ensue, following an epidural abscess formation. Cervical osteomyelitis may lead to a retropharyngeal abscess formation, causing dysphagia. A nonhealing foot ulcer, especially if >2 cm in diameter, must alert one to the possibility of underlying osteomyelitis. This is almost a certainty if the underlying bone is palpable with a probe (9).

5. DIAGNOSIS

Early diagnosis of a septic joint or osteomyelitis is of utmost importance, as early intervention will prevent or minimize bone necrosis or destruction of the affected joint. This can be challenging in the elderly population, because of the often more indolent, nonspecific, and at times asymptomatic course of these infections (4). In addition to these challenges, other factors such as the location of the infection, precipitating conditions, or preexisting illnesses can impose difficulties in diagnoses. For example, infection in some sites such as hip and shoulder joints and vertebrae or pelvis may manifest with few symptoms and signs; the radiological abnormalities in contiguous focus osteomyelitis may be identical to those due to precipitating conditions such as penetrating injuries or cellulitis; and in rheumatoid arthritis it may be difficult to distinguish the pain in a septic joint from an acutely inflamed joint (15).

As always a careful and thorough history, physical examination may not only reveal the diagnosis but also shed some light on the etiology, chronicity, and pathogenesis of these diseases. Routine laboratory tests are for the most part very nonspecific. Leukocytosis is present in most acute osteomyelitis and septic arthritis. However, in chronic osteomyelitis the WBC count may be normal.

Erythrocyte sedimentation rate (ESR) and C-reactive protein may be elevated or normal in early infection or in chronic osteomyelitis but are more useful for monitoring treatment and detecting relapses. In the absence of renal failure or nephrotic syndrome, a diabetic patient with a foot ulcer and an ESR >100 mm/hr is highly specific but not sensitive for the diagnosis of osteomyelitis (16). Blood cultures are an easy and inexpensive way of identifying the pathogenic organisms. They are positive in 30% of the cases of hematogenous osteomyelitis, 25% in vertebral infections, and 50% in acute cases of osteomyelitis (13).

A definitive diagnosis of septic arthritis is made with the identification of the organism(s) in the infected tissues by microscopy and culture. Examination, including Gram stain, leukocyte count, and culture, of the synovial fluid is a key to the diagnosis of a septic joint. Arthrocentesis must be performed prior to antibiotic use, to increase the culture yield of organisms. If arthrocentesis by closed needle aspiration is not possible, the joint should be aspirated under imaging guidance. Magnetic resonance imaging (MRI) and computed tomography (CT) scans can detect effusions in joints that are difficult to identify on physical examination, especially the hip and the sacroiliac joints. Hip joints may require surgical arthrotomy for diagnostic microbiology. The gross appearance of an infected synovial fluid may be turbid, serosanguinous, or even of frank pus, with an average leukocyte count (most of which are neutrophils) of 50,000–150,000 cells/mm^3. The synovial fluid chemistry values may be normal or the total protein and lactic dehydrogenase values may be elevated, while glucose levels may be depressed. Synovial fluid must be examined under polarized light microscopy to exclude crystal arthropathy, which may have a very similar presentation as septic arthritis. Gram stain of synovial fluid is positive in 75% of patients infected with *S. aureus* and 50% with gram-negative bacteria. In suspected tuberculous arthritis the synovial fluid should be examined for acid-fast bacilli (AFB) and for mycobacteria. The AFB smear is positive in 30%, and the culture is positive in 80% of cases of tuberculous arthritis (2,15).

Osteomyelitis is often a difficult disease to diagnose. Studies that have evaluated different combinations of clinical criteria, radiographic findings, and culture methods for the diagnosis have not been for the most part prospective and are subject to much controversy. The diagnostic tests must be individualized to the clinical scenario (9). The gold standard for the diagnosis of osteomyelitis is an open bone biopsy. Percutaneous needle aspiration, percutaneous biopsy, and debridement bone biopsy are the techniques of obtaining tissue samples, but it is important to obtain the culture samples through uninfected tissues to avoid contamination. Although bone biopsy is the gold standard in the diagnosis of osteomyelitis, radiologic tests are important in the evaluation of a patient with suspected bone infections. No single imaging technique has 100% specificity and sensitivity for every case of musculoskeletal infection. Depending on the age of the patient, presence of orthopedic hardware, location of infection, underlying bone or joint, and systemic conditions, the choice of imaging modalities must be individualized to the patient's condition. Plain radiographs are performed first and may be sufficient to diagnose osteomyelitis, especially if chronic, but are frequently unhelpful in early osteomyelitis or in the diagnosis of septic arthritis. They may reveal joint space narrowing, soft tissue swelling and at later stages show destructive changes or osteomyelitis in the underlying bone. Plain films are frequently normal in the early stages of osteomyelitis and changes may not appear until days later. Generally, MRI scan has been used most often clinically to diagnose acute osteomyelitis when plain radiographs were normal. Table 4 examines the advantages and pitfalls of different radiologic methods used to diagnose osteomyelitis (9,13).

6. ANTIBIOTIC TREATMENT

Optimal therapy of infections in the elderly requires treating much more than the organ system affected by the disease. An effort should be made to improve the patient's overall health and functional status including improvement of the patient's nutritional, metabolic, cognitive, and emotional status. It is also important to optimally treat any underlying conditions such as diabetes mellitus and poor vascular flow to facilitate healing. Successful management of bone and joint infections requires an early diagnosis and prompt antimicrobial therapy and, when necessary, surgical intervention. It is vital to identify the pathogens in order to select an appropriate antibiotic regimen, and this is best achieved by obtaining a sample of the infected tissues or surrounding pus or fluids. However, in chronic osteomyelitis organisms isolated from the sinus tract drainage may not accurately reflect the organisms present in the bone (12).

In osteomyelitis, obtaining a bone biopsy for culture is very important unless typical radiographic changes are accompanied by a positive blood culture. Surgical debridement of infected bone and soft tissues provides specimens for culture and aids eradication of the infection. In septic arthritis, after culture specimens are obtained, empirical antibiotics must be initiated immediately to cover the most likely pathogens, based on the clinical scenario or Gram-stain findings. The antibiotics selected must penetrate the bone and joints in adequate concentrations. It is not necessary to inject antibiotics into the joint as adequate levels of the drugs are usually achieved in the synovial fluid and the surrounding tissues (15). Drainage of the infected joint prevents destruction of the cartilage and postinfectious arthritis and is associated with a better outcome. Repeated needle aspirations, arthroscopic drainage or open arthrotomy, and lavage may be necessary. The choice of procedure depends on the accessibility of the joint and the ease of drainage of pus and necrotic tissues. Hip joints and loculated effusions with abundant necrosis of the cartilage, synovium, and bone, and those who have failed repeated needle aspirations usually require an arthrotomy and open surgical drainage. Most rheumatologists advise repeated closed needle aspirations, whereas orthopedic surgeons usually prefer an arthrotomy (4). Weight bearing on the affected joint should be avoided until inflammation decreases; however, early mobilization with the help of analgesics must be encouraged to avoid contractures and functional limitations (4,15,17,18).

The duration of antimicrobial therapy cannot be generalized for all patients and must be individualized to each patient. Empirical treatment in joint infections is based on the Gram-stain smear results, age, and the clinical scenario. In the elderly, if the Gram stain is negative and the patient is sexually active, it is important to administer an antibiotic that covers for *N. gonorrhoeae* and *S. aureus* and to culture the urethra and the cervix. Infection by the gonococcus is much less common in the elderly but cannot be overlooked. As a general rule, joint infections secondary to *Hemophilus influenzae*, streptococci and gram-negative cocci are treated with 2 weeks of IV antibiotics, while infections due to staphylococci and gram-negative bacilli are generally treated for a minimum of 3 weeks with parenteral drugs. Serial synovial fluid analysis should be performed after antibiotic treatment is initiated in

Table 4 Diagnostic Tests

Test	Findings	Advantages	Disadvantages
C-reactive protein, ESR	Elevated or normal	In acute phase mostly elevated When elevated on presentation it is used to monitor treatment and relapse In diabetic foot ulcer, if ESR >100 mm/hr, it is very specific but insensitive for OM	Nonspecific May be normal in early stages
Plain radiographs	Soft tissue swelling Periosteal reaction Lytic bone changes Brodie's abcess	Readily available. Inexpensive Helps exclude other conditions, such as gas. Fairly specific May aid in interpreting other studies in chronic OM	In early stages of acute OM, may be normal Insensitive for the diagnosis of OM Cannot exclude if negative, then must proceed to other studies, given later
99 mTc, three-phase bone scan	Labeled phosphorus, accumulates in areas of increased osteoblastic activity Three phases: 0 min, 15 min, 4 hr Significantly increased uptake in all three phases, with OM	95% sensitive and specific Positive within 24 hr of symptoms Test of choice for acute OM if plain films are normal When hardware in place, it is the test of choice	False negative if there is obstruction to blood flow, e.g., chronic OM False positives with fractures, tumors, following surgery, septic arthritis, healed OM, diabetic foot, and Paget's disease Poor anatomic detail
67 gallium citrate	Radioactive gallium accumulates at sites of inflammation	Great specificity for inflammation May help distinguish infectious from noninfectious processes, so used after 99 mTc scan	Poor anatomic detail
111Indium-labeled leukocyte scan	Labeled WBCs accumulate at the sites of inflammation or infection and in the bone marrow	Useful at sites of fracture nonunion Better sensitivity and specificity than bone scan in diabetic feet Used in combination with three-phase bone scan in hands and feet	Poor anatomic detail Nonspecific for bone Less sensitive for axial skeleton
Bone marrow scan	99-Tc labeled sulfur taken up by the reticuloendothelial system Allows imaging of the marrow	Used in combination with indium scan to rule out axial skeleton OM, especially when hardware in place	Poor anatomic detail

Ultrasound scan	Subperiosteal fluid collection. Soft tissue abscesses adjacent to the bone Periosteal thickening and elevation >2 mm	Good for guided percutaneous aspiration	Insufficient information about this method for diagnosis of OM
MRI scan	T1 weighted image: decrease signal intensity in the disk and adjacent vertebral bodies Loss of endplate definition T2 weighted image: increase signal intensity in the disk and adjacent vertebral bodies. Gadolinium enhances the disk, adjacent vertebral bodies involved paraspinal and epidural soft tissues	95% sensitivity Very good anatomic resolution. Provides detailed information about activity and extent of infection, spinal cord impingement, epidural abscesses, and soft tissues Particularly helpful in evaluation of vertebrae and infected feet Helps plan surgical debridement. Imaging of choice in diabetic foot ulcer (more specific than bone scan)	Does not always distinguish OM from a healing fracture or tumors Cannot be used with metal implants
CT scan		More sensitive in chronic OM Good for guided percutaneous aspiration Detects cortical destruction, intraosseous gas, and soft tissue extension	Metal interferes with images
Biopsy	Histopathologic features: necrotic bone, inflammatory exudates, and bone resorption	Open bone biopsy is the gold standard for diagnosis of OM Cultures must be obtained through uninvolved tissue Bone biopsy is the best way of diagnosing chronic OM	Invasive procedure Needle biopsy only Sensitivity 87%; specificity 93%

Abbreviations: OM, osteomyelitis; ESR, erythrocyte sedimentation rate; TC, technesium; WBCs, white blood cells; MRI, magnetic resonance imaging; CT, computed tomography.

order to demonstrate that the fluid has become sterile and that the WBC count is decreasing. If improvement does not occur, then after open drainage is performed, appropriate parenteral antibiotics should be administered for an additional week or longer depending on clinical response. When prosthesis and the surrounding musculoskeletal tissues are infected, cure can only be achieved by removal of the prosthesis and debridement of all surrounding infected tissues (3). Table 5 lists recommended antibiotics according to the organisms isolated or suspected.

Acute osteomyelitis can usually be treated solely with antibiotics; however, the treatment of chronic osteomyelitis often requires complete surgical debridement of the necrotic and infected soft tissues. In chronic osteomyelitis, antibiotics can be withheld depending on the stability of the patient's clinical condition and until surgical debridement can be performed and culture samples are obtained. Empirical antibiotics are started intraoperatively—after tissues for microbiology are obtained—until culture and sensitivity results are obtained. Then, specific treatment based on microbiology data is continued for 4–6 weeks following surgery. Empirical therapy in bone and joint infections should consist of IV administration of bactericidal agents and later modified based on in vitro susceptibility of the identified organisms. Because osteomyelitis is traditionally treated with 4–6 weeks of parenteral antibiotics, this requires long periods of hospitalization and is very expensive. This can be particularly problematic in the elderly. Outpatient parenteral antibiotic

Table 5 Antibiotic Treatment

Clinical scenario/identified organism by Gram stain or culture	Antibiotic options (IV, unless stated)
Streptococci, staphylococci (penicillin sensitive)	Penicillin G
Staphylococcus aureus (methicillin sensitive)	Oxacillin or nafcillin or cephalosporin, e.g., cefazolin, or vancomycin (if penicillin allergic)
S. aureus (methicillin resistant)	Vancomycin, linezolid, and quinipristin-dalfopristin
Pseudomonas aeruginosa	Aminoglycoside and either broad-spectrum β-lactam, e.g., ticarcillin, ceftazidime, and aztreonam or fluoroquinolone, especially ciprofloxacin
Gram-negative organism (other than *P. aeruginosa*)	Third-generation cephalosporin or aminoglycoside or fluoroquinolone or aztreonam
Community-acquired septic arthritis with a negative Gram-stain smear	Third-generation cephalosporin
Contiguous osteomyelitis with vascular insufficiency	Mild disease: oral amoxicillin–clavulanate Severe disease: imipenem or ticarcillin/clavulanate or ampicillin/sulbactam or trovafloxacin or cefepime and metronidazole or aztreonam and metronidazole and vancomycin
Sternal osteomyelitis	Vancomycin and rifampin oral
Salmonella species	Fluoroquinolones or third-generation cephalosporin

administration is possible with the placement of long-term IV access (12). Oral quinolones can be used after the initial 2 weeks of IV antibiotics to treat gram-negative osteomyelitis, with ciprofloxacin offering the best coverage against *Pseudomonas aeruginosa*; however, the current quinolones have variable activity against staphylococci, streptococci, enterococci, and anaerobic bacteria. Resistance among staphylococci is emerging against the β-lactams and the quinolones; however, in some cases oral clindamycin or amoxicillin-clavulanate may be used instead. Ciprofloxacin also has poor activity against streptococci, enterococci, and anaerobes, while levofloxacin and sparfloxacin have very good activity against streptococci species.

In patients with vascular insufficiency, the patient can be managed with long-term oral suppressive antibiotic therapy, if debridement or amputations are not an option. The level of vascularity determines the extent of the amputation. The length of antibiotic treatment after an amputation depends on the amount of residual infection in the area. If the infected bone and soft tissues are completely removed, then the patient is only given 7–10 days of antibiotics (to treat any residual distant infected sites resulting from the osteomyelitis). The choices of antibiotics and the duration of treatment should be individually decided (Table 4) (3,12–15).

7. PREVENTION

Patients with prosthetic joints should receive antibiotic prophylaxis before any invasive medical or dental procedures resulting in bacteremia.

REFERENCES

1. Kaandorp CJE, van Schaardenburg D, Krijnen P, Moens HJB. Risk factors for septic arthritis in patients with joint disease. Arthritis Rheum 1995; 38:1819–1825.
2. Goldenberg DL, Sexton DJ. Bacterial (nongonococcal) arthritis. Accessed, May 2004. http://www.utdol.com/application/topic.asp?file=st_b_inf/7197&type=A&selected Title=1~27.
3. Smith JW, Shahbaz, Hasan M. Infectious arthritis. In: Mandell GL, Bennett JE, Dolin R, eds. Principles and Practice of Infectious Diseases. 5th ed. Philadelphia, PA: Churchill Livingston, 2000:1175–1181.
4. Wright V. Diseases of the joints. In: Pathy MSJ, ed. Principles and Practice of Geriatric Medicine. Vol. 105. 3rd ed. Chichester, New York: John Wiley and Sons Ltd, 1998: 1133–1163.
5. Kaandorp CJE, Kriknen P, Moens HJB, Habbema JD, van Schaardenburg D. The outcome of bacterial arthritis. A prospective community-based study. Arthritis Rheum 1997; 40:884–892.
6. Cunha BA. Osteomyelitis in elderly patients. Clin Infect Dis 2002; 35:287–293.
7. Morgan DS, Fisher D, Marianos A, Currie BJ. An 18 year clinical review of septic arthritis from tropical Australia. Epidemiol Infect 1996; 117:423–428.
8. Paluska S. Osteomyelitis. Clin Fam Pract 2004; 6:127–147.
9. Ghiorzi T, Mackowiak P. Diagnosis of osteomyelitis. Accessed May 2004. http://www.utdol.com/application/topic.asp?file=st_b_inf/2049&type=A&selected Title=2~81.
10. Mader JT, Du Y, Simmons D, Calhoun JH. Pathogenesis of osteomyelitis. Accessed May 2004. http://www.utdol.com/application/topic.asp?file=st_b_inf/5849&type=A & selected Title=6~81.

11. Bremell T, Lange S, Yacoub A, Ryden C, Tarkowski A. Experimental *Staphylococcus aureus* arthritis in mice. Infect Immun 1991; 59:2615–2623.

12. Mader JT, Calhoun J. Osteomyelitis. In: Mandell GL, Bennett JE, Dolin R, eds. Principles and Practice of Infectious Diseases. 5th ed. Philadelphia, PA: Churchill Livingston, 2000:1182–1196.

13. Maguire JH. Osteomyelitis. In: Braunwald E, Fauci AK, Kasper DL, Hauser SL, Longo DL, Jameson JL, eds. Harrison's Principles of Internal Medicine. 15th ed. New York: McGraw-Hill, 2001:825–828.

14. Mader JT, Du Y, Simmons D, Calhoun JH. Clinical features and microbiology of osteo-myelitis. Accessed Oct 2003. http://www.utdol.com/applicatin/topic/topicText.asp.../ 6279&tye=A&selectedTitle=1∼7.

15. Thaler SJ, Maguire JH. Infectious arthritis. In: Braunwald E, Fauci AS, Kasper Dl, Hauser SL, Longo DL, Jameson JL, eds. Harrison's Principles of Internal Medicine. 15th ed. New York: McGraw-Hill, 2001:1998–2002.

16. Newman LG, Waller J, Palestro CJ, Schwartz M, Klein MJ, Hermann G, Harrington E, Harrington M, Roman SH, Stagnaro-Green A. Unsuspected osteomyelitis in the diabetic foot ulcers. Diagnosis and monitoring by leukocyte scanning with indium In-111 oxyqui-noline. J Am Med Assoc 1991; 266:1246–1251.

17. Mader JT, Shirtliff ME, Bergquist S, Calhoun JH. Principles of the management and treatment of osteomyelitis. Accessed Oct 2004. http://www.utdol.com/applicatin/ topic/print.asp?file=s_b_inf/6029.

SUGGESTED READING

Cunha BA. Osteomyelitis in elderly patients. Clin Infect Dis 2002; 35:287–293.
Kortekangas P. Bacterial arthritis in the elderly. Drugs Aging 1999; 14:165–171.
Yoshikawa TT. Aging and bacterial arthritis. Infect Dis Clin Pract 1996; 5:548–550.

40

Prosthetic Device Infections in the Elderly

Robert S. Urban and Steven L. Berk
Texas Tech University Health Sciences Center School of Medicine,
Amarillo, Texas, U.S.A.

Key Points:

- The pathogenesis of prosthetic device infection, an increasing problem due to the expanding use of implanted devices in the elderly, involves microbial virulence factors as well as impairment in host defenses.
- Central nervous system shunt infections usually require removal of the device, reimplantation (often after a period of external drainage), and prolonged antibiotic administration.
- The diagnosis of prosthetic joint infection is suggested by clinical, radiographic, and laboratory features; standard treatment (two-stage exchange arthroplasty) may be modified to debridement and long-term antibiotic therapy in selected elderly patients.
- Prosthetic valve endocarditis can be difficult to diagnose in the elderly. Curative treatment always requires prolonged antibiotic therapy and often replacement of the prosthetic valve; transesophageal echocardiography provides improved diagnostic accuracy in selected patients.
- Infected vascular grafts, pacemakers, and defibrillators may involve either endovascular or extravascular aspect of the device and provide unique challenges in diagnosis and treatment.

1. INTRODUCTION

The use of prosthetic devices, shunts, and grafts increases year by year and because of their increasing use in degenerative conditions such as calcific aortic stenosis, conduction system disease, and aortic aneurysm (to name a few), their use is increasing disproportionately in the elderly. In 2001, 152,000 total hip prostheses, 299,000 total knee prostheses, and 921,000 pacemakers were implanted; over 70% were inpatients aged ≥65 years. Although infection caused by the use of these devices is rare (usually <1%), when it occurs, the consequences can be devastating. Removal or revision of the device, the usual optimal therapy, can be difficult and antibiotic administration may be of long duration and complex. Age, with its comorbidities and contraction of life expectancy, complicates therapeutic decisions further. This chapter reviews the relevant concerns and issues involved in infection of the most common prosthetic devices.

While each type of prosthetic device has its own pattern of pathogens, staphylococci are particularly important. A balance between bacterial virulence factors and host resistance accounts for the frequency of these infections. Virulence factors include tissue and microbial adherence molecules and foreign body surface biofilm formation. *Staphylococcus aureus* has been well studied in this regard. It produces several adhesins which attach to fibrinogen (important in endovascular infections) and fibronectin (important in tissue infections). The specific gene cluster for adhesin production has been described and is shared by several strains (1). Biofilm is a mixture of microbial products (mostly carbohydrates) and host proteins and is largely responsible for the failure of antimicrobials and host defenses to clear organisms from the infected device.

Host response to device infection is abnormal in that neutrophil and monocyte function are inhibited by contact with the device surface. Endothelialization of endovascular devices (a process which usually takes 1–3 months) appears to decrease the likelihood of infection. T-cell function and platelet adherence may be abnormal when exposed to grafts or devices. Whether or not the waning of host immunity with aging increases the likelihood and virulence of device infections in the elderly is unknown. It is possible that the frequency of such infections in the elderly is simply a reflection of the increasing use of devices for degenerative diseases.

All of these factors emphasize the importance of optimal antibiotic therapy for prosthetic device infections in the elderly. The clinical aspects of these device infections, including their diagnosis, treatment, and prevention, are described. When possible, comparisons between infections in adults vs. the elderly are included.

2. SHUNT INFECTIONS

2.1. Epidemiology and Clinical Relevance

Central nervous system (CNS) shunts are often used in older patients in the treatment of hydrocephalus, including normal pressure hydrocephalus. The neonate and the elderly are at increased risk of shunt infection of the CNS. While the prevalence of shunt infections varies, the infection rate in elderly patients may be as high as 16%. Previous shunt revision and a prior drainage device are risk factors for infection. Both ventricular peritoneal (VP) shunts and ventricular atrial (VA) devices may become infected. Ventricular atrial device infection is more likely to cause infective endocarditis and shunt nephritis, particularly in older patients (2).

2.2. Etiologic Pathogens

The organisms causing these CSF shunt infections are the same in both elderly patients and younger adults. Coagulase-negative staphylococci cause 50% or more infections. *S. aureus* is the second most common pathogen. However, gram-negative bacilli and diphtheroids cannot be ignored as they are responsible for 5–10% of infections. Etiologic agents will vary with the nosocomial pattern of infection in different hospitals.

2.3. Clinical Manifestations

Shunts usually become infected following colonization after surgery. Infection may ascend from the distal end in a VP shunt or may occur through hematogenous spread, especially with VA shunts. The patient may present with headache, vomiting, or fever; the presentation is less acute and the systemic toxicity generally less severe than in typical bacterial meningitis. VP shunt infection may present with abdominal pain at the distal end of the shunt. As a general rule, shunt infection in older patients is more commonly associated with mental status changes and less fever than in younger patients.

2.4. Diagnosis

The definitive diagnosis of shunt infection is made by aspiration of the shunt to examine cerebrospinal fluid (CSF). Lumbar punctures are not useful. CSF aspirates will show a mild to moderate leukocytosis. The elderly often display fewer white cells in the CSF than younger patients. Blood cultures are positive in 90% of patients with VA shunts but <25% of patients with VP shunts (2).

2.5. Antibiotic Treatment

The management of shunt infections varies between individuals and surgeons. Gram stain and culture of CSF should be obtained from the shunt reservoir; blood cultures should also be obtained. Cultures should be held for at least 7 days.

There are three options for the treatment of a shunt infection. The first entails removing the shunt, utilizing an external drainage device, and instituting systemic antibiotics. The second involves removal of the infected shunt, replacing it immediately with a new indwelling device, and instituting antibiotic therapy. The third alternative is to leave the shunt in place and treat with systemic and/or intraventricular antibiotics.

Gardner, Lepzig, and Saigh (2) noted that 94% of infections treated with shunt removal and external drainage were cured, compared with 71% of patients treated with immediate shunt replacement (2,3). Usually, after removal of all the shunt components, the surgeon places an external ventricular drainage device. If complete removal of the device is not feasible, an alternative (but less satisfactory) approach is to exteriorize the distal end of a VP shunt. A course of effective systemic and/or intraventricular antibiotics is given. Once cultures have been documented to be sterile for 3–5 days, the external device is removed, and the new shunt is replaced at a different site. The treatment is continued for 10–14 days. A 21-day total course of antibiotics has been recommended depending on the organism, particularly if a new shunt is reimplanted at the same time as removal of the infected shunt. If the shunt is not removed, 3–6 weeks of treatment is generally advised.

Empirical therapy requires coverage of staphylococci with vancomycin and the occasional nosocomial gram-negative bacilli with a third-generation cephalosporin. Rifampin is sometimes added to vancomycin for synergy against gram-positive bacteria, particularly if full removal and delayed replacement of the device are not possible. Specific therapy is guided by sensitivity of the individual organism. If vancomycin or gentamicin is given intraventricularly, a "preservative-free" preparation should be used. If vancomycin is given intraventricularly, usually 10 mg is an appropriate starting dose. When vancomycin is given systemically, trough levels should be monitored as the drug can accumulate. Successful treatment with linezolid has recently been reported (3).

2.6. Prevention

Recent studies have suggested that rifampin-impregnated silicon catheters (4) or other antibiotic impregnated shunt systems (5) may be effective in preventing CNS shunt infections.

3.   PROSTHETIC JOINT INFECTION

3.1. Epidemiological Clinical Relevance

The prevalence of infection of prosthetic hip joints is 1.5–5%. Current studies have estimated the mortality from surgical intervention to be 0.4–2% in patients ≥65 years of age and 2–7% in >80 years of age (6). Prosthetic knee joints have a prevalence of infection of 1.3–9%. The infection risk of shoulder, wrist, or ankle replacement is 1–2%, whereas the risk in elbow replacements may be as high as 9%. Both total hip arthroplasty and total knee arthroplasty have become safer with aggressive prophylactic measures such as laminar flow rooms, body exhaust suits, and preoperative antibiotics (6).

3.2. Etiologic Pathogens

Aspirated material reveals visible organisms on Gram stain, usually gram-positive cocci, in 30% of cases, and pathogens are recovered by culture in 85–98% of cases, depending on prior antibiotic therapy. Infection criterion on histology or frozen section is defined by 5–10 white blood cells of light microscopy per high-powered field. The sensitivity is about 85% using this criterion, and the specificity is 99% when 10 white blood cells per high-powered field are noted.

Staphylococci are isolated from 41% to 60% of patients with infected prosthetic joints, with *S. aureus* as the most common pathogen, particularly if hematogenous infections are included (7). In a series of elderly patients, coagulase-negative staphylococci and *S. aureus* were isolated in nearly equal frequency; enterococci were the third most common isolate (8). Gram-negative bacteria, including *Pseudomonas aeruginosa*, are present in 8–28% of cases. Fastidious bacteria or mycobacterium can cause indolent infections (9). Polymicrobial infection has been increasingly reported (up to 19% of cases in some studies).

3.3. Clinical Manifestations

Most patients with an infected joint develop symptoms (usually increasing pain at rest and with activity) within 3 months of surgery (10). Another 30–35% of the patients present from several months to a year postoperatively with joint pain. In addition to pain, decreased mobility is a common complaint. Signs of systemic toxicity or fever are less dramatic in the elderly. Only 40–45% of elderly patients with prosthetic joint infection will have fever (8). Drainage or erythema may occasionally be present at the site of the incision, but infections can be quite indolent (9). Older patients who require hip replacement are more likely to have suffered a fall with subsequent fracture. This situation is typically associated with osteoporosis, gait disorder, polypharmacy, decreased sensory input (visual and proprioceptive), and general frailty—all conditions which can complicate postoperative care and recovery.

The average age of patients with an infected prosthetic hip is 67 years. Elderly patients with rheumatoid arthritis have a greater risk of infection than those with degenerative disease (8). Advanced age per se (independent of comorbid factors such as diabetes mellitus or malignancy) has not generally been shown to be a risk factor for infection. The presence of other foci of infection, especially urinary tract infections or pressure ulcers, does increase the risk of subsequent infection.

3.4. Diagnosis

Radiology plays an important role in the diagnosis of prosthetic joint infection, particularly in the elderly. Radiographic signs of loosening of the prosthesis are seen in two-thirds of late infections but in <50% of early infections. Arthography (after hip aspiration) may be helpful in detecting loosening of the cemented components by showing penetration of the dye between cement and bone. Radiography and even bone scans may fail to distinguish between a low-grade infection and aseptic loosening of the prosthesis. A bone scan following hip surgery may take as long as 6 months to become normal in the area of the lesser trochanter. The area around the acetabulum and the tip of the prosthesis may show increased activity for up to 2 years. The bone scan in infection generally shows a more diffuse pattern of abnormality along the prosthetic shaft and is usually positive on the two early phases of the scan. False-positive scans may occur in up to 40% and false-negative findings in 5–10% of cases. A gallium scan would suggest osteomyelitis by a focal uptake. However, any inflammatory bone process may cause increased uptake. White blood cell scans are more specific for making a definitive diagnosis of infection but may be less sensitive.

Magnetic resonance image scan and even positron emission tomography (PET) are increasingly used to make the definitive diagnosis. For prosthetic hip infections, PET scans have a sensitivity of 90% and specificity of 89% in one recent study (6), but are less accurate in knee infections.

The erythrocyte sedimentation rate (ESR) is elevated in >85% of the patients with infection. If 30–35 mm/hr is used as the threshold for infection, then the sensitivity rate will range from 61% to 88%. It is a nonspecific measure of inflammation. With ESR <30 mm/hr, prosthetic joint infections are unlikely, and the specificity rate will range from 96% to 100%. However, the ESR may not accurately diagnose those patients with an infection in the early postoperative period (9). The C-reactive protein (CRP) is an acute phase protein that can be used to follow the course of acute infections. It rises and falls faster than the ESR. If a CRP of 10 is used as the threshold for a total hip infection, the specificity and sensitivity for CRP are both about 90%. The CRP should return to normal in about 2–3 weeks after hip replacement.

3.5. Antibiotic Treatment

The standard approach to the infected prosthetic hip is a two-stage exchange arthroplasty. The prosthesis, debris, and cement are removed and 6 weeks of antibiotics based on culture results are given. For some organisms such as gram-negative bacilli, longer periods of antibiotic therapy may be necessary. The patient is unable to bear weight for weeks to months before a new prosthesis is reimplanted. A long rehabilitation period is required, but cure rates are reported as >80%. Obviously, such a treatment plan is a difficult undertaking for a debilitated, elderly patient.

A less aggressive approach—open debridement with retention of the hip prosthesis, followed by 6 weeks of intravenous antibiotics—may be considered in well-chosen elderly patients. This approach has been recommended for elderly patients with staphylococcal or streptococcal infections, who do not have a loosened prosthesis. It is not used in patients with major skin, soft tissue, or bone defects.

Fishman et al. (11) recently used a computer model to compare the two procedures in elderly patients with infected total hip arthroplasty. While the study is not definitive, it does suggest that the less aggressive procedure may provide a survival advantage because of decreased initial surgical mortality rates. However, the relapse rate after debridement and retention is about 30% per year. With oral antibiotic suppressive therapy, this rate may be lower. For *S. aureus* infection that has been delayed in diagnosis, relapse rate is much higher and retention of the device is not recommended.

In some elderly, debilitated patients, removal of the prosthesis is extremely difficult. When removal of an infected prosthesis is not possible, chronic suppressive oral antibiotic therapy is sometimes successful (success rate ≈60%) (12). The use of oral agents such as ciprofloxacin combined with rifampin can be beneficial in some cases of prosthetic joint infection (13). The functional outcomes for elderly patients are poor with the majority unable to walk without assistance. Forty percent may show persistent or recurrent infection (14). Chronic antimicrobial suppression is appropriate when removing the prosthesis is not feasible, the organism is of low virulence and highly susceptible to antibiotics, there is no systemic infection, the device has not come loose, and the patient is compliant.

For total knee arthroplasty (TKA) revisions, recommendations are even more subjective. Two-stage procedures seem to be more effective than one stage, but not in all studies. Debridement with retention of the TKA can be done with arthroscopic surgery. Results are best when patients have been symptomatic for <7 days and have no radiographic signs of prosthetic loosening. In one study, however, only 24% of patients were cured by the debridement (6).

3.6. Prevention

Clinical studies suggest that antibiotic prophylaxis is useful at the time of joint replacement. Agents directed against staphylococci and streptococci, such as first-generation cephalosporins, are usually recommended. The use of antibiotic impregnated cement is also useful. Antimicrobial prophylaxis for patients with prosthetic joints who undergo dental procedures and other invasive procedures (such as cystoscopy and endoscopy) has been recommended by the American Dental Association and the American Academy of Orthopedic Surgeons (15).

4. PROSTHETIC HEART VALVES

4.1. Epidemiology and Clinical Relevance and Microbiology

The incidence of prosthetic valve endocarditis (PVE) is about 1.5–3% within 1 year after valve surgery. This increases from 5.7% after 5 years (7). Coagulase-negative staphylococci are the predominant agent of PVE during the initial 2 months after surgery and, in fact, are the most common organisms for the first year after a valve replacement. Thereafter, viridans streptococci, enterococci, *S. aureus*, and fastidious gram-negative coccobacilli (the typical causes of native valve endocarditis) increase in prevalence (7). Gram-negative bacilli or fungal PVE, though uncommon, is usually nosocomial and therefore most often presents in the initial 2 months after surgery.

The incidence of PVE in the elderly has increased in the past decade as more degenerative and less rheumatic valvular disease is being treated with valve replacement. Furthermore, surgeons are becoming more comfortable with valve replacement surgery in octogenarians and above. Finally, the use of invasive interventions such as indwelling intravenous lines, dialysis catheters, and even pacemakers increases the incidence of bacteremia and PVE in patients with prosthetic valves. In some studies over 20% of endocarditis in the elderly is PVE (16).

4.2. Clinical Manifestations

The clinical features of PVE are similar to those of native valve endocarditis except that new murmurs are more frequent among those infected with prosthetic valves. Patients with PVE may develop congestive heart failure and systemic emboli. These symptoms are common in the general elderly population but should alert the clinician to the possibility of PVE. Any prolonged fever in a patient with a prosthetic valve should be viewed as possible PVE (7). Symptoms and signs of PVE are otherwise similar to those of native valve endocarditis. Numerous studies have compared the clinical manifestations endocarditis in elderly patients vs. younger adults. While studies differ, in general elderly patients have less fever and fewer systemic complaints (see also chapter, "Infective Endocarditis"). The elderly tend to present with nonspecific symptoms such as malaise and anorexia; in one-third, CNS changes such as confusion of lethargy predominate. Classic stigmata of endocarditis, such as Roth spots or Osler nodes, occur in fewer than 10% of the elderly. Delays in diagnosis are common in the elderly patient population since murmurs may be attributed to aortic sclerosis and mental status changes and focal neurologic signs to cormorbid disease (16). Mortality from PVE in elderly patients is twice as high as in young adults. However, valve replacement surgery can be performed with acceptable mortality rates even in the very elderly (17).

4.3. Diagnosis

The use of transesophageal echocardiogram (TEE) has greatly improved the diagnosis of both native valve endocarditis and PVE. Kemp and colleagues (18) reviewed the use of TEE in diagnosing PVE and found a range of sensitivity from 77% to 100% and a negative predictive value of 90%. Table 1 illustrates conditions for which TEE might be especially helpful diagnostically.

TEE may be of particular importance in the diagnosis of endocarditis in some elderly patients. In one study, Werner et al. (19) reported that transthoracic echocardiography identified only 45% of vegetations in patients >70 years of age, as compared with 75% of patients <45 years of age. TEE increased the sensitivity to >90% in both groups. Hence, there may be an increased value of TEE in the elderly patient with small vegetations. TEE may also better distinguish preexisting valvular abnormalities from true vegetations.

Table 1 Indications for Transesophageal Echocardiography for Suspected Infective Endocarditis

---

Prosthetic cardiac valves
Left-sided infective endocarditis (IE)
Staphylococcus aureus IE
Fungal IE
Previous IE
Prolonged clinical symptoms (3 months) consistent with IE
Cyanotic congenital heart disease
Systemic to pulmonary shunts
Poor clinical response to antimicrobial therapy for IE

4.4. Antibiotic Treatment

Treatment for PVE requires prolonged antibiotic therapy (Table 2). Antibiotic recommendations are the same for elderly patients as for younger adults and are based on isolation of the etiologic agent (7). In elderly patients taking coumadin, drug interaction with rifampin must be anticipated. Also, nephrotoxicity with gentamicin is increased in the elderly and in patients taking concurrent nephrotoxins. Table 2 provides antibiotic regimens of choice and alternate regimens.

For patients who have contraindications to vancomycin or who develop neutropenia or other complications, linezolid and quinupristin/dalfopristin offer treat-

Table 2 Prosthetic Valve Endocarditis Treatment

Streptococci:
Highly penicillin-susceptible viridans streptococci or *S. bovis* (MIC < 0.1 µg/mL) and
   patients whose infection involves prosthetic valves or other prosthetic materials: a 6-week
   regimen of penicillin recommended together with gentamicin for at least the first 2 weeks

Streptococci with an MIC >0.1 µg/mL:
It may be desirable to administer the aminoglycoside for more than 2 weeks (4–6 weeks)
Vancomycin can be used in penicillin-allergic patients

Enterococci and nutritionally variant streptococci:
Ampicillin or vancomycin plus gentamicin or streptomycin for 6–8 weeks

Methicillin-sensitive *Staphlococcus aureus*:
Nafcillin (or a first-generation cephalosporin or vancomycin if allergic) plus rifampin for
   6 weeks plus gentamicin for 2 weeks. Rifampin plays a unique role in the eradication of
   staphylococcal infection involving prosthetic material; combination therapy is essential
   to prevent emergence of rifampin resistance

Methicillin-resistant *Staphylococcus aureus*:
Vancomycin plus rifampin for 6 weeks plus gentamicin for 2 weeks

Coagulase-negative staphylococci:
Vancomycin plus rifampin for 6 weeks plus gentamicin for 2 weeks

HACEK (*Haemophilus parainfluenzae, Haemophilus aphrophilus, Actinobacillus,
   Cardiobacterium, Eikonella, Kingella*):
Third-generation cephalosporin for 6 weeks or ampicillin plus gentamicin for 6 weeks

For culture-negative or empirical treatment:
Vancomycin plus gentamicin plus ceftriaxone or ampicillin–sulbactam plus gentamicin

---

Abbreviations: MIC, minimum inhibitory concentration.

ment options, but only when vancomycin cannot be used. Linezolid, although bacteriostatic for most gram-positive cocci, has been used successfully in a few cases of endocarditis.

More than half of all patients with PVE may be candidates for surgical valve replacement. The most common indication for surgery is moderate to severe heart failure due to dysfunction of the prosthesis. Uncontrolled bacteremia, fever persisting for >10 days during appropriate antibiotic treatment, recurrent arterial emboli, evidence of myocardial or valve ring abscess, and relapse after appropriate antimicrobial therapy are other indications for surgery. In addition, infections caused by fungi, *S. aureus*, and gram-negative bacteria often require surgical intervention. Surgical indications in the elderly are the same as in younger patients, although comorbid conditions do need to be assessed preoperatively.

4.5. Prevention

Prosthetic valves may become infected because of bacteremia resulting from invasive procedures (7). Elderly patients often undergo dental, gastrointestinal (GI), or genitourinary (GU) procedures that may cause transient bacteremia. Table 3 reviews the dental procedures for which endocarditis prophylaxis is recommended. The indications for endocarditis prophylaxis for GI procedures are noted in Table 4, and the indications for PVE prophylaxis for GU and respiratory procedures are noted in Table 5. Note that prophylaxis is considered "optional" for some procedures but is recommended for high-risk patients such as those with prosthetic valves, a previous history of infective endocarditis, cyanotic congenital heart disease, ventricular septal defect, aortic valve disease, and mitral regurgitation. Moderate-risk cardiac conditions include mitral valve prolapse with regurgitation, tricuspid valve disease,

Table 3 Endocarditis Prophylaxis and Dental Procedures

Prophylaxis is recommended for patients with high- and moderate-risk cardiac
  conditions and receiving the following dental procedures:
Dental extractions
  Periodontal procedures including surgery, scaling and root planning, probing,
  and recall maintenance
  Dental implant placement and reimplantation of avulsed teeth
  Endodontic (root canal) instrumentation or surgery only beyond the apex
  Subgingival placement of antibiotic fibers or strips
  Initial placement of orthodontic bands but not brackets
  Intraligamentary local anesthetic injections
  Prophylactic cleaning of teeth or implants where bleeding is anticipated
Prophylaxis not recommended for these dental procedures:
  Restorative dentistry (operative and prosthodontic) with or without retraction cord
  Local anesthetic injections (nonintraligamentary)
  Intracanal endodontic treatment; postplacement, and buildup
  Placement of rubber dams
  Postoperative suture removal
  Placement of removable prosthodontic or orthodontic appliances
  Taking oral impressions
  Fluoride treatments
  Orthodontic appliance adjustment
  Shedding of primary teeth

Table 4 Endocarditis Prophylaxis and GI Procedures

Prophylaxis is recommended for patients with high- and moderate-risk
  cardiac conditions:
Indicated:
  Sclerotherapy for esophageal varices
  Esophageal stricture dilation
  Endoscopic retrograde cholangiography with biliary obstruction
  Biliary tract surgery
  Surgical operations that involve intestinal mucosa
Not indicated:
  Transesophageal echocardiography
  Endoscopy with or without gastrointestinal biopsy (prophylaxis is optional
  for high-risk patients such as prosthetic valves)

---

mitral stenosis, and degenerative valve disease of the elderly. The regimens used for
prophylaxis for patients allergic to penicillin include clindamycin or azithromycin.

5. VASCULAR GRAFT INFECTIONS

5.1. Epidemiology, Clinical Relevance, and Microbiology

The frequency of graft infections ranges from 1% to 6%. The majority of infections
are thought to occur at the time of implantation. Staphylococci are the most common pathogens. Early infections are usually caused by *S. aureus*, whereas infections
presenting later are usually caused by the more coagulase-negative staphylococci.
Rarely, gram-negative bacilli may also cause infections of grafts. Risk factors include
groin incisions, emergency surgery, multiple interventions, and contiguous infection

Table 5 Prosthetic Valve Endocarditis Prophylaxis and Respiratory and Genitourinary
Procedures

Prophylaxis is recommended for patients with high- and moderate-risk cardiac conditions
  and undergoing the following procedures:
Respiratory
  Tonsillectomy and/or adenoidectomy
  Surgical operations that involve respiratory mucosa
  Bronchoscopy with a rigid bronchoscope
  Endotracheal intubation
  Bronchoscopy with a flexile bronchoscope, with or without biopsy
  Tympanostomy tube insertion
Genitourinary
  Prostatic surgery
  Cystoscopy
  Urethral dilation
Prophylaxis is not recommended for these procedures:
  Vaginal hysterectomy
  Vaginal delivery
  Cesarean section
  In uninfected tissue
  Urethral catheterization
  Insertion or removal of intrauterine devices

---

in the graft area. Elderly patients with diabetes mellitus, chronic renal disease, and immunosupression are at particular risk.

5.2. Clinical Manifestations

Graft infections, especially those involving coagulase-negative staphylococci, may not become evident for months to years. Clinical diagnosis may be particularly difficult in the elderly patient. In an elderly patient with vascular graft, nausea, malaise, anorexia, and weight loss may be symptoms of graft infection. Significant upper GI bleeding in a patient with a prior aortofemoral graft raises great concern for an aortoenteric fistula. Physical examination findings in the elderly will often be diagnostic. Signs of infection depend on graft site but include a localized inguinal mass or a graft-cutaneous sinus tract (1). Evidence of a wound infection adjacent to a nonfunctional graft, false aneurysm, thrombosis, or anastamotic bleeding suggests graft infection. A sinus tract to a graft and a graft imbedded in infected tissue are, of course, other clues on physical examination.

5.3. Diagnosis

Computed tomography (CT) scan can show graft inflammation, fluid collections, or abscess surrounding the graft, or air fluid levels. Magnetic resonance imaging may also be useful; arteriography is less helpful unless occlusion of the graft is suspected. Sinography can establish a fistula tract in connection with an infected graft.

5.4. Antibiotic Treatment

For management of graft infections, the infected prosthesis needs to be removed and devitalized tissue debrided. Vascular flow must be re-established to the distal bed. Revascularization should be followed by an appropriate course of antibiotics (20,21). Generally, patients with graft infections are treated for a minimum of 6 weeks with parenteral therapy, depending on microorganism. A longer course of antibiotics may be required if the newly implanted graft appears to have been contaminated at the anastomotic site or if the arterial stump was closed proximal to the infected site. The clinician may need to consider lengthy, perhaps lifelong, suppressive regimens of oral antibiotics.

5.5. Other Infections

Endovascular stents are now commonly used with percutaneous angioplasty of carotid, renal, and peripheral vessels. Stent infections are extremely rare, perhaps as low as one in 10,000 cases. Infection, when it does occur, typically arises 1–4 weeks after a placement and presents with complications such as aneurysm, abscess formation, arterial necrosis, or septic emboli. CT scan and angiography will show an inflammatory reaction around the stent. Excision with revascularization is required as well as intensive antibiotic therapy directed against the offending organism, usually a staphylococcus (1).

Percutaneous coronary artery intervention with stent placement has become extremely common even in elderly, debilitated patients. Fortunately, the incidence of infection, even in debilitated patients with comorbid disease, is very low. There are only a few reports of intracoronary stent infection, all from either *S. aureus* or

P. aeruginosa. Findings included localized abscess, pericarditis, and pericardial empyema.

Other types of rare device infection include vascular closure device infection, Dacron carotid patches, and vena cava filters. These are reviewed by Baddour et al. (1).

6. PACEMAKER INFECTIONS

6.1. Epidemiology and Clinical Relevance

A pacemaker consists of essentially two components. The pulse generator is the power source that generates the electrical stimulus. This is conducted to a pacing electrode, usually via an endocardial or occasionally an epicardial lead. Elderly patients seem to be especially prone to pacemaker infections. The average age of patients with pacemaker endocarditis is 72 years.

Pacemaker infections may appear as a localized infection and/or abscess in the pulse-generator pocket (7). Erosion of the skin in the pacing system may lead to pocket infection. There may be fever with positive blood cultures in the patient who has a pacemaker and no obvious focus of infection. Generally, pulse-generator pocket infections result from contamination at the time of implantation of the pacemaker. Those infections, involving the conducting system, may occur secondary to bacteremic spread. There is an approximate prevalence of 0.13–12% of pacemaker infections reported in the literature (1,7). It has been demonstrated that endothelialization of the leads becomes evident at 6–8 weeks. Implantable cardioverter-defibrillators cause similar types of infection.

6.2. Microbiology, Clinical Manifestations, and Diagnosis

The clinical manifestations of pacemaker infections include fever or related complications such as erosion of the pulse-generator pocket, sepsis, pericarditis, or even mediastinitis. Generally, bacteremia from a pacemaker infection is from infection of the pacer pocket or related to extension of infection along the wire into the vascular system. Hematogenous colonization of the pacemaker conducting system resulting from bacteremia from a distant source has been documented, but is fortunately rare. *S. aureus* and coagulase-negative staphylococci account for >75% of pacemaker infections. Rarely, gram-negative bacilli and fungi may be involved as well. Diagnosis is made by positive blood cultures or by echocardiogram which shows vegetations on the pacemaker site. TEE is more sensitive than TTE and may detect 95% of wire vegetations.

6.3. Antibiotic Treatment

The management of the pacemaker infection varies according to the clinical scenario (1,7). Removal of the pacemaker is optimal treatment. Most patients require at least 4 weeks of antibiotic therapy. If the infectious process has been clearly localized to the pulse-generator pocket only, the generator should be removed and another one implanted at a distant site. The situation becomes more complicated if the conducting system or leads are infected. It is generally necessary to try to remove the entire pacemaker system at that point. This may be somewhat difficult in elderly patients with a limited life expectancy and a high operative risk. The failure to remove an infected lead can result in mortality as high as 65%. If the infected lead is retained, complications occur in as many as 50% of patients. Various techniques for lead extraction have been described in detail in the literature (1,7) and are complex. Under some circumstances, cardiopulmonary bypass must be used to remove the infected material (22).

6.4. Prevention

There have been no well-controlled studies that allow firm conclusions regarding prevention of infection during pacemaker replacement or implantation. A recent meta-analysis favors antibiotic prophylaxis (23).

REFERENCES

1. Baddour LM, Bettmann MA, Bolger AF, Epstein AE, Ferrieri P, Gerber MA, Gewitz MH, Jacobs AK, Levison ME, Newburger JW, Pallasch TJ, Wilson WR, Baltimore RS, Falace DA, Shulman ST, Tani LY, Taubert KA. Nonvalvular cardiovascular device-related infections. Circulation 2003; 108:2015–2031.
2. Gardner P, Leipzig TJ, Sadigh M. Infections of mechanical cerebrospinal fluid shunts. Curr Clin Top Infect Dis 1988; 9:185–214.
3. Gill CJ, Murphy MA, Hamer DH. Treatment of Staphylococcus epidermidis ventriculo-peritoneal shunt infection with linezolid. J Infect Dis 2002; 45:129–132.
4. Hampl JA, Weitzel A, Bonk C, Kohnen W, Roesner D, Jansen B. Rifampin-impregnated silicone catheters: a potential tool for prevention and treatment of CSF shunt infections. Infection 2003; 31:109–111.
5. Govender ST, Nathoo N, vanDellen JR. Evaluation of an antibiotic-impregnated shunt system for the treatment of hydrocephalus. J Neurosurg 2003; 99:831–839.
6. Lentino JR. Prosthetic joint infections: bane of orthopedists, challenge for infectious disease specialists. Clin Infect Dis 2003; 36:1157–1161.
7. Karchmer AW, Longworth DL. Infections of intracardiac devices. Cardiol Clin 2003; 21:253–271.
8. Powers KA, Terpenning MS, Voice RA, Kauffman CA. Prosthetic joint infections in the elderly. Am J Med 1990; 88:5-9N–5-13N.
9. Gillespie WJ. Prevention and management of infection after total joint replacement. Clin Infect Dis 1997; 25:1310–1317.
10. Stecklbert JM, Osmon DR. Prosthetic joint infections. In: Bisno AL, Waldvogel FA, eds. Infections Associated with Indwelling Medical Devices. 2nd ed. Washington, DC: American Society for Microbiology, 1994:259–290.
11. Fisman DN, Reilly DT, Karchmer AW, Goldie SJ. Clinical effectiveness and cost-effectiveness of 2 management strategies for infected total hip arthroplasty in the elderly. Clin Infect Dis 2001; 32:419–430.
12. Sergreti J, Nelson JA, Trenholme GM. Prolonged suppressive antibiotic therapy for infected orthopedic prostheses. Clin Infect Dis 1998; 27:711–713.
13. Zimmerli W, Widmer AF, Blatter M, Frei R, Ochsner PE. Role of rifampin for treatment of orthopedic implant-related staphylococcal infections: a randomized controlled trial. Foreign-Body Infection (FBI) Study Group. J Am Med Assoc 1998; 279:1537–1541.
14. Norman DC, Yoshikawa TT. Infections of the bone, joint, and bursa. Clin Geriatr Med 1994; 10:703–718.
15. American Dental Association and American Academy of Orthopaedic Surgeons Advisory Statement. Antibiotic prophylaxis for dental patients with total joint replacements. J Am Dent Assoc 1997; 128:1004–1008.

16. DiSalvo G, Thuny F, Rosenberg V, Pergola V, Belliard O, Derumeaux G, Cohen A, Larussi D, Giorgi R, Casalta JP, Caso P, Habib G. Endocarditis in the elderly: clinical, echocardiographic, and prognostic features. Eur Heart J 2003; 24:1576–1583.
17. Gregoratos G. Infective endocarditis in the elderly: diagnosis and management. Am J Geriatr Cardiol 2003; 12:183–189.
18. Kemp WE Jr, Citrin B, Byrd BF III. Echocardiography in infective endocarditis. South Med J 1999; 92:744–754.
19. Werner GS, Schulz R, Fuchs JB, Andreas S, Prange H, Ruchowski W, Kreuzer H. Infective endocarditis in the elderly in the era of transesophagel echocardiography: clinical features and prognosis compared with younger patients. Am J Med 1996; 100:90–97.
20. Yeager RA, Porter JM. The case against the conservative nonresectional management of infected prosthetic grafts. Adv Surg 1996; 29:33–39.
21. Earnshaw JJ. Conservative surgery for aortic graft infection. Cardiovasc Surg 1996; 4:570–572.
22. Vogt PR, Sagdic K, Lachat M, Candinas R, von Segesser LK, Turina MI. Surgical management of infected permanent transvenous pacemaker systems: ten year experience. J Card Surg 1996; 11:180–186.
23. DaCosta A, Kirkorian G, Cucherat M, Delahaye G, Chevalier P, Cerisier A, Isaaz K, Touboul P. Antibiotic prophylaxis for permanent pacemaker implantation: a meta-analysis. Circulation 1998; 97:1796–1801.

SUGGESTED READING

Baddour LM, Bettmann MA, Bolger AF, Epstein AE, Ferrieri P, Gerber MA, Gewitz MH, Jacobs AK, Levison ME, Newburger JW, Pallasch TJ, Wilson WR, Baltimore RS, Falace DA, Shulman ST, Tani LY, Taubert KA. Nonvalvular cardiovascular device-related infections. Circulation 2003; 108:2015–2031.
Karchmer AW, Longworth DL. Infections of intracardiac devices. Cardiol Clin 2003; 21: 253–271.
Lentino JR. Prosthetic joint infections: bane of orthopedists, challenge for infectious disease specialists. Clin Infect Dis 2003; 36:1157–1161.

41
Human Immunodeficiency Virus Infection

Allen S. Funnyé
Divisions of General Internal Medicine and Geriatrics, Department of Internal Medicine, Charles R. Drew University of Medicine and Science, Martin Luther King, Jr.–Charles R. Drew Medical Center, Los Angeles, California, U.S.A.

Key Points:

- Older adults have had one of the highest rates of increase for human immunodeficiency virus (HIV) infection and are at risk of developing acquired immune deficiency syndrome (AIDS).
- HIV infection may be more severe and progressive in older adults, but they respond well to highly active antiretroviral treatment.
- HIV infection may go unsuspected and unrecognized leading to presentations at diagnosis of more advanced disease.
- HIV dementia may mimic Alzheimer's disease, which generally lacks ataxia and motor impairment.
- Related comorbidities such as coronary artery disease, diabetes mellitus, depression, and hyperlipidemia may impact the choices of antiretroviral therapy.

1. INTRODUCTION

Acquired immune deficiency syndrome (AIDS) was first reported in 1981, and in 1983 the virus causing AIDS was identified. In the United States the virus was called humanT-lymphotrophic virus (HTLV-III) and in France, lymphadenopathy-associated virus (LAV). In 1986, the name was changed to human immunodeficiency virus (HIV) (1,2).

AIDS is a syndrome of immunodeficiency affecting primarily the CD4+ T-lymphocytes and has a disease spectrum ranging from primary infection or acute retroviral syndrome to asymptomatic infection, which may last for years, early symptomatic infection, and advanced HIV disease (3). HIV has affected primarily younger individuals and it has been known as a disease of the young; however, it is the ninth leading cause of death in those aged 45–64 years. Prevention efforts and most literature reports have focused on this younger age group. Studies involving older individuals that could clarify the effect of HIV and aging on the response to treatment are sparse. With the increasing aging of the population, AIDS is likely to be encountered more often in individuals >55 years of age. Thus, it is important

Table 1 AIDS Cases >50 Years by Male Sex, Age at Diagnosis, and Race/Ethnicity, Reported Through December 2001, United States

Male age at diagnosis (years)	White, not Hispanic		Black, not Hispanic		Hispanic		Grand total	
	No.	Male grand total (%)	No.	(%)	No.	(%)	No.	(%)
50–54	17,498	23.16	12,959	17.15	5,861	7.76	36,318	48.07
55–59	9,337	12.36	6,987	9.25	3,242	4.29	19,566	25.90
60–64	5,139	6.80	3,819	5.05	1,769	2.34	10,727	14.20
65 or older	4,249	5.62	3,242	4.29	1,455	1.93	8,946	11.84
Male total	36,223	47.94	27,007	35.74	12,327	16.31	75,557	100.00

Table 2 AIDS Cases >50 Years by Female Sex, Age at Diagnosis, and Race/Ethnicity, Reported Through December 2001, United States

Female age at diagnosis (years)	White, not Hispanic		Black, not Hispanic		Hispanic		Grand total	
	No.	Female grand total (%)	No.	(%)	No.	(%)	No.	(%)
50–54	1,309	9.27	3,447	24.42	1,245	8.82	6,062	42.94
55–59	816	5.78	1,865	13.21	750	5.31	3,479	24.64
60–64	519	3.68	1,103	7.81	411	2.91	2,069	14.66
65 or older	1,044	7.40	1,073	7.60	355	2.51	2,507	17.76
Female total	3,688	26.12	7,488	53.04	2,761	19.56	14,117	100.00

Source: From Ref. 5.

that clinicians are aware of the clinical approach and management of HIV infection in this age group.

2. EPIDEMIOLOGY IN OLDER ADULTS

Through December 2000 the percentage of AIDS cases reported in the United States in those >50 years of age at the time of diagnosis was approximately 11%. During the mid-1990s, the rate of increase in AIDS cases in the >50 years age group was among the highest in the United States. Older African–American males and females are disproportionately affected by AIDS, representing 50% of female cases >50 years and 35% of male cases >50 years while representing only 12% of the population (4) (see Tables 1 and 2) (5). Rates in older men who have sex with men decreased nearly 50% since 1989 while heterosexual transmission has doubled from 6% in 1992 to 13% in 1997. Drug abuse and its association with HIV infection in older adults have not been frequently appreciated. The percentage of those >50 years old with HIV infection related to drug abuse was 8% in 1988, 11% in 1991, and 17% in 2000 (4).

The number of older people living with HIV infection is difficult to ascertain. Older people at risk do not get tested as often as younger people. This coupled with the fact that HIV infection has not been a reportable disease in many states may underestimate the true prevalence of disease. It is possible that as many as 60,000 people >60 years old are now living with HIV infection. By the year 2030 the projected number of individuals aged ≥65 years will double to more than 70 million, which would constitute 20% of the population. This may result in an even higher prevalence of HIV infection in the older age group (6).

3. PATHOGENESIS OF HIV IN THE ELDERLY

The pathogenesis of HIV may differ according to genetic type. The two genetic types of HIV (HIV-1 and HIV-2) differ in pathogenesis and geographic predilection. HIV-1 is predominantly found in the United States, Asia, and Europe, whereas HIV-2 is found mainly in Africa. HIV-1 is the most common cause of AIDS in the world. HIV-1 has pathophysiological differences from HIV-2, which include: (1) a higher initial viral load set point, (2) higher rates of infection and progression, (3) a significantly faster decline of CD4+ lymphocytes, (4) higher rates of transmission than HIV-2, and (5) higher rates of perinatal transmission than HIV-2. The subtypes (clades) of HIV-1 also have important geographic differences. HIV-1 subtype B predominates in the United States and Europe and appears less heterosexually transmitted than subtype E, which occurs more in Thailand, central Africa, and Asia (7). Genetic types and subtypes of HIV have not been characterized as to the pathogenesis and geographic location in older adults. The discussions which follow relate to infection with HIV-1.

Studies from the late 1980s and early 1990s showed that older people with HIV did not do as well as younger individuals. They had lower CD4+ cell counts, a more advanced stage at initial diagnosis, more comorbidities, and a more aggressive clinical course (8). Older age was related to a more rapid progression of HIV disease and higher rates of death and opportunistic diseases (9). In 1995, prior to highly active and retroviral treatment (HAART), older age showed a linear correlation with an increased probability of death, with an estimated risk of progression to AIDS or death of 2% per year of age (10). This difference in progression has been explained by the decline in immune function that accompanies aging, and to delayed diagnosis and comorbidities (8,9).

In a study involving 1216 HIV-infected hemophiliacs varying in ages from 8 to 79, Darby et al. investigated the role of age in the progression of HIV infection. They showed that age at infection had a substantial effect on survival. Eighty-six percent of patients who seroconverted before the age of 15 survived for 10 years after infection, compared with only 12% of patients who seroconverted at or after age 55 (11). AIDS may progress more rapidly in older individuals and they may also present at a more advanced stage of disease at diagnosis. Causes of more rapid progression include higher viral set point; preferential infection of memory T cells which increase proportionally in the elderly; more rapid destruction of T cells; progressive increase in T cells with shortened telomeres, which may be destroyed faster; impaired replacement of HIV-infected CD4 T cells; and less effective anti-HIV cytotoxic T-lymphocyte activity than in younger persons (12).

A study by Perez et al. showed that persons over 50 have a blunted CD4 cell recovery when treated with HAART, and CD4 recovery was negatively correlated with age. Nevertheless, there was a 72% decrease in the hazard ratio for older treated individuals compared with older untreated individuals. The effect of HAART substantially improved the survival rate for older individuals and supports the importance of treatment in this group (13). A retrospective study by Wellons et al. involving 101 older patients, mean = 56.7 years (range 50–79), and 202 younger patients, mean = 32.8 years (range 21–39), compared immunologic and virologic outcomes of older vs. younger patients on HAART. Older HIV-infected patients responded well to HAART with a significantly greater percentage achieving a plasma HIV RNA level below detectable limits. The greater viral suppression may have been secondary to the greater rate of adherence in older people (8).

Most studies on the progression of HIV disease in older individuals were done before the advent of HAART. In order to determine whether or not the progression of HIV disease in older persons had been altered since the advent of HAART, Grimes et al. studied 52 HIV-infected men ≥50 years old and used a control group of 52 HIV-infected men aged <50 years (9). The mortality rate was higher among patients who were ≥50 years of age than among those who were <50 years of age (18% vs. 6%; $p = 0.06$), but when the data were examined according to cause of death, there were no significant differences in the number of AIDS-related deaths or opportunistic diseases. Older patients had increases in CD4+ T-lymphocyte counts that were comparable to those in younger patients. These results provided evidence that there should be no difference in the management of older and younger HIV-infected patients (9). Manfredi et al. compared outcomes in 66–84-year-olds vs. 55–65-year-olds (10). Mean drop in viremia was nearly 1 log 10 among the younger group and 0.5 log 10 among older patients, even after 12 months of therapy. CD4 level was comparable between the two groups at baseline, whereas immune recovery was significantly slower and blunted in patients aged ≥65 years. The older group had a tendency toward a more frequent diagnosis of AIDS, an increased rate of patients naive to antiretroviral therapy (ART), and a less rapid and effective virologic response and complete viral suppression over time.

4. CLINICAL MANIFESTATIONS

Time to AIDS diagnosis and death is more rapid in older persons and advanced age is associated with decreased survival following an AIDS diagnosis. Rapid progression in the elderly may be secondary to an increased viral set point or decreased host immune response. Those with an extremely low set point may eventually be found to be long-term progressors. The percentages of long-term progressors in the elderly is not known. There are several important HIV-related conditions of significant importance in the overall assessment and management of older adults with HIV infection.

4.1. Geriatric Syndromes

Older persons, especially frail older persons, may present with nonspecific problems such as failure to thrive, malnutrition, falls, confusion, dizziness, lethargy, and incontinence. These problems may be the manifestation of several conditions. For example, dizziness can be associated with anxiety, depression, impaired balance, impaired hearing, postural hypotension, past myocardial infarction, and use of more than five medications. Several conditions or associations may be present with one manifestation or syndrome. This is in contrast to younger individuals or traditional syndromes in which a specific defect may cause the clinical manifestations. Geriatric syndromes, then, may be defined as a set of lost specific functional capacities potentially caused by a multiplicity of pathologies in multiple organ systems (14). The advanced AIDS patient may share several clinical features seen in the elderly with geriatric syndromes. Some of the more important or prevalent syndromes include dementia, delirium, frailty, failure to thrive, dizziness, and syncope. AIDS patients may develop HIV dementia, and frailty from the wasting aspects of the disease and sarcopenia. Patients may be delirious from infections or central nervous system causes and may have dizziness and syncope for similar reasons. This makes the recognition and management of potentially frail elderly with HIV infection especially challenging.

4.2. Acute HIV-1 Infection

Symptomatic acute HIV infection (acute retroviral syndrome) occurs in 40–90% of patients. The frequency in older patients is not known. The main symptoms are fever (96%), lymphadenopathy (74%), pharyngitis (70%), rash (erythematous maculopapular or mucocutaneous ulcerations) (70%), and myalgias/arthralgias (54%). Neurologic symptoms include meningoencephalitis or aseptic meningitis, peripheral neuropathy, and cognitive impairment or psychosis (15). The set point for plasma viremia occurs during acute infection and influences the progression of HIV. Patients with high viral set points may progress more rapidly.

HIV acute infection often goes unrecognized, especially in older people, and is often attributed to a viral syndrome. It is important to recognize acute HIV infection because early intervention can theoretically decrease the severity of the disease, alter the initial viral set point, reduce the rate of viral mutations, preserve immune function, and reduce the risk of viral transmission. However, major questions regarding drug therapy in acute HIV infection remain. These include: what is the risk–benefit ratio and the length of therapy? Risks of treatment include drug toxicities, resistance, and possible indefinite treatment. Whether acute treatment is truly beneficial is a controversial and an unresolved point of contention. Ongoing clinical trials are addressing these issues, but the author knows of no specific studies involving clinical presentations, viremia, CD4 counts, treatment, and other issues of acute HIV infection in the elderly.

4.3. Dementia

Between 15% and 20% of people with advanced HIV disease eventually develop HIV-associated dementia. Older age at AIDS diagnosis is a significant risk factor for HIV dementia. HIV-associated dementia typically develops late in HIV disease after other AIDS-related illnesses have been diagnosed. It is characterized by disabling cognitive, behavioral, and motor impairments. Among the cognitive symptoms of HIV-associated dementia are decreased short-term memory and concentration, increased distractibility, loss of spontaneity, and mental slowing down. Behavioral changes include personality changes, apathy, withdrawal, irritability, and depression. Clumsiness, tremor, and leg weakness are motor impairments linked to this dementia (6).

HIV dementia may mimic Alzheimer's disease or vascular dementia. Some important differences should be noted. HIV dementia is associated with ataxia, reflex abnormalities, weakness, and peripheral neuropathy, whereas Alzheimer's disease is not generally associated with these. Patients with Alzheimer's disease may have aphasia, a language disorder, which is not present in HIV dementia. In addition, HIV dementia often responds to antiviral therapy, whereas Alzheimer's does not (16). Although HAART may increase the length of survival for people with HIV, the inability of protease inhibitors (PIs) to cross the blood–brain barrier may increase the risk of developing HIV-associated dementia.

The impact of HIV-associated cognitive decline on psychosocial interactions, adherence to medications, and ability to benefit from educational intervention can be profound. HIV-infected adults with significant neurocognitive compromise are at risk of poor medication adherence, particularly if they have been prescribed a complex dosing regimen. Hinkin et al. (17) studied the effect of cognitive dysfunction and regimen complexity on medication adherence in 137 HIV-infected patients aged 25–69 years with 25% being >50 years of age. The presence of cognitive dysfunction was found to confer a twofold or greater risk of poor adherence. Older age without cognitive decline was associated with better adherence. Patients aged ≥50 years were 2.9 times more likely to adhere than were younger subjects. Postulated reasons for better adherence included the following: patients were >50 years of age but most were <60 years old, and most cognitive decline occurs after the seventh decade; older patients were already used to taking medications; and taking medications interrupts lifestyle less in the elderly.

4.4. Opportunistic Infections

The range of opportunistic infections (OIs) are similar in the young and the elderly. They may progress more rapidly in older patients and they may be frequently misdiagnosed. Symptoms such as fatigue, anorexia, weight loss, and memory impairment may be attributed to old age. The same symptoms frequently occur in OIs such as tuberculosis, cryptococcal meningitis, and *Pneumocystis carinii* pneumonia (PCP). As in younger individuals the most frequent OIs include PCP and candida esophagitis. Treatment and prophylaxis are essentially the same, taking into account altered pharmacokinetics, drug interactions, and comorbidities.

4.5. Comorbid Diseases

Many chronic diseases such as diabetes mellitus, hypertension, coronary artery disease (CAD), and congestive heart failure occur in older HIV-infected patients. Significant and frequent comorbidities also include depression, chronic airway diseases, and osteoarthritis. HIV-infected patients >55 years old have four times more comorbid conditions than those <45 years old, and average at least 2.4 comorbidities per person. When these diseases occur on the backdrop of HIV infection, the clinical presentation and treatment may be significantly impacted. For example, the concern with lactic acidosis resulting from nucleoside reverse transcriptase inhibitors (NRTIs) is magnified in diabetic patients who have the potential to develop diabetic ketoacidosis. Lipid abnormalities become more prevalent with age and also with diabetes mellitus, which is frequently associated with dysplipidemia and an increase in triglycerides. The potential for HAART to increase lipids and produce metabolic dysfunction is well known. This, coupled with the fact that increased triglycerides and decreased cholesterol concentrations were noted in advanced HIV infection even before the advent of HAART, highlights the importance of HIV as a direct cause of metabolic dysfunction and magnifies the interrelationships of comorbidities such as CAD, hypertension, and diabetes mellitus (6).

5. TREATMENT OF HIV INFECTION

Treatment of HIV infection in the elderly should include assessing functional capacity, the potential for polypharmacy and adherence, altered pharmokinetics, and the effect of comorbidities. The elderly frequently take multiple medications for comorbid conditions. Adherence has been thought to be a problem for older patients because of the large number of pills, side effects, and drug–drug interactions related to PIs. Recent studies have shown that adherence in older patients is as good as or better than in younger patients (6,8,18).

Age-related pharmacodynamic changes can result in increased therapeutic effect of drugs and potential toxicity. Decreased hepatic mass as well as hepatic blood flow may cause as much as 25% reduction in hepatic metabolism. Regional blood flow to the liver at age 65 years is reduced by 40–45% compared with a 25-year-old. This may also affect drugs cleared by first-pass metabolism. There is a linear decrease in renal function as one grows older. The glomerular filtration rate (GFR), as measured by the creatinine clearance, decreases by up to a third and at a rate of 8 mL/min/decade after age 40 years. Blood urea nitrogen (BUN) and creatinine may not adequately reflect the decrease in GFR. The BUN may be low because of decreased protein intake and the serum creatinine may be lower because of decreased muscle mass. These changes magnify the potential for adverse drug interactions in the elderly.

5.1. HIV Drug Classes

There are currently five major classes of antiretroviral drugs: nucleoside analog reverse transcriptase inhibitors, nucleotide reverse transcriptase inhibitors, nonnucleoside reverse transcriptase inhibitors (NNRTIs), PIs, and fusion inhibitors.

5.1.1. Nucleoside Analog Reverse Transcriptase Inhibitors

NRTIs were the first drugs approved for the treatment of HIV infection. They inhibit the synthesis of DNA by reverse transcriptase, which results in the decrease or prevention of HIV replication. Nucleoside analogs resemble the natural building blocks of DNA and are triphosphorylated within the cell. Reverse transcriptase does not distinguish between the phosphorylated NRTIs from their natural building blocks and uses the nucleoside analogs in the synthesis of viral DNA. This results in incorporation of a false nucleoside analog into a strand of DNA with the resultant prevention of the production of a full-length copy of DNA. NRTIs may cause mitochondrial toxicity with a potentially fatal syndrome of lactic acidosis and hepatic steatosis (19).

5.1.2. Nonnucleoside Analog Reverse Transcriptase Inhibitors

NNRTIs also inhibit the synthesis of viral DNA but do so by a mechanism different from that of NRTIs, which act as false nucleotide analogs. They bind to reverse transcriptase and inhibit the reverse transcriptase directly. They may induce or inhibit cytochrome P450 (CYP). Resistance develops rapidly and cross-resistance is common in this class. NRTI- and PI-resistant HIV isolates remain sensitive to NNRTI (19).

5.1.3. Nucleotide Reverse Transcriptase Inhibitors

These are phosphorylated nucleosides and consequently do not require intracellular phosphorylation. They inhibit reverse transcriptase and viral replication and function the same way as NRTIs (19).

5.1.4. Protease Inhibitors

PIs prevent the processing of viral proteins into functional forms by binding the viral protease enzyme. This prevents cleavage of precursor proteins necessary for HIV maturation, infection of new cells, and viral replication. Viral particles are still produced but are ineffective in infecting new cells. PIs are metabolized by CYP and may cause hepatotoxicity, lipodystrophy, gastrointestinal distress, increased bleeding, and insulin resistance with hyperglycemia and hyperlipidemia (19).

5.1.5. Fusion Inhibitors

HIV fuses into the target cell by utilizing the HIV envelop protein gp41. This protein undergoes a conformational change (folds), which allows HIV to fuse into the target cell membrane. Fusion inhibitors bind to this protein and interfere with the conformational change, thereby preventing the entry of HIV into target cells. Enfuvirtide (Fuzeon) was the first HIV fusion inhibitor. There has been no reported resistance to enfuvirtide in enfuvirtide-naive patients. Enfuvirtide is active against HIV strains that are resistant to other classes of antiretrovirals. It must be given by subcutaneous injections twice a day and there is a high incidence of local reactions (20).

5.2. Principles of HIV Treatment in the Elderly

In general, the elderly should be treated like the young with knowledge of important comorbidities. ART should be started in all those with symptomatic HIV infection, with CD4+ T cells less than 200, and individualized in those with CD4 counts between 200 and 350. Plasma viremia, a strong prognostic indicator for HIV infection, should be used to help determine initiation of therapy for CD4 counts between 200 and 350. The advantages and disadvantages of antiretroviral drug classes as initial treatment are given in Table 3 (21).

Patient understanding, willingness to adhere to treatment, their current and future pill burden, severity of HIV infection, potential adverse drug reactions and interactions, and comorbidities are significant factors in deciding whether to initiate treatment. The patient's current drugs should be reviewed and the potential for drug–drug interactions assessed. Most antiretroviral drug interactions are mediated through inhibition or induction of hepatic enzymes. All PIs and NNRTIs are metabolized in the liver by the CYP system. Lipid-lowering statins, calcium channel blockers, sildenafil (Viagra), and St. John's Wort may have significant interactions. These drugs are frequently used in older patients with comorbidities and their interactions should be determined. St. John's Wort, an over-the-counter medication used for depression, may have significant interactions with all of the PIs and NNRTIs and should not be used. Bepridil, a type 4 calcium channel blocker indicated for chronic angina pectoris, should not be used with the PIs ritonavir, amprenavir, and atazanavir. Peak concentrations and half-life are markedly increased in the elderly (>74 years). The risk of cardiotoxicity, including arrhythmias, heart block, and prolonged QT interval on electrocardiogram, would be significant. Simvastatin and lovastatin should not be used with any of the PIs or with the NNRTI, delavirdine, which would result in large increases in statin levels and increased risk of myopathy and rhabdomyolysis. Sildenafil may significantly increase levels of the PIs. Use of sildenafil in patients aged $\geq$65 years is associated with increased serum levels of the drug and thus an even greater tendency for toxicity including myocardial ischemia when used with PIs.

Substrates are drugs or xenobiotic substances that are acted on by the CYP enzymes. Induction refers to increased synthesis or decreased degradation of these enzymes resulting in decreased plasma levels and pharmacodynamic effect(s) of the substrate. Inhibition refers to enzyme inactivation or the process of substrates competing for the same catalytic site, which results in a decrease in drug (substrate) metabolism and increased levels of the drug. All PIs are substrates and inhibitors of CYP3A4. Using a CYP3A4 substrate with a potent CYP3A4 inhibitor may lead to markedly prolonged elimination half-life ($t_{1/2}$) and drug toxicity. Coadministration of PIs or NNRTIs with a potent CYP3A4 inducer may lead to lower drug concentrations and reduced therapeutic efficacy of the antiretroviral agents. For example, the rifamycins (rifampin and rifabutin) are CYP3A4 inducers that can reduce plasma concentrations of most PIs and NNRTIs. Rifabutin is a less potent inducer, and is considered an alternative to rifampin for the treatment of tuberculosis when it is used with a PI- or NNRTI-based regimen. NRTIs do not undergo hepatic transformation through the CYP metabolic pathway.

Once-daily therapy improves patient convenience and adherence; however, there are few long-term trials comparing once- vs. twice-daily regimens. Missing a once a day drug may have significant consequences related to the development of drug resistance depending on the pharmacokinetics of the antiretroviral.

Some agents or combinations of agents are generally contraindicated due to suboptimal antiviral potency, unacceptable toxicity, or pharmacological concerns. Monotherapy is contraindicated except zidovudine (ZDV) monotherapy as part of the Pediatric AIDS clinical trial group 076. Dual nucleoside therapy has not

Table 3 Advantages and Disadvantages of Antiretroviral Components Recommended as Initial Antiretroviral Therapy

ARV class	Antiretroviral agent(s)	Advantages	Disadvantages
NNRTIs		Less fat maldistribution and dyslipidemia than PI-based regimens Save PI options for future use	Low genetic barrier to resistance Cross resistance among NNRTIs Skin rash Potential for CYP450 drug interactions
	Efavirenz	Potent antiretroviral activity Low pill burden and frequency (1 tablet per day)	Neuropsychiatric side effects Teratogenic in nonhuman primates; contraindicated in pregnancy; avoid use in women of child bearing years
	Nevirapine	More safety experience in pregnant women No food effect	Higher incidence of rash than with other NNRTIs, including rare serious hypersensitivity reaction Higher incidence of hepatotoxicity than, with other NNRTIs, including serious cases of hepatic necrosis
PIs		NNRTI options saved for future use Longest prospective study data including data on survival benefit	Metabolic complications—fat maldistribution, dyslipidemia, insulin resistance CYP3A4 inhibitors and substrates—potential for drug interactions (esp. with ritonavir-based regimens)
	Lopinavir/ritonavir	Potent antiretroviral activity Co-formulated as Kaletra®	Gastrointestinal intolerance Hyperlipidemia Little experience in pregnant women Food requirement
	Amprenavir/ritonavir	No food effect FDA-approved once-daily regimen	Less extensive experience Frequent skin rash High pill burden and capsule size
	Atazanavir	Less adverse effect on lipids than other PIs Once daily dosing Low pill burden	Hyperbilirubinemia (indirect) PR interval prolongation—generally inconsequential unless combined with another drug with similar effect

	Advantages	Disadvantages
Indinavir	Long-term virologic and immunologic efficacy experience	Interaction with tenofovir and efavirenz—avoid concomitant use unless combined with RTV (ATV 300 mg qd + RTV 100 mg qd) Food requirement 3-times-daily dosing and food restriction reduced adherence High fluid intake required (1.5–2 L per day) Nephrolithiasis
Indinavir/ritonavir	Low-dose ritonavir Indinavir $T_{1/2}$ and C_{min} allows for twice-daily instead of 3-times-daily dosing Eliminates food restriction of indinavir	Possibly higher incidence of nephrolithiasis than with IDV alone High fluid intake required (1.5–2 L per day)
Nelfinavir	More extensive experience in pregnant women than with other PIs	Diarrhea Higher rate of virologic failure than with other PIs in comparative trials Food requirement
Saquinavir (hgc or sgc) + ritonavir	Low-dose ritonavir reduces saquinavir daily dose and frequency—C_{max}, C_{min}, and $T_{1/2}$	Gastrointestinal intolerance (sgc worse than hgc)
NRTIs	Established backbone of combination antiretroviral therapy	Rare but serious cases of lactic acidosis with hepatic steatosis reported with most NRTIs
Triple NRTI regimen	Abacavir + zidovudine (or stavudine) + lamivudine only	Abacavir + zidovudine + lamivudine co-formulated as Trizivir® Minimal drug-drug interactions Low pill burden Saves PI and NNRTI for future option	Inferior virologic response when compared to efavirenz based and indinavir-based regimens Potential for abacavir hypersensitivity reaction
Dual NRTIs backbone of three or more drug combination therapy	Zidovudine + lamivudine	Most extensive and favorable virological experience Co-formulated as Combivir® – ease of dosing No food effect Lamivudine – minimal side effects	Bone marrow suppression with zidovudine Gastrointestinal intolerance

(Continued)

Table 3 Advantages and Disadvantages of Antiretroviral Components Recommended as Initial Antiretroviral Therapy (*Continued*)

ARV class	Antiretroviral agent(s)	Advantages	Disadvantages
	Stavudine + lamivudine	No food effect Once-daily dosing (when extended release stavudine formulation becomes available)	**Adverse effects associated with stavudine:** Peripheral neuropathy, lipoatrophy, hyperlactatemia and lactic acidosis, reports of progressive ascending motor weakness, potential for hyperlipidemia Higher incidence of mitochondrial toxicity with stavudine than with other NRTIs
	Tenofovir + lamivudine	Good virologic response when used with efavirenz Well tolerated Once-daily dosing	Data lacking for tenofovir use in patients with renal insufficiency Tenofovir—reports of renal impairment Tenofovir—food requirement
	Didanosine + lamivudine	Once-daily dosing	Peripheral neuropathy, pancreatitis—associated with didanosine Food effect—needs to be taken on an empty stomach
	NRTI + emtricitabine	Long half-life of emtricitabine allows for once daily dosing (of emtricitabine)	

Source: From Ref. 21.

demonstrated potent and sustained antiviral activity compared to three-drug combination regimens and is contraindicated. A three-NRTI regimen with abacavir + tenofovir + lamivudine has a high rate of significant early virologic nonresponse as does the three-NRTI regimen of didanosine + tenofovir + lamivudine. Didanosine + stavudine may result in a high incidence of toxicities such as peripheral neuropathy, pancreatitis, and lactic acidosis.

Stavudine antagonizes ZDV and should not be used with it; in addition, the combination may cause lactic acidosis and severe hepatomegaly with steatosis. Zalcitabine plus stavudine or zalcitabine plus didanosine have increased rates and severity of peripheral neuropathy. Atazanavir and indinavir can cause grade 3–4 hyperbilirubinemia, which may be additive when used together. Hydroxyurea promotes the toxicity of didanosine with increased rates of peripheral neuropathy and pancreatitis.

Combinations should always be used and include:

- An NNRTI with two NRTIs (NNRTI-based regimens that are PI sparing)
- A PI with low-dose ritonavir and two NRTIs (PI-based regimens that are NNRTI sparing)
- Three NRTIs (triple-NRTI regimens that are both PI and NNRTI sparing)
- An NNRTI with two NRTIs is a preferred regimen that avoids pill burden and potential side effects of PI-based regimens. A disadvantage is that a single mutation in the gene for reverse transcriptase can produce resistance to all NNRTIs (21).

5.3. Important Side Effects of HAART in Older Adults

5.3.1. Lactic Acidosis/Hepatic Steatosis

Chronic hyperlactatemia can occur with NRTIs. Cases of severe lactic acidosis with hepatomegaly and steatosis are rare but associated with a high mortality rate. This may be related to mitochondrial toxicity. Nevirapine, an NNRTI, has the greatest potential for causing clinical hepatitis.

5.3.2. Hyperglycemia

Hyperglycemia has been reported in 3–17% of patients receiving HAART. Brambilla et al. (22), in a retrospective study involving 1011 HIV-positive patients, found that older age and regimens including stavudine or indinavir were associated with a higher risk of developing diabetes mellitus. Insulin resistance associated with PI use results in hyperglycemia, diabetes mellitus, worsening of preexisting diabetes mellitus, and diabetic ketoacidosis.

5.3.3. Fat Maldistribution

HIV infection and ART have been associated with altered fat distribution. There may be fat wasting (lipoatrophy) or fat accumulation (hyperadiposity).

These changes have been called lipodystrophy. Lipodystrophy may be associated with dyslipidemias, glucose intolerance, or lactic acidosis. There is no clear effective therapy for lipodystrophy.

5.3.4. Hyperlipidemia

Dyslipidemia can be the direct result of HIV infection or a consequence of ART (23). Cardiovascular risk factors associated with HIV infection and HAART include plasma lipid abnormalities (decreased high-density lipoprotein cholesterol, increased low-density lipoprotein, cholesterol-increased triglycerides), increased visceral fat, insulin resistance, chronic inflammation, and endothelial dysfunction/atherosclerosis (24). Before HAART, cachexia, low total cholesterol, and high triglyceride levels were reported in HIV patients. Several features of the metabolic syndrome overlap with common features of HIV treatment-associated lipodystrophy such as hyperinsulinemia, glucose intolerance, an atherogenic lipoprotein phenotype, a prothrombotic state, and central obesity (23).

Hypertriglyceridemia is common and severe in patients taking ritonavir. Lipid abnormalities tend to be most marked with ritonavir and lopinavir–ritonavir. NNRTs cause alterations in lipid profiles but less than with PIs (23). However, the dyslipidemia associated with PIs may not be class specific. The PI atazanavir has little effect on lipids (24). Patients with risk factors for hyperlipidemia should be monitored closely. Statins may be necessary but one should use agents less affected by CYP such as pravastatin. Switching from a PI to nevirapine or abacavir results in improved total cholesterol and triglycerides. PIs have been associated with myocardial infarctions; consequently, clinicians must weigh the risks of hyperlipidemia including myocardial infarction vs. the risks and benefits of switching therapy or initiating statin therapy. PI-associated insulin resistance and altered expression of apolipoprotein C-III gene may mediate PI-associated dysplipidemia (23). Another potential mechanism for PI- associated hyperlipidemia has been described, which consists of PI-induced protection of apolipoprotein B degradation by the proteasome (25). In HIV-infected patients with elevated cholesterol or triglyceride levels, nonpharmacologic interventions should be tried first unless the patient has existing coronary heart disease or total cholesterol levels >400 mg/dL (24).

5.3.5. Osteonecrosis, Osteopenia, and Osteoporosis

Avascular necrosis and osteonecrosis have been associated with HIV infection. Earlier studies have linked osteonecrosis to PI therapy; however, recent case–control studies have not shown HAART to be a consistent risk factor for the development of osteonecrosis (26). Osteoporosis has been associated with PI use, and this has been documented by dual-energy x-ray absorptiometry (DEXA) scans. PIs may inhibit conversion of 25-hydroxy vitamin D to 1,25-di-hydroxy vitamin D, which may contribute to the development of osteoporosis. Patients should have adequate intake of calcium and vitamin D. In patients at risk of osteoporosis, such as the older patient, a DEXA scan should be performed. Alendronate should be prescribed if the DEXA scan is consistent with osteopenia and there are no contraindications (27).

5.3.6. Skin Rash

Rashes range from mild to severe, including Stevens–Johnson syndrome and toxic epidermal necrosis. NNRTIs are more prone to cause skin rashes and should prompt permanent discontinuation of NNRTI or other offending agents. Nevirapine in particular causes more frequent and severe skin rashes; however, rashes are NNRTI class specific and may occur with other NNRTIs. Abacavir, an NRTI, is associated with a systemic hypersensitivity reaction. Therapy should be discontinued and not restarted. Aprenavir is the PI that causes skin rashes most frequently. It is a sulfonamide and has the potential for cross-reactivity with sulfur drugs and should be used with caution in cases of sulfur allergies.

6. PREVENTION

Older people with HIV infection have significant emotional distress and thoughts of suicide, suggesting a need for targeted interventions to improve mental health and prevent suicide. In addition, interventions are needed for both primary and secondary prevention of HIV infection. There is a stereotypical view that the elderly are not at risk of acquiring HIV. In one survey of 100 senior center directors in Illinois and Southern California, only seven said they provided their clients with HIV/AIDS information. Anonymous testing studies have shown an unanticipated prevalence of HIV among the elderly. Older heterosexuals average two to four sexual contacts per month and infected elders may continue to act as a source of infection. At least 1 million homosexual males aged ≥65 years may continue high-risk behaviors into old age. Mucosal disruption from thinned anal and vaginal mucosa increases the risk of HIV transmission. Elderly at-risk Americans >50 years old are less likely to use a condom during sex and one-fifth as likely to have been tested for HIV antibodies (28).

The magnitude of mortality due to undiagnosed and unrecognized HIV infection in the elderly is not known. Providers may be reluctant to consider AIDS as a possibility in older individuals until late in the course of the disease. Unsuspected HIV infection was identified (by testing discarded serum) in 5% of patients >60 years old who died in one New York City hospital (6).

HIV infection may be more common among elderly patients in certain communities with high HIV seroprevalence, the majority of which have no identifiable risk factor. Elderly women appear to be at particularly high risk. Long-term care providers will be increasingly more likely to encounter elderly people living with AIDS in need of their services (16). Prevention programs may be more difficult in the face of cognitive, visual, and auditory declines that occur with age. An individualized approach may be necessary to address such challenging issues in the elderly. Prevention efforts which are done individually have been found to be more effective. This allows for questions and concerns to be more readily answered, and the patient's response and alertness monitored (29).

REFERENCES

1. Sepkowitz KA. AIDS—the first 20 years. N Engl J Med 2001; 344:1764–1772.
2. Gold J, Dwyer J. A short history of AIDS. Med J Aust 1994; 160:251–252.
3. Fauci AS. Multifactorial nature of human immunodeficiency virus disease: implications for therapy. Science 1993; 262(5136):1011–1018.
4. Centers for Disease Control and Prevention. AIDS among persons aged ≥50 years—MMWR United States, 1991–1996. MMWR 1998; 47:21–27.
5. Centers for Disease Control and Prevention. U.S. HIV and AIDS cases reported through December 2001. Surveillance Report. Year-end edition. Vol. 13, No. 2.
6. Shah SS, McGowan JP, Smith C, Blum S, Klein RS. Comorbid conditions, treatment, and health maintenance in older persons with human immunodeficiency virus infection in New York City. Clin Infect Dis 2002; 35:1238–1243.

7. Hu DJ, Buve A, Baggs J, van der Groen G, Dondero TJ. What role does HIV-1 subtype play in the transmission and pathogenesis? An epidemiological perspective. AIDS 1999; 13:873–871.

8. Wellons MF, Sanders L, Edwards LJ, Bartlett JA, Heald AE, Schmader KE. HIV infection: treatment outcomes in older and younger adults. J Am Geriatr Soc 2002; 50: 603–607.

9. Grimes RM, Otiniano E, Rodriguez-Barradas MC, Lai D. Clinical experience with human immunodeficiency virus infected older patients in the era of effective antiretroviral therapy. Clin Infect Dis 2002; 34:1530–1533.

10. Manfredi R, Calza L, Davide C, Chiodo F. Antiretroviral treatment and advanced age: epidemiologic, laboratory, and clinical features in the elderly. J Acquir Immune Defic Syndr 2003; 33:112–120.

11. Darby SC, Ewart DW, Giangrande PL, Spooner RJ, Rizza CR. Importance of age at infection with HIV-1 for survival and development of AIDS in UK haemophilia population. Lancet 1996; 347:1573–1579.

12. Bender BS. HIV and aging as a model for immunosenescence. J Gerontol A Biol Sci Med Sci 1997; 52A(5):M261–M263.

13. Perez JL, Moore RD. Greater effect of highly active antiretroviral therapy on survival in people aged ≥50 years compared with younger people in an urban observational cohort. Clin Infect Dis 2003; 36:212–218.

14. Tangaroran GL, Kerins GJ, Besdine RW. Clinical approach to the older patient: an overview. In: Cassel CK, Leipzig RM, Cohen HJ, Larson EB, Meier DE, Capello CF, eds. Geriatric Medicine: An Evidence-Based Approach. New York: Springer-Verlag, 2003:149–162.

15. Niu MT, Stein DS, Schnittman SM. Primary human immunodeficiency virus type 1 infection: review of pathogenesis and early treatment intervention in humans and animal retrovirus infections. J Infect Dis 1993; 168(6):1490–1501.

16. Genke J. HIV/AIDS and older adults. The invisible ten percent. Care Manag J 2000; 2:196–205.

17. Hinkin CH, Castellon SA, Durvasula RS, Hardy DJ, Lam MN, Mason KJ, Thrasher D, Goetz MB, Stefaniak M. Medication adherence among HIV+ adults, effects of cognitive dysfunction and regimen complexity. Neurology 2002; 59:1944–1950.

18. Adeyemi OM, Badri SM, Max B, Chinomona N, Barker D. HIV infection in older patients. Clin Infect Dis 2003; 36:1347.

19. Drugs for HIV infection. Med Lett 2001; 43(1119):103–108.

20. Enfuvirtide (Fuzeon) for HIV infection. Med Lett 2003; 45(1159):49–50.

21. Department of Health and Human Services. Guidelines for the Use of Antiretroviral Agents in HIV-1 Infected Adults and Adolescents. November 10, 2003;1-94.

22. Brambilla AM, Novati R, Calori G, Meneghini E, Vacchini D, Luzi L, Castagna A, Lazzarin A. Stavudine or indinavir-containing regimens are associated with an increased risk of diabetes mellitus in HIV-infected individuals. AIDS 2003; 17:1993–1995.

23. Dubé MP, Stein JH, Aberg JA, Fichtenbaum CJ, Gerber JG, Tashima KAT, Henry WK, Currier JS, Sprecher D, Glesby MJ. Guidelines for the evaluation and management of dyslipidemia in human immunodeficiency virus (HIV)—infected adults receiving antiretroviral therapy: recommendations of the HIV Medicine Association of the Infectious Disease Society of America and the Adult AIDS Clinical Trials Group. Clin Infect Dis 2003; 37:613–627.

24. Currier JS. Cardiovascular risk associated with HIV therapy. J Acquir Immune Defic Syndr 2002; 31:S16-S23.

25. Domingo P, Sambeat MA, Peréz A, Ordoñez J. Effect of protease inhibitors on apolipoprotein b levels and plasma lipid profile in HIV-1-infected patients on highly active antiretroviral therapy. J Acquir Immune Defic Syndr 2003:114–116.

26. Allison GT, Bostrom MP, Glesby MJ. Osteonecrosis in HIV disease: epidemiology, etiologies, and clinical management. AIDS 2003; 17:1–9.

27. Montessori V, Press N, Harris M, Akagi L, Montaner JSG. Adverse effects of antiretro-
     viral therapy for HIV infection. Can Med Assoc J 2004; 170(2):229–238.
28. Newcomer V. Human immunodeficiency virus infection and acquired immunodeficiency
     syndrome in the elderly. Arch Dermatol 1997; 133:1311–1312.
29. Williams E, Donnelly J. Older Americans and AIDS: some guidelines for prevention.
     Social Work 2002; 47:105–111.

SUGGESTED READING

Funnyé AS, Akhtar AJ, Biamby G. Acquired immunodeficiency syndrome in older African
     Americans. J Natl Med Assoc 2002; 94:209–214.
Kilby JM, Eron JJ. Novel therapies based on mechanisms of HIV-1 cell entry. N Engl J Med
     2003; 348:2228–2238.
Nichol JE, Speer DC, Watson BJ, Watson MR, Vergon TL, Vallee CM, Meah JM. Aging with
     HIV: psychological, social, and health issues. San Diego, CA: Academic Press, 2002.
Tinetti ME, Williams CS, Gill TM. Dizziness among older adults: a possible geriatric
     syndrome. Ann Intern Med 2000; 132:337–344.

42
Septic Shock in the Elderly

Burke A. Cunha
Infectious Disease Division, Winthrop-University Hospital, Mineola and Department of Medicine, State University of New York School of Medicine, Stony Brook, New York, U.S.A.

Key Points:

- Sepsis and septic shock occurs when an organism overcomes host defenses resulting in a cascade of physiological events and ultimate organ/failure or death.
- Septic shock or severe sepsis occurs disproportionately more often in older adults; as many as two-thirds of all cases in the United States are persons aged ≥65 years.
- Septic shock is not commonly associated with pneumonia, meningitis, osteomyelitis, septic arthritis, infective endocarditis, and cellulitis, which are important infections in the elderly.
- Older patients with septic shock should be evaluated for urosepsis, intravenous-line sepsis, or intra-abdominal sepsis as the most frequent sources of sepsis.
- Antimicrobial therapy, hemodynamic stabilization, treating the primary cause of infection, and surgical intervention as appropriate are hallmarks of therapy.

1. EPIDEMIOLOGY AND CLINICAL RELEVANCE

Septic shock may be defined as multiple major organ dysfunction that is due to an infectious process accompanied by hypotension and bacteremia (1,2). For sepsis to occur in a patient, there must be impairment or breaching of host defenses due to a large inoculum of a relatively avirulent organism or a small inoculum of a highly virulent organism. Sepsis and its most severe manifestation, septic shock, is a relatively uncommon occurrence given the constant interplay between the host and the microbial world. Septic shock in the elderly that fulfills this description is limited to relatively few clinical situations. Compared with other age groups, septic shock is more common among the elderly patients admitted to the hospital than in younger adults.

The most common disorders associated with septic shock in the elderly include urosepsis, intravenous-line sepsis, and intra-abdominal/pelvic sepsis. These are the main clinical scenarios with septic shock potential (3–6). Septic shock is more common in the elderly because of the age-related increase in the disorders that predispose to sepsis and septic shock. Urosepsis, for example, is most common in elderly men who have urinary tract abnormalities, or who have had urological instrumentation.

Urological abnormalities of the urinary tract that predispose to sepsis include relative obstruction due to benign prostatic hypertrophy, relative or total obstruction due to tumor, renal stone disease, or urological instrumentation. Elderly individuals are more likely to have intra-abdominal disorders that predispose to septic shock (e.g., diverticulitis with perforation/abscess, colon cancer with obstruction/perforation). Intravenous-line sepsis is more frequent among the elderly because more elderly patients are admitted to hospitals and are more likely to have prolonged intravenous (IV) therapy, particularly via peripherally inserted central catheter (PICC) lines. Central venous access devices that may be complicated by IV-line infection. Although host defenses wane with increasing age, decreased B and T lymphocyte function per se, do not account for septic shock being more common in the elderly (4–7).

The therapy of septic shock depends on correcting the underlying cause. Surgical interventions, e.g., abscess drainage, removal of stones, decompression of obstructed urinary tract, relief of an obstructed biliary tract, removal of infected an central/PICC lines, all are life-saving modalities. Together with surgical interventions, antimicrobial therapy remains the cornerstone of effective treatment for septic shock. The results are optimal when appropriate antimicrobial therapy is coupled with early surgical intervention in the treatment of septic shock.

The cornerstone of nonsurgical therapy for septic shock remains early and appropriate antimicrobial therapy directed against the flora of the organ system involved, which is the pathogenic flora causing septic shock (8–10). Many non-antibiotic antisepsis therapies have been tried and have failed.

2. ETIOLOGIC PATHOGENS

Most cases of septic shock are due to gram-negative aerobic bacilli or gram-positive aerobic cocci. Microorganisms associated with septic shock are the resident microflora from the site of infection.

Aerobic gram-negative bacilli and gram-positive cocci (e.g., group B streptococci or enterococci) are the most common pathogens in urinary tract infections in the elderly. The same organisms cause septic shock in the elderly when the normal anatomical/host defenses of the genitourinary tract are altered. Urinary instrumentation in the elderly, i.e., voiding cystometrograms, diagnostic procedures, transurethral resection of the prostate, bladder, ureteral or renal stones, and ureteral stent placement/removal all have uroseptic potential due to aerobic gram-negative bacilli or gram-positive cocci organisms. Importantly, *Staphylococcus aureus*, *Bacteroides fragilis*, and *Streptococcus pneumoniae* are not usual uropathogens (Table 1) (4,6,11–13).

3. CLINICAL MANIFESTATIONS

There is an ongoing equilibrium maintained between host defenses and the host's microbial environment. Infection occurs when this balance is disrupted by impairment bypass of host defenses, an increase in virulence of pathogens, or numbers of infecting microorganisms. The structure of the human body and all host defense mechanisms are designed to prevent sepsis in the microbially laden host environment. Because sepsis requires a major disruption of this relationship—which

Table 1 Microorganisms and Organ System Correlates in Septic Shock

Source of sepsis	Usual pathogens	Usual nonpathogens
Urosepsis	E. coli/aerobic gram-bacilli	S. pneumoniae
	Group B streptococci	S. aureus
	Enterococci	B. fragilis
Intravenous-line sepsis	S. epidermidis (CoNS)	S. pneumoniae
	S. aureus (MSSA>MRSA)	B. fragilis
	K. pneumoniae	Pseudomonas aeruginosa
	Enterobacter sp.	
	Serratia sp.	
Intra-abdominal/pelvic sepsis	E. coli/aerobic gram-bacilli	Enterococci
	B. fragilis	S. aureus
		S. pneumoniae

occurs under relatively few circumstances—sepsis occurs less frequently than might be expected.

Adults with functional or anatomical asplenia are predisposed to overwhelming sepsis. However, most adults reaching advanced age have some degree of splenic function, and for this reason overwhelming sepsis secondary to asplenia is rare in elderly adults. T- and B-lymphocyte function wane with age and predispose to infection, but not septic shock. Even human immunodeficiency virus patients with little or no T-lymphocyte function die from a variety of infections, e.g., disseminated *Mycobacterium avium-intracellulare* infection or malignancies, but septic shock is uncommon in this subset of compromised hosts. Similarly, in patients with febrile neutropenia receiving chemotherapy for hematologic malignancies, septic shock is relatively uncommon. Patients with intact host defenses and who experience febrile bacteremia caused by gram-negative bacilli or gram-positive cocci secondary to venous devices do not usually present with septic shock. If host defenses are bypassed, overwhelmed or compromised, then patients of any age, including elderly patients, can develop sepsis/septic shock (6,11).

Appendicitis may occur at any age, and may be complicated by gangrene or perforation. Children and young adults can usually survive such an insult; however, septic shock is not an uncommon sequela of a perforated appendix in elderly patients. Gallbladder disease increases with age and elderly patients are more likely than younger adults to develop cholangitis due to malignant/benign obstruction or biliary stones. Diseases of the colon, particularly diverticulitis and colon cancer, are important predisposing factors in elderly patients (6,12,13).

The most common cause of septic shock in elderly patients is urosepsis. Urosepsis is defined as sepsis of urinary tract origin when the urinary isolate and the organism in the bloodstream are the same. In adult elderly men, enlargement of the prostate is a normal phenomenon of aging, and predisposes to relative urinary tract obstruction due to prostate enlargement. Elderly women have altered genitourinary tracts because of a relaxed pelvic musculature, which is a function of age, and often have cystocele or rectocele, which predisposes to bacteriuria. Bacteriuria alone is insufficient to cause sepsis and additional factors are necessary to make the patient septic, e.g., compromised host defenses. For this reason, elderly women with diabetes mellitus or systemic lupus erythematosus may develop bacteremia, sepsis, or septic shock from cystitis (4,6,12,13).

It is important to appreciate that there are only a few conditions associated with septic shock in the elderly, and it is equally important to recognize that certain conditions do not cause septic shock in the elderly. Community-acquired pneumonia (CAP) and nursing home-acquired pneumonia (NHAP) are not associated with septic shock. Such patients commonly present with hypotension and a "septic picture," but in fact, most of these patients do not have sepsis but have a noninfectious cause of fever, leukocytosis, and hypotension. Most patients with apparent CAP and septic shock in reality have acute myocardial infarction, congestive heart failure, pulmonary embolism, gastrointestinal (GI) hemorrhage, or an exacerbation of chronic obstructive pulmonary disease that causes a decrease in blood pressure/an increase in the peripheral white blood cell count with a shift to the left mimicking sepsis. These conditions may be referred to as "pseudosepsis" since they mimic sepsis with clinical features in common with sepsis (14–19) (Table 2).

4. DIAGNOSIS

4.1. Intravenous-Line Sepsis

IV lines are common in elderly hospitalized patients and certain types of IV devices are more likely to result in sepsis. PICC lines and short-term/long-term central lines, e.g., Hickman and Broviac catheters, may be associated with sepsis in adults as well as elderly patients. Peripheral IV lines and arterial lines are rarely associated with sepsis. Because central lines are inserted through the skin and are usually in place for extended periods of time, the likelihood of skin organisms being introduced/ gaining access to the bloodstream via the catheter lumen/tunnel, is greater with central than with peripheral IV lines, which are usually in for a shorter duration. Therefore, the most common pathogens associated with central IV lines are the *Staphylococcus epidermidis* [coagulase-negative staphylococci (CoNS)] or *S. aureus*

Table 2 Disorders Associated with Septic Shock in the Elderly

Infectious diseases associated with septic shock	Infectious diseases generally not associated with septic shock
Urinary tract infections	Meningitis
Obstruction (relative/complete)	Encephalitis
Foreign bodies/stents (obstructed)	Dental infections
Urinary tract stones	CAP
IV line infections	NHAP
PICC lines	Gastritis/duodenitis
Central IV lines	Cholecystitis
Septic thrombophebitis	Diarrhea
Intra-abdominal/pelvic infections	Cellulitis
Cholangitis (biliary obstruction	Osteomyelitis
secondary to tumor, benign stricture,	Septic arthritis
or stones)	Endocarditis
Appendicitis (gangrene/perforation	Febrile neutropenia
abscess)	
Diverticulitis (perforation/abscess)	
Colon cancer (perforation/abscess)	
Colitis (ischemic/*Clostridium difficile*)	

[both methicillin-sensitive *S. aureus* (MSSA) and methicillin-resistant *S. aureus* (MRSA)]. Gram-negative organisms may cause IV-line infections if introduced into the IV fluid by medical personnel injecting medications into the line, or via junctional disconnects. Gram-negative aerobic bacilli may also be involved in line infections if there is a contaminated infusate. Gram-negative aerobic bacilli, regardless of the mechanism of introduction, are uncommon causes of intravenous-line sepsis compared to gram-positive organisms (20,21).

4.2. Intra-abdominal/Pelvic Sepsis

The distal GI tract is the organ system that contains the greatest concentration of microorganisms. The upper GI tract distal to the stomach is often colonized with aerobic gram-negative bacilli in low numbers. The normal flora of the terminal ileum and colon is composed predominantly of anaerobic gram-negative bacilli, e.g., *B. fragilis*. Three-quarters dry weight of feces is made up of *B. fragilis* species with the remainder being due to aerobic gram-negative bacilli, e.g., coliforms Any process that releases a high concentration of these organisms locally or into the bloodstream, may result in local or systemic infectious complications including septic shock. The intra-abdominal conditions most often associated with septic shock are cholangitis due to an obstructed biliary tract, perforated/obstructed colon, or colitis. The organisms associated with cholangitis are the same as with cholecystitis, i.e., *Escherichia coli*, *Klebsiella pneumoniae*, or enterococci, usually *Enterococcus faecalis*. Biliary tract obstruction may be due to benign or malignant stricture, occluded stents, or gallbladder stones/sludge obstructing the common biliary duct. Appendicitis at any age, but particularly in the elderly, if complicated with perforation/abscess, has the potential to eventuate in septic shock in elderly patients (6,12,13).

Colon cancer and diverticular disease are common in the elderly. Colon cancer may cause obstruction/perforation resulting in the release of large numbers of organisms locally and in the circulation, which predispose to septic shock. Similarly, diverticulitis with pericolonic/peridiverticular abscess with perforation is another frequent septic shock scenario in individuals with advanced age. Perforation of the colon may result from colonoscopy itself or complications of colonic biopsy or polyp

Table 3 Empirical Antimicrobial Therapy of Septic Shock

	Monotherapy	Combination therapy
Urosepsis	Antipseudomonal penicillin or fluroquinolone or carbapenem[a]	Third-/fourth-generation cephalosporin plus ampicillin
Intravenous-line sepsis	Carbapenem or third-/fourth-generation cephalosporin	Antipseudomonal penicillin plus aminoglycoside
Intra-abdominal/ pelvic sepsis	Carbapenem or antipseudomonal penicillin	Third-/fourth-generation cephalosporin plus either metronidazole or clindamycin

[a]Antipseudomonal penicillin: ticarcillin, piperacillin; fluoroquinolone: ciprofloxacin, levofloxacin, gatifloxacin; carbapenem: imipenem, meropenem, ertapenem.
Abbreviations: PICC, peripherally inserted central catheter; CoNS, coagulase-negative staphylococci; VRE, vancomycin-resistant enterococci; IV, Intravenous-line.

removal. The mechanism of injury is not as important as the magnitude of the insult. Enterococci are permissive pathogens between the gallbladder and the urinary bladder, e.g., in the abdomen or pelvis. Enterococci, being permissive pathogens, will not cause infection in this area in the absence of copathogens, i.e., either aerobic gram-negative coliform bacilli or *B. fragilis*. For this reason, coverage for intra-abdominal or pelvic septic shock is based on providing antimicrobial therapy with a high degree of anticoliform/*B. fragilis* activity, which does not necessarily include antienterococcal activity (4,7,9,13).

5. THERAPY

Because septic shock is so frequently associated with an infected foreign body, obstruction, infected stones, or perforation of a viscus, these surgical evaluation and intervention are critical in the management of these conditions. In addition to volume replacement and pressors, the critical component of therapy is directed at correcting the underlying cause. Patients with intravenous-line sepsis should have the IV line removed and appropriate antibiotic therapy initiated. Therapy is directed against the pathogens usually associated with intravenous-line sepsis, i.e., gram-positive cocci and, less commonly, aerobic gram-negative bacilli. Antimicrobial therapy without removal of the IV device may result in some clinical improvement, but not cure. However, failure to remove an infected device in a patient in shock can result in a fatal outcome. In critically ill patients, if the diagnosis of IV-line infection is likely, then the line should be removed and replaced. For urosepsis, therapy is directed against the common uropathogens. Community-acquired uropathogens include the common gram-negative aerobic bacilli, i.e., coliforms, group B streptococci, and enterococci. In the hospital setting, half the cases of nosocomial urinary tract infections are also caused by the aerobic gram-negative bacilli and the remaining half are infections caused by enterococci. The majority of enterococcal infections are due to *E. faecalis* ($\approx$90%), and the remaining are due to *Enterococcus faecium* ($\approx$10%). Virtually all strains of *E. faecium* are vancomycin resistant and therefore it is proper to consider *E. faecium* strains as being vancomycin-resistant enterococci (VRE). In most institutions, *E. faecalis* (non-VRE) enterococci are the predominant organism in the gut and pathogen. If the VRE are common in the institution or isolate from clinical specimens, then specific anti-VRE therapy should be instituted with linezolid, daptomycin, or quinupristin–dalfopristin. If the patient has urinary tract obstruction, the obstruction should be relieved. If the patient has infected stones, they should be removed if clinically possible, or if the patient has obstructed stents, they should be replaced. Appropriate antimicrobial therapy should be done simultaneously with the surgical procedure, and should not be used as an excuse to delay a potentially life-saving surgical decompression or corrective procedure (4,6,7).

5.1. Antimicrobial Therapy of Intra-abdominal/Pelvic Infections

If the patient is in septic shock due to cholangitis, the gallbladder should be emergently removed and the biliary tract surgically decompressed. Without relief of obstruction, antimicrobial therapy is ineffective in cholangitis. Whether the patient has an obstructed biliary stent, benign stricture, malignant obstruction, or an occluded common bile duct due to stones, surgical decompression of the biliary tract should be done as soon as possible and is critical to the survival of the patient. Antimicrobial therapy should be initiated and should be directed against the usual biliary pathogens, i.e., *E. coli*, *K. pneumoniae*, and enterococci (*E. faecalis*). Removal of the gallbladder/relief of obstruction brings prompt clinical improvement to the patient in septic shock due to cholangitis. Antimicrobial therapy is normally continued for at least 1 week postoperatively. There is no preferred antimicrobial regimen providing the antibiotics chosen are effective against the presumed pathogens. Monotherapy is preferred to combination therapy. Monotherapy has the advantages of lower cost, simplicity of use, decreased potential for drug–drug interactions, and is less expensive than combination therapy (7,22).

Excluding the biliary tract, intra-abdominal sources of sepsis include perforation of the colon, which may be due to any one of a variety of causes. The cause of the perforation is of less importance than the magnitude of the perforation and degree of peritoneal spillage of fecal content. Patients with intestinal obstruction need to have the obstruction relieved and antimicrobial therapy initiated as soon as possible. Patients with an intestinal perforation or abscess which has ruptured should have exploratory laparotomy and perforation sealed/peritoneum lavaged. Antimicrobial therapy is directed against the common aerobic gram-negative coliforms as well as *B. fragilis*, the primary anaerobe of the lower abdomen/pelvis. Monotherapy or combination therapy may be utilized if the antibiotics selected provide activity against both the common aerobic gram-negative bacilli associated with intra-abdominal/pelvic infection and *B. fragilis*. Antienterococcal coverage may be included but is not essential. In septic shock, antibiotics that minimize endotoxin release may confer a therapeutic advantage over those with the same spectrum that increase endotoxin release. For this reason, carbapenems may be preferable to β-lactams in the treatment of intra-abdominal/pelvic infections, particularly serious ones, e.g., septic shock, which not only will contain the infection but will also minimize the cytokine-mediated end-organ damage. The duration of therapy of postsurgical procedure is ordinarily 1–2 weeks (4,6,23,24).

6. PREVENTION

Currently, there is no role for anticytokine or antiendotoxin therapy in the treatment of septic shock. Over the past two decades, many different approaches have been used to minimize organ damage due to cytokine-mediated end-organ damage. These results have largely failed because the host defense array is complex and interfering with one or two branches of a complex system does not affect the overall outcome. Studies showing some anticoagulant sepsis therapies have not been of convincing benefit. Drugs based on this approach assume that the fundamental pathophysiological defect in sepsis is microthrombi, which may not be the case. Studies showing the efficacy of such regimens were heavily weighted with patients with urosepsis, which in nonelderly patients without septic shock is rarely fatal. These studies lack sufficient patients with serious sepsis due to intra-abdominal or pelvic origin. The bleeding side effects associated with such agents is not inconsequential. Before such therapy can be recommended as adjunctive therapy in septic shock, more data in seriously ill patients with intra-abdominal or pelvic sepsis need to be obtained (25,26).

REFERENCES

1. Bone RC, Balk RA, Cerra FB, Dellinger RP, Fein AM, Knaus WA, Schein RM, Sibbald WJ. Definitions for sepsis and organ failure and guidelines for the use of innovative therapies in sepsis. Chest 1992; 101:1644–1655.
2. Vincent JL. Sepsis: the magnitude of the problem. In: Vincent JL, Carlet J, Opal S, eds. The Sepsis Text. New York: Kluwer Academic Publishers, 2001:1–10.
3. Diep D, Tran A, Johan B. Age, chronic disease, sepsis, organ system failure, and mortality in a medical intensive care unit. Crit Care Med 1990; 18:474–479.
4. Hines DW, Lisowski JM, Bone RC, Bartlett JG. Sepsis. In: Gorbach SL, Bartlett JG, Blacklow NR. Infectious Diseases. 3rd ed. Philadelphia, PA: Lippincott Williams & Wilkins, 2004:561–568.
5. Levy B, Bollaert P-E. Clinical manifestations and complications of septic shock. In: Dhainaut J-F, Thijs LG, Park G, eds. Septic Shock. London: WB Saunders Company Limited, 2000:339–354.
6. Chintanadilok J, Bender BS. Sepsis. In: Yoshikawa TT, Norman DC, eds. Infectious Disease in the Aging. Totowa, NJ: Humana Press, 2001:33–52.
7. Norman DC, Yoshikawa TT. Intraabdominal infections in the elderly. J Am Geriatr Soc 1983; 31:677–684.
8. Winn T, Tayback M, Israel E. Mortality due to septicemia in the elderly: factors accounting for a rapid rise. Md Med J 1991; 40:803–807.
9. Cruz K, Dellinger RP. Diagnosis and source of sepsis: the utility of clinical findings. In: Vincent JL, Carlet J, Opal S, eds. The Sepsis Text. New York: Kluwer Academic Publishers, 2001:11–28.
10. Rello J, Quintana E, Mirelis B, Gurgui M, Net A, Prats G. Polymicrobial bacteremia in critically ill patients. Intensive Care Med 1993; 19:22–25.
11. Rackow EC, Astiz ME. Pathophysiology and treatment of septic shock. J Am Med Assoc 1991; 266:548–554.
12. Meyers BR, Sherman E, Mendelson MH, Velasquez G, Srulevitch-Chin E, Hubbard M, Hirschman SZ. Bloodstream infections in the elderly. Am J Med 1989; 86:379–386.
13. Brun-Buisson C, Doyon F, Carlet J, Dellamonica P, Govin F, LePoutre A, Mercier JC, Offenstadt G, Regnier B. Incidence, risk factors, and outcome of severe sepsis and septic shock in adults A multicenter prospective study in intensive care units. A Med Assoc 1995; 274:968–974.
14. Groeneveld ABJ, Thijs LG. Diagnosis: from clinical to haemodynamic evaluation. In: Dhainaut J-F, Thijs LG, Park G, eds. Septic Shock. London: WB Saunders Company Limited, 2000:355–388.
15. Redl H, Spittler A, Strohmaier W. Markers of sepsis. In: Vincent JL, Carlet J, Opal S, eds. The Sepsis Text. New York: Kluwer Academic Publishers, 2001:47–66.
16. Parker MM, Parillo JE. Septic shock Hemodynamics and pathogenesis. J Am Med Assoc 1983; 250:3324–3327.
17. Mieszczanska H, Lazar J, Cunha BA. Cardiovascular manifestations of sepsis. Infect Dis Pract 2003; 27:183–186.
18. Cunha BA. Mimics of sepsis. In: Cunha BA, ed. Infectious Diseases in Critical Care Medicine. New York: Marcel Dekker, Inc., 1998:57–66.
19. Harris RL, Musher DM, Bloom K, Gathe J, Rice L, Sugarman B, Williams TW Jr, Young EJ. Manifestations of sepsis. Arch Intern Med 1987; 147:1895–1906.
20. Cunha BA. Urosepsis. In: Cunha BA, ed. Infectious Diseases in Critical Care Medicine. New York: Marcel Dekker, Inc., 1998:501–508.
21. Cunha BA. Intravenous line infections. Crit Care Clin 1998; 8:339–346.
22. Cunha BA. Antibiotic treatment of sepsis. Med Clin North Am 1995; 79:551–558.
23. Cunha BA, Gill MV. Antimicrobial therapy of sepsis. In: Fein AM, Abraham EM, Balk RA, Bernard GR, Bone RC, Dantzker DR, Fink MP, eds. Sepsis and Multiorgan Failure. Baltimore, MD: Williams & Wilkins, 1997:483–493.

24. Norrby-Teglund A, Low DE. Treatment of sepsis. In: Finch RG, Greenwood D, Ragnar Norrby S, Whitley RJ, eds. Antibiotic and Chemotherapy. New York: Churchill Livingstone, 2003:513–526.
25. Wenzel RP, Pinsky MR, Ulevitch RJ, Young L. Current understanding of sepsis. Clin Infect Dis 1996; 22:407–412.
26. Abraham E. Anti-cytokine therapy. In: Vincent JL, Carlet J, Opal S, eds. The Sepsis Text. New York: Kluwer Academic Publishers, 2001:719–728.

SUGGESTED READING

Cunha BA. Infectious Diseases in the Elderly. Littleton, MA: PSG Publishing Company, Inc., 1988.
Cunha BA. Sepsis. In: Cunha BA, ed. Emedicine. infectious diseases.com, 2005.
Dhainaut J-F, Thijs LG, Park G. Septic Shock. London: WB Saunders Company Limited, 2000.
Nobel Symposium No. 124. Septicemia and shock: pathogenesis and novel therapeutic strategies. Scand J Infect Dis 2003; 35:529–696.
Vincent J-L, Carlet J, Opal SM. The Sepsis Text. New York: Kluwer Academic Publishers, 2001.

43

Antibiotic-Resistant Bacterial Infections

Thomas T. Yoshikawa
Department of Internal Medicine, Charles R. Drew University of Medicine and Science,
Martin Luther King, Jr.–Charles R. Drew Medical Center, Los Angeles, California, U.S.A.

Key Points:

- The elderly are at the greatest risk of death due to infections caused by antibiotic-resistant bacteria.
- Methicillin–resistant *Staphylococcus aureus* (MRSA) causes primarily colonization, but serious infections can occur in any body site.
- The drug-of-choice for MRSA infections is vancomycin; alternative agents include quinupristin–dalfopristin and linezolid.
- Vancomyin–resistant enterococci (VRE) are opportunistic bacteria that most commonly infect the genitourinary tract and gastrointestinal tract but can also cause infective endocarditis and skin and soft tissue infections.
- VRE infection is best treated with quinupristin–dalfopristin for *Enterococcus faecium* (ineffective against *Enterococcus faecalis*) and linezolid for either *E. faecium* or *E. faecalis*.

Bacterial infections comprise the most common and important infections in older adults. Because the elderly are at a higher risk for many types of infections including those due to bacteria, there is a higher rate of prescribing antibiotics in this population. Thus, the risk and prevalence of developing antimicrobial-resistant organisms greatly increase in the elderly. Bacteria that are resistant to antibiotics pose a special problem for older patients since these organisms are the most frequently isolated pathogens in life-threatening or serious infections. With age as a risk factor for death in serious infections, the lack of availability of effective antibiotics against infecting pathogens greatly increases the mortality from infections in the elderly population. In this chapter, the discussion will focus on two of the most frequently encountered antibiotic-resistant bacteria in infected older adults, i.e., methicillin-resistant *Staphylococcus aureus* (MRSA) and vancomycin (glycopeptide)-resistant enterococci (VRE).

1. METHICILLIN-RESISTANT *STAPHYLOCOCCUS AUREUS*

1.1. Epidemiology and Clinical Relevance

MRSA was first recognized in the United States in the 1960s as a nosocomial pathogen, and the earliest report of this infection in nursing home residents appeared in
1970 (1). Since then, MRSA has become the predominant cause of hospital-acquired
staphylococcal infections (2), and rates of isolation (colonization and infection) of
this organism from residents in nursing homes range from 5% to 34% (3). Moreover,
there is evidence that community-acquired staphylococcal infections due to MRSA
are increasing in incidence (4).

The infections caused by MRSA are the same as those due to methicillin-
sensitive *S. aureus* (MSSA). Because of the propensity for staphylococci to colonize
the skin and enter the bloodstream, virtually any organ or tissue can become infected
with MSSA or MRSA. In older adults, the sites most often infected with staphylococci are skin and soft tissue, bone, joint, muscle, lung, heart valve, pericardium,
kidney, and central nervous system. The clinical severity of infection in MRSA-
infected patients appears to be similar to that of MSSA-infected patients. The vast
majority of nursing home residents who are culture-positive for MRSA are colonized
rather than infected with this organism. It is estimated that only 3–10% of nursing
home residents colonized with MRSA develop frank infection (3). However, MRSA-
colonized residents have a greater risk of developing infection with MRSA than non-
colonized nursing home residents. Risk factors for colonization and/or infection with
MRSA in nursing home residents include poor functional status, prior antimicrobial
therapy, presence of invasive devices, and skin breakdown.

1.2. Microbiology

Staphylococci are ubiquitous in nature and are found primarily in skin, skin glands,
and at times mucous membranes (e.g., nose, mouth).

Staphylococci morphologically on Gram stain appear as gram-positive cocci in
singles, pairs, tetrads, chains, or "grape-like" clusters. There are 35 species of staphylococci. They are nonmotile, nonsporeforming, usually catalase positive, facultatively anaerobic (except a few species), and typically unencapsulated (5). *S. aureus*
is differentiated from all other staphylococci by its coagulase-positive test.

Methicillin resistance is defined by a minimum inhibitory concentration (MIC)
of 16 µg/mL or more of methicillin or 4 µg/mL or more of oxacillin. As a general rule
resistance to methicillin by staphylococci confers resistance to most other β-lactam
antibiotics (e.g., penicillins, cephalosporins, carbapenems). Most clinical strains of
MRSA contain the *mecA* gene (6); some strains of MRSA are due to hyperproduction
of penicillinase. Currently available antimicrobial agents shown to be effective against
MRSA include vancomycin, quinupristin–dalfopristin, and linezolid. In a small
number of strains of MRSA, they may have limited susceptibility to clindamycin
or trimethoprim–sulfamethoxazole. Partial resistance to vancomycin has now been
reported for *S. aureus* [vancomycin-intermediate *S. aureus* (VISA)] (5).

1.3. Clinical Disease

Table 1 summarizes the most common and important types of infections caused by
both MSSA and MRSA in elderly patients. In addition to those infections listed in

Table 1 Clinical Infections with MRSA and MSSA in the Elderly

Site	Types of infections
Skin	Cellulitis; abscesses (furuncles, carbuncles); postoperative wound
Skeletal	Acute and chronic osteomyelitis; septic arthritis
Pulmonary	Pneumonia (community and institutionally acquired); empyema; lung abscess
Heart	Endocarditis; pericarditis
Central nervous system (CNS)	Meningitis; brain abscess; subdural empyema; epidural abscess
Genitourinary	Intrarenal abscess; perinephric abscess
Devices	Hemodialysis shunts; prosthetic heart valves, joints, CNS shunts; IV catheters

Abbreviations: MRSA, methicillin-resistant *Staphylococcus aureus*; MSSA, methicillin-sensitive *Staphylococcus aureus*; IV, intravenous.

the table, conjunctivitis and postoperative wound infections caused by MRSA have been reported (7,8).

1.4. Diagnosis

The diagnosis of MRSA infection requires compatible clinical manifestations (history and physical examination), radiological findings, and a culture of the infected site yielding MRSA. Standard procedures for obtaining body fluids, purulent material, infected tissue, and blood should be used. Laboratory isolation of *S. aureus* follows routine procedures; susceptibility testing or subculture onto antibiotic-containing media specifically to detect MRSA should be routinely performed. In nursing home residents, a determination should be made whether aggressive diagnostic (and thus therapeutic) interventions should be instituted through advance directives and/or discussions with the resident and family members before proceeding with tests or treatments.

1.5. Antibiotic Treatment

It should be first determined if the recovery of MRSA by culture is colonization or true infection. Isolation of MRSA on skin, mucosal surfaces, and rectum may be simply colonization and does not require antimicrobial therapy unless an outbreak is identified in a closed setting (e.g., nursing home). In cases of an outbreak of MRSA in an institution, application of mupirocin ointment to skin, mucosa, or wounds will temporarily eradicate the organism; however, long-term use of mupirocin will result in decreased efficacy and resistance to the antibiotic (3,9).

Table 2 describes the most appropriate antibiotics for infections caused by MRSA. Vancomycin is the most frequently prescribed drug for MRSA. Instances in which the patient is intolerant of vancomycin, oral treatment (e.g., outpatient setting) of MRSA infection is desired, or vancomycin resistance to MRSA (VISA) is identified, linezolid may be an alternative agent to prescribe (10). Quinupristin–dalfopristin is available only in parenteral form [intravenous (IV)] and can be used

Table 2 Recommended Antibioties for MRSA

Antibiotics	Dosage	Route	Comment
Vancomycin	500–1000 mg q 12 hr	IV	Adjust dosage for renal function and severity of infection
Quinupristin-dalfopristin	75 mg/kg q 8 hr	IV	Effective also against MSSA
Linezolid	400–600 mg q 12 hr	IV, PO	Use 400 mg for skin infection; 600 mg for all other infections; effective also against MSSA

Abbreviations: MRSA, methicillin-resistant *Staphylococcus aureus*; IV, intravenous; O, oral (per os); MSSA, methicillin-sensitive *Staphylococcus aureus*.

as an alternative agent to vancomycin (see also chapters discussing these two drugs). The duration of therapy is dependent on site of infection and severity of infection.

1.6. Prevention

The fundamental principle in preventing antibiotic-resistant pathogens is to reduce the prescribing of inappropriate administration of antibiotics (11). Treating colonization or nonbacterial infections (e.g., viral respiratory tract infection) are examples of inappropriate use of antibiotic therapy. Excessive use of prophylactic antibiotics also risks development of resistance to antimicrobial agents and should be discouraged. Careful hand washing; wearing of gloves when in direct contact with patients; and proper wearing of gowns and/or masks when handling infected purulent material/body fluids or exposure to aerosolized infected material (e.g., suction of lung secretions) should be strictly enforced (3).

2. VANCOMYCIN-RESISTANT ENTEROCOCCI

2.1. Epidemiology and Clinical Relevance

Enterococci are important causes of nosocomial urinary tract and wound infections as well as nosocomial bacteremia. Approximately 10% of enterococci isolates, including those recovered from the bloodstream, are resistant to vancomycin, a glycopeptide antibiotic (teicoplanin is the another glycopeptide that is not presently available in the United States and thus will not be discussed further in this chapter) (12). Vancomycin-resistant enterococci (VRE) are also being found with increasing frequency in long-term care facilities (13,14).The rates of colonization of nursing home residents with VRE vary from 10% to 47%. The risk factors for colonization and infection with VRE include advanced age, prior antibiotic use—especially vancomycin and cephalosporins, recent hospitalization, poor functional status, severe underlying diseases, and use of indwelling devices (13,15,16). Despite some controversy, recent data suggest that vancomycin resistance is an independent risk factor for death in patients with enterococcal bacteremia (17,18).

Thus, enterococci including VRE are considered opportunistic pathogens that infect persons who are debilitated, immunocompromised, hospitalized, and have been exposed recently to prolonged antibiotic therapy.

2.2. Microbiology

Enterococci are commonly found in soil, water, food, plants, and mammals including humans. They are predominantly inhabitants of the gastrointestinal tract but occasionally are found in the genitourinary tract and oral cavity (19). Previously, enterococci were classified within the genus *Streptcoccus*, with its primary differentiation from other streptococci determined by their group D serological response and higher resistance to commonly prescribed antibiotics. *Streptococcus faecalis* and *Streptococcus faecium* were the primary isolates within group D streptococci that had clinical relevance. However, molecular studies warranted that *S. faecalis* and *S. faecium* be classified into a separate genus, i.e., *Enterococcus*. There are approximately 20 different *Enterococcus* species; however, *E. faecalis* and *E. faecium* remain the most clinically relevant isolates.

Enterococci are catalase-negative, gram-positive cocci that morphologically appear singly, in pairs, or as short chains. They are facultatively anaerobic, grow in broth containing 6.5% NaCl, hydrolyze esculin in the presence of 40% bile salts, and ferment glucose without producing gas (19). *E. faecalis* is generally the most frequently isolated enterococci from human infections (80–90%) with *E. faecium* being recovered in 5–10% of clinical specimens.

Intrinsic resistance to many antibiotics is common among enterococcal species; these include β lactams and aminoglycosides. Acquired resistance through acquisition of various genetic determinants is also quite common with enterococci. High-level acquired resistance to aminoglycosides (20) and glycopeptides such as vancomycin is now well known to occur in a variety of settings including nursing homes.

Vancomycin resistance in *E. faecalis* and *E. faecium* is caused by production of modified cell-wall precursors that decrease the affinity for vancomycin. These modified cell-wall precursors are a result of gene clusters that alter the bacterial ligases—enzymes that are involved in the early stage of synthesis of cell-wall precursors. VanA ligase and VanB ligase are the clinically relevant enzyme alterations. VanA-type strains of enterococci are highly resistant to both vancomycin (MIC $\geq$64 µg/mL) and teicoplanin (MIC $\geq$16 µg/mL or greater); VanB-type strains are resistant to vancomycin but susceptible to teicoplanin (MIC $\leq$4 µg/mL) (21). Although *E. faecalis* is the predominant cause of enterococcal infections, <3% are resistant to vancomycin; however, *E. faecium* is the major strain associated with VRE (16).

2.3. Clinical Disease

Similar to MRSA, VRE acquisition by elderly persons may simply represent colonization. Thus, careful clinical assessment should be performed to determine if a true infection is present when VRE is isolated from a clinical specimen or site.

Table 3 summarizes the major sites of infection associated with VRE.

2.4. Diagnosis

In the presence of compatible clinical manifestations of infection, the isolation of VRE from culture will make the diagnosis. The clinical specimens should be handled

Table 3   Common Infections Caused by Enterococci in the Elderly

Site	Comment
Genitourinary	Urinary tract infection (UTI) is common, especially with long-term bladder catheters
Gastrointestinal	May be cause of cholecystitis or biliary sepsis; intra-abdominal abscess and peritonitis may be caused by enterococci (usually found with other bowel microflora)
Heart valves	Endocarditis may be secondary to coexisting UTI or occasionally from enterococci in oral cavity or other gastrointestinal site
Skin and soft tissue	Pressure ulcer and postoperative abdominal or genitourinary wounds are common sites; intravenous catheters may be a source of infection

in the usual and routine manner including blood cultures, infected wound sites, and collection of drainage or purulent material. Appropriate radiological tests, i.e., plain radiographs, imaging scans, and radionuclide scans, should be obtained. However, in a nursing home setting, evaluations may be tempered by advance directives; both the resident and family member should be involved with decisions about diagnostic and therapeutic interventions before they are initiated.

3. ANTIBIOTIC TREATMENT

In the unusual circumstance of a VRE strain being susceptible to penicillin or ampicillin, these antibiotics would be recommended for treating mild to moderately severe infections caused by enterococci resistant to vancomycin. For serious or life-threatening VRE infections, an aminoglycoside should be added to penicillin or ampicillin provided there is no high-level resistance to the aminoglycoside. On occasions VRE may be susceptible to such agents as nitrofurantoin, quinolones, tetracyclines, and chloramphenicol (22). However, the adequacy of response of VRE to these drugs is unclear and thus they should be reserved for milder or less severe infections (e.g., lower urinary tract infection).

The drugs most commonly prescribed for serious VRE infections are quinupristin–dalfopristin and linezolid (10,16). However, quinupristin–dalfopristin is active against only *E. faecium* but not *E. faecalis*. Linezolid, an oxazolidinone, is active against both species of VRE and has the advantage of being formulated in both oral and IV forms. The dosage of these agents is described in Table 2. Duration of therapy will vary depending on the site and severity of infection (see also chapters discussing quinupristin–dalfopristin and linezolid).

4. PREVENTION

Preventing development of enterococci resistant to vancomycin can only occur by reducing the prescribing practice of this antibiotic.

Reduction of transmission of VRE in hospitals and nursing homes will require education of all staff interacting with patients and residents on infection control principles, policies, and procedures. A detailed description of strategies and procedures for infection control of VRE is beyond the scope of this chapter. However, appropriate surveillance cultures, isolation of infected/colonized persons when indicated, hand washing, use of gloves and gowns when in contact with body fluids, environmental disinfection, and judicious use of antibiotics are cornerstones of controlling acquisition and transmission of VRE (16).

REFERENCES

1. O'Toole RD, Drew WL, Dahlgren BJ, Beaty HN. An outbreak of methicillin-resistant *Staphylococcus aureus* infection: observations in hospital and nursing home. J Am Med Assoc 1970; 213:257–263.
2. Kelley M, Weber DJ, Dooley KE, Rutala WA. Healthcare-associated methicillin-resistant *Staphylococcus aureus*. Semin Infect Control 2001; 1:157–171.
3. Strausbaugh LJ. Methicillin-resistant *Staphylococcus aureus*. In: Yoshikawa TT, Ouslander JG, eds. Infection Management for Geriatrics in Long-Term Care Facilities. New York: Marcel Dekker Inc., 2002:383–409.
4. Johnston BL. Methicillin-resistant *Staphylococcus aureus* as a cause of community-acquired pneumonia—a critical review. Semin Respir Infect 1994; 9(3):199–206.
5. Bannerman TL. *Staphylococcus*, *Micrococcus*, and other catalase-positive cocci that grow aerobically. In: Murray PR, Baron EJ, Jorgensen JH, Pfaller MA, Yolken RH, eds. Manual of Clinical Microbiology. 8th ed. Washington, DC: ASM Press, 2003:384–404.
6. de Lencastre H, de Jonge BLM, Matthews PR, Tomasz A. Molecular aspects of methicillin resistance in *Staphylococcus aureus*. J Antimicrob Chemother 1994; 33:7–24.
7. Brennen C, Muder RR. Conjunctivitis associated with methicillin-resistant *Staphylococcus aureus* in long-term-care facility. Am J Med 1990; 88:5-14N–7-14N.
8. Manian FA, Meyer PL, Setzer J, Senkel D. Surgical site infections associated with methicillin-resistant *Staphylococcus aureus*: do postoperative factors play a role?. Clin Infect Dis 2003; 36:863–868.
9. Mody L, Kauffman CA, McNeil SA, Galecki AT, Bradley SF. Mupirocin-based decolonization of *Staphylococcus aureus* in residents of 2 long-term care facilities: a randomized, double-blind, placebo-controlled trial. Clin Infect Dis 2003; 37:1467–1474.
10. Babcock HM, Fraser V. Clinical experience with linezolid: a case series of 53 patients. Infect Dis Clin Pract 2002; 11:198–204.
11. Yoshikawa TT. Antimicrobial resistance and aging: beginning of the end of the antibiotic era? J Am Geriatr Soc 2002; 50:S226–S229.
12. Sahm DF, Marsilio MK, Piazza G. Antimicrobial resistance in key bloodstream bacterial isolates: electronic surveillance with the Surveillance Network Database—USA. Clin Infect Dis 1999; 298:259–263.
13. Elizaga ML, Weinstein RA, Hayden MK. Patients in long-term care facilities: a reservoir for vancomycin-resistant enterococci. Clin Infect Dis 2002; 34:441–446.
14. Strausbaugh LJ, Sukumar SR, Joseph CL. Infectious disease outbreaks in nursing home: an unappreciated hazard for frail elderly persons. Clin Infect Dis 2003; 36:870–876.
15. Joshi N, Milfred D, Caputo G. Vancomycin-resistant enterococci: a review. Infect Dis Clin Pract 1996; 5:528–537.
16. Mody L, McNeil SA, Bradley SF. Vancomycin (glycopeptide)-resistant enterococci. In: Yoshikawa TT, Ouslander JG, eds. Infection Management for Geriatrics in Long-Term Care Facilities. New York: Marcel Dekker, Inc., 2002:411–428.
17. Edmond MB, Ober JF, Dawson JD, Weinbaum DL, Wenzel RP. Vancomycin-resistant enterococcal bacteremia: natural history and attributable mortality. Clin Infect Dis 1996; 23:1234–1239.
18. Vergis EN, Hayden MK, Chow JW, Snydman DR, Zervos MJ, Linden PK, Wagener MM, Schmitt B, Muder RR. Determinants of vancomycin resistance and mortality rates in

enterococcal bacteremia. A prospective multicenter study. Ann Intern Med 2001; 135: 484–492.

19. Teixeira LM, Facklam RR. Enterococcus. In: Murray PR, Baron EJ, Jorgensen JH, Pfaller MA, Yolken RH, eds. Manual of Clinical Microbiology. Washington, DC: ASM Press, 2003:422–433.
20. Chenoweth CE, Bradley SF, Terpenning MS, Zarins LT, Ramsey MA, Schaberg DR, Kauffman CA. Colonization and transmission of high-level gentamicin-resistant enterococci in a long-term care facility. Infect Control Hosp Epidemiol 1994; 15:703–709.
21. Leclercq R, Courvalin P. Resistance to glycopeptides in enterococci. Clin Infect Dis 1997; 24:545–556.
22. Morris JG, Roghmann M-C, Schwalbe R. Management of patients with vancomycin resistant enterococci. Infect Dis Clin Pract 2000; 9:10–16.

SUGGESTED READING

Babcock HM, Fraser V. Clinical experience with linezolid: a case series of 53 patients. Clin Infect Dis Pract 2002; 11:198–204.
Elizaga ML, Weinstein RA, Hayden MK. Patients in long-term care facilities: a reservoir for vancomycin-resistant enterococci. Clin Infect Dis 2002; 34:441–446.
Mody L, McNeil SA, Bradley SF. Vancomycin (glycopeptide)-resistant enterococci. In: Yoshikawa TT, Ouslander JG, eds. Infection Management for Geriatrics in Long-Term Care Facilities. New York: Marcel Dekker, Inc., 2002:411–428.
Strausbaugh LJ. Methicillin-resistant *Staphylococcus aureus*. In: Yoshikawa TT, Ouslander J, eds. Infection Management for Geriatrics in Long-Term Care Facilities. New York: Marcel Dekker, Inc., 2002:383–409.

44
Fungi

Carol A. Kauffman

*Division of Infectious Diseases, University of Michigan Medical School,
Infectious Diseases Section, Veterans Affairs Ann Arbor Healthcare System, Ann Arbor,
Michigan, U.S.A.*

Key Points:

- Successful treatment of denture stomatitis (chronic atrophic candidosis) requires removal of the denture at night, thorough cleaning and disinfection of the appliance, and use of an antifungal agent, usually fluconazole.
- Onychomycosis cannot be treated with local creams, but requires several months' treatment with systemic antifungal agents (itraconazole or terbinafine).
- In most patients, candiduria represents colonization and not urinary tract infection, and does not need to be treated with an antifungal agent.
- Histoplasmosis, blastomycosis, and coccidioidomycosis in older adults may represent new infection or reactivation of infection acquired years before.
- Chronic necrotizing pulmonary aspergillosis and sino-orbital aspergillosis are more common in older adults than in younger persons.

The most common fungal infections that occur in older adults are local infections of skin and mucous membranes. Dermatophytes, superficial colonizers of skin and hair structures, and *Candida* species, colonizers of the gastrointestinal (GI) and genito-urinary tracts are the prominent pathogens. Invasive fungal infections are much less common. Environmental molds, such as *Aspergillus*, cause disease almost entirely in those who are immunosuppressed. Infections with opportunistic fungi appear to be increasing in older adults. Reasons for this include an expansion of the donor trans-plant pool to include older adults, greater use of aggressive chemotherapy for cancer in older adults, and the increasing role of immunosuppressive drugs, such as tumor necrosis factor inhibitors, for chronic illnesses that are common with aging. The endemic mycoses, such as histoplasmosis and blastomycosis, can cause either new infection or reactivation infection years after the initial exposure in older adults.

1. DERMATOPHYTE INFECTIONS

Tinea infections are exceedingly common, regardless of age, and there appears to be no obvious propensity to increase with aging. Many older men will have tinea corporis, tinea cruris, or tinea pedis, which they have had all of their life. Onychomycosis, on the other hand, does appear to increase with increasing age, with as many as 30% of patients >60 years of age demonstrating onychomycosis (1).

1.1. Epidemiology

Transmission of dermatophytes directly from person to person is uncommon although outbreaks have been described in long-term care facilities (2). Dogs and cats have been documented as a source for dermatophyte infections, especially those due to *Microsporum canis*. When this occurs, the animal must be treated, as well as the patient, in order to eliminate the infection. Tinea pedis is frequently contracted in bathing facilities, such as pools and showers. The ability of dermatophytes to remain viable on wet floors until they subsequently adhere to the feet undoubtedly helps the propagation of these organisms to new hosts.

1.2. Microbiology

The genera of dermatophytes that most commonly cause tinea infections and onychomycosis are *Trichophyton*, *Microsporum*, and *Epidermophyton*. Different species vary in their host specificity. Many cause disease only in humans and other species have been associated with animals, as well as humans.

1.3. Clinical Disease

Dermatophytes normally infect only the keratinized layers of the skin, the hair shafts, and the nails (3). On the trunk and extremities, they characteristically produce annular lesions that have prominent edges and contain pustules, central clearing, and scaling. Pruritus is often mild, and the rash can mimic contact dermatitis, eczema, and psoriasis. In men, tinea cruris presents as a sharp-edged, erythematous, pustular, scaling rash in the groin and on the anterior thighs.

Although similar to intertrigenous candidiais, there are no satellite lesions, which are prominent with candidiasis.

Tinea pedis usually starts in the web spaces of the toes producing maceration and fissures and then extends to the soles and lateral borders of the feet, which become erythematous and scaly; pruritus is a prominent symptom. Superinfection of tinea pedis by bacterial pathogens may lead to cellulitis. Patients who have recurrent lower-extremity cellulitis should be examined carefully for signs of tinea pedis as this is a frequent point of ingress of streptococci and staphylococci into the dermis.

Fungal infection of the toenails is predominantly caused by dermatophytes. Most patients with onychomycosis also have chronic tinea pedis. The nail becomes thickened and opaque and assumes a white, yellow, or brown hue. The distal part of the nail can completely crumble, and it may be impossible for the patient to trim this nail. Fingernails are much less commonly involved than toenails.

1.4. Diagnosis

The diagnosis of most dermatophyte infections can be made clinically. However, the diagnosis can easily be verified and should be done to ensure that noninfectious causes of rash are not treated inappropriately. After scraping the border of a lesion with a scalpel blade, the scrapings are collected on a piece of dark paper, transferred to a microscopic slide on which is added a drop of potassium hydroxide, and examined with a microscope for hyphae. For onychomycosis, full-thickness nail clippings taken as close to the nail bed as possible are collected as above, treated with potassium hydoxide on a slide, and viewed with a microscope for fungal elements. Frequently, direct microscopic examination is not helpful with onychomycosis. Culture of the nail clippings may help direct the choice of antifungal agent.

1.5. Treatment

Tinea infections usually respond to topical therapy with creams (4). Lotions or sprays are easier to apply to large or hairy areas. Particularly for tinea cruris and tinea pedis, the affected area should be kept as dry as possible to hasten resolution. For patients who have extensive skin lesions, oral itraconazole, 200 mg daily, or terbinafine, 250 mg daily, can be used. Terbinafine has fewer drug–drug interactions than itraconazole and for that reason should be used first for older adults who require systemic therapy. However, both drugs have the potential for hepatotoxicity and should be used with caution in older adults (see also chapter "Antifungal Drugs").

Onychomycosis does not respond to topical therapy. The rationale for treating onychomycosis should extend beyond simple aesthetic reasons. Pain associated with the nail thickening, inability to trim the nail, secondary bacterial infection, and the presence of diabetes mellitus, which predisposes to serious foot infections, are valid reasons for treating onychomycosis. Either itraconazole, 200 mg daily, or terbinafine, 250 mg daily, both of which accumulate in the nail plate, can be given for 3 months to treat onychomycosis. Itraconazole can be given as pulsed therapy, 200 mg twice daily, 1 week out of each month for 3–4 months, and there are some data suggesting that pulsed therapy also is effective using terbinafine (5) (see also chapter "Antifungal Drugs").

1.6. Prevention

Avoidance of public showers and pools helps prevent spread of dermatophyte infections. Drying the feet well after bathing, wearing clean socks daily, and avoiding maceration are important in preventing tinea pedis recurrences. Routine visits to a podiatrist can help improve care of toenails and lead to early diagnosis and appropriate therapy. Prophylactic systemic antifungal agents have no role to play in preventing dermatophyte infections. However, treating the first signs of tinea infection with application of antifungal creams or lotions will help keep the infection in remission.

2. MUCOCUTANEOUS *CANDIDA* INFECTIONS

These are common fungal infections in older adults. Generally, local factors and alterations of the normal physiology that occur with aging are responsible for the occurrence of most of these infections in older adults.

2.1. Epidemiology

Candida species are yeasts that colonize the GI and genitourinary tracts of humans. As many as 84% of veterans residing in a long-term care facility were shown to be colonized with *Candida* (6). Most mucocutaneous *Candida* infections are acquired as the result of overgrowth and subsequent local invasion of mucous membranes or epithelium by the yeast. This is often related to the use of broad-spectrum antimicrobial agents, local physiologic changes, or much less commonly diminished cell-mediated immunity, which controls the growth of *Candida* on mucosal surfaces.

2.2. Microbiology

Candida albicans is the most common colonizing species and the cause of most infections. *Candida glabrata*, *Candida parapsilosis*, and *Candida tropicalis*, although found less frequently, also cause infection. These organisms are readily grown in the microbiology laboratory on standard media. Exudate, purulent material, or body fluids stained with Gram stain reveal budding yeast that is characteristic for *Candida* species.

2.3. Clinical Disease

Oropharyngeal candidiasis or thrush in older adults does not occur because of increasing age alone. Other factors must be present. These include inhaled corticosteroids, radiation therapy to the head and neck areas, xerostomia, and the presence of upper dentures (7). Rarely, broad-spectrum antibiotic therapy, without other factors, is associated with thrush. The possibility of underlying immunosuppression due to cancer or acquired immunodeficiency syndrome should be explored in an older adult who develops thrush and has no obvious risk factors.

Oropharyngeal candidiasis appears as nonpainful white plaques on the buccal, palatal, and oropharyngeal mucosa. The plaques can be scraped off with a tongue depressor revealing underlying erythematous mucosa. Perleche or angular cheilitis due to *Candida* is usually painful and can appear with or without oropharyngeal lesions.

Denture stomatitis, also called chronic atrophic candidosis, is a variant of oral candidiasis that has been noted in as many as 65% of patients who wear dentures and occurs particularly in those with full upper dentures (8). Lower dentures are rarely linked to the development of candidiasis. This form of candidiasis is associated with poor oral hygiene and the practice of not removing the denture at night. Patients often complain of pain and irritation associated with their dentures. The usual finding is diffuse erythema on the hard palate; plaques are uncommon.

In patients who are immunosuppressed, *Candida* can cause esophagitis, with or without oropharyngeal involvement. The prominent symptom is odynophagia, and the patient can almost always pinpoint precisely the area of retrosternal pain.

Intertrigenous candidiasis occurs in warm moist areas, such as in the perineum and under large breasts and pannus. The lesions are erythematous, pustular, and pruritic and have a distinct border and smaller satellite lesions beyond the border. The main differential diagnosis is tinea cruris or corporis due to dermatophytes.

Candida also can cause paronychia and onychomycosis, especially on the hand. The nails become thickened, opaque, and wrinkled, and onycholysis is frequent. This occurs most often in persons who have their hands immersed in water for long periods of time.

Candida vulvovaginitis becomes less common after the menopause, perhaps related to diminished estrogen levels. Among older women with *Candida* vulvovaginitis, risk factors include diabetes mellitus, corticosteroid therapy, and broad-spectrum antibiotic therapy (9). Infection is manifest primarily as vaginal discharge that may be curd-like or thin and watery. External burning on urination and vulvar pruritus are common. The labia are erythematous and swollen, the vagina shows erythema, and white plaques and discharge usually are evident.

2.4. Diagnosis

Mucocutaneous candidiasis is usually diagnosed clinically. Scrapings of skin lesions can be treated with potassium hydroxide and examined for yeast cells. Samples of oropharyngeal plaques or vaginal discharge can be easily obtained with a cotton swab, smeared onto a microscope slide, and then stained with Gram stain or viewed as a wet preparation for the presence of budding yeasts and pseudohyphae. Culture is not necessary unless there is a poor response to therapy or multiple recurrent episodes. In a patient who has symptoms suggesting esophagitis, empirical systemic antifungal therapy is usually given, and only if the patient does not respond within 3–4 days of therapy is endoscopy performed.

2.5. Treatment

Oropharyngeal candidiasis should be treated with clotrimazole troches four to five times daily or nystatin suspension, which is swished around in the mouth and swallowed four times daily. Generally, patients tolerate the troches better than the nystatin suspension. Oral fluconazole tablets, 100 mg daily, or itraconazole suspension, 100–200 mg daily, should be reserved for patients with more severe disease, such as might occur following radiation therapy. Treatment of denture stomatitis requires a multipronged approach (7). The dentures must be removed nightly and aggressively cleaned with an agent, such as chlorhexidine. Nystatin suspension or clotrimazole troches can be tried as initial therapy, but frequently systemic therapy with oral fluconazole is required. *Candida* esophagitis always requires systemic therapy, and fluconazole, 100–200 mg daily, is the drug-of-choice.

Candida infections of the skin usually respond to topical therapy with creams or lotions, such as clotrimazole or nystatin. In the case of intertrigenous candidiasis, an antifungal powder is often more effective because it helps to keep the area dry, which promotes healing. For patients who have extensive skin lesions, oral itraconazole, 200 mg daily, or fluconazole, 200 mg daily, should be used (see also Chapter 25).

Candida vaginitis can be treated with any of the myriad of topical antifungal creams or suppositories (e.g., clotrimazole, miconazole) that are available or a single-dose 150 mg fluconazole tablet (9). Topical agents may be difficult to apply for older women, and single-dose fluconazole is preferred by many women. Removing any precipitating factors is important to prevent recurrence, but even then a small number of women will continue to have recurrent infection. For these women, suppressive treatment with fluconazole, 150 mg weekly, may be necessary.

2.6. Prevention

Avoiding drugs that cause xerostomia, decreasing the use of inappropriate broad-spectrum antibiotics, and emphasizing good dental hygiene will help to decrease the risk of thrush in older adults. Dentures should always be removed at night and should be cleaned daily by brushing with a denture brush and soaking in chlorhexidine or a commercially available denture cleanser. Cutaneous yeast infections are best prevented by good personal hygiene and avoidance of maceration of tissues under pendulous structures. Prevention of vaginal candidiasis involves removal of risk factors, such as broad-spectrum antimicrobial agents, and controlling underlying diseases, especially diabetes mellitus.

3. *CANDIDA* URINARY TRACT INFECTIONS

Candiduria is a frequent finding in older adults, especially those in hospital or in a long-term care setting. Candiduria itself is merely a laboratory finding and is seen both with colonization and urinary tract infection. Indeed, the major problem is discerning which patient has infection of the urinary tract and which patient merely has colonization. Current thinking is that most patients who have candiduria are colonized and should not be treated with antifungal agents.

3.1. Epidemiology

The source of *Candida* in the urine is almost always from the perineum. Thus, it is the patient's own colonizing *Candida* species that colonize and infect the urinary tract. Although nosocomial spread of *Candida* has been described, this mode of acquisition accounts for a very small proportion of cases of candiduria. Factors predisposing to candiduria include diabetes mellitus, use of broad-spectrum antibiotics, presence of an indwelling urethral catheter, and genitourinary tract abnormalities, especially those causing obstruction (10,11). Many patients have concomitant or prior bacterial urinary tract infections.

3.2. Microbiology

The organisms causing candiduria are the same as those colonizing normal humans. *C. albicans* is the most common species, followed by *C. glabrata*, *C. tropicalis*, and other species.

3.3. Clinical Disease

Most patients with candiduria are asymptomatic and probably do not have infection. Patients with lower urinary tract infection can have symptoms, such as suprapubic discomfort, dysuria, and frequency, that are indistinguishable from those seen with bacterial cystitis. Patients who have upper urinary tract infection may develop fever, flank pain, nausea, and vomiting, symptoms indistinguishable from those seen with bacterial pyelonephritis. Uncommonly, a fungus ball composed of fungal hyphae may form and cause symptoms of obstruction of bladder or kidney.

3.4. Diagnosis

The major diagnostic dilemma arises in determining whether yeasts in a urine sample represent contamination, colonization, or infection (10,11). Contamination is the easiest to exclude by obtaining a second sample of urine for culture. In older women, catheterization of the urethra may be needed to obtain an uncontaminated urine specimen. Differentiating between colonization and infection is more difficult. The presence of an indwelling urinary catheter in most patients with candiduria means that pyuria will be present and cannot be used as a marker for infection. Quantitation of yeast in the urine has not been shown to separate infection from colonization. A urine sample containing 10,000 colonies of yeast per microliter can be found with upper tract infection, and a sample containing greater than 100,000 colonies of yeast per microliter often occurs with colonization of the bladder. The presence of pseudohyphae, although once thought to indicate urinary tract infection, has been shown to be of no benefit. Thus, evaluation of a urine sample is less helpful in patients with candiduria than in those with bacteriuria.

For patients suspected of having upper tract infection, imaging studies are necessary. Ultrasonography, computerized tomography (CT), or retrograde pyelography can be used to ascertain the presence of hydronephrosis; fungus balls are seen as masses obstructing the collecting system or filling the bladder and definitely indicate infection.

3.5. Treatment

If it has been decided that a *Candida* urinary tract infection is present, the treatment is relatively straightforward. An important initial step is to remove, if at all possible, the risk factors that led to the infection. Thus, obstruction should be relieved, the chronic indwelling urethral catheter removed, and broad-spectrum antibiotics stopped. The treatment of choice is fluconazole, given as an initial loading dose of 400 mg, then 200 mg daily for 2 weeks (12). Bladder irrigation with amphotericin B also has been used as a treatment for *Candida* urinary tract infection (13). However, this maneuver, which requires placing an indwelling triple-lumen catheter, will only be useful for lower tract infection, and it is likely that all it does is eradicate colonization transiently. The practice has fallen out of favor because the benefit appears to be transient and not worth the risk of placing the catheter.

The most difficult treatment problem is the patient who has *C. glabrata* urinary tract infection, and who has failed therapy with fluconazole because the organism is resistant to this agent. Possibilities for treatment include single-dose or low-dose short-course amphotericin B, short-course flucytosine, or possibly use of an extended spectrum azole or an echinocandin. Consultation with an infectious diseases specialist is important in these recalcitrant cases.

3.6. Prevention

The simplest means to prevent candiduria and *Candida* urinary tract infections is to avoid the use of indwelling urethral catheters and broad-spectrum antibiotics and to ensure that there is no obstruction to urine flow.

4. INVASIVE OR DISSEMINATED CANDIDIASIS AND CANDIDEMIA

In acute care hospitals, *Candida* species are the fourth leading cause of nosocomial bloodstream infections and are responsible for 10% of hospital-acquired bloodstream infections. The attributable mortality from candidemia approaches 40% and is highest in older adults (14,15). *C. glabrata* is an important cause of candidemia in older adults (16). Risk factors for candidemia in older adults include broad-spectrum antibiotics, central vascular catheters, parenteral nutrition, acute renal failure with dialysis, and surgical procedures involving the GI tract. Although candidemia and invasive candidiasis are serious and life-threatening infections in older adults, they are almost always seen in patients in hospital for another problem, and diagnostic tests and treatment modalities are generally managed by an infectious diseases or other specialist. (The reader is referred to an infectious diseases text for further information.)

5. CRYPTOCOCCOSIS

Cryptococcosis is seen predominantly among patients who are immunosuppressed. However, approximately 20–25% of patients have no overt immunosuppression, and older adults figure prominently in this group. The disease manifestations can be subtle, and treatment, which extends for months, can be difficult.

5.1. Epidemiology

Cryptococcal infection is acquired from the environment. Growth of the organism appears to be enhanced by droppings from birds. The organism is aerosolized and inhaled, leading to pulmonary infection, which is usually asymptomatic. Only rarely is the source and time of exposure to the environment actually established. In many patients, it is likely that primary infection occurs years earlier, and then as cell-mediated immunity wanes, because of intercurrent disease, immunosuppressive therapy, or simply aging itself, the infection reactivates and presents as meningitis.

5.2. Microbiology

Cryptococcus neoformans is a heavily encapsulated yeast that reproduces by budding in tissues. In the environment it is nonencapsulated and is easily aerosolized and inhaled. It is highly neurotropic. The organism is readily grown on standard laboratory media in a few days.

5.3. Clinical Disease

Cryptococcosis is noted most often in older adults who have been treated with corticosteroids, have received an organ transplant, or who have diabetes mellitus, renal failure, liver dysfunction, or chronic obstructive pulmonary disease. However, ≈20–25% of patients, most of whom are older, have no identified risk factors (17). A recent retrospective review of 316 patients who did not have concomitant human immunodeficiency virus infection noted that mortality rates for patients with meningitis or pulmonary crytococcosis were higher for those patients aged >60 years (17).

The classic presenting symptoms of cryptococcal meningitis are headache, fever, focal neurological findings, and confusion. However, in older adults the only symptom may be mental status changes (18). Headache may be mild or quite severe. When increased intracranial pressure occurs, the headache is accompanied by vomiting and visual complaints. Pulmonary cryptococcosis, presenting as nodules or infiltrates and less often as cavitary lesions, occurs more often in older adults than in their younger counterparts. Every patient with pulmonary cryptococcosis should have a spinal tap performed to exclude concomitant meningitis.

5.4. Diagnosis

A patient suspected of having cryptococcal meningitis should have a lumbar puncture performed as soon as possible. Obtaining an opening pressure is extremely important as this is often elevated in cryptococcal meningitis, and efforts must be made to lower the pressure quickly to normal. Findings in the cerebrospinal fluid (CSF) are those of a lymphocytic meningitis with 50–500 white blood cells usually noted; the protein is elevated (usually 90–200 µg/dL) and the glucose is decreased (usually 20–40 µg/dL). An India ink preparation, which highlights the organism's capsule, and cultures should be performed. Cryptococcal polysaccharide capsular antigen should be sought in CSF and serum by use of a latex agglutination test that is available in almost every hospital laboratory. This assay is very sensitive and specific for cryptococcal infection. Because discrete ring-enhancing lesions, either single or multiple, can occur along with meningeal involvement, a contrast-enhanced CT or magnetic resonance imaging scan should be obtained on all patients with cryptococcal meningitis.

5.5. Treatment

Cryptococcal meningitis requires induction treatment with intravenous amphotericin B and oral flucytosine. In older adults, because of the risk of nephrotoxicity, a lipid formulation of amphotericin B should be used; the usual dosage is 5 mg/kg daily (see also chapter "Antifungal Drugs"). Flucytosine should never be used at a dosage >100 mg/kg daily, and the dosage must be reduced in patients with a reduced creatinine clearance. Combination therapy should continue for at least 2 weeks; the CSF cultures should be negative and clinical improvement noted before changing to oral fluconazole consolidation therapy at 400 mg daily (19). The total length of fluconazole therapy is a minimum of 10 weeks, but many patients require therapy for months depending on their response and underlying illness. Pulmonary cryptococcosis without evidence of disseminated infection can be treated with fluconazole, 400 mg daily. The treatment should continue until all lung lesions have resolved.

5.6. Prevention

Cryptococcosis is acquired from the environment and usually no discrete point source can be identified. There are no effective preventive measures that can be taken.

6. ENDEMIC MYCOSES: HISTOPLASMOSIS, BLASTOMYCOSIS, COCCIDIOIDOMYCOSIS

Infection with these fungi is acquired from the environment. Each has its own ecological niche, and people become infected when they encounter these organisms during various occupational or recreational activities or just in the course of their activities of daily living. All of these mycoses have a variety of distinctive clinical syndromes, and treatment varies with the host and the extent of disease. Only the manifestations that appear to be more common in older adults and the treatment of those syndromes will be discussed in this chapter.

6.1. Epidemiology

The desert southwest, especially Arizona and southern California, constitute the major endemic area for coccidioidomycosis. In contrast, histoplasmosis and blastomycosis are primarily seen along the Mississippi and Ohio River valleys, with smaller areas of endemicity noted elsewhere in the East and Midwest. In the endemic areas for histoplasmosis and coccidioidomycosis, most people are infected in childhood and experience only a "viral-like illness" without any suspicion that a fungal infection has occurred. Infection in older adults is frequently a manifestation of reactivation of this infection that was acquired years before. Reactivation may be linked to an immunosuppressive illness or drugs that suppress cellular immunity. However, for some patients, the only risk factor appears to be older age with the accompanying decrease in cell-mediated immunity. It is not clear to what extent primary infection with blastomycosis occurs in childhood, but it is thought to be less than that noted with the other two endemic mycoses. Reactivation infection has been seen with blastomycosis, but seems to be less frequent than that reported with histoplasmosis.

A recently described trend is that the primary infection with *C. immitis* appears to be occurring more often in older adults. Indeed, the highest rate of infection with *C. immitis* in Arizona is now among those aged ≥65 years (20). This is likely related to the influx of older adults into the desert southwest endemic areas for *C. immitis*. Most of these older adults have not had prior exposure to *C. immitis* and are thus at risk of developing primary infection, which is likely to be more severe than when it occurs in childhood.

6.2. Microbiology

All of the endemic mycoses are dimorphic, meaning that they exist in the contagious mold form in the environment and then undergo transformation after infection has occurred and assume either a yeast or a spherule form in tissues. The reader is referred to an infectious disease text for a discussion of the microbiology of each of these fungi.

6.3. Clinical Disease

Among the endemic mycoses, histoplasmosis is unique in that several manifestations of infection are seen almost entirely in older adults (21). Chronic cavitary pulmonary histoplasmosis is seen almost entirely in older men who have chronic obstructive pulmonary disease and chronic progressive disseminated histoplasmosis also is noted mostly in older adults. Manifestations of chronic cavitary pulmonary histoplasmosis mimic those of reactivation tuberculosis. Patients have fever, night sweats, anorexia, weight loss, cough with sputum production, hemoptysis, and shortness of breath. Unilateral or bilateral upper lobe cavitary infiltrates and lower lobe scarring are seen on chest radiograph.

Patients with chronic progressive disseminated histoplasmosis have intense infection of macrophages, which are unable to kill the organism, and dissemination becomes widespread. Patients have fever, night sweats, anorexia, weight loss, and fatigue. Pancytopenia and elevated alkaline phosphatase reflect involvement of bone marrow and liver. Lymphadenopathy and mucocutaneous ulcerations are common; infiltration of the adrenal glands leads to Addison's disease manifested by weakness, orthostatic hypotension, hyperkalemia, and hyponatremia. Diffuse infiltrates are noted on chest radiograph.

Blastomycosis in older adults is similar to that in younger individuals. Pulmonary disease can mimic tuberculosis or present as a mass-like lesion resembling lung cancer. Skin lesions are the most common extrapulmonary manifestation of disease and are usually heaped-up nodules with discrete borders and microabscesses in the interior of the lesion. Genitourinary and osteoarticular involvement often accompany cutaneous lesions.

Coccidioidomycosis is primarily a pulmonary infection, and the manifestations are protean in older adults as well as younger individuals. However, older individuals are more likely than younger persons to develop more severe pulmonary disease when infected with *C. immitis*. Nodules, cavities, and diffuse infiltrates are all noted with coccidioidomycosis. The clinical manifestations of disseminated coccidioidomycosis include nodular, ulcerative, and granulomatous skin lesions, destructive bony lesions, and subcutaneous abscesses and sinus tracts. Meningitis is the most feared complication and appears to occur more often in older adults. The usual presenting symptoms are headache, fever, and confusion.

6.4. Diagnosis

The diagnosis of an endemic mycotic infection is definitively established with the growth of the organism from tissue samples, body fluids, or exudates. However, this is the slowest diagnostic test, and often, an initial diagnosis can be made by the distinctive histopathological features seen with each organism. Serology is useful for coccidioidomycosis and histoplasmosis, and the detection of *H. capsulatum* antigen in urine from patients with disseminated infection has become a valuable diagnostic tool. It is essential that a firm diagnosis be established because therapy will continue for months to years, and use of antifungal agents is often accompanied by serious adverse effects or drug–drug interactions.

6.5. Treatment

Treatment of all the endemic mycoses is similar, with a few nuances that differ depending on the organism and the site of infection. Both chronic progressive disseminated histoplasmosis and chronic cavitary pulmonary histoplasmosis must be treated or the patient will die of the infection. For patients who are moderately ill, the agent of choice is itraconazole, 200 mg once or twice daily. Patients who are severely ill with either form of histoplasmosis should be treated initially with intravenous amphotericin B at a dosage of 0.7–1 mg/kg daily. In older adults, it is preferable to use a lipid formulation of amphotericin B at a dosage of 3–5 mg/kg/day. Treatment should be changed to itraconazole, 200 mg twice daily, after the patient's condition has improved. Therapy should continue for at least a year and sometimes longer for these forms of histoplasmosis. Fluconazole is less active against *H. capsulatum* and remains a second-line agent that must be given at a higher dosage of 400–800 mg daily. Treatment of other forms of histoplasmosis will not be discussed here (see also chapter "Antifungal Drugs").

All older adults with blastomycosis should be treated. Itraconazole is the drug-of-choice for non-life-threatening blastomycosis. The dosage is 200 mg either once or twice daily for a minimum of 6 months; when osteomyelitis is present, treatment should continue for at least a year. Severe life-threatening blastomycosis, which often is manifested as the adult respiratory distress syndrome, should be treated with amphotericin B at a dosage of 1 mg/kg daily. After the patient has improved, therapy can be changed to itraconazole, 200 mg twice daily. Fluconazole is a second-line drug and must be given at a dosage of 400–800 mg daily.

Older adults who are moderately ill with pulmonary or disseminated coccidioidomycosis can be treated either with itraconazole or fluconazole, at a dosage of 400 mg daily, For those with severe infection, amphotericin B is the agent of choice, with step-down to an azole after the patient is stabilized. Treatment is given for 1–2 years for most patients.

For patients with meningitis, fluconazole is the drug-of-choice because of its superior CSF levels (22). Although the initial studies used 400 mg daily, many clinicians use 800 mg for the treatment of meningitis. Chronic suppressive fluconazole therapy must be continued life-long to prevent relapse of infection. Unfortunely, not all patients respond to fluconazole; nonresponders require intrathecal administration of amphotericin B.

6.6. Prevention

Older adults living in the area endemic for *C. immitis* should be cautioned about the risks of acquiring this infection especially during windstorms that blow in from the desert. However, it is impossible to ensure that infection with *C. immitis* will not occur when people live in the endemic area. Histoplasmosis is extremely common in the endemic area. Avoiding certain activities, such as demolishing old buildings, landscaping areas in which large numbers of birds have roosted, and cleaning old farm buildings and attics, decreases one's risk of acquiring histoplasmosis. Avoiding decaying wood and vegetation may help prevent infection with *B. dermatitidis*.

7. OPPORTUNISTIC MOLD INFECTIONS: ASPERGILLOSIS, ZYGOMYCOSES

Although opportunistic mold infections are uncommon in older adults, they carry an exceedingly high mortality rate. Early recognition and aggressive therapy are essential. *Aspergillus* species most commonly cause infection in patients who are immunocompromised because of neutropenia, chemotherapy, corticosteroids, or a transplantation procedure. However, two forms of aspergillosis are subacute in presentation and occur more often in older adults, and these will be discussed (23,24). The zygomycetes cause infection in immunocompromised patients similar to those described as at high risk of aspergillosis, but these molds also cause infection in diabetics in ketoacidosis and in patients on iron chelators (25), many of whom are older adults.

7.1. Epidemiology

Aspergillus species and the zygomycetes, the molds that most often cause infection in older adults, are ubiquitous in the environment, and reach enormous numbers in decaying organic material. Exposure occurs during the course of everyday living. For most individuals, exposure never leads to infection because of a robust host defense against these opportunists. However, immunocompromised individuals and those with other underlying illnesses are unable to prevent invasion, which is usually through the upper or lower respiratory tract.

7.2. Microbiology

Over a thousand species of *Aspergillus* are known; most are harmless environmental saprophytes. The most common pathogenic species are *Aspergillus fumigatus* and *Aspergillus flavus*. The zygomycetes constitute a class of molds that are characterized by large nonseptate hyphae and the ability to invade quickly through tissue leading to necrosis. The most common genera causing human infection are *Rhizopus*, *Rhizomucor*, and *Mucor*.

7.3. Clinical Disease

Two forms of aspergillosis, sino-orbital infection and chronic necrotizing pulmonary infection, occur more commonly in older adults than in younger adults. Older adults who have these forms of aspergillosis are usually not overtly immunocompromised, but in many instances, corticosteroids have been given. Often, the steroids were given after the disease began for treatment of presumed inflammatory ocular disease. Patients with chronic necrotizing pulmonary aspergillosis almost always have chronic obstructive pulmonary disease and have often received corticosteroids for this disease.

Symptoms of orbital aspergillosis include pain in the eye and face, proptosis, ophthalmoplegia, and loss of vision. The infection often arises in an adjacent sinus and then extends behind the orbit and into the brain (24).

Patients with chronic necrotizing pulmonary aspergillosis generally present with pneumonia that is unresponsive to antibacterial agents (23). They have fever, cough productive of purulent sputum, pleuritic chest pain, increasing dyspnea, weight loss, and fatigue. The chest radiograph shows pulmonary infiltrates, usually in the upper lobes that progress to cavitation; pleural involvement is common.

The zygomycetes cause a variety of different syndromes. The most common is rhinocerebral infection involving the sinuses and orbit with extension into the cavernous sinus and brain. Other patients have necrotizing pulmonary infection or cutaneous lesions. This infection is seen in older adults who have poorly controlled diabetes mellitus. Of special concern are older patients, who have myelodysplastic syndrome for which they receive repeated transfusions and then require chelation therapy with deferoxamine (25). The deferoxamine is used by *Rhizopus* species for growth enhancement, and acute overwhelming invasive pulmonary and/or rhinocerebral zygomycosis is the result.

7.4. Diagnosis

The opportunistic molds usually are easily grown from sputum or tissue samples. The problem arises in differentiating contaminants or colonizing organisms from those causing tissue invasion. Histopathological evidence of tissue invasion is extremely helpful in establishing a diagnosis of infection with an invasive mold, and the culture results then define the specific organism causing disease. Serological techniques are of no benefit for the diagnosis of opportunistic mold infection.

7.5. Treatment

The treatment of aspergillosis has been revolutionized by the introduction of the second-generation azoles. Voriconazole has become the initial treatment choice for invasive aspergillosis and is much better tolerated by older adults than amphotericin B, the previous mainstay of therapy. Generally, initial therapy will be with intravenous voriconazole at a dosage of 4 mg/kg twice daily, and then therapy can be changed to the oral formulation, 200 mg twice daily as soon as the patient is able to swallow tablets (see chapter "Antifungal Drugs"). Amphotericin B may still be required for some patients, and caspofungin is an alternative agent for patients who fail or cannot tolerate voriconazole. In patients with sino-orbital aspergillosis, antifungal therapy stops the progression of the infection, but vision frequently does not return (24). Surgical decompression is an important adjunct to antifungal therapy. In patients with chronic necrotizing pulmonary aspergillosis, most experience has been with amphotericin B, but voriconazole will likely become the drug-of-choice. Resolution occurs in some individuals, but others experience a relapsing and remitting course even with antifungal therapy (23).

Patients with zygomycoses are treated with a lipid formulation of amphotericin B given in high dosages (5–10 mg/kg). The zygomycetes are resistant to all other antifungal agents. Correction of underlying risk factors, such as ketoacidosis, removing growth factors, such as deferoxamine, and aggressive surgical debridement of all necrotic tissue are all essential for cure of this infection.

7.6. Prevention

There is little that can be done to prevent exposure to the ubiquitous environmental molds. However, preventing exposure of immunocompromised patients to large numbers of conidia is important; they should be warned to avoid compost piles, other decaying vegetation, and renovations on buildings that can easily lead to dispersal of conidia.

REFERENCES

1. Heikkila H, Stubb S. The prevalence of onychomycosis in Finland. Br J Dermatol 1995; 133:699–703.
2. Lewis SM, Lewis BG. Nosocomial transmission of *Trichophyton tonsurans* tinea corporis in a rehabilitation hospital. Infect Control Hosp Epidemiol 1997; 18:322–325.
3. Weitzman I, Summerbell RC. The dermatophytes. Clin Microbiol Rev 1995; 8:240–259.
4. Rezabek GH, Friedman AD. Superficial fungal infections of the skin. Diagnosis and current treatment recommendations. Drugs 1992; 43:674–682.
5. Tosti A, Piraccini BM, Stinchi C, Venturo N, Bardazzi F, Colombo MD. Treatment of dermatophyte infections: an open randomized study comparing intermittent terbinafine therapy with continuous terbinafine treatment and intermittent itraconazole therapy. J Am Acad Dermatol 1996; 34:595–600.
6. Hedderwick SA, Wan JY, Bradley SF, Sangeorzan JA, Terpenning MS, Kauffman CA. Risk factors for colonization with yeast species in a Veterans Affairs long-term care facility. J Am Geriatr Soc 1998; 46:849–853.
7. Shay K, Truhlar MR, Renner RP. Oropharyngeal candidosis in the older patient. J Am Geriatr Soc 1997; 45:863–870.
8. Budtz-Jorgensen E. Oral mucosal lesions associated with the wearing of removable dentures. J Oral Pathol 1981; 10:65–80.
9. Sobel JD. Candidal vulvovaginitis. Clin Obstet Gynecol 1993; 36:153–165.
10. Kauffman CA, Vazquez JA, Sobel JD, Gallis HA, McKinsey DS, Karchmer AW, Sugar AM, Sharkey PK, Wise GJ, Mangi R, Mosher A, Lee JY, Dismukes WE, the NIAID Mycoses Study Group. Prospective multicenter surveillance study of funguria in hospitalized patients. Clin Infect Dis 2000; 30:14–18.

11. Lundstrom T, Sobel J. Candiduria: a review. Clin Infect Dis 2001; 32:1602–1607.
12. Sobel JD, Kauffman CA, McKinsey D, Zervos M, Vazquez JA, Karchmer AW, Lee J, Thomas C, Panzer H, Dismukes WE, the NIAID Mycoses Study Group. Candiduria: a randomized, double-blind study of treatment with fluconazole and placebo. Clin Infect Dis 2000; 30:19–24.
13. Jacobs LG. Fungal urinary tract infections in the elderly: treatment guidelines. Drugs Aging 1996; 8:89–96.
14. Gudlaugsson O, Gillespie S, Lee K, Vande Berg J, Hu J, Messer S, Herwaldt L, Pfaller M, Diekema D. Attributable mortality of nosocomial candidemia, revisited. Clin Infect Dis 2004; 37:1172–1177.
15. Nucci M, Colombo AL, Silveira F, Richtmann R, Salomao R, Branchini ML, Spector N. Risk factors for death in patients with candidemia. Infect Control Hosp Epidemiol 1998; 19:846–850.
16. Malani PN, Bradley SF, Little RA, Kauffman CA. Trends in species causing fungemia in a tertiary care medical center over 12 years. Mycoses 2001; 44:446–449.
17. Pappas PG, Perfect JR, Cloud GA, Larsen RA, Pankey GA, Lancaster DJ, Henderson H, Kauffman CA, Haas DW, Saccente M, Hamill RJ, Holloway MS, Warren RM, Dismukes WE. Cryptococcosis in HIV-negative patients in the era of effective azole therapy. Clin Infect Dis 2001; 33:690–699.
18. Steiner I, Polacheck I, Melamed E. Dementia and myoclonus in a case of cryptococcal encephalitis. Arch Neurol 1984; 41:216–217.
19. Saag MS, Graybill JR, Larsen RA, Pappas PG, Perfect JR, Powderly WG, Sobel JD, Dismukes WE. Practice guidelines for the management of cryptococcal disease. Clin Infect Dis 2000; 30:710–718.
20. Leake JAD, Mosley DG, England B, et al. Risk factors for acute symptomatic coccidioido-mycosis among elderly persons in Arizona, 1996–1997. J Infect Dis 2000; 181:1435–1440.
21. Kauffman CA. Fungal infections in older adults. Clin Infect Dis 2001; 33:550–555.
22. Galgiani JN, Catanzaro A, Cloud GA, et al. Fluconazole therapy for coccidioidal meningitis. Ann Intern Med 1993; 119:28–32.
23. Denning DW, Riniotis K, Dobrashian R, Sambatakou H. Chronic cavitary and fibrosing pulmonary and pleural aspergillosis: case series, proposed nomenclature change, and review. Clin Infect Dis 2003; 37(suppl 3):S265–S280.
24. Washburn RG, Kennedy DW, Begley MG, Henderson DK, Bennett JE. Chronic fungal sinusitis in apparently normal hosts. Medicine (Baltimore) 1988; 67:231–247.
25. Daly AL, Bradley SF, Velaquez LA, Kauffman CA. Mucormycosis: association with deferoxamine therapy. Am J Med 1989; 87:468–471.

SUGGESTED READING

Chapman SW, Bradsher RW, Campbell GD, et al. Practice guidelines for the management of patients with blastomycosis. Clin Infect Dis 2000; 30:679–683.
Galgiani JN, Ampel NM, Catanzaro A, et al. Practice guidelines for the treatment of coccidioidomycosis. Clin Infect Dis 2000; 30:658–661.
Pappas PG, Rex JH, Sobel JD, Filler SG, Dismukes WE, Walsh TJ, Edwards JE. Guidelines for the treatment of candidiasis. Clin Infect Dis 2004; 36:161–189.
Wheat J, Sarosi G, McKinsey D, et al. Practice guidelines for the management of patients with histoplasmosis. Clin Infect Dis 2000; 30:688–695.

45
Common Viral Infections

Ann R. Falsey
University of Rochester School of Medicine and Dentistry, Department of Medicine, Rochester General Hospital, Rochester, New York, U.S.A.

Key Points:

- The common respiratory viruses are major causes of morbidity and mortality in older persons, particularly individuals with chronic heart and lung disease.
- Together, influenza and respiratory syncytial virus infections lead to over 50,000 deaths annually in people ≥65 years of age in the United States.
- Influenza vaccination is both efficacious and cost-effective in elderly persons.
- Viral gastroenteritis in frail older persons can lead to death due to complications of dehydration.

1. INTRODUCTION

Of the viral diseases which effect older people, the common respiratory viruses are the most frequent. Although the incidence of viral respiratory infections decreases with advancing age their impact increases substantially. Primary infections with these viruses (Table 1) occur in young childhood with reinfections occurring throughout adulthood. Viral gastroenteritis also occurs less frequently in elderly persons, yet it causes significant morbidity and mortality in institutional settings. Frail older persons are particularly susceptible to the complications of dehydration. Systemic herpes viruses such as Epstein Barr virus and cytomegalovirus are relatively rare in the elderly adult but are important to consider in the differential diagnosis of puzzling cases of fever of unknown origin, jaundice, or refractory diarrhea.

2. RESPIRATORY VIRUSES

2.1. Influenza

Despite the availability of an effective vaccine, influenza remains the most important viral infection in older persons. Pneumonia and influenza together constitute the fifth leading cause of death in persons aged ≥65 years (1). Influenza viruses are RNA viruses in the orthomyxovirus family and are classified as either type A or

Table 1 Respiratory Viral Infections

Virus	Peak season	Incubation (days)	Clinical clues	Antiviral therapy
Influenza A	Winter	1–3	High fever, headache, myalgias	Amantadine, Rimantadine, Oseltamivir, Zanamivir
Influenza B	Winter	1–3	High fever, headache, myalgias	Oseltamivir, Zanamivir
Respiratory syncytial virus	Winter	2–8	Rhinorrhea, wheezing	Ribavirin
Parainfluenza	Fall–spring	2–3	Pharyngitis, hoarseness	None
Rhinovirus	All	1–2	Rhinorrhea	None
Coronavirus	Winter–spring	2–5	Nonspecific	None
Human metapneumovirus	Winter	4–5	Nonspecific	None

B, on the basis of stable internal viral proteins. Influenza A viruses are further classified by their major surface glycoproteins, hemagglutinin (H) and neuraminidase (N). As with other RNA viruses, influenza viruses mutate frequently. Minor changes known as "drift" are due to spontaneous mutations in the H or N genes and occur in both A and B viruses leading to yearly influenza epidemics. Major antigenic changes, known as "shift," occur when the segmented viral genomes of unrelated influenza A viruses reassort and result in a virus with a completely different H or N protein. When these new viruses emerge, pandemics occur in nonimmune populations. Currently, two influenza A viruses, H1N1 and H3N2, in addition to influenza B, are circulating in the United States. H1N1 viruses generally do not cause serious problems in older persons, possibly due to immunity acquired in younger life.

2.1.1. Epidemiology and Clinical Relevance

Each winter, the introduction of influenza into the community typically results in a bell-shaped increase in acute respiratory illnesses lasting 6–8 weeks with infection rates highest in preschool and school age children and lowest in older adults (2). Despite a lower incidence of infection, the rates of complications, such as pneumonia and hospitalizations, are highest in persons aged ≥65 years. Rates of pneumonia are generally under 10% in persons 5–50 years old, but rise steadily after age 50, reaching over 70% in persons >70 years (2). The overall number of influenza-associated hospitalizations in the United States has ranged from 16,000 to 220,000 in the last two decades with 43% occurring among persons aged ≥65 years (3). Recent estimates from the Centers for Disease Control and Prevention (CDC) indicate that there are approximately 44,000 deaths annually in persons aged ≥65 years attributable to influenza (4). Additionally, influenza-associated deaths have increased significantly over the past 20 years, which is felt in part due to the aging population. The presence of one high-risk medical condition (cardiovascular, pulmonary, renal, metabolic, neurologic, or malignant disease) increases the risk of influenza-related deaths 39-fold. The highest death rates (870 per 100,000) due to influenza occur in persons with both chronic cardiac and pulmonary disease.

The impact of influenza outbreaks in long-term care facilities can be devastating. A number of reports document high rates of pneumonia and death during H3N2 and influenza B outbreaks in nursing homes. Attack rates of 20–30% are not unusual, and rates of pneumonia and hospitalization may be as high as 50% and 30%, respectively. Additionally, case fatality rates may reach 30% in frail institutionalized persons. Risk factors for infection in nursing home residents include nonvaccinated status, low preinfection influenza-specific antibody titers, and increased functional status (5). Paradoxically, higher attack rates are sometimes observed in more functional ambulatory residents, possibly due to increased exposure.

2.1.2. Clinical Manifestations

Influenza-infected patients of any age typically present with the abrupt onset of fever, chills, headache, and myalgias. Dry cough, sore throat, and ocular symptoms are also common (3). Rhinorrhea occurs but is usually not profuse and is frequently overshadowed by constitutional symptoms. Fever remains a frequent finding in older persons with influenza but the height of the fever may be lower than that in children and young adults. It is important to remember that not all older persons will present with "classic" flu-like symptoms. This is particularly true in persons where cognitive impairment prevents patients from offering specific complaints. Infection may be characterized by increased lethargy, confusion, anorexia, or unexplained fever. In addition, increased respiratory difficulties may be ascribed to worsening of underlying medical conditions such as congestive heart failure or chronic obstructive pulmonary disease (COPD) rather than a viral infection. Primary influenza pneumonia may occur in persons of all ages, most often during pandemics (1). Influenza-related pneumonia in older persons is frequently due to secondary bacterial or mixed viral–bacterial infection. The illness is usually characterized by classic influenza symptoms followed by a 3–4 day period of improvement, then sudden recrudescence of fever with the development of worsening respiratory symptoms.

2.1.3. Diagnosis

Influenza infection can be diagnosed by a variety of methods including clinical features, viral culture, rapid antigen detection, reverse transcription polymerase chain reaction (RT-PCR), and serology. The use of clinical symptoms and signs such as fever, myalgias, and cough are relatively specific for the diagnosis of influenza in young healthy adults when influenza is epidemic in the community (3). Unfortunately, clinical features are less helpful in older patients, particularly in nonepidemic periods. Several studies have shown that the constellation of fever, cough, and short duration of symptoms is predictive of influenza in elderly and chronically ill adults, yet still do not provide adequate discrimination from other pathogens to be clinically useful.

Since the clinical features may be indistinguishable from other respiratory viruses which circulate during the winter months, laboratory confirmation is essential for appropriate therapeutic decisions and infection control policies. The traditional method of influenza diagnosis is isolation of the virus in cell culture. Nasopharyngeal swabs and washes, as well as sputum and bronchioalveolar lavage fluid, can be cultured for influenza. Influenza virus is reasonably hardy and will survive overnight if specimens are kept on ice; therefore, viral culture is a useful diagnostic tool even in nursing home settings (2). Clinical utility of viral culture, which typically provides results after 3–7 days, is limited because patient management issues frequently require more rapid answers. Early in epidemics, it is important to obtain viral isolates for strain typing. However, particularly in closed populations where explosive epidemics may occur, the rapid diagnosis of influenza is highly desirable.

A number of diagnostic techniques including RT-PCR, immunofluorescent assay (IFA), and enzyme immunoassay (EIA) on direct patient specimens have been developed and offer same-day results. Although both sensitive and specific, RT-PCR is expensive and is not widely commercially available. Rapid tests for the direct detection of influenza viral proteins although not as sensitive as culture or RT-PCR are appealing because results can be available in <1 hr and are easy to perform (Table 2) (1,6). Sensitivity of commercial tests in elderly inpatients is approximately 50%, yet specificity remains good and results can be used to guide antiviral therapy and appropriate isolation. Rapid testing has been evaluated in the nursing home setting and when used in combination with viral culture is associated with lower institutional attack rates than when viral culture alone is used for diagnosis. The use of rapid testing followed by viral culture on negative specimens provides rapid results without sacrificing sensitivity. Point-of-care testing can now be done in outpatient settings, and questions have arisen regarding the cost-effectiveness of this practice. Outpatient influenza testing should be individualized according to the complexity of the patient and the degree of influenza activity in the community.

Influenza infection can be confirmed serologically by complement fixation, hemaglutination inhibition assay, or EIA (2). Since nearly all adults have antibodies against influenza due to previous infections and/or vaccination, a single elevated titer is not useful for the diagnosis of acute infection. Demonstration of a fourfold or greater rise in influenza-specific IgG in paired acute and convalescent sera can confirm the diagnosis retrospectively.

Table 2 Diagnostic Tests for Influenza

Test	Manufacturer	Specimen	Type of flu detected	Discriminates A and B	CLIA waived[a]
Directigen flu A	Becton, Dickinson & Co.	a,w,s,t	A	—	N
Directigen flu A & B	Becton, Dickinson & Co.	a,w,s,t,bal	A and B	Y	N
Flu OIA	Thermo BioStar	a,s,t, sputum	A and B	N	N
Zstate flu	Zyme Tx, Inc.	t	A and B	N	Y
Quick vue	Quidel Corp.	a,w,s	A	—	Y
Now flu A	Binax, Inc.	w,s	A	—	N
Now flu B	Binax, Inc.	w,s	A	—	N

[a]CLIA waiver—test may be performed in a physician's office.
Abbreviations: a, nasal aspirate; N, no; w, nasal wash; Y, yes; s, nasal swab; t, throat swab; bal, bronchoalveolar lavage; CLIA, Clinical Laboratory Improvement Act.
Source: Adapted from Ref. 6.

Table 3 Antiviral Agents Available for Treatment and Prophylaxis of Influenza

Drug	Form	Indication	Dosage
Amantadine	Oral	Treatment or prophylaxis	100 mg/day[a]
Rimantadine	Oral	Treatment or prophylaxis	100 mg/day
Zanamivir	Inhaled	Treatment	10 mg twice daily
Oseltamivir	Oral	Treatment or prophylaxis	75 mg twice daily[a]

[a]Requires adjustment in renal failure.

2.1.4. Treatment

Four antiviral agents, amantadine, rimantadine, zanamivir, and oseltamivir, are approved in the United States for the treatment and prophylaxis of influenza A infection (Table 3). When administered prophylactically, these drugs are 70–90% effective in preventing influenza illness (3). These agents can also reduce illness severity, duration of symptoms, and days of viral shedding if they are given within 48 hr of symptom onset. Indications for treatment and prophylaxis are outlined in Table 4 (see Chapter 24: Antiviral Drugs).

2.1.5. Prevention and Infection Control

Because outbreaks of influenza in long-term care facilities are associated with significant morbidity and mortality, prevention of influenza in the nursing home setting is critical. Outbreaks tend to be explosive in nature and difficult to control because influenza is spread by small-particle aerosol and residents may be infectious prior to the onset of symptoms. Therefore, the cornerstone of an effective infection control program is yearly vaccination for all staff and residents (3). Consent for annual influenza vaccination should be obtained from guardians or residents upon admission to a long-term care facility. When influenza activity has been confirmed in the community, resident furloughs should be restricted to those that are medically necessary and visitors with respiratory illnesses should be discouraged. Symptomatic residents should be restricted to their rooms with the doors closed, and employees should use gloves and masks when entering the rooms. If possible, residents and staff from affected wards should be cohorted and vaccination should be offered again to all

Table 4 Indications for Influenza Antivirals

Considered antiviral use:
  Prophylaxis (usually reserved for epidemic periods)
    Unvaccinated persons
    Recently vaccinated persons awaiting antibody response (2–4 weeks)
    High-risk subjects when vaccine is a poor antigenic match
    High-risk household exposures regardless of vaccination status (5–7 days)
    Residents of long-term care facilities during outbreaks until (1 week after last case)
  Treatment
    Persons with influenza within 48 hr of symptoms
    Persons with complicated influenza (pneumonia, severe disease or hospitalized)
      even if symptom duration is >48 hr

unvaccinated staff and residents. Many authorities, including the CDC, recommend antiviral prophylaxis once influenza A has been documented within an institution (3). Chemoprophylaxis should be given to all residents regardless of their vaccination status and should be continued until 1 week after the onset of the last case of presumed influenza has occurred.

Influenza vaccine is an effective measure for reducing the impact of influenza infection in elderly persons and is recommended for all persons aged ≥65 years. At present, inactivated influenza vaccine is the only vaccine available for elderly adults. The vaccine contains three strains of influenza (H3N2, H1N1, and B) representing the viruses likely to circulate in the upcoming winter. Because vaccine virus is initially grown in eggs, individuals with egg hypersensitivity should not receive vaccine (3). A number of studies have shown that serum antibody response to influenza vaccination is more variable in older persons. However, many of these studies suffered from methodological flaws which fail to control for the presence of chronic diseases, prevaccination antibody titers, and previous influenza vaccination status. Overall, the protective efficacy of influenza vaccine depends on the age and immunocompetence of the subjects, as well as the match of vaccine to the circulating epidemic strain. Only one randomized double-blind, placebo-controlled study of influenza vaccine has been reported (7). In this study the investigators found a 50% reduction in serologically proven influenza and a 53% reduction in clinical influenza among vaccinated persons. Most other studies examining vaccine efficacy have been case–control retrospective analyses and all have shown influenza vaccine to be both efficacious and cost-effective (8). In a 3-year case–control study of 25,000 older persons, vaccination was associated with a reduction in hospitalization by 48–57%. In addition, during the 3 years of study, vaccination was associated with a decrease in mortality from all causes of 39–54%. When older persons are stratified by chronic medical conditions, influenza vaccine is found to be beneficial in all groups with the highest absolute risk reduction demonstrated in high-risk subjects. Lastly, vaccination is associated with reductions in risk of hospitalizations for cardiac disease and stroke.

For residents of nursing homes, influenza vaccine is most effective in preventing serious complications of influenza rather than in preventing infection itself (3). In this population vaccination reduces uncomplicated influenza infection by only 30–40%. However, it has been shown to prevent 50–60% of influenza-related pneumonias and hospitalizations and has reduced death rates by 80%. Furthermore, high rates of vaccination in nursing homes may induce herd immunity and thus benefit unvaccinated residents.

2.2. Respiratory Syncytial Virus

Respiratory syncytial virus (RSV) ranks second only to influenza as a major viral pathogen in elderly persons (4,9). RSV is an enveloped, single-stranded, nonsegmented RNA virus belonging to the paramyxovirus family. It is well recognized as the leading cause of lower respiratory tract disease in infants and young children, and infection by age 2 years is universal. However, immunity to RSV is incomplete and reinfections occur throughout adult life, typically causing mild upper respiratory tract infections (URTI) (10).

2.2.1. Epidemiology and Clinical Relevance

RSV was first recognized as a problem in the elderly in institutionalized older persons. Since 1977 there have been numerous reports of RSV outbreaks in nursing homes and several prospective studies in which RSV was identified as a common pathogen (9). Although attack rates as high as 90% have been reported in outbreaks, infection rates are more commonly in the range of 2–12% in prospective studies. Complication rates of RSV among frail older persons have been variable with rates of pneumonia ranging from 5% to 67% and death rates from 0% to 20%. The variability is likely due to case definitions, methods of diagnosis, and the frailty of the residents studied. A reasonable estimate is that RSV will infect 5–10% of residents per year, with rates of pneumonia and death of 10–20% and 2–5%, respectively. Similar to children, elderly persons who attend senior daycare programs also appear to be at increased risk of RSV infection. In one study investigators found 10% of 165 elderly and 5% of the 113 staff members developed respiratory infections proven to be RSV during a 15-month period and it was among the most commonly identified viruses (11).

RSV infection is also a cause of serious disease in community-dwelling older persons. Although the precise incidence is unknown, recent estimates indicate that RSV is a cause of excess morbidity and mortality in persons aged ≥65 years at rates similar to influenza. A study from the CDC using a national database of deaths and viral activity estimated that approximately 12,000 deaths occur annually in persons aged ≥65 years compared with 335 deaths in children under 1 year of age (4). In a study of elderly persons in upstate New York admitted during three winters with acute cardiopulmonary conditions, RSV was identified in 10% of patients compared with 13% with influenza (9). The impact of RSV illness in those persons requiring hospitalization was significant as 18% were admitted to an intensive care unit, 10% required ventilatory support, and 10% died. Of note, 14% of those surviving required a higher level of care at discharge. Although 44% had a discharge diagnosis of pneumonia, much of the RSV morbidity was associated with other diagnoses, including COPD exacerbation (19%) and congestive heart failure (CHF) (20%). RSV was also found to be the third most common identifiable cause of pneumonia in 1195 adults with community-acquired pneumonia (12). RSV was found in 4.4% of cases compared with 6.2% due to *Streptococcus pneumoniae* and 5.4% due to influenza virus. A reasonable estimate using data from a number of studies during the past 30 years is that RSV accounts for 2–9% of pneumonias throughout the year and 5–15% during the winter (9).

Published studies evaluating the outpatient burden of RSV disease in community-dwelling older persons are limited. In a prospective study of respiratory infections in elderly persons in the United Kingdom, RSV accounted for 3% of the illnesses among 533 persons followed for two winter seasons (13). It is estimated that RSV also accounts for approximately 15% of physician visits for respiratory illnesses during the winter months compared with 30% for influenza. RSV infection is also felt to be a cause of COPD exacerbations, although the percentage of illnesses caused by RSV has ranged widely from 0% to 17.4% in the series published to date (9). Risk factors for severe disease include the presence of chronic pulmonary disease, poor functional status, and low serum-neutralizing antibody titers.

2.2.2. Clinical Manifestations

The clinical manifestations of RSV in older persons can be quite variable, ranging from a mild upper respiratory infection to severe pneumonia (9). Data from

Table 5   Clinical Manifestations of RSV Infections in Older Persons

	%
Symptoms	
Nasal congestion	73
Sore throat	57
Hoarse	39
Cough	77
Sputum	63
Dyspnea	37
Constitutional	57
Signs	
Fever $T > 38°C$	32
Rhinorrhea	60
Rales	8
Wheezing	24
Laboratory	
Chest X-ray infiltrates	4

prospective studies, where both healthy and frail elderly were evaluated, provide the best information on the spectrum of disease. In these studies, the most common symptoms include nasal congestion, cough, sputum production, and constitutional symptoms (Table 5). Dyspnea and wheezing are more common in patients with COPD but can occur in healthy older people as well (9). RSV and influenza frequently cocirculate and are difficult to distinguish clinically. While no feature is diagnostic, certain symptoms and signs may be helpful. Nasal discharge and wheezing are more typical of RSV illness whereas gastrointestinal (GI) complaints, high fevers, and prominent myalgias are more characteristic of influenza.

2.2.3. Diagnosis

Diagnosis of RSV infection may be accomplished by culture, direct antigen detection, RT-PCR, or serologic analysis. In older persons, diagnosis during acute infection has been problematic. Although viral culture is the gold standard of diagnosis in children, adults shed considerably less virus (1000-fold less) and for a shorter period of time. In addition, RSV is thermolabile and does not survive prolonged transit times, which can be a particular problem in long-term care facilities (9). At best, viral culture is approximately 50% sensitive compared with serology even when optimal conditions are used. Direct antigen detection by IFA or commercial EIA has been used successfully on nasal wash specimens in children with sensitivities of 75–95%. In contrast, EIA is much less sensitive than culture in adults. When three rapid diagnostic tests (DFA and EIA—Directigen and VIDAS) were compared with culture, RT-PCR, and retrospective serology, all methods were very insensitive in elderly persons. RT-PCR is a valuable new tool that is over 70% sensitive and 99% specific when compared with serology but is presently used primarily in research settings.

   Infection with RSV can be demonstrated by a four-fold or greater rise in RSV-specific IgG by either EIA or complement fixation. Since RSV infection in the adult always represents reinfection, a single elevated titer is not reliable evidence of acute RSV infection. Serology by EIA has been found to be both sensitive and specific for RSV infection (9). RSV-specific IgM has been detected in older subjects with RSV;

however, its utility for early diagnosis is limited since antibody response generally requires 5–7 days, and rheumatoid factor may interfere with the assay.

2.2.4. Treatment

Treatment of RSV infection in the elderly adult is generally supportive with fluids, oxygen, bronchodilators, and/or corticosteroids as appropriate. Antibiotics may also be reasonable in selected patients with pneumonia and bacterial pathogens isolated in sputum. Ribavirin, a nucleoside analog with activity against RSV, is approved for young children infected with RSV. Clinical efficacy has been demonstrated in this group with little toxicity (10). No controlled trials have been done in adults; however, anecdotal reports in immunocompromised patients and elderly adults suggest that it may be beneficial in selected cases. Because early diagnosis is infrequent, therapy is not usually possible. The approved method of administration for ribavirin is 20 mg/mL reservoir concentration, delivered by continuous aerosol for 12–18 hr a day for 3 days. In the agitated or confused elderly patient, this regimen can be difficult to administer. More recent data from infants indicate that high-dose (60 mg/mL) short-duration therapy given over 2 hr three times a day is equally effective as standard therapy (9). Clearly, more information in this age group is needed before any general recommendation can be made.

2.2.5. Prevention

At the present time there is no licensed RSV vaccine; however, as vaccine candidates become available, older persons are a logical target population for immunization. Recent trials with subunit and live attenuated vaccines have demonstrated variable immunogenicity (9). Since an effective vaccine and treatment in this age group remain elusive, the best management is prevention. It is believed that RSV is spread by large droplets and fomites, and thus close contact or contact with contaminated environmental surfaces or skin is necessary for transmission (10). In contrast to influenza, which tends to cause explosive outbreaks, nursing home outbreaks of RSV are usually a steady trickle of cases over several weeks. It is probable that RSV is introduced into the long-term care facility by staff members or visitors. Hand washing is the single most important infection control measure for limiting the spread of RSV in the nursing home. Because compliance with hand washing is sometimes poor, some authorities have advocated the use of gloves in addition to strict hand washing. Since transmission is not by small-particle aerosol, respiratory isolation is not necessary.

2.3. Parainfluenza Viruses

The parainfluenza viruses (PIV) are members of the paramyxovirus family with four serotypes and two subgroups (1, 2, 3, 4a, 4b). Infection is almost universal by age 5 years and in young children, PIV infection causes croup, bronchiolitis, and pneumonia. Peak activity of PIV-1 and PIV-2 occurs during the fall months whereas PIV-3 occur year-round (10). Reinfections occur throughout life, and epidemiological studies indicate that PIV infections account for ≈1–15% of acute respiratory tract infections in adults. Parainfluenza infections in healthy young adults are generally manifest as mild URTI.

Comprehensive studies of parainfluenza in community-dwelling older persons using sensitive techniques are lacking, but current data indicate that, although not commonly identified, elderly persons may develop serious illness with PIV infection.

In the United Kingdom between 1972 and 1986, 2% of the total of 5781 reports of PIV disease were in persons ≥65 years of age (14). Most of the infections were PIV-1 (32%) and PIV-3 (65%). In a 15-month prospective study of 165 frail seniors attending daycare, PIV-1 or -3 accounted for only 1% of all acute respiratory illnesses (11). The most recent study of PIV as a cause of lower respiratory disease in adults was performed during 1991–1992 in the United States and identified PIV-1 in 2.5% and PIV in 3.1% of cases during epidemic periods (15). PIV-2 was very uncommon.

The impact of PIV is more well defined in institutionalized older persons. Prospective studies of respiratory illnesses in nursing homes have documented PIV infection in 4–14% of cases of respiratory illnesses (14,16). In addition, several outbreaks of PIV infection in long-term care facilities have been described with high attack rates and substantial morbidity and mortality. Five outbreaks of PIV in nursing homes were reported in the United Kingdom between 1976 and 1982 and were characterized by "chest infections," fever, coryza, and malaise. During one outbreak, four persons died of bronchopneumonia (14). Clusters of PIV types 1 and 3 have also been described in U.S. nursing homes where illnesses were characterized by fever, rhinorrhea, sore throat, and cough with several cases of pneumonia and death. Most recently, an outbreak of PIV-3 occurred in a Canadian nursing home, affecting 31% of residents and 6% of staff (16). Lower respiratory tract involvement occurred most commonly in residents requiring extended care (82%), compared with those who were in residential care (27%). Thirty-one percent were febrile and one resident was hospitalized with pneumonia. Last, infection with PIV may predispose to bacterial infection and was felt to be an indirect cause of a recent outbreak of invasive pneumococcal disease in a nursing home.

Diagnosis of PIV infection can be accomplished by viral culture of the nasopharyngeal secretions or sputum. Adults typically shed fewer viruses than do children (10). Serologic analysis of acute and convalescent blood by complement fixation or EIA can establish a diagnosis retrospectively. However, as is true of most other respiratory viral infections, a single elevated titer is not felt to be diagnostic. PIV-1 and PIV-3 infections result in heterologous antibody responses, and therefore it is not possible to distinguish the two infections serologically. Currently, there are no commercially available rapid antigen tests for the diagnosis of PIV.

Treatment of parainfluenza infection is supportive. At the present time there are no available antiviral agents with proven clinical effectiveness against PIV. Ribavirin has activity in vitro and in vivo, but to date there have not been randomized, controlled trials in humans.

An effective PIV vaccine has not yet been developed. Therefore, the prevention of PIV infection can only be accomplished by interruption of virus transmission. Although most studies suggest direct person-to-person transmission of parainfluenza, the precise mechanism is unknown. Similar to influenza virus, PIV is stable in small-particle aerosols at low humidities found in hospitals; yet outbreaks tend to proceed more slowly than influenza or other aerosol-spread infections. In the long-term care facility, infection control policies are similar to those recommended for RSV with an emphasis on hand washing, gloves, and cohorting, if possible.

2.4. Rhinovirus

Rhinoviruses are ubiquitous RNA viruses and members of the picornavirus family with over 100 antigenic types identified. These viruses account for ≈25–50% of URTI and are the most commonly identified cause of the "common cold." Rhinovirus infections occur sporadically throughout the year, but peaks of activity are seen in the fall and spring. Illnesses in healthy young adults are generally mild and self-limited but may be more severe in older adults as well as those with COPD (17,18). Rhinoviruses are rarely implicated as a cause of pneumonia, which is believed to reflect their biologic characteristics. However, recent data suggest that infection of the lower airways is possible.

Although there are few studies addressing the issue of rhinovirus infection in independent elderly persons, it would appear to be a common event. A prospective surveillance study of respiratory illnesses in the elderly living in the community using RT-PCR for diagnosis detected rhinoviruses in 121/497 (24%) respiratory illnesses, a rate six times greater than influenza A or B (13). Patients were moderately disabled with a median duration of illness of 16 days with 19% confined to bed, and 26% unable to perform their activities of daily living. Forty-three percent consulted their doctors and one patient died. Chronic ill health and smoking increased the likelihood of lower respiratory complications. Seniors living in congregate settings such as long-term care facilities or attending senior daycare centers also appear to be at risk of infection (11,19). In prospective studies of acute respiratory illnesses in nursing homes, rhinoviruses have been isolated in 6–9% of illnesses (19). In addition, rhinoviruses have been isolated from 7% of ill seniors attending daycare (20).

Rhinovirus illnesses in frail elderly persons are characterized most frequently by cough (71–94%), nasal congestion (79–89%), constitutional symptoms (43–91%), and sore throat (21–51%). Studies focusing on rhinovirus infections in frail older persons have produced conflicting data on the severity of infections in these populations (11,19). In general, rhinovirus infections are mild with low rates of pneumonia, hospitalization, and death (11). However, patients may have lower respiratory tract symptoms and persons with underlying lung disease are at highest risk for severe illness (19).

Two studies have evaluated patients hospitalized for acute respiratory illnesses for evidence of rhinovirus infection (21,22). In a study of 1198 illnesses in patients of all ages, rhinoviruses were isolated by viral culture in 3.8% of the cases. Of subjects >35 years of age, 73% had asthma, COPD, or CHF (21). Five rhinovirus infections were identified by RT-PCR in a more recent study of 100 elderly adults hospitalized with respiratory illnesses during the winter months (22). All patients had significant underlying disease and four had radiographic evidence of pneumonia and one had respiratory failure. Despite prolonged illnesses all eventually recovered and were discharged.

In the past, diagnosis of rhinovirus infection was limited to viral culture, which is felt to be insensitive. Because of many serotypes, serologic diagnosis of rhinovirus is not practical. The development of RT-PCR has improved the ability to detect rhinoviruses by approximately two- to fivefold over standard viral culture. Thus, it is likely that the true impact of rhinoviruses in older people has been underestimated and further studies are needed (13).

Since treatment is supportive and aimed toward patient comfort, specific viral diagnosis is not usually critical to the practicing physician. Particular care should be used when recommending "cold" medications to older persons, which frequently contain combinations of drugs. Antihistamines and sympathomimetics may cause adverse side effects such as confusion, urinary retention, hypertension, and tachyarrhythmias in elderly persons.

Clustering of rhinovirus infections in long-term care facilities suggests that nosocomial transmission occurs (19). Rhinoviruses are hardy viruses, surviving up to 3 hr on environmental surfaces and skin. Virus can be efficiently transferred to hands and infection produced by autoinoculation. Hand washing is the best method to interrupt transmission and the use of virucidal preparations, such as 2% iodine, may offer additional benefit.

2.5. Coronaviruses

After rhinoviruses, coronaviruses are the most frequent cause of the common cold syndrome, accounting for approximately 5–30% of upper respiratory infections (23). Coronaviruses are RNA viruses with three major serotypes, 229E, OC43, and severe acute respiratory syndrome (SARS) CoV presently identified. The recently discovered SARS coronavirus, which causes a devastating respiratory infection, will be described in another chapter (see chapter "New and Emerging Pathogens"). Peak viral activity of 229E and OC43 occurs in winter and early spring. Coronavirus primary infection typically occurs in school-age children with reinfections common throughout life.

Similar to rhinovirus infections, infections with coronaviruses generally do not result in serious illness in healthy adults. Symptoms are usually mild and include malaise, headache, sore throat, and nasal congestion (23). As with many of the respiratory viruses, exacerbations of asthma and COPD have been linked with coronavirus infection in adults (17).

Few data are available on the impact of coronavirus infections in the elderly, but two studies indicate that infection with this virus can also be more severe in frail older persons. In a prospective study by Nicholson et al. of acute respiratory illnesses in 11 nursing homes in the United Kingdom, 13 of 119 episodes were associated with coronavirus OC43 and 229E infections (24). Illnesses were described as similar to influenza and 25% had lower respiratory tract complications defined as dyspnea, wheezing, severe or productive cough. In a study of frail older persons attending daycare, 8% of respiratory infections were serologically documented to be due to coronavirus 229E or OC43 (11). Illnesses typically lasted 2 weeks and almost half of the ill persons received antibiotics. Despite being relatively debilitated, all the patients recovered without significant sequelae. Similar to rhinovirus, coronaviruses appear to account for a small number of hospitalizations in adults (21,22).

Unfortunately, the diagnosis of coronavirus infection can only be accomplished in research settings. The organism is extremely fastidious and requires tracheal organ culture for isolation (23). Complement fixation and EIA may be used to diagnose coronavirus infection serologically. RT-PCR is a sensitive tool that has been increasingly used in research settings but is also not commercially available.

No antiviral compounds are available for the treatment of coronavirus infections and management is based on providing symptomatic relief. The transmission of coronavirus is unknown and, although no specific comments on infection control policies can be made, good hand washing is recommended.

2.6. Human Metapneumovirus

Human metapneumovirus (hMPV) is a newly discovered respiratory pathogen first described by investigators in the Netherlands in 2001. This new RNA virus is genetically most closely related to RSV and belongs to the *Pneumovirinae* subfamily. Serologic analyses indicate that infection with hMPV is nearly universal by age 5 years and that the virus has been circulating for at least 50 years undetected. In temperate climates, the virus circulates predominantly in winter months overlapping with other seasonal respiratory pathogens such as influenza and RSV. Similar to RSV, primary hMPV is common in young children, accounting for approximately 12% of respiratory illnesses (25). Serologic evidence and limited clinical data indicate that reinfection with hMPV occurs throughout life. In a prospective study from New York during two winter seasons, hMPV was identified by RT-PCR or serology in 4.5% of illnesses (26). Infections were noted in all groups studied; young adults (6.6%), healthy elderly (1.7%), high-risk adults (2.9%), and residents of long term care facilities (5.4%). Additionally, hMPV accounted for 1.4% and 10.8% of hospitalizations for acute cardiopulmonary conditions in elderly and adults with high-risk conditions during two winters, respectively.

Clinical manifestations of hMPV in children are similar to RSV and range from upper respiratory infection to bronchiolitis and pneumonia (25). Young adults may be asymptomatic, whereas older adults appear to have more severe illness (26,27). When elderly outpatients were compared with young adults, the elderly experienced wheezing and dyspnea more often than did young adults. In addition, adults with chronic cardiopulmonary conditions were ill twice as long as healthy young adults and sought medical attention more commonly (26). The demographics of those requiring hospitalization appear very similar to patients hospitalized with RSV or influenza. In studies of hospitalized subjects, small numbers of patients have required intensive care and mechanical ventilation and deaths have been reported (26,27). Immunosuppression and the presence of chronic pulmonary and cardiac conditions are risk factors for poor outcome.

At the present time, diagnosis of hMPV is primarily in research settings. Isolation of hMPV in cell culture is difficult and, thus, many investigators have relied on RT-PCR and serology. Treatment of hMPV infection is supportive as antivirals for the treatment or prevention of hMPV infection are not available. The mode of transmission of hMPV is unknown but given its close relationship with RSV it likely has a similar mode of spread. Nosocomial transmission of hMPV has been documented in two pediatric studies and as with other respiratory viruses, careful hand washing is felt to be of primary importance in the prevention of spread.

2.7. Gastroenteritis Viruses

After respiratory viruses, GI viruses are the leading causes of serious viral illnesses in the elderly. Although deaths related to diarrhea have traditionally been thought to be a problem of young children in developing countries, 51% of the 28,000 diarrhea-related deaths in the United States from 1979 to 1987 occurred in adults >74 years of age compared with 11% in children <5 years old (28). The odds ratio of dying during a hospitalization involving gastroenteritis for adults aged >70 years was 52.6 compared with children <5 years of age. Residents of nursing homes are at particular risk of infectious diarrhea illness because of the potential for spread in closed populations. The majority of nursing home outbreaks of gastroenteritis are probably viral in origin since bacterial causes are not usually identified. These agents include rotavirus, enteric adenoviruses, calicivirus, Norwalk-like virus (NLV), Snow Mountain agent, and small round viruses (29). NLV are a group of antigenically distinct RNA viruses of the Caliciviridae family. Recent reports indicate that NLV have a major role in the etiology of gastroenteritis in nursing homes and are implicated in 59–86% of outbreaks. Rotaviruses are the second most commonly identified gastroenteritis virus in older persons and have been implicated in several outbreaks in elderly residents of long-term care facilities (30). The mode of transmission is assumed to be fecal–oral for most viruses, and viruses are relatively resistant to common disinfectants facilitating nosocomial dissemination. Attack rates have ranged from 36% to 66% with mortality rates of 1–10%. The typical illness includes voluminous vomiting and watery diarrhea with low-grade fever. Bloody stools are not usually seen and diarrhea typically lasts 2–3 days. Death may result from dehydration, progressing to oliguria and acidosis (28,30). A commercial rapid EIA test is available for the diagnosis of rotavirus and is available in many microbiology laboratories. Most often the diagnosis of viral gastroenteritis is made based on clinical features. However, it is important to exclude bacterial pathogens and antibiotic-associated diarrhea which may require specific antimicrobial treatment. The mainstay of treatment for viral gastroenteritis is replacement of fluid losses. In the absence of vomiting, oral rehydration therapy may be used with intravenous fluids reserved for those unable to take oral fluids.

REFERENCES

1. Cox NJ, Subbarao K. Influenza. Lancet 1999; 354:1277–1282.
2. Treanor JJ. Influenza virus. In: Mandell GL, Bennett JE, Dolin R, eds. Principles and Practices of Infectious Diseases. 5th ed. Philadelphia: Churchill Livingston, 2000: 1823–1849.
3. Centers for Disease Control and Prevention. Prevention and control of influenza. MMWR 2001; 50(RR04):1–46.
4. Thompson WW, Shay DK, Weintraub E, Brammer L, Cox N, Anderson LJ, Fukuda K. Mortality associated with influenza and respiratory syncytial virus in the United States. J Am Med Assoc 2003; 289:179–186.
5. Hall WN, Goodman RA, Noble GR, Kendal AP, Steece RS. An outbreak of influenza B in an elderly population. J Infect Dis 1981; 144:297–302.
6. Storch GA. Rapid tests for influenza. Curr Opin Pediatr 2003; 15:77–84.
7. Govaert TME, Thijs CTMCN, Masurel N, Sprenger MJW, Dinant GJ, Knottnerus JA. The efficacy of influenza vaccination in elderly individuals. A randomized double-blind placebo-controlled trial. J Am Med Assoc 1994; 272:1661–1665.
8. Nichol KL. The efficacy, effectiveness and cost-effectiveness of inactivated influenza vaccines. Vaccine 2003; 21:1769–1775.
9. Falsey AR, Walsh E. Respiratory syncytial virus infection in adults. Clin Microbiol Rev 2000; 13:371–384.
10. Hall CB. Respiratory syncytial virus and parainfluenza virus. N Engl J Med 2001; 334:1917–1928.
11. Falsey AR, McCann RM, Hall WJ, Tanner MA, Criddle MM, Formica MA, Irvine CS, Kolassa JE, Barker WH, Treanor JJ. Acute respiratory tract infection in daycare centers for older persons. J Am Geriatr Soc 1995; 43:30–36.
12. Dowell SF, Anderson LJ, Gary HE Jr, Erdman DD, Plouffe JF, File TM Jr, Marston BJ, Breiman RF. Respiratory syncytial virus is an important cause of community-acquired lower respiratory infection among hospitalized adults. J Infect Dis 1996; 174:456–462.
13. Nicholson KG, Kent J, Hammersley V, Esperanza C. Acute viral infections of upper respiratory tract in elderly people living in the community: comparative, prospective, population based study of disease burden. Br Med J 1997; 315:1060–1064.
14. Public Health Laboratory Service Communicable Disease Surveillance Centre. Parainfluenza infections in the elderly 1976–82. Br Med J 1983; 287:1619.
15. Marx A, Gary HE, Martston BJ, Erdman DD, Breiman RF, Torok TJ, Plouffe JF, File TM Jr, Anderson LJ. Parainfluenza virus infection among adults hospitalized for lower respiratory tract infection. Clin Infect Dis 1999; 29:134–140.

16. Glasgow KW, Tamblyn SE, Blair G. A respiratory outbreak due to parainfluenza virus type 3 in a home for the aged—Ontario. Can Commun Dis Rep 1995; 21:57–61.

17. Glezen WP, Greenberg SB, Atmar RL, Piedra PA, Couch RB. Impact of respiratory virus infections on persons with chronic underlying conditions. J Am Med Assoc 2000; 283:499–505.

18. Nicholson KG, Kent J, Hammersley V, Cancio E. Risk factors for lower respiratory complications of rhinovirus infections in elderly people living in the community: prospective cohort study. Br Med J 1996; 313:1119–1123.

19. Wald TG, Shult P, Krause P, Miller BA, Drinka P, Gravenstein S. A rhinovirus outbreak among residents of a long-term care facility. Ann Intern Med 1995; 123:588–593.

20. Falsey AR, McCann RM, Hall WJ, Criddle MC, Formica MA, Wycoff D, Kolassa JE. The "common cold" in frail older persons: impact of rhinovirus and coronavirus in a senior daycare center. J Am Geriatr Soc 1997; 45:706–711.

21. El-Sahly HM, Atmar RL, Glezen WP, Greenberg SB. Spectrum of clinical illness in hospitalized patients with "common cold" virus infections. Clin Infect Dis 2000; 31: 96–100.

22. Falsey AR, Walsh EE, Hayden FG. Rhinovirus and coronavirus infection-associated hospitalizations among older adults. J Infect Dis 2002; 185:1338–1341.

23. Larson HE, Reed SE, Tyrrell DAJ. Isolation of rhinoviruses and coronaviruses from 38 colds in adults. J Med Virol 1980; 5:221–229.

24. Nicholson KG, Baker DJ, Farquhar A, Hurd D, Kent J, Smith SH. Acute upper respiratory tract viral illness and influenza immunization in homes for the elderly. Epidemiol Infect 1990; 105:609–618.

25. Williams JV, Harris PA, Tollefson SJ, Halburnt-Rush LL, Pingsterhaus JM, Edwards KM, Wright PF, Crowe JE Jr. Human metapneumovirus and lower respiratory tract disease in otherwise healthy infants and children. N Engl J Med 2004; 350(5):443–450.

SUGGESTED READING

Falsey AR, Walsh EE, Hayden FG. Rhinovirus and coronavirus infection-associated hospitalizations among older adults. J Infect Dis 2002; 185:1338–1341.

Green KY, Belliot G, Taylor JL, Valdesuso J, Lew JF, Kapikian AZ, Lin FY. A predominant role for Norwalk-like viruses as agents of epidemic gastroenteritis in Maryland nursing homes for the elderly. J Infect Dis 2002; 185:133–146.

Nichol KL. The efficacy, effectiveness and cost-effectiveness of inactivated influenza vaccines. Vaccine 2003; 21:1769–1775.

Thompson WW, Shay DK, Weintraub E, Brammer L, Cox N, Anderson LJ, Fukuda K. Mortality associated with influenza and respiratory syncytial virus in the United States. J Am Med Assoc 2003; 289:179–186.

46

Parasites

Shobita Rajagopalan
*Department of Internal Medicine, Division of Infectious Diseases, Charles R. Drew
University of Medicine and Science, Martin Luther King, Jr.–Charles R. Drew Medical
Center, Los Angeles, California, U.S.A.*

Key Points:

- Parasitic infections and infestations are common in countries of Asia, Africa, Central and South America but are relatively rare in developed nations. The environment in such developing countries, i.e., overcrowding, malnutrition, contamination of food and water sources, and the presence of appropriate vectors is more conducive to the transmission of parasitic illnesses.
- The increased trend of international tourism to exotic tropical and subtropical destinations, particularly among the elderly, enhances the risk of acquiring parasitic illnesses in this older population.
- The age-associated alteration in T-cell function increases morbidity and mortality due to parasitic illnesses.
- Such risks can often be readily minimized by taking simple measures to decrease exposure, i.e., vaccine and chemoprophylaxis as recommended, following the simple principles of "boil it, peel it, cook it, or forget it" and using insect repellant when necessary.
- This review addresses the parasitic differential diagnoses of common clinical manifestations, i.e., fever, eosinophilia, and rash, affecting returning travelers including the elderly. More detailed information regarding specific parasitic infections can be reviewed from the suggested reading provided at the end of this chapter.

Parasitic diseases are common in developing nations but are relatively rare elsewhere. The environment in such countries, i.e., overcrowding, malnutrition, pollution, contamination of food and water sources, and the presence of appropriate vectors, facilitates the transmission of parasitic illnesses. From the perspective of industrialized countries, international travel to exotic tropical and subtropical destinations, especially among the elderly, enhances the risk of acquiring parasitic illnesses. The age-associated relative alteration in the T-cell population and function in addition places elderly travelers at a higher risk of more serious illnesses (1). Such risks can often be easily minimized by advocating simple measures to decrease exposure, i.e., vaccine and chemoprophylaxis as recommended, drinking bottled water, eating properly cooked meals, and using insect repellant when necessary. Casual visitors from endemic countries are less likely to spread parasitic diseases because the environmental requirements, vectors, or intermediate hosts needed for transmission are often not present in industrialized countries. However, transmission of imported infections may occur via the fecal–oral route, blood transfusion or organ transplant, or suitable local vectors.

In this selective review, we will emphasize the parasitic differential diagnoses of common clinical manifestations, i.e., fever, eosinophilia, and rash, affecting individuals including the elderly who have recently traveled to the developing world. Detailed information regarding specific parasitic diseases may be reviewed from the suggested reading section provided at the end of this chapter. Although the incidence of many of these parasitic illnesses among older travelers is unknown, surveillance systems, i.e., GeoSentinel, from the International Society of Travel Medicine and the Centers for Disease Control and Prevention, and TropNetEurop, the European Network on Imported Infectious Disease Surveillance, are beginning to yield more information. The pharmacotherapy of parasitic infections is discussed in Chapter 26: Antiparasitic Drugs.

1. ILLNESS AFTER INTERNATIONAL TRAVEL

Between 20% and 70% of the 50 million people who travel from industrialized nations to the developing world each year report some illness associated with their travel (2,3). Although most illnesses reported by travelers are mild, 1–5% of travelers become ill enough to seek medical attention either during or immediately after travel, 0.01–0.1% require medical evacuation, and 1 in 100,000 die. Individuals visiting family and friends while abroad and adventure travelers are at particularly increased risk of illness during travel. Such individuals may not perceive risks in the travel environment and may forgo recommended vaccines and chemoprophylactic regimens (4).

2. FEVER

Approximately 3% of people traveling internationally for short periods of time report fever, the presence of which requires prompt attention (5,6). The initial evaluation must focus on infections that are life-threatening, treatable, or transmissible. Careful assessment of the travel history, likely incubation period, exposure history, associated symptoms and signs, duration of fever, immunization status, use or nonuse of antimalarial chemoprophylaxis, and degree of compliance with a chemoprophylactic regimen, if used, helps to establish the diagnosis. Determining an approximate incubation period can be especially helpful in excluding possible causes of fever (Table 1). As indicated by the exposure history, time course of illness, and associated symptoms and signs, initial investigations for febrile travelers may include prompt evaluation of peripheral blood for malaria; complete and differential blood counts; liver-function tests; urinalysis; culture of blood, stool, and urine; chest radiography; and specific serologic assays.

2.1. Undifferentiated Fever

2.1.1. Malaria

Malaria is the most important cause of fever among returning travelers. Malaria caused by *Plasmodium falciparum* can be rapidly fatal and must be immediately

Table 1 Common Parasitic Causes of Fever, Distribution, and Mode of Transmission

Disease	Distribution	Mode of transmission
Incubation <14 days		
Undifferentiated fever		
Malaria	Tropics and subtropics	Bite of female anopheles mosquito
East African trypanosomiasis	Sub-Saharan East Africa	Bite of tse-tse fly
Fever with CNS involvement		
Angiostrongyloidiasis, eosinophilic meningitis	East and Southeast Asia, Jamaica	Ingestion of slug slime
East African trypanosomiasis	Sub-Saharan East Africa	Bite of tse-tse fly
Incubation 14 days to 6 weeks		
Malaria		
Acute schistosomiasis (Katayama fever)	Parts of Africa, Asia, Latin America	Skin penetration by cercariae
Amebic liver abscess		
East African trypansomiasis	Most developing countries As above	
Incubation >14 days to 6 weeks		
Malaria	Worldwide: Asia, Africa, Latin America	Bite of female anopheles mosquitoes

diagnosed or excluded in all febrile persons who have recently visited an area where malaria is endemic (7). Approximately 90% of *P. falciparum* infections are acquired in sub-Saharan Africa, and 90% of travelers who are infected begin to have symptoms within 1 month after their return (8,9). In contrast, more than 70% of cases of malaria due to *Plasmodium vivax* infection are acquired in Asia or Latin America, and only 50% of travelers infected with *P. vivax* begin to have symptoms within 1 month after their return; in approximately 2%, fever develops more than 1 year afterward. Persons who visit relatives and friends while traveling abroad are at particular risk and account for approximately 40% of reported cases of malaria in the United States. Resistance to antimalarial drugs is widespread and increasing. Although currently recommended antimalarial drugs are efficacious, they do not guarantee protection against malaria, and malaria remains an important diagnostic consideration in febrile travelers, regardless of any previous use of antimalarial agents. Although a history of fever is typically present, 10–40% of persons with malaria may be afebrile when first examined (10,11). Patterns of fever are rarely diagnostic, but fevers occurring at regular intervals of 48–72 hr are virtually pathognomonic of *P. vivax*, *Plasmodium ovale*, and *Plasmodium malariae* infections. Other symptoms at presentation, including headache, cough, and gastrointestinal problems, may mimic the constellation of symptoms in other conditions, so malaria should be considered in all febrile travelers regardless of their clinical presentation.

Examination of blood films should be repeated at least once within 12–24 hr after the first evaluation, if initial blood films are negative for malaria and if malaria is still suspected. Thrombocytopenia without leukocytosis is a characteristic feature. Splenomegaly may be present. The clinical course of malaria due to *P. falciparum* is unpredictable, and nonimmune travelers with this type of malaria should generally be admitted to the hospital to facilitate prompt therapy and to allow monitoring for complications (including hypoglycemia). Antimalarial drugs should be administered parenterally if there is evidence of severe malaria (including renal failure, respiratory distress, altered consciousness, seizures, shock, or severe anemia) or if the level of

P. falciparum in the blood exceeds 4% of the visible erythrocytes in a nonimmune patient.

2.2. Fever Associated with Involvement of the Central Nervous System

In addition to the cosmopolitan processes that may cause fever associated with neurologic changes, special considerations in travelers include malaria. Eosinophilic meningitis should prompt consideration of angiostrongyliasis; the latter is caused by invasion of the meningeal space by the rat lungworm (*Angiostrongylus cantonensis*) and was the cause of a recently reported outbreak among travelers who had visited the Caribbean (12). A number of tourists visiting game parks in northern Tanzania recently acquired East African trypanosomiasis, which is transmitted through the bite of the tsetse fly (13). This illness manifests as an erythematous swelling or chancre at the site of the fly bite, fever, headache, and myalgia, before it progresses to meningoencephalitis. During the acute phase of the disease, trypanosomes are often detectable on smears of peripheral blood.

2.3. Fever Associated with Respiratory Findings

Respiratory symptoms in a febrile traveler should suggest the presence of common respiratory pathogens such as *Streptococcus pneumoniae*, influenza viruses, and other respiratory viruses, mycoplasma, and *Legionella pneumophila*. *L. pneumophila* infection has been acquired by travelers in spas on cruise ships and in hotels. Cough, nonspecific pulmonary infiltrates, and peripheral eosinophilia should prompt consideration of Löffler's syndrome, which results from transient migration of larval helminths (ascaris, hookworm, or strongyloides) through the alveolar spaces (14).

2.4. Fever Associated with Eosinophilia

Although fever in association with peripheral eosinophilia (eosinophil count ≥400 per cubic millimeter) may be due to hematologic conditions or acute allergic reactions, the presence of both fever and eosinophilia in a traveler should prompt consideration of an infectious cause (15). Peripheral eosinophilia is characteristically associated with helminthic infections in which the worms dwell or migrate through tissues (Table 2). Diagnoses to be considered in febrile travelers with eosinophilia include acute hookworm, ascaris, or strongyloides infection; acute schistosomiasis (Katayama fever); visceral larva migrans (toxocariasis); lymphatic filariasis; and acute trichinosis (16–18). The initial evaluation of travelers with fever and eosinophilia should include examination of a stool specimen for ova and parasites; serologic tests for strongyloidiasis, schistosomiasis, or other helminthic infections; and examination of blood smears or skin snips to detect microfilariae, depending on the geographic areas of travel and the clinical findings.

3. DIARRHEA

Many travelers to developing countries report diarrhea. Most episodes of traveler's diarrhea resolve during or shortly after travel, often in response to antimicrobial and

Table 2 Parasitic Causes of Fever and Eosinophilia

Parasitic diseases	Eosinophilia[a]
Dientamoeba fragilis infection[b]	Absent or mild
Trichuriasis (whipworm infection)	Absent or mild
Enterobiasis (pinworm infection)	Absent or mild
Schistosomiasis	Absent or mild; may be moderate to high in acute schistosomiasis (Karayama fever)
Cysticerosis (*Taenia solium* infection, larva stage)	Absent or mild; may be moderated if encysted larvae die and release antigen
Echinococensis (hydarid disease)	Absent or mild; may increase in severity if cyst rupture or leak
Chronic clonorchiasis and opisthorchiasis (liver fluke infection)	Absent or mild; may be moderate or marked in early infection
Isosporiasis[b]	Absent (in immunocompromised persons) or mild
Paragonimiasis	Absent or mild; moderate or marked during larval migration
Hookworm infection	Absent or mild, moderate or marked during larval migration
Sparganosis	Absent or mild
Strongylodiasis	Absent (in disseminated infection), mild, or moderate
Ascaris lumbricoides infection (larval stage)	Mild or moderate
Angioserongyliasis (*Angiostrongylus cantonensis* infection)	Mild or moderate
Gnathostomiasis onchocerciasis	Mild, moderate, or marked
Fascioliasis (*Fasciola hepatica* or liver fluke infection)	Mild, moderate, or marked during larval migration
Lymphatic filariasis	Mild, moderate, or marked
Loiasis	Moderate or marked
Toxocariasis	Moderate or marked
Acute trichinosis	Moderate or marked
Tropical pulmonary eosinophilia (occult lymphatic filariasis)	Marked

[a]Eosinophilia is considered absent when there are less than 400 eosinophils per cubic millimeter of peripheral blood, mild when there are 400–1000 eosinophils per cubic millimeter of peripheral blood, moderate if there are 1000–3000 eosinophils per cubic millimeter of peripheral blood, and marked when there are greater than 3000 eosinophils per cubic millimeter of peripheral blood.
[b]Only protozoal infections associated with eosinophilia.

antimotility agents. Five to ten percent of the travelers report diarrhea that lasts for 2 weeks or longer, and 1–3% report diarrhea that lasts 4 weeks or longer (19). Causative bacterial or viral agents may be identified in 50–75% of travelers with diarrhea that lasts less than 2 weeks (20). As the duration of diarrhea increases, the likelihood of identifying a specific infectious cause decreases, although the likelihood of diagnosing a parasitic infection increases (21) (Table 3). *Giardia lamblia*, *Cryptosporidium parvum*, *Entamoeba histolytica*, and *Cyclospora cayetanensis* are the most frequently identified parasites, although they are detected in fewer than one-third of travelers with chronic diarrhea and in only 1–5% of travelers with acute diarrhea (22,23).

Table 3 Parasitic Causes of Diarrhea

Duration of diarrhea	Parasitic differentials
Acute (duration < 2 weeks)	
	G. lamblia
	C. parvum
	E. histolytica
	C. cayatenensis
	Isospora belli
	Balantidium coli
	Trichinella spiralis
Chronic or persistent (duration 2–4 weeks)	
Microsporidial	*Enterocytozooan bineusi*,
	Encephalitozooan intestinalis
Protozoal	*G. lamblia*
	E. histolytica
	C. parvum
	C. cayetenensis
	Dientameba fragilis
Helminthic	*Trichuris trichura*
	S. stercoralis
	Schistosoma
	Capillaria philippinensis
	Fasciolopsis buski
	Metagonimus yokogawai

Source: Modified from Ryan ET, Wilson ME, Kain KC. N Engl J Med 2002; 347:505–516.

Amebic dysentery, which is caused by *E. histolytica*, often presents insidiously (over a period of days) and may be complicated by hepatic abscess formation. If no causative agent is identified, persons with chronic inflammatory enteropathy should be further evaluated for possible inflammatory bowel disease or cancer.

Prolonged traveler's diarrhea with malabsorption should prompt consideration of a protozoal infection of the small bowel (especially infection with *G. lamblia*) and tropical sprue (24). Though pathologically indistinguishable from nontropical sprue (i.e., gluten-sensitive enteropathy or celiac disease), tropical sprue is not associated with antigliadin and antiendomysial serum antibodies and does not respond to the removal of gluten from the diet; it does respond to a prolonged course of oral tetracycline and folate. Common noninfectious causes of chronic diarrhea in travelers include postinfectious disaccharidase deficiency and irritable bowel syndrome. Diarrhea that begins more than 1 month after travel is probably not due to exposure during travel.

In persons with diarrhea, a specimen of stool should be cultured for enteric pathogens and examined microscopically for ova and parasites if there is evidence of an invasive enteropathy, the diarrhea is persistent, the diarrhea is unresponsive to empirical therapy, or the infected person is immunocompromised. The sensitivity of microscopical examination of a single stool specimen for the detection of ova and parasites varies, depending on the parasite, but it generally exceeds 80% (25). The likelihood of identifying a parasite may be increased by examining additional stool samples or by performing immunofluorescence or enzyme immunoassays for specific parasites, including *G. lamblia, C. parvum*, and *E. histolytica*. Analysis of serum for antibodies against *E. histolytica*, *Strongyloides stercoralis*, and schistosoma may also be useful diagnostic aids.

In many cases of persistent diarrhea, no known causative agent is identified (26). In these cases, some experts recommend an empirical course of an antimicrobial agent such as a fluoroquinolone or a macrolide for suspected bacterial diarrhea or metronidazole (or a related agent) for presumed giardiasis, since *G. lamblia* is the most commonly identified intestinal parasite in travelers. Multiple courses of antimicrobial agents should be avoided. Persons whose diarrhea does not improve may benefit from more extensive evaluation, such as endoscopic examination and biopsy, to exclude entities such as tropical sprue and inflammatory bowel disease.

4. DERMATOLOGIC CONDITIONS

Dermatologic conditions are common among persons who have traveled recently (27–29). The location of lesions, their pattern (maculopapular, nodular, ulcerative, or linear), and the presence or absence of associated symptoms (such as pain, pruritus, and fever) are useful in establishing the diagnosis.

4.1. Papules

Bites from insects (such as bedbugs and fleas) cause pruritic, papular lesions that generally occur in clusters or in a linear distribution (Fig. 1, panel A). Scabies (due to *Sarcoptes scabiei* infection) is common in the developing world, and adventurous backpackers and sexually active travelers are those most commonly infected. Seabather's eruption is a pruritic, papular rash that tends to be confined to the skin that is covered by a bathing suit; however, it can occur elsewhere as well (Fig. 1, panel B) (30). It is caused by larval forms of sea anemones (e.g., *Edwardsiella lineata*) and jellyfish (e.g., *Linuche unguiculata*) that become trapped under bathing-suit fabric after exposure to salt water. In contrast, cercarial dermatitis usually involves exposed skin and results from penetration of the skin by schistosomal cercariae in freshwater (in cases of swimmer's itch) (Fig. 1, panel C) or coastal water (in cases of clam digger's itch). In expatriates and long-term travelers, particularly those returning from Africa, a pruritic papular rash may be due to onchocerciasis (caused by *Onchocerca volvulus*) (31). The clinician should note that drug reactions may also manifest as maculopapular, urticarial, or fixed eruptions on the skin.

4.2. Subcutaneous Swellings and Nodules

Common causes of fixed, painful subcutaneous swellings include myiasis, tungiasis, and furuncles. Myiasis is caused by invasion of the skin by the larvae of diptera (flies), including *Cordylobia anthropophaga* (the tumbu fly) in Africa and *Dermatobia hominis* (the botfly) in Latin America. Myiasis lesions resemble boils but have a central opening through which serosanguinous material oozes and through which the larvae may emerge (Fig. 1, panel D). Patients often report intermittent pain and a sensation of movement in the area of the lesion. Tungiasis (also known as jiggers), seen in travelers returning from Latin America, Africa, or India, develops after the female sand flea, *Tunga penetrans*, invades the skin, often around the toenails and soles (Fig. 1, panel E). Infection with *Loa loa* may become evident years after exposure as eyeworm or as migratory areas of angioedema (Calabar swellings),

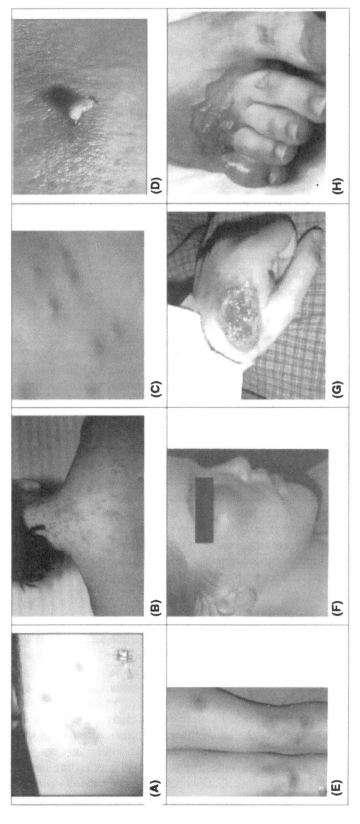

Figure 1 Dermatological manifestations of infections in returned travelers. (**A**) Bed bug bites linear and grouped papular lesions. *Source:* www.firstcoast-news.com/health/news. (**B**) Seabathers eruption. *Source:* http://www.fau.edu/safe/sealice4.jpg. (**C**) Cercarial dermatitis. *Source:* http://dermatlas.med.jh-mi.edu/derm/result.cfm?Pattern=1524359377. (**D**) Myiasis. *Source:* http://www.medizin.unituebingen.de/~webitm/myiasis.jpg. (**E**) Tungiasis. *Source:* http://forlag.fadl.dk/sample/derma/images/472.jpg. (**F**) Calabar swelling face. *Source:* http://www.medicine.mcgill.ca/ tropmed/txt/lecture4.htm. (**G**) Cutaneous leishmaniasis. *Source:* http://www3.baylor.edu/~Charles_Kemp/hand.jpg. (**H**) Cutaneous larva migrans. *Source:* http://www.emedicine.-com/ped/topic1278.htm.

thought to be inflammatory reactions to adult worms (Fig. 1, panel F) (32). Acute East African trypanosomiasis is characterized by a relatively painless, erythematous, indurated, fixed swelling that may ulcerate; it may be mistaken for a focal cellulitis.

4.3. Ulcers

Although less common, ulcers due to cutaneous leishmaniasis are important to recognize (33). These painless ulcers typically enlarge slowly, with a granulomatous or crusted base and raised margins (Fig. 1, panel G). New World leishmaniasis due to *Leishmania (Viannia) braziliensis* complex may progress to form destructive localized recrudescences on mucosal surfaces. Leishmaniasis is occasionally manifested as isolated lymphadenopathy or as lymphocutaneous changes resembling sporotrichosis or *Mycobacterium marinum* infection.

4.4. Linear and Migratory Lesions

Cutaneous larva migrans is the most frequent serpiginous lesion among travelers (Fig. 1, panel H). It results from the migration of animal hookworms (e.g., *Ancylostoma braziliense* and *Ancylostoma caninum*) in superficial tissues. It is usually acquired after direct contact of the skin with soil or sand contaminated with dog or cat feces. The lesions, which may initially be papular or vesicular, are pruritic and are commonly found on the foot or buttock. *S. stercoralis* larvae may be rapidly mobile (moving at approximately 5 cm/hr) and produce a cutaneous track (larva currens) that is often perianal. Phytophotodermatitis results from exposure of the skin to psoralen-containing compounds, such as those present in limes. Phytophotodermatitis results when the psoralens are exposed to ultraviolet light, resulting in painless, nonpruritic, hyperpigmented streaks that generally do not expand or migrate after presentation.

REFERENCES

1. Humphreys NE, Richard KG. Effects of ageing on the immunoregulation of parasitic infection. Infect Immun 2002; 70:5148–5157.
2. Steffen R, Rickenbach M, Wilhelm U, Helminger A, Schar M. Health problems after travel to developing countries. J Infect Dis 1987; 156:84–91.
3. Hill DR. Health problems in a large cohort of Americans traveling to developing countries. J Travel Med 2000; 7:259–266.
4. Ryan ET, Kain KC. Health advice and immunizations for travelers. N Engl J Med 2000; 342:1716–1725.
5. MacLean J, Lalonde R, Ward B. Fever from the tropics. In: Mabley P, Jong EC, Keystone JS, eds. Travel Medicine Advisor. Vol. 5. Atlanta: American Health Consultants, 1994:27.2–27.14.
6. Doherty JF, Grant AD, Bryceson AD. Fever as the presenting complaint of travellers returning from the tropics. QJM 1995; 88:277–281.
7. World Health Organization. Severe falciparum malaria. Trans R Soc Trop Med Hyg 2000; 94(suppl 1):S1–S90.
8. Newman RD, Barber AM, Roberts J, Holtz T, Steketee RW, Parise ME. Malaria surveillance—United States, 1999. MMWR CDC Surveill Summ 2002; 51:15–28.
9. Kain KC, Harrington MA, Tennyson S, Keystone JS. Imported malaria: prospective analysis of problems in diagnosis and management. Clin Infect Dis 1998; 27:142–149.

10. Svenson JE, MacLean JD, Gyorkos TW, Keystone J. Imported malaria: clinical presentation and examination of symptomatic travelers. Arch Intern Med 1995; 155:861–868.

11. Dorsey G, Gandhi M, Oyugi JH, Rosenthal PJ. Difficulties in the prevention, diagnosis, and treatment of imported malaria. Arch Intern Med 2000; 160:2505–2510.

12. Slom TJ, Cortese MM, Gerber SI, Jones RC, Holtz TH, Lopez AS, Zambrano CH, Sufit RL, Sakolvaree Y, Chaicumpa W, Herwaldt BL, Johnson S. An outbreak of eosinophilic meningitis caused by Angiostrongylus cantonensis in travelers returning from the Caribbean. N Engl J Med 2002; 346:668–675.

13. Jelinek T, Bisoffi Z, Bonazzi L, Van Thiel P, Bronner U, De Frey A, Gundersen SG, McWhinney P, Ripamonti D. Cluster of African trypanosomiasis in travelers to Tanzanian national parks. Emerg Infect Dis 2002; 8:634–635.

14. Habib NA, Behrens RH. Respiratory infections in the traveler. Curr Opin Pulm Med 2000; 6:246–249.

15. Schulte C, Krebs B, Nothdurft HD, von Sonnenburg F, Loscher T. Diagnostic significance of blood eosinophilia in returning travelers. Clin Infect Dis 2002; 34:407–411.

16. Doherty JF, Moody AH, Wright SG. Katayama fever: an acute manifestation of schistosomiasis. Br Med J 1996; 313:1071–1072.

17. Harries AD, Myers B, Bhattacharrya D. Eosinophilia in Caucasians returning from the tropics. Trans R Soc Trop Med Hyg 1986; 80:327–328.

18. Libman MD, MacLean JD, Gyorkos TW. Screening for schistosomiasis, filariasis, and strongyloidiasis among expatriates returning from the tropics. Clin Infect Dis 1993; 17:353–359.

19. Castelli F, Pezzoli C, Tomasoni L. Epidemiology of travelers' diarrhea. J Travel Med 2001; 8(suppl 2):S26–S30.

20. Ericsson CD. Travelers' diarrhea: epidemiology, prevention, and self-treatment. Infect Dis Clin North Am 1998; 12:285–303.

21. Von Sonnenburg F, Tornieporth N, Waiyaki P, Lowe B, Peruski LF Jr, DuPont HL, Mathewson JJ, Steffen R. Risk and aetiology of diarrhoea at various tourist destinations. Lancet 2000; 356:133–134.

22. DuPont HL, Capsuto EG. Persistent diarrhea in travelers. Clin Infect Dis 1996; 22:124–128.

23. Okhuysen PC. Traveler's diarrhea due to intestinal protozoa. Clin Infect Dis 2001; 33:110–114.

24. Thielman NM, Guerrant RL. Persistent diarrhea in the returned traveler. Infect Dis Clin North Am 1998; 12:489–501.

25. Senay H, MacPherson D. Parasitology: diagnostic yield of stool examination. Can Med Assoc J 1989; 140:1329–1331.

26. Donowitz M, Kokke FT, Saidi R. Evaluation of patients with chronic diarrhea. N Engl J Med 1995; 332:725–729.

27. Caumes E, Carriere J, Guermonprez G, Bricaire F, Danis M, Gentilini M. Dermatoses associated with travel to tropical countries: a prospective study of the diagnosis and management of 269 patients presenting to a tropical disease unit. Clin Infect Dis 1995; 20:542–548.

28. Kain KC. Skin lesions in returned travelers. Med Clin North Am 1999; 83:1077–1102.

29. Wilson ME. Skin problems in the traveler. Infect Dis Clin North Am 1998; 12:471–488.

30. Freudenthal AR, Joseph PR. Seabather's eruption. N Engl J Med 1993; 329:542–544.

31. McCarthy JS, Ottesen EA, Nutman TB. Onchocerciasis in endemic and nonendemic populations: differences in clinical presentation and immunologic findings. J Infect Dis 1994; 170:736–741.

32. Klion AD, Massougbodji A, Sadeler BC, Ottesen EA, Nutman TB. Loiasis in endemic and nonendemic populations: immunologically mediated differences in clinical presentation. J Infect Dis 1991; 163:1318–1325.

33. Herwaldt BL, Stokes SL, Juranek DD. American cutaneous leishmaniasis in U.S. travelers. Ann Intern Med 1993; 118:779–784. (Erratum, Ann Intern Med 1993; 119:173.)

SUGGESTED READING

Centers for Disease Control and Prevention Parasitic Disease Division. http://www.dpd.
cdc.gov/dpdx/.
Ryan ET, Wilson ME, Kain KC. Illness after international travel. N Engl J Med 2002;
347:505–516.

47

New and Emerging Pathogens

Mark Loeb

Departments of Pathology and Molecular Medicine and Clinical Epidemiology and Biostatistics, McMaster University, Hamilton, Ontario, Canada

Key Points:

- Clinical presentation of severe acute respiratory syndrome (SARS) is nonspecific.
- Diagnosis of emerging infections remains an important clinical challenge.
- Older adults are at high risk of complications of SARS and West Nile virus (WNV) infection.
- At present, there is no effective therapy for these infections.
- Although efforts are under way, there are presently no effective vaccines for SARS or WNV.

The Institute of Medicine in 1992 defined emerging infections as "New, reemerging or drug resistant infections whose incidence in humans has increased within the past two decades or whose incidence threatens to increase in the near future" (1). Recently, it has become evident that severe acute respiratory syndrome (SARS) and West Nile virus (WNV), two such emerging infections, pose an important threat to the health of older adults. This chapter will focus on these agents and will summarize available evidence of the impact of these infections on older adults. The first section of this chapter will review SARS and the second section will discuss WNV.

1. SEVERE ACUTE RESPIRATORY SYNDROME

1.1. Epidemiology and Clinical Relevance

SARS has been documented in over 8400 persons globally with cases in Asia, Europe, and North America. A novel coronavirus has been identified as the etiologic agent. The first cases of SARS arose from Guandong province, in the south of China in November 2002. The outbreak was officially recognized by the World Health Organization February 13, 2003, based on initial reports from the Chinese government. Unfortunately, many more deaths ensued over the next 5 months.

Both the global and the local spread of SARS are related to so-called "super-spreading" events. A critical event for the global spread of SARS occurred at the Hotel Metropol in Hong Kong in late February 2003. A physician who had treated hospitalized patients in the city of Guangzhou and who was symptomatic with SARS during his stay in Hong Kong became the source of infection for 12 people, the majority of whom were staying on the same floor as him. These individuals, also tourists, eventually sought medical care in hospitals in Hong Kong, Vietnam, Singapore, Ireland, the United States, and Canada. There was secondary spread in all these countries with the exception of United States and Ireland.

Spread of SARS occurred primarily within the healthcare setting. The secondary spread that occurred, predominantly in acute care hospitals, was largely due to a failure to recognize a new respiratory syndrome along with the associated delay in assuming appropriate infection control precautions soon enough. Fortunately, spread of SARS to elderly residents of long-term care facilities was limited. However, transfer of patients to a nursing home did lead to secondary spread in Hong Kong (2). The incubation period of SARS, estimated to range from 2 to 10 days with a mean incubation period of 6 days, is sufficiently long enough for some people to be presymptomatic on admission and develop symptoms later. Importantly, there is no evidence that individuals who are asymptomatic can transmit the virus. The incidence of asymptomatic infection appears to be very low. In fact, in the Toronto outbreak <2% of healthcare workers with multiple exposures to SARS patients developed serological evidence of infection.

The reproductive number of the SARS coronavirus, that is, the expected number of infectious secondary cases generated by an average infectious case in a completely susceptible population, has been estimated to range from 2.2 to 3.7 (3). This figure is not particularly high compared to the reproductive numbers of other respiratory viruses spread by respiratory droplet aerosol, such as influenza or measles. The clinical experience with SARS reflects this, i.e., once appropriate infection control precautions are instituted, the virus can promptly be contained and transmission can be stopped. The fact that SARS, unlike influenza, for example, is not efficiently transmitted in the community supports this as well. The notable exception to the lack of community transmission was the spread at the Hotel Metropol, where it is hypothesized that virus detected by polymerase chain reaction (PCR) in vomit near the index case's room or elevator may have been the source of environmental transmission. Community spread also occurred at Amoy garden in Hong Kong, an apartment complex where the leading hypothesis is that sewage contaminated with small virus-containing droplets entered bathrooms of the apartment complex through dried-up U traps (4).

The epidemiologic evidence suggests that within hospitals, the transmission mode was by droplet, although limited aerosol transmission may also have played a role. Superspreading events, defined as spread from one source patient to many others, played an important role. In one report of SARS transmission in a Beijing hospital, patients linked to superspreading tended to be older, were more ill, had more contacts, and were more efficient at spreading the virus compared to other source patients not linked to superspreading (5).

To date, there have been a number of studies that have addressed risk factors for acquiring SARS. There is no evidence to suggest that the elderly are prone to infection with SARS; however, there is ample evidence that outcomes are worse. A consistent finding is that exposure to aerosol-generating procedures is a high risk. For example, a retrospective cohort study in a Toronto hospital revealed that assisting with intubation as well as suctioning prior to intubation was associated with a fourfold risk of acquiring SARS among critical care nurses (6). Manipulation of an oxygen mask resulted in a ninefold increased risk to nursing staff. Studies to further define risk factors among household contacts and hospitalized patients are ongoing.

1.2. Microbiology

SARS is caused by a novel strain of coronovirus (SARS-CoV) believed to have originated from an animal in southern China, such as a masked palm civet. Corono viruses are single-stranded RNA viruses known to cause illness in both animals and humans. The virus belongs to a new group within the coronavirus family. An important feature of the SARS-CoV is that, unlike other respiratory viruses, the viral load increases until about the 10th day of illness and then it diminishes (4). This has implications for both infection control precautions as well as clinically. The chance of secondary transmission if a case is put into isolation before the viral load has peaked can be lessened. Clinically, one often sees worsening of symptoms after the first week of illness. Molecular epidemiologic studies reveal that the SARS-CoV from outbreaks in Hong Kong, Vietnam, Singapore, Toronto, and Taiwan are clonally related whereas those from Guangdong province are more diverse genetically (4). This may imply that some molecular lineages are more likely to be transmitted than others.

1.3. Clinical Disease

At presentation, SARS is characterized by fever, myalgia, cough, chills, or rigors. Unfortunately, this syndrome is nonspecific and the clinical features cannot be used to distinguish it from other viral or bacterial respiratory syndromes. The most common symptom is fever, occurring in virtually all cases. Shortness of breath occurs later in the illness. Some patients have diarrhea and the others have nausea and vomiting. In the elderly, SARS may present as an afebrile illness, where malaise and decreased appetite are the main features (7). Alternatively, it can present with a low-grade fever with few respiratory symptoms (8). When compared to younger patients with SARS, older patients are less likely to present with fever, chills, and diarrhea (7). This pattern is similar to community-acquired pneumonia, where symptoms and signs of pneumonia are less distinct in older adults.

There are a number of factors associated with a poor prognosis in SARS. An important factor is older age. Studies have shown that older patients are at substantially higher risk of death (7). In a study from China, the mortality rate among patients aged ≥ 50 years was 13 times that for patients aged < 50 years (9). In another study, every 10-year increase in age was associated with a twofold increase in death (10). In a study from Hong Kong, multivariate analysis revealed that age > 60 years and serum lactate dehydrogenase level > 3.8 μkat/L at presentation were independent predictors of mortality (11). Comorbidity, especially diabetes mellitus but heart disease also, has been repeatedly demonstrated to be a risk factor for adverse outcomes in SARS (4). The aforementioned risk factors were noted in a Toronto study of 196 patients with SARS (12). Thirty-eight (19%) SARS patients became critically ill (12). The interquartile range age of the 38 patients was 57.4 (39.0–69.6) years. The median duration between initial symptoms and admission to the intensive care unit was 8 (5–10) days. Twenty-nine (76%) required mechanical ventilation. Mortality at 28 days was 13 (34%) of 38 patients and for those requiring mechanical ventilation, mortality was 13 (45%) of 29 patients. Six patients (16%) remained mechanically ventilated at 28 days. Two of these patients had died by 8 weeks' follow-up. Patients who died were more often older, had preexisting diabetes mellitus, and on admission to hospital were more likely to have bilateral radiographic infiltrates (12).

Along with increased lactate dehydrogenase, elevated serum creatinine kinase and alanine aminotransferase are often seen in SARS. However, these laboratory indices cannot discriminate SARS from other respiratory infections. The chest radiograph is abnormal in the majority of patients with SARS, the most common abnormalities being ground-glass opacifacations. Again, these findings are not specific for SARS.

1.4. Diagnosis

One of the most important challenges of SARS has been making the diagnosis. The lack of an accurate real-time diagnostic test allowed SARS to be spread in hospitals around the world. SARS can be diagnosed very accurately retrospectively using serology. That is, antibodies to the virus will appear in >95% of infected patients at least 21 days (but preferably 28 days) or longer after onset of symptoms. Although this is of important epidemiologic value, it is not helpful to the front-line clinician who must decide whether a patient has SARS. A number of groups are working on developing nucleic acid amplification tests, such as reverse transcriptase-PCR; however, none of these tests have a sufficiently high positive or negative predictive value to date. Although SARS-CoV is readily cultured, the infection control risks to laboratory workers do not make routine culturing of the virus an attractive option. Other types of assays being studied, including immunoblot assays and radioimmunoassays, are still in a developmental phase. The utility of clinical symptoms in diagnosing SARS is nondiagnostic.

1.5. Treatment

There are a number of agents that have been proposed as therapy for SARS. However, there have not been any randomized, controlled trials of therapy to document efficacy. Ribavirin, a synthetic nucleoside antiviral agent with inhibitory activity against both DNA and RNA viruses, was commonly used during the SARS outbreak. Usually in an aerosolized form, it has been used for the treatment of respiratory syncytial virus pneumonitis in both adults and children. The combination of oral ribavirin and interferon has also been shown to be efficacious in the treatment of chronic hepatitis C. High-dose intravenous ribavirin has been used in the treatment of Lassa fever and hemorrhagic fever with renal syndrome. The theoretical rationale for using this agent was its in vitro activity against other respiratory viruses, including respiratory syncytial virus and influenza, and its use began before the agent of SARS was fully defined. There are no systematic evaluations of efficacy of ribavirin for SARS. However, there are reports of toxicity. In Toronto, 61% of the patients with SARS who were treated with ribavirin developed hemolytic anemia. Hypocalcemia and hypomagnesemia were reported in 58% and 46% of patients, respectively (13).

There have been reports of benefit with treatment from high-dose corticosteroids; however, there have been no randomized, controlled trials to substantiate efficicacy (14). One concern about these regimens is long-lasting adverse reactions, such as avascular necrosis and neuromuscular sequelae.

There are theoretical and limited clinical data to suggest a role for interferon-alpha (IFNα) in the treatment of SARS. Evidence exists that prophylactic treatment of SARS coronavirus-infected macaques with the pegylated IFNα significantly reduces viral replication and excretion, viral antigen expression by type 1 pneumocytes, and pulmonary damage when compared with untreated macaques (15). In a study of 22 patients with probable SARS, IFN treatment was associated with a shorter time to resolution of radiologic infiltrates, better oxygen saturation, less of an increase in creatine kinase, and more rapid resolution of lactate dehydrogenase (16).

1.6. Prevention

There are many groups that are presently working on a vaccine against the SARS-CoV. One of the obstacles has been the inability to find an animal model where the disease manifestations are reliably reproduced when the animal is challenged with the virus. Once an animal model is found, testing where these animals are vaccinated, then challenged with the SARS-CoV can begin. Research groups are currently working on vaccines using inactivated virus, recombinant virus, or plasmid DNA.

In the absence of a vaccine, surveillance measures are an important strategy for preventing the spread of SARS. Use of personal protective equipment is also important. Evidence exists suggesting that use of a mask can reduce the relative risk of SARS by 80% in critical care units (6).

2. WEST NILE VIRUS

2.1. Epidemiology and Clinical Relevance

Since the 1999 outbreak in New York City, WNV has emerged as an important human pathogen in North America. There has been a steady increase in the annual incidence of human cases of WNV infection in the United States and Canada. This reached epidemic proportions in the summer of 2003. Given the low background of immunity in the population, the spread of WNV through migrating birds will likely result in continued future human epidemics.

Few studies have addressed risk factors of infection with WNV. In a study from Ontario, it was found that time spent outside at dusk or dawn on a nonworkday was a significant risk factor for WNV infection (17). This is consistent with the findings of the New York City investigation, where univariate analysis revealed an increased risk of infection in individuals who spent ≥ 2 hr outdoors with the risk increasing if no insect repellent was used (18). There is no evidence that older adults are at increased risk of infection than younger individuals; however, outcomes are clearly worse in older people, as described later.

2.2. Microbiology

Phylogenetic analysis done on nucleic acid sequence data from a number of full-length genomes has demonstrated two distinct lineages of WNV strains (19). Complete genome sequences performed on WNV strains in North America have revealed little genetic variability. This suggests that host response may play a key role in pathogenesis.

2.3. Clinical Disease

The pathological changes within the central nervous system (CNS) due to WNV, an enveloped RNA virus, appear to be due to several factors, including the direct result of viral proliferation within neuronal and glial cells, cytotoxic immune response to infected cells, diffuse perivascular inflammation, and microglial nodule formation (20). However, the range of clinical manifestations of WNV infection is highly variable. Of infected persons, ≈20% develop mild symptoms (West Nile fever, e.g., fever, malaise, headache, myalgia, and rash), and about 1 in 150 develop meningitis or encephalitis (21). The incidence of severe neurological syndromes increases with age and includes encephalitis, meningitis, acute flaccid paralysis, peripheral neuropathy, polyradiculopathy, optic neuritis, and acute demyelinating encephalitis.

Although there is no evidence that older adults are at higher risk of infection (proportion of people infected ranges from 2% to 6% for various age groups), there is consistent evidence to support the fact that older adults are at higher risk of complications due to WNV infection (21). The incidence of neuroinvasive disease, defined by meningitis, encephalitis, or acute flaccid paralysis, increases with age. Individuals ≥65 years of age who are infected have a 1 in 50 chance of developing a complication as compared to 1 in 150 infected aged <65 years. In one study of 32 elderly patients with WNV, mortality was 22% with all deaths occurring in those ≥78 years of age (22).

Limited data suggest that there may be substantial long-term morbidity among patients with severe WNV infection. One follow-up survey conducted by the New York City Department of Health found that at 12 months postdischarge, patients had frequent persistent symptoms including fatigue (67%), memory loss (50%), difficulty in walking (49%), muscle weakness (44%), and depression (38%). Three case series have noted substantial morbidity at hospital discharge. Of 19 patients hospitalized in New York and New Jersey in 2000, 10 (53%) had recovered but not to previous functional status (22). Upon discharge, seven (37%) were fully ambulatory, five (26%) were ambulatory with assistance, and two (11%) were bedridden. A case series of patients in southern Ontario with severe WNV infection revealed that only 13 of 47 (28%) were discharged home without support (23). In these retrospective studies, no standardized measures of functional, neurological, or cognition were used. A recently reported prospective case series by investigators at the Center for Disease Control and Prevention described 8-month outcomes in 16 patients with neurological manifestations of WNV infection (24). Of the 15 surviving patients, four (27%) were either dependent or undergoing rehabilitation at 8 months. Five patients, including all three with acute flaccid paralysis, described continuing difficulties with daily activities such as grooming, housekeeping, and mobility. Ten (67%) of surviving patients reported persistent fatigue at 8 months while four (27%) had persistent cognitive deficits including memory, short-term recall, and slowness of thought. While neurological status was assessed, no standardized measures of health-related quality of life, limb strength, fatigue severity, or functional scores were reported. Nevertheless, these data suggest that patients with acute flaccid paralysis may have a worse prognosis.

Interestingly, in a study of 32 older patients, of the 25 survivors, 22 returned to premorbid baseline function at 3 months. In contrast to other viral infections, chronic conditions had no impact on outcome (22).

2.4. Diagnosis

The diagnosis of WNV infection is usually made using serology. Acute infection is diagnosed by detecting IgM antibody in serum or cerebrospinal fluid (CSF) using an enzyme-linked immunosorbent assay. The presence of IgM antibodies in the CSF indicates infection of the CNS. False-positive WNV IgM antibody results can occur from recent infection with another flavivirus such as dengue. Confirmation of an acute WNV infection is done using a plaque reduction neutralization test. It is important to note that IgM antibodies can persist for over a year, so that a positive IgM test may be unrelated to current illness under investigation (25).

2.5. Treatment

There is no effective treatment for WNV infection. There have been no reported trials of efficacy of antiviral agents. Agents that have been considered for therapy include ribavin, interferon, gamma globulin, and corticosteroids.

2.6. Prevention

Although animal vaccines exist, there are presently no human vaccines available. Personal protection can reduce the risk of WNV infection by 50% (17). This is particularly important for the elderly, where the risk of complications is increased.

REFERENCES

1. Lederberg J, Shope RE, Oaks SC Jr, eds. Emerging Infections: Microbial Threats to Health in the United States. Committee on Emerging Microbial Threats to Health, Institute of Medicine. Washington: National Academy Press, 1992.
2. Ho WW, Hui E, Kwok TC, Woo J, Leung NW. Outbreak of severe acute respiratory syndrome in a nursing home. J Am Geriatr Soc 2003; 51:1504–1505.
3. Lipsitch M, Cohen T, Cooper B, Robins JM, Ma S, James L, Gopalakrishna G, Chew SK, Tan CC, Samore MH, Fisman D, Murray M. Transmission dynamics and control of severe acute respiratory syndrome. Science 2003; 300:1966–1970.
4. Peiris JS, Yuen KY, Osterhaus AD, Stohr K. The severe acute respiratory syndrome. N Engl J Med 2003; 18(349):2431–2441.
5. Shen Z, Ning F, Zhou W, He X, Lin C, Chin DP, Zhu Z, Schuchat A. Superspreading SARS events, Beijing, 2003. Emerg Infect Dis 2004; 10:256–260.
6. Loeb M, McGeer A, Henry B, Ofner M, Rose D, Hlywka T, Levie J, McQueen J, Smith S, Moss L, Smith A, Green K, Walter SD. SARS among critical care nurses, Toronto Emerg. Infect Dis 2004; 10:251–255.
7. Chan TY, Miu KY, Tsui CK, Yee KS, Chan MH. A comparative study of clinical features and outcomes in young and older adults with severe acute respiratory syndrome. J Am Geriatr Soc 2004; 52:1321–1325.
8. Cheng HM, Kwok T. Mild SARS in elderly patients. Can Med Assoc J 2004; 16(170):927.
9. Zou Z, Yang Y, Chen J, Xin S, Zhang W, Zhou X, Mao Y, Hu L, Liu D, Chang B, Chang W, Liu Y, Ma X, Wang Y, Liu X. Prognostic factors for severe acute respiratory syndrome: a clinical analysis of 165 cases. Clin Infect Dis 2004; 38:483–489.
10. Lee N, Hui D, Wu A, Chan P, Cameron P, Joynt GM, Ahuja A, Yung MY, Leung CB, To KF, Lui SF, Szeto CC, Chung S, Sung JJ. A major outbreak of severe acute respiratory syndrome in Hong Kong. N Engl J Med 2003; 348:1984–1986.
11. Choi KW, Chau TN, Tsang O, Tso E, Chiu MC, Tong WL, Lee PO, Ng TK, Ng WF, Lee KC, Lam W, Yu WC, Lai JY, Lai ST. Outcomes and prognostic factors in 267 patients with severe acute respiratory syndrome in Hong Kong. Ann Intern Med 2003; 139:715–723.
12. Fowler RA, Lapinsky SE, Hallett D, Detsky AS, Sibbald WJ, Slutsky AS, Stewart TE. Critically ill patients with severe acute respiratory syndrome. J Am Med Assoc 2003; 290:367–373.

13. Knowles SR, Phillips EJ, Dresser L, Matukas L. Common adverse events associated with the use of ribavirin for severe acute respiratory syndrome in Canada. Clin Infect Dis 2003; 37:1139–1142.

14. So LK, Lau AC, Yam LY, Cheung TM, Poon E, Yung RW, Yuen KY. Development of a standard treatment protocol for severe acute respiratory syndrome. Lancet 2003; 361:1615–1617.

15. Kanchan A, Ziebuhr J, Wadhwani P, Mesters JR, Hilgenfeld R. Coronavirus main proteinase (3CL^{pro}) structure: basis for design of anti-SARS drugs. Science 2004; 300: 1763–1767.

16. Loutfy MR, Blatt LM, Siminovitch KA, Ward S, Wolff B, Lho H, Pham DH, Deif H, LaMere EA, Chang M, Kam KC, Farcas GA, Ferguson P, Latchford M, Levy G, Dennis JW, Lai EK, Fish EN. Interferon alfacon-1 plus corticosteroids in severe acute respiratory syndrome: a preliminary study. J Am Med Assoc 2003; 290:3222–3228.

17. Loeb M, Elliott S, Gibson B, Nosal R, Fearon M, Drebot M, Harrington D, Smith S, George P, Eyles J. Ontario seroprevalence study for West Nile virus: a 2002 "hotspot". 2004. International Conference on Emerging Infectious Diseases, Atlanta, GA, 2004.

18. Mostashari F, Bunning ML, Kitsutani PT, Singer DA, Nash D, Cooper MJ, Katz N, Liljebjelke Ka, Biggersaff BJ, Fine AD, Layton MC, Mullin SM, Johnson AJ, Martin DA, Hayes EB, Campbell GL. Epidemic West Nile encephalitis. New York, 1999: results of a house-hold based seroepidemiologic study. Lancet 2001; 358:261–264.

19. Lanciotti RS, Roehrig JT, Deubel V, Smith J, Parker M, Steele K, Crise B, Volpe KE, Crabtree MB, Scherret JH, Hall RA, MacKenzie JS, Cropp CB, Panigrahy B, Ostlund E, Schmitt B, Malkinson M, Banet C, Weissman J, Komar N, Savage HM, Stone J, McNamara T, Gubler DJ. Origin of the West Nile virus responsible for an outbreak of encephalitis in the northeastern United States. Science 1999; 286:2333–2337.

20. Shieh WJ, Guarner J, Layton M, Fine A, Miller J, Nash D, Campbell GL, Roehrig JT, Gruber DJ, Zaki SR. The role of pathology in an investigation of an outbreak of West Nile encephalitis in New York, 1999. Emerg Infect Dis 2000; 6:370–372.

21. Peterson LR, Marfin A, Gubler DJ. West Nile virus. J Am Med Assoc 2003; 290: 524–528.

22. Berner YN, Lang R, Chowers MY. Outcome of West Nile fever in older adults. J Am Geriatr Soc 2002; 50:1844–1846.

23. Weiss D, Carr D, Kellachan TC, Phillips M, Bresnitz E, Laytom M, West Nile Virus Outbreak Response Working Group. Clinical findings of West Nile virus infection in hospitalized patients, New York and New Jersey, 2000. Emerg Infect Dis 2001; 7:654–658.

24. Pepperell C, Rau N, Krajden S, Kern R, Humar A, Mederski B, Simor A, Low DE, McGeer A, Mazzulli T, Burton J, Jaigobin C, Feason M, Artsob H, Drebot MA, Halliday W, Brunton J. West Nile virus infection in 2002: morbidity and mortality among patients admitted to hospital in southcentral Ontario. Can Med Assoc J 2003; 168:1399–1405.

25. Sejvar JJ, Haddad MB, Tierney BC, Campbell GL, Marfin AA, Van Gerpen JA, Fleischauer A, Leis AA, Stokie DS, Petersen LR. Neurological manifestations and outcome of West Nile Virus infection. J Am Med Assoc 2003; 290:511–515.

26. Roehrig JT, Nash D, Maldin B, Labowitz A, Martin DA, Lanciotti RS, Campbell GL. Persistence of virus-reactive serum immunoglobulin M antibody in confirmed West Nile virus encephalitis cases. Emerg Infect Dis 2003; 9:376–379.

SUGGESTED READING

Davis J, Lederburg J, eds. Emerging Infectious Diseases from the global to the local perspective. Workshop Summary. Institute of Medicine. Washington: National Academy Press, 2001.

Mclean A, May R, Pattison J, Weiss R, eds. SARS as a case study in emerging infections. London: Oxford University Press, 2005.

48

Unique Aspects in the Nursing Home Setting

Chesley L. Richards, Jr.
Division of Healthcare Quality Promotion, National Center for Infectious Diseases, Centers for Disease Control and Prevention, Atlanta, Georgia, U.S.A. and Division of Geriatric Medicine and Gerontology, Department of Medicine, Emory University School of Medicine, Atlanta, Georgia, U.S.A.

Joseph G. Ouslander
Geriatric Research, Education, and Clinical Center (GRECC), Atlanta, Georgia, U.S.A.

Key Points:

- Infections and antimicrobial prescription are common among nursing home residents.
- Nursing home residents are often frail, cognitively or functionally impaired, and may present atypically. However, contemporary nursing homes are heterogenous and clinicians should recognize that younger, postacute residents may be receiving therapy [e.g., intravenous (IV) medications, physical therapy, and wound care] or IV equivalent to many acute care hospitals.
- Clinicians are rarely on-site to evaluate residents with suspected infection and most antimicrobials are prescribed empirically by telephone order.
- Few diagnostic studies are available in nursing homes and results may not be optimally communicated to clinicians.
- Guidelines, specific for nursing homes, to optimize the evaluation of fever and infection and for optimizing antimicrobial prescription have been published and may be helpful in guiding clinicians.

Long-term care has been defined as "an array of health, personal care, and social services provided over a sustained period of time to persons with chronic conditions and with functional limitations" (1). These services can be provided in the home in community settings or in institutions. The primary institutional setting for the provision of long-term care is the nursing home. In nursing homes, health or medical services are provided along with personal care and social services. This differentiates nursing homes from community settings such as assisted living facilities or personal care homes in which primarily personal care and social services are provided and residents seek medical care through physician's ambulatory practices. On the opposite end of the spectrum, the fundamental difference between nursing homes and acute care hospitals is that nursing homes are as much a place to live in as an environment for providing medical care. Although the traditional nursing home resident is a cognitively or functionally impaired elderly adult, recent trends in nursing homes have increased the number and proportion of residents who are receiving postacute care following acute care hospitalization. These residents may be receiving rehabilitation following a surgical operation or acute illness, or may be receiving skilled nursing services such as intravenous (IV) antimicrobials, parenteral or enteral nutrition, or aggressive wound care. In contrast, nursing homes may also provide care for residents with advance directives to limit medical care such as residents receiving hospice care or residents who have severe cognitive or functional impairment. This chapter will review the characteristics of nursing homes and their residents, some of the important differences between acute care hospitals and nursing homes and clinicians practicing in the nursing home setting. Finally, key guidelines regarding the general approach to evaluation of fever and suspected infection and to antimicrobial prescribing in nursing homes will be discussed.

1. CHARACTERISTICS

1.1. Nursing Home Characteristics

In the United States >40% of adults will reside in a nursing home at some point during their life. The majority (53%) of residents in nursing homes will spend ≥1 year (2,3). Nursing homes may include a heterogenous mix of facilities variably called skilled nursing facilities, postacute rehabilitation facilities, or chronic care facilities. From the most recent national data in the United States (1999), there were 1.6 million residents in nursing homes of which 90% were aged ≥65 years (4). The majority of nursing homes (67%) have proprietary ownership with smaller proportions owned by nonprofit organizations (27%) or government (6%). Both Medicare and Medicaid certify ≈80% of nursing homes.

In 1999, the average base charge for private-pay residents ranged from $101 for residential care to $146 for skilled care (4). In comparison, average per diem rates for Medicare and Medicaid were $213 and $105, respectively. The primary expected source of payment for the majority (59%) of residents was Medicaid, although Medicaid covered only 40% residents on initial admission to the nursing home (Fig. 1). Thus, most long-stay residents will come to depend on Medicaid as a source of continued funding for nursing home care.

1.2. Nursing Home Staffing

Nursing home staffing is lower than staffing in acute care hospitals. Although there are nearly three times as many nursing homes as acute care hospitals (16,000 vs. 5800) and more than 50% more nursing home beds (1.6 million vs. 987,000), nursing homes have one-third of the number of full- or part-time employees (1.9 million vs. 5.3 million) as acute care hospitals (5). On average, nursing homes have 80 full-time equivalent (FTE) employees per 100 beds although this differs by type of nursing home ownership, region, total nursing home beds, and occupational category (Table 1) (4). The majority of nursing home employees (64%) provide nursing services. Nursing staff includes registered nurses (RN) (7.6 FTEs per 100 beds), licensed practical nurses (LPN) (10.6 FTEs per 100 beds), and nurse's aides (32.9 FTEs

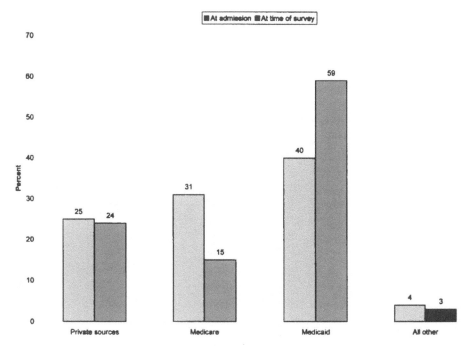

Figure 1 Percentage distribution of primary expected source of payment at admission and at time of survey: United States, 1999. *Source*: From Ref. 4.

per 100 beds) (4). These FTE distributions represent the entire staff not just staffing per shift. Consequently, these data emphasize that nurse's aides provide the bulk of direct resident care in nursing homes. Especially during evening/night shifts or on weekends, a typical 100-bed nursing home may have only one or two RNs or LPNs on duty. Improving the ratio of nursing staff to residents and expanding the presence of RNs has been proposed as an important steps toward improving the quality of care in nursing homes (1).

1.3. Resident Characteristics

Of 1.6 million nursing home residents in 1999 in the United States, most were female (72%), ≥75 years (78%), widowed (57%), and residing in nursing homes in the Midwest and South (63%) (4). Prior to nursing home admission, most residents came from a hospital (46%) or a private residence (30%). Impairments suffered by nursing home residents were most commonly visual (32%), hearing (21%), walking (59%), or continence (67%). Overall, the overwhelming majority of all nursing home residents (94%) required some type of mechanical aid. The most frequent aids used by nursing home residents were eyeglasses (62%), wheelchairs (62%), and walkers (25%). As one might expect, >90% of nursing home residents received medical or nursing services. Less commonly, restorative services such as occupational therapy (19%), physical therapy (27%), or speech/hearing therapy (8%) were used. Hospice services were provided to 1.8% of nursing home residents. The population of residents in nursing homes is highly dependent on staff for activities of daily living (ADLs). Of the five ADLs (bathing, dressing, eating, transferring, or toileting), most residents (64%)

Table 1 Number and Rate per 100 Beds of FTE Employees by Occupational Categories and Selected Nursing Home Characteristics

Facility characteristic	All full-time equivalent employees	Number	Administrative medical and therapeutic	Total rate per 100 beds	Nursing				All other staff
					RN	LPN	Nurse's aides		
All facilities	1,512,200	80.5	5.1	51.1	7.6	10.6	32.9		24.2
Ownership									
Proprietary	920,000	74.4	4.9	48.3	6.8	10.4	31.1		21.2
Voluntary nonprofit	457,300	91.6	5.8	56.0	9.1	11.0	35.9		29.7
Government and other	134,900	93.5	5.1	58.1	9.1	11.2	37.7		30.3
Beds									
<50 beds	64,500	93.2	10.3	61.5	12.0	12.8	36.7		24.4
50–99	400,500	82.7	5.9	51.9	7.5	10.5	33.9		20.1
100–199	742,400	78.0	4.7	50.0	7.2	10.8	29.8		22.8
200 or more	304,800	81.6	4.3	51.0	8.0	9.8	29.6		25.7
Geographic region									
Northeast	382,100	92.6	5.2	59.2	10.1	10.6	38.5		28.1
Midwest	445,100	74.4	4.7	45.5	7.4	9.3	28.8		24.2
South	481,100	78.2	5.0	50.6	5.7	12.1	32.9		22.6
West	203,800	80.4	6.4	52.5	8.7	10.2	33.6		21.5
Affiliation									
Chain	861,700	66.4	4.5	42.8	6.1	9.3	27.4		19.0
Independent	648,700	111.6	6.5	69.5	11.0	13.5	45.0		35.7

Source: From Ref. 4.

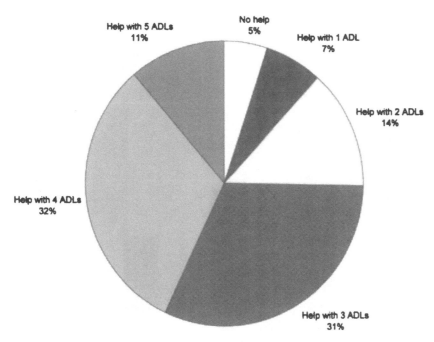

Figure 2 Percentage distribution of residents with dependencies in ADLs and number of dependencies: United States, 1999. *Source*: From Ref. 4.

require assistance with three or four ADLs (Fig. 2). The most common ADL requiring assistance is bathing (94%) (Fig. 3).

While these data reinforce the notion of the stereotypical nursing home resident who is a female, ≥ 80 years of age, cognitively or functionally impaired, and living with several underlying medical conditions, this description of a nursing home resident does not adequately portray the broad diversity of residents in contemporary facilities. In 1999, 2.5 million residents were discharged from nursing homes (4). The majority of residents discharged had a length of stay of ≤ 3 months (68%). While many of these discharges after relatively short nursing homes stays were because the resident died (16%) or was transferred to a hospital (24%), many occurred in residents who stabilized (27%) or recovered (18%). Of the 423,000 nursing home discharges occurring in residents with nursing home stays of 1 year or longer, the most common reasons for these discharges were because the resident died (49%) or was transferred to a hospital (37%). Factors associated with a lower likelihood of hospitalization include female sex, a do not resuscitate order, and cognitive impairment while factors associated with higher risk of hospitalization are Medicare payment, a diagnosis of congestive heart failure or cancer, and residents who had impaired functional ability (6).

Regarding resident-level risk factors for infection, immunologic senescence, malnutrition, chronic diseases, medications (e.g., immunosuppressants and central nervous system agents that diminish cough reflex), cognitive deficits that may complicate resident compliance with basic sanitary practices (e.g., hand hygiene), or functional impairments (e.g., fecal and urinary incontinence, immobility, and diminished cough reflex) are all associated with increased risk of infection (7–10)

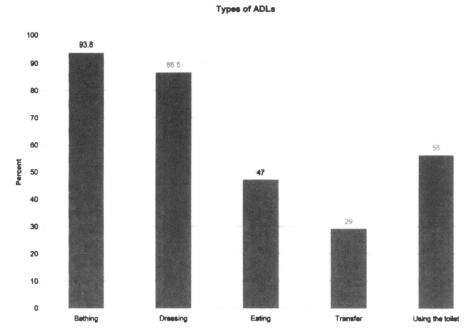

Figure 3 Percentage of nursing home residents with dependencies in ADL and percentage distribution of residents by number of dependencies: United States, 1999. *Source*: From Ref. 4.

(Table 2). Medical interventions may also increase the risk of infection. Indeed, with the growth of subacute or postacute care, many nursing homes now have residents receiving interventions or therapy (e.g., central venous catheters, hemodialysis, parenteral antimicrobial or nutrition therapy, and mechanical ventilation) equivalent in complexity to interventions performed in many acute care hospitals.

1.4. Clinician Characteristics

Direct medical care is rarely provided by physicians in the nursing home setting. The majority of physicians (77%) do not spend time caring for nursing home residents

Table 2 Nursing Home Resident-Level Risk Factors for Infection

---

Immunologic senescence

Lack of vaccination (e.g., influenza and pneumococcal)

Malnutrition

Chronic diseases (e.g., cancer and diabetes mellitus)

Medications (e.g., immunosuppressants and central nervous system agents that diminish cough reflex)

Cognitive deficits that may complicate resident compliance with basic sanitary practices (e.g., hand hygiene)

Functional impairments (e.g., fecal and urinary incontinence, immobility, diminished cough, and reflex)

Medical interventions (e.g., central venous catheters, hemodialysis, parenteral antimicrobial or nutrition therapy, mechanical ventilation)

---

(11). For physicians who provide nursing home care, the median effort is 2 hr/week or ≈4% of the physicians' overall practice. Very few physicians (3%) spend more than 5 hr/week providing medical care in nursing homes. Family physicians are more likely to provide medical care in nursing homes than physicians from other specialties. More physicians in solo practice (27%), partnerships (26%), or group practices (23%) provide medical aid in nursing homes than physicians in medical schools (9%) or hospital-based practices (11%). Consequently, nonphysician clinicians often provide direct medical care in nursing homes. Models using both physician assistants and nurse practitioners have been described and represent an increasingly prevalent practice style. In previous reports, the use of nonphysician clinicians has resulted in fewer hospitalizations of nursing home residents and decreased overall costs. For example, regular nursing home visits (three to four visits per week) by a physician assistant in a 92-bed facility were associated with reduced hospitalizations (38%) and total hospital days (62%) among nursing home residents (12). Annual Medicare charges for physician or physician assistant services increased by $22,304 per year but hospital diagnosis related group reimbursements decreased by $96,043. The Evercare program, a national Medicare-funded, capitated, and for-profit program of United Healthcare recently demonstrated that on-site medical care provided by nurse practitioners reduces overall hospitalizations and preventable hospitalizations among nursing home residents and results in annual savings in hospital costs of $103,000 per nurse practitioner (13). In a national survey of nursing homes, 63% reported having nurse practitioners with a median of two nurse practitioners per facility (14).

In addition to practicing clinicians, each nursing home is required to have a medical director. The medical director is responsible for providing oversight, participating in drug utilization review and quality assurance programs, and working with attending physicians on appropriate drug therapies and medical care issues (1). Most medical directors are either internists or family physicians and on average spend 10–20 hr/month performing medical director responsibilities. At a national level, the American Medical Director's Association (AMDA) is the primary professional organization for medical directors and provides training and certification for medical directors (15).

Finally, most nursing homes have on their staff or through contract consultant pharmacists who can assess the quality of care regarding medication prescriptions and provide consultation regarding drug therapy issues. In most long-term care facilities (LTCFs), consultant pharmacists perform mandatory medication reviews and provide feedback to the LTCF administrator and medical director. Consultant pharmacists may offer an important on-site perspective and expertise in improving the management of a wide range of medications, including antimicrobials, and should be seen as a potential resource for clinicians and medical directors regarding antimicrobial management (16). During disease outbreaks in nursing homes, consultant pharmacists may also provide valuable resident and family counseling regarding medication side effects or support regarding distribution of prophylactic antimicrobials (e.g., oseltamivir) (17).

1.5. Nursing Home Characteristics and Infection Risk

A fundamental difference between nursing homes and acute care facilities is the residential nature of nursing homes. As residential facilities, nursing homes typically promote activities and policies that foster socialization of residents through group activities, both inside and outside the nursing home. While these activities are important for promoting good physical and mental health for residents, they may also increase the risk of exposure to and transmission of communicable infectious diseases (7–10). Occupational and physical therapy activities, while vital toward restoring or maintaining physical and mental function, may increase risk of person-to-person transmission or exposure to contaminated environmental surfaces (e.g., physical or occupational therapy equipment). In nursing homes, group bathing facilities or whirlpool therapy units may be potential sources of infection with water-borne pathogens. Finally, group dining is generally encouraged for nursing home residents. A common dining area may used for all nursing home residents or for residents of a specific ward, hall, or wing in a large facility. Group dining may be an avenue for person-to-person transmission of infectious diseases and for food-borne disease outbreaks (7–10). Low rates of healthcare worker immunization in nursing homes have been associated with outbreaks caused by vaccine-preventable respiratory infections (e.g., influenza, *Streptococcus pneumoniae*) (10,18–20). Finally, specific institutional characteristics have been associated with disease outbreaks. In a study of outbreaks among New York nursing homes, institutional risk factors for respiratory or gastrointestinal infection outbreaks included larger homes and nursing homes with a single nursing unit or with multiple units but shared staff (21). Risk of outbreaks was lower in nursing homes with paid employee sick leave.

1.6. Infections with Antimicrobial-Resistant Pathogens

The introduction or emergence of antimicrobial-resistant bacteria in nursing homes has resulted in both regional outbreaks of antimicrobial-resistant infections and increasing prevalence of such resistant organisms (22,23). In addition to the individual and institutional risk factors for infection discussed previously, colonization with antimicrobial-resistant pathogens (e.g., methicillin-resistant *Staphylococcus aureus*, vancomycin-resistant *Enterococcus*, multidrug resistant *Escherichiae coli*, *Acinetobacter*, *Enterobacter*, or *Pseudomonas aeruginosa*) increases the likelihood of both epidemics and high rates of endemic disease with antimicrobial-resistant pathogens in LTCFs (24). Risk factors for the development of infection with multidrug resistance include exposure to antimicrobials, lack of handwashing sinks, and lower levels of registered nurse staffing (25).

2. UNIQUE CHALLENGES AND GUIDELINES FOR ANTIMICROBIAL USE IN NURSING HOMES

For clinicians in nursing homes, several unique challenges complicate the evaluation of residents with suspected infection and the appropriate use of antimicrobial therapy (Table 3). These challenges include the myriad of risk factors in a nursing home population, the often subclinical or atypical presentation of residents with infection, the lack of on-site clinician evaluation, and the lack of diagnostics and the limited follow-up residents receive the following empirical antimicrobial prescription. Recently, guidelines have been published for infection evaluation and antimicrobial prescriptions specifically aimed at nursing home residents; these are discussed later.

Table 3 Challenges for Infection Evaluation and Antimicrobial Prescription in Nursing Home Residents

---

Nursing home residents
  Multiple chronic conditions
  Malnutrition and poor oral intake
  Atypical or subclinical presentation
    Fever without localization
    Altered mental status without fever
    Failure to thrive without fever or localization
  Poor or altered response to antimicrobial therapy
  Increased risk of toxicity
  Cognitive, speech or functional deficits that limit communication of symptoms
Nursing home staff
  Limited or no availability of on-site clinician evaluation of residents with suspected infection
  Nursing staffing
    Limited training among nurses aides to recognize infection
    Limited availability of licensed nurses to evaluate and monitor residents
Diagnostic studies
  Few studies available
  Results reporting may be too slow to impact clinical decision making
  Few facilities have institution level antimicrobial susceptibility data to guide empirical therapy
Antimicrobial therapy
  Limited availability of IV therapy
  Difficult to have clinician reassessment of residents (e.g., 48–72 hr) to either confirm need for continued antimicrobial therapy or narrow the spectrum of therapy

---

2.1. Guideline for Infection Evaluation in Nursing Home Residents

In an effort to improve the evaluation of nursing home residents with fever or suspected infection, recommendations outlining the minimum evaluation for infection in nursing home residents have been published (26). The guideline specifies tasks appropriate for nursing assistants and licensed nurses during the evaluation of infection. For residents with suspected infection, the guideline recommends that nurse's aides measure vital signs (e.g., temperature, blood pressure, pulse, respiratory rate, and presence of pain), identify residents with fever or suspected infection, and relay this information to licensed nursing staff. Next, the LPN or RN performs an initial clinical assessment on residents with fever or suspected infection, and significant findings are relayed to clinicians (26). Nursing homes should have training and procedures in place to ensure that residents with suspected infection are quickly identified by nursing staff and the appropriate information relayed to clinicians.

The guideline also suggests appropriate diagnostic testing for febrile or potentially infected residents. When diagnostic evaluation is performed, only limited tests are available in many nursing homes. In the overwhelming majority of nursing homes, laboratory testing is not performed in an on-site laboratory but is performed in a hospital or in a commercial laboratory. The delay between obtaining specimens and actual laboratory processing may be substantial. When combined with delays in getting reports back to clinicians in nursing homes, suboptimal timeliness of reporting is the norm and, in some situations, may lead to poor decisions regarding empirical or continued antimicrobial use. Medical directors should work with nursing home administrators, directors of nursing, and laboratory providers in both improving specimen collection and reporting results. Where possible, laboratory providers should provide a facility-specific antibiotic susceptibility testing profile (i.e., antibiogram), either for the individual facility or for the network of nursing homes. The availability of a specific antibiogram may improve the initial selection of empirical antimicrobial therapy. Furthermore, improving the availability of accurate microbiological results may allow clinicians to re-evaluate the resident at 48–72 hr with the goal of individualizing antimicrobial therapy to the identified pathogen and antimicrobial susceptibility profile. Acutely ill residents or those residents who require diagnostic studies not available in nursing homes may be transferred to acute care hospitals for further evaluation and therapy. Residents with presumed infections account for one-quarter of all hospital transfers from nursing homes (27).

Minimum appropriate laboratory evaluation for fever and various presumed infections varies depending on the type of suspected infection (26). First, clinicians should be cognizant that many nursing home residents may present atypically when developing infection. For example, altered mental status or a decline in oral intake without fever may be the initial presentation for pneumonia or urinary tract infection (UTI) in some residents. In addition, residents with cognitive or speech impairment may not be able to communicate symptoms related to infection and may instead develop agitation or combativeness. All residents with a presumed infection should have a complete blood count performed. Leukocytosis [white blood cell (WBC) count >14,000], even in the absence of left shift, warrants further careful assessment for infection. In many nursing homes, residents with fever and no symptoms referable to the urinary tract often receive antimicrobial therapy for UTIs based on positive urine cultures only. Urinalysis and urine culture should be reserved for residents with symptoms of UTI without indwelling urinary catheters. In residents with chronic indwelling urinary catheters, urinalysis and urine culture should be obtained only for symptoms or signs referable to the urinary tract or for presumed sepsis. Specimens should be collected preferably following replacement of catheter. For residents with suspected pneumonia and tachypnea (respiratory rate >25 per minute), the minimum evaluation should include determining oxygen saturation using pulse oximetry and obtaining a chest radiograph. Sputum Gram stain and culture should be obtained only if purulent sputum is available and if the sample can be transported to the clinical laboratory within ≤2 hr of collection. In addition to the recommended tests, the guideline also makes recommendations on tests that may not be appropriate in nursing home residents. For example, blood cultures should probably not be obtained in most nursing home residents because of the high likelihood of contamination, the low yield, and the recognition that residents with presumed sepsis or bacteremia should probably be transferred to acute care facilities for evaluation and management. If blood cultures are obtained, nursing home medical directors should ensure that staff members (e.g., nurses) collecting the blood samples have been trained in proper antisepsis and collection technique. Working with the hospital or commercial laboratory to monitor for probable contaminants in blood culture results (e.g., coagulase-negative *Staphylococcus*) may provide early clues when collection techniques are suboptimal. Similarly, surface cultures from infected wounds are not recommended because of the high likelihood of contamination and the low yield from these cultures.

Table 4 Minimum Criteria for the Initiation of Antimicrobial Therapy in Nursing Home Residents

---

Skin and soft tissue infections
New or increasing purulent drainage at the wound, skin, or soft tissue site or two of the following
   Fever[a]
   Redness
   Warmth
   Tenderness
   New or increasing swelling at the affected site
Lower respiratory infections
For residents with fever >38.9°C and at least one of the following
   >25 breaths per minute
   Productive cough
Fever >37.9 but <38.9
   Cough and at least one of the following
      Pulse >100
      Delirium
      Rigors
      Respiratory rate >25
Afebrile with COPD and age ≥65
   New or increased cough with purulent sputum production
Afebrile without COPD
   New cough with purulent sputum
   And >25 breaths per minute or delirium
UTI
No in-dwelling catheter
   Acute dysuria alone or fever[a]
   And at least one of the following: new or worsening urgency, frequency, suprapubic pain, gross hematuria, costovertebral angle tenderness, and urinary incontinence
With chronic in-dwelling catheter
   And at least one of the following: fever,[a] new costovertebral angle tenderness, rigors, and new onset of delirium
Fever[a] with unknown focus of infection
Fever[a] and new onset of delirium or rigors

---

[a] Fever defined as >37.9 (100.0) or 1.5°C increase over baseline.
Abbreviations: COPD, chronic obstructive pulmonary disease.
Source: From Ref. 27.

2.2. Antimicrobial Use in Nursing Homes

Empirical antimicrobial use is widespread in nursing homes. In Maryland, 8% of nursing home residents were receiving antibiotic therapy at a given time, and over a year, 54% received at least one course of antibiotic therapy (28). In four nursing homes in New York State, the percentage of patient-days during which antibiotics were given ranged from 2.7% to 6.8% (29). The majority of patient febrile episodes resulted in antibiotic therapy, with upper respiratory illnesses, bronchitis/pneumonia, and UTIs accounting for the majority of indications (30). Following diagnostic evaluation, 39% of patients continued to receive antibiotics despite negative laboratory and radiographic studies for bacterial infections. In a study of Canadian nursing homes, 66% of the residents received an antibiotic over a 12-month period with the majority being prescribed for either respiratory infections or UTIs (31). Among residents treated for UTIs, one-third actually had asymptomatic bacteriuria and should not have been treated with antibiotics. In general, previous studies have found substantial inappropriate use of antibiotics in nursing homes, ranging from 25% to 75% (30). Categories of inappropriate use included continued antimicrobial exposure despite no clinical evidence of infection, antimicrobial therapy with agents to which organisms from appropriate clinical cultures were not susceptible, and use of antimicrobials in residents with known allergies to the agent or with significant drug–drug interactions. Inappropriate use of an antimicrobial agent adds to patient care costs, may place the patient at risk of adverse medication reactions, and increases the risk of infections with antibiotic-resistant organisms (30).

In an effort to improve antimicrobial prescribing, minimum criteria for the initiation of antimicrobial therapy in LTCF residents have been proposed (32). These criteria are summarized in Table 4. These recommendations were not meant as strict management guidelines for clinically complex residents; the resident's overall status must be considered by the clinician before decisions are made on treatment. The recommendations are useful in attempting to provide a rationale and a guide for empirical antimicrobial therapy in otherwise stable residents. The guideline was based on expert opinion and remains to be tested in clinical trials. An important action that would potentially make a significant impact on antimicrobial prescribing in nursing homes is a re-evaluation of residents with suspected infection within 48–72 hr after initial empirical antimicrobial prescription. For those residents in whom the clinical course (e.g., afebrile, no change in baseline functional status) and diagnostic study results (e.g., normal WBC count and negative culture results) do not suggest infection, clinicians should consider discontinuing antimicrobial therapy.

3. CONCLUSION

Nursing homes represent an increasingly important site of medical care for older adults. While most physicians do not provide direct medical in nursing homes, they will encounter nursing home residents at some point in either primary practice or specialty consultants. Infections and antimicrobial use are relatively common in nursing homes. There are substantial barriers to effective diagnosis and prescribing in the nursing home environment including the lack of direct physician evaluation of residents with suspected infection, limited availability of diagnostic tests, widespread empiric antimicrobial prescribing without the facility of antimicrobial susceptibility reports (antibiograms) to guide therapy, and limited ability to reassess residents after antimicrobial prescription. Clinicians should remain cognizant of the many challenges in providing optimal antimicrobial therapy in this environment and individualize the evaluation and management of nursing home residents accordingly. Hospitalists, consultants, and specialists should recognize that residents coming from nursing homes may have received multiple courses of empirical antimicrobial therapy for suspected infection without supporting microbiological cultures and should consider evaluating residents for antimicrobial-resistant organisms, especially in the context of antimicrobial treatment failures. An extensive research agenda has been proposed for infections and antimicrobial use in nursing homes to advance the epidemiologic and clinical science underpinning treatment. Hopefully, new knowledge from this research will be forthcoming to help clinicians improve antimicrobial prescribing in this population and setting (33).

REFERENCES

1. Institute of Medicine. In: Wunderlich GS, Kohler P, eds. Improving the Quality of Long-Term Care. Washington, DC: National Academy Press, 2001:1–20, 199–201.
2. Kemper P, Murtaugh CM. Lifetime use of nursing home care. N Engl J Med 1991; 324:595–600.
3. Murtaugh CM, Kemper P, Spillman BC, Carlson BL. The amount, distribution, and timing of lifetime nursing home use. Med Care 1997; 35:204–218.
4. Jones A. The national nursing home survey: 1999 Summary. National Center for Health Statistics. Vital Health Stat 2002; 13(152).
5. Eberhardt MS, Ingram DD, Makuc DM. Urban and Rural Chartbook. Health, United States 2001. Hyattsville, MD: National Center for Health Statistics, 2001.
6. Intrator O, Castle NG, Mor V. Facility characteristics associated with hospitalization of nursing home residents: results of a national study. Med Care 1999; 37:228–237.
7. Ouslander JG, Osterweil D, Morley J. Medical Care in the Nursing Home. New York: McGraw-Hill Co., 1997.
8. Ouslander JG, Schnelle JF. Nursing home care. In: Hazzard WR, Blass JP, Ettinger WH, Halter JB, Ouslander JG, eds. Principles of Geriatric Medicine and Gerontology. New York: McGraw-Hill, 1999.
9. Nicolle LE, Strausbaugh LJ, Garibaldi RA. Infections and antibiotic resistance in nursing homes. Clin Microbiol Rev 1996; 9:1–17.
10. Nuorti JP, Butler JC, Crutcher JM, Guevara R, Welch D, Holder P, Elliott JA. An outbreak of multidrug resistant pneumococcal pneumonia and bacteremia among unvaccinated nursing home residents. N Engl J Med 1998; 338:1861–1868.
11. Katz PR, Karuza J, Kolassa J, Hutson A. Medical practice with nursing home residents: results from the national physician professional activities census. J Am Geriatr Soc 1997; 45:911–917.
12. Ackermann RJ, Kemle KA. The effect of a physician assistant on the hospitalization of nursing home resisdents. J Am Geriatr Soc 1998; 46:610–614.
13. Kane RL, Keckhafer G, Flood S, Bershadsky B, Siadaty MS. The effect of Evercare on hospital use. J Am Geriatr Soc 2003; 51:1427–1434.
14. Rosenfeld P, Kobayahsi M, Barber P, Mezey M. Utilization of nurse practitioners in long-term care: findings and implications of a national survey. J Am Med Dir Assoc 2004; 51:9–15.
15. American Medical Directors Association. www.amda.com.
16. Harjivan C, Lyles A. Improved medication use in long-term care: building on the consultant pharmacist's drug regimen review. Am J Managed Care 2002; 8:318–326.
17. Bowles SK, Kennie N, Ruston L, Simor A, Louie M, Collins V. Influenza outbreak in a long-term-care facility: considerations for pharmacy. Am J Health Syst Pharm 1999; 56:2303–2307.
18. Potter J, Stott DJ, Roberts MA, Elder AG, ODonnell B, Knight PV, Carman WF. Influenza vaccination of health care workers in long-term care hospitals reduces the mortality of elderly patients. J Infect Dis 1997; 175:1–6.
19. Nichol KL, Grimm MB, Peterson DC. Immunizations in long-term care facilities: policies and practice. J Am Geriatr Soc 1996; 44:349–355.
20. Carman WF, Elder AG, Wallace LA, McAulay K, Walker A, Murray GD, Stott DJ. Effects of influenza vaccination of health-care workers on mortality of elderly people in long-term care: a randomized controlled trial. Lancet 2000; 355:93–97.
21. Li J, Birkhead GS, Strogatz DS, Coles FB. Impact of institution size, staffing patterns, and infection control practices on communicable disease outbreaks in New York state nursing homes. Am J Epidemiol 1996; 143:1042–1049.
22. Bonomo RA. Multiple antibiotic-resistant bacteria in long-term care facilities: an emerging problem in the practice of infectious disease. Clin Infect Dis 2000; 31:1414–1422.

23. Wiener J, Quinn JP, Bradford PA, Goering RV, Nathan C, Bush K, Weinstein RA. Multiple antibiotic-resistant Klebsiella and *Escherichia coli* in nursing homes. J Am Med Assoc 1999; 281:517–523.
24. Strausbaugh LJ, Crossley KB, Nurse BA, Thrupp LD. Antimicrobial resistance in long-term care facilities. Antimicrobial use in long-term care facilities. Infect Control Hosp Epidemiol 1996; 17:129–140.
25. Loeb MB, Craven S, McGeer AJ, Simor AE, Bradley SF, Low DE, Armstrong-Evans M, Moss LA, Walter SD. Risk factors for resistance to antimicrobial agents among nursing home residents. Am J Epidemiol 2003; 157:40–47.
26. Bentley DW, Bradley S, High K, Schoenbaum S, Taler G, Yoshikawa TT. Practice guidelines for evaluation of fever and infection in long-term care facilities. Clin Infect Dis 2000; 31:640–653.
27. Irvine PW, Van Buren N, Crossley K. Causes for hospitalization of nursing home residents: the role of infection. J Am Geriatr Soc 1984; 32:103–107.
28. Warren JW, Palumbo FB, Fitterman L, Speedie SM. Incidence and characteristics of antibiotic use in aged nursing home patients. J Am Geriatr Soc 1991; 39:963–972.
29. Mylotte JM. Antimicrobial prescribing in long-term care facilities. Infect Control Hosp Epidemiol 1999; 27:10–19.
30. Nicolle LE, Bentley D, Garibaldi R, Neuhaus E, Smith P. Antimicrobial use in long-term care facilities. Infect Control Hosp Epidemiol 2000; 21:537–545.
31. Loeb M, Simor AE, Landry L, Walter S, McArthur M, Duffy J, Kwan D, McGeer A. Antibiotic use in Ontario facilities that provide chronic care. J Gen Intern Med 2001; 16:376–383.
32. Loeb M, Bentley DW, Bradley S, Crossley K, Garibaldi R, Gantz N, McGeer A, Muder RR, Mylotte J, Nicolle LE, Nurse B, Paton S, Simor A, Smith P, Strausbaugh L. Development of minimum criteria for the initiation of antibiotics in residents of long-term care facilities: results of a consensus conference. Infect Control Hosp Epidemiol 2001; 22: 120–124.
33. Richards C. Infections in residents of long-term care facilities: an agenda for research. Report of an expert panel. J Am Geriatr Soc 2002; 50:570–576.

SUGGESTED READING

Bentley DW, Bradley S, High K, Schoenbaum S, Taler G, Yoshikawa TT. Practice guidelines for evaluation of fever and infection in long-term care facilities. Clin Infect Dis 2000; 31:640–653.

Nicolle LE, Bentley D, Garibaldi R, Neuhaus E, Smith P. Antimicrobial use in long-term care facilities. Infect Control Hosp Epidemiol 2000; 21:537–545.

Loeb M, Bentley DW, Bradley S, Crossley K, Garibaldi R, Gantz N, McGeer A, Muder RR, Mylotte J, Nicolle LE, Nurse B, Paton S, Simor A, Smith P, Strausbaugh L. Development of minimum criteria for the initiation of antibiotics in residents of long-term care facilities: results of a consensus conference. Infect Control Hosp Epidemiol 2001; 22:120–124.

Richards C. Infections in residents of long-term care facilities: an agenda for research. Report of an expert panel. J Am Geriatr Soc 2002; 50:570–576.

Strausbaugh LJ, Crossley KB, Nurse BA, Thrupp LD. Antimicrobial resistance in long-term care facilities. Antimicrobial use in long-term care facilities. Infect Control Hosp Epidemiol 1996; 17:129–140.

49

Common Infections in the Nursing Home Setting

Suzanne F. Bradley
Geriatric Research Education and Clinical Center, Veterans Affairs Ann Arbor Healthcare System, and Divisions of Infectious Diseases and Geriatric Medicine, University of Michigan Medical School, Ann Arbor, Michigan, U.S.A.

Key Points:

- Infections are as common in nursing homes as in a hospital.
- The clinical presentation of infection in nursing home residents can be atypical.
- Diagnosis of infection should focus on the most common clinical syndromes.
- The diagnostic evaluation for infection is based primarily on the clinical assessment of symptoms and signs rather than laboratory and diagnostic testing.
- Treatment should focus on the most common organisms causing the suspected infection.

1. INTRODUCTION

1.1. Epidemiology and Clinical Relevance

On average, 4.1 infections per 1000 patient-care days (range 0.8–9.5 infections per 1000 patient-care days) occur in skilled nursing facilities) (1). Infections in nursing homes are as common as in hospital but are thought to be less severe. The broad range of infection rates may reflect the heterogeneity of the populations that require chronic care today and the wide variety of healthcare services provided. Patients with the most severe nursing home-acquired infections are typically transferred to hospital because of the increased need for monitoring, nursing care, diagnostic evaluation, and treatment, which are not traditionally available in most skilled nursing facilities. Even now, infection rates in the nursing home approach those seen in the acute-care setting. With the expansion of rehabilitative and subacute care services, more chronic care facilities are providing a wider range of services for an increasingly ill patient population (see also chapter "Unique Aspects in the Nursing Home Setting"). In the current environment, it is likely that the severity of infections cared for in chronic care facilities will continue to increase.

In the nursing home, infections of the urinary and respiratory tracts occur most commonly followed by skin and soft tissue infections (SSTI) (1,2). Together, these three clinical syndromes account for the majority of infections seen in the chronic-care setting. Gastrointestinal (GI) and bloodstream infections (BSI) are less commonly seen or, perhaps, documented. Cultures of blood are rarely obtained in the nursing home because BSI is a common premorbid event and patients are either rapidly transferred to acute care before the diagnosis can be made or advanced directives preclude intensive evaluation (1,3).

1.2. Etiologic Pathogens

The exact prevalence of specific infectious agents in the nursing home is difficult to ascertain. The most likely sites of infection, the ease of specimen collection and diagnostic testing, and the likelihood that the results will alter treatment greatly influence the prevalence of infections diagnosed in the nursing home. Urinary tract infection (UTI) is typically mentioned as the most common infection, yet it is often overdiagnosed. Cultures of urine are easily obtained, and bacteria and yeast are easily grown (4,5).

In contrast, less is known about lower respiratory tract infections (LRTI) even though they may be just as common. Collection of adequate sputum specimens in frail patients is difficult. Many common bacterial respiratory pathogens are fastidious and difficult to grow. Detection of respiratory viruses is difficult, infection control procedures are already initiated, and results rarely influence treatment decisions (6–8).

Diagnosis of SSTI is also fraught with problems. Without blood cultures, the cause of cellulitis is rarely known. Without culture of deep tissue obtained by biopsy, differentiation between infection and superficial colonization of wounds is difficult (9,10). Among nursing home residents, diarrhea is common, frequently self-limited, and care is supportive. Fecal samples are readily obtainable but rarely are sent for diagnosis of viral, parasitic, or invasive or toxin-producing bacteria infections, other than *Clostridium difficile* (11,12).

Other mitigating factors such as the prevalence of device use, acquisition in hospital prior to admission, antecedent use of antibiotics, and the state of the host immune system also influence the pathogens present in the nursing home. Antibiotic-resistant bacteria are more common in hospitals and nursing homes than in the community. Infections are considered to be nursing home-acquired if a patient becomes infected after ≥ 72 hr in the facility (2). The organisms that cause specific clinical syndromes will be discussed under each entity below.

Colonization with antibiotic-resistant bacteria appears to be common in the nursing home setting. It is less clear that colonization with these resistant bacteria invariably leads to infection. However, knowledge of rates of resistance in a given facility may alter antimicrobial prescribing practices. In a few studies, asymptomatic colonization with methicillin-resistant *Staphylococcus aureus* (MRSA) has been found to be more than 20% and vancomycin-resistant enterococci in approximately 10% of nursing home residents. Quinolone resistance is becoming increasingly common nationwide, particularly among MRSA isolates, and resistance among gram-negative bacilli (GNB) is increasing (13,14).

Outbreaks of GNB resistant to third-generation cephalosporins and aztreonam have been described, and these bacteria will likely become an increasing and endemic problem. Resistance to these antibiotic classes suggests that the organism may be a producer of extended-spectrum β-lactamases (ESBL). The presence of an ESBL is associated not only with resistance to all cephalosporins, but also potentially with all penicillins, monobactams, and many other antibiotics (13).

1.3. Clinical Manifestations

Localization of infection by history and physical examination in nursing home residents is difficult. Many residents with impaired cognitive or communication abilities cannot provide a reliable history. In addition, impairment of the host inflammatory response by age or drug effect may blunt focal symptoms or physical findings. As a result, findings suggestive of a specific clinical syndrome may be subtle or absent. Focal physical findings and laboratory results may be misinterpreted in nursing home residents with multiple comorbid illnesses and dysfunction of organ systems due to noninfectious diseases (1,3). The symptoms and signs associated with specific clinical syndromes will be discussed separately.

Detection of infection in nursing home residents often requires a more generalized approach. Acute change in the ability to perform basic activities of daily living such as new or worsening incontinence, impairment in mobility, or ability to feed or dress oneself is a very sensitive indicator of infection in nursing home residents (1,3).

Fever in nursing home residents is also a very sensitive indicator of infection if it is present and appropriately defined. Only 40% of infected nursing home residents will have a temperature $\geq 101°F$. The use of $100°F$ ($37.8°C$) for detection of fever in nursing home residents is much more sensitive, detecting 70% of infections with a specificity of 90%. More than half the nursing home residents who meet this definition of fever will have infection. Other proposed definitions of fever include a $2°F$ ($1.1°C$) increase over baseline temperature or $>99°F$ ($37.2°C$) orally or $99.5°F$ (37.5 C) rectally (1,3) (see also chapter "Clinical Manifestations of Infections").

Dehydration may accompany fever and suggest possible infection in this population. In addition, decreased oral intake, dry mucous membranes and tongue, or furrowed tongue may provide clues that fever and infection are present (1).

1.4. Diagnosis

Criteria for hospital-based diagnosis of infection from the Centers for Disease Control and Prevention (CDC) rely heavily on laboratory results and diagnostic procedures. McGeer et al. have developed definitions for nursing home infection based primarily on readily available clinical criteria from history and physical examination; these criteria are commonly used but have not been validated (2).

Few studies have assessed what laboratory or diagnostic procedures are useful in establishing the diagnosis of infection in nursing home residents. A complete blood count can be a useful diagnostic tool in this setting. A white blood cell count $>14,000$ cells/mm^3, neutrophils $\geq 90\%$, and elevated total band count $>6\%$ or ≥ 1500 cells/mm^3 predict a high likelihood of infection in older adults (1). Dehydration may be confirmed by the presence of hypernatremia and prerenal azotemia; 60% of febrile nursing home residents may have these abnormalities (1). Therefore, an abnormal complete blood count or serum chemistry might provide an important clue that infection and associated dehydration a present.

1.5. Antibiotic Treatment

The decision to begin antibiotic therapy should be based on the patient's clinical condition (15). All nursing home patients do not require urgent treatment. If urgent treatment is needed, then the choice of antibiotic should be based on the most likely clinical syndrome and the most likely organisms causing that infection. Geographic and institutional variation in pathogens and their antimicrobial susceptibilities does occur. Consultation with the nursing home infection control practitioner can be useful in determining what organisms and antibiotic resistance patterns are common in that facility.

The route of antibiotic administration is also influenced by the severity of the patient's clinical condition. Intravenous (IV) or intramuscular therapy may be preferred in the patient with a GI tract that is not functioning well and in whom absorption of an oral antibiotic is not guaranteed. In the severely nursing home ill patient, if IV therapy is available, broad-spectrum penicillins, second-generation cephalosporins, and carbapenems treat a wide array of streptococci, MRSA, enterococci, and aerobic and anaerobic GNB (see also Chapters 7: Penicillins, 8: Cephalosporins, and 9: Carbapenems).

If and when the organism is known, treatment can be altered based on antimicrobial susceptibilities. Duration of therapy should be based on the presumed clinical syndrome to be treated and the organism isolated. Oral therapy can be considered for some clinical syndromes and pathogens, especially if the medication is 100% bioavailable or if the patient is clinically stable and has a functional GI tract. Cost, drug interactions, and toxicity are other factors that should be considered when choosing an antibiotic. Appropriate adjustments in dose and frequency of administration should also be made for renal and hepatic dysfunction if present.

1.6. Prevention

Prevention should focus on minimizing risk factors for infection. Increased risk of infection may relate to residence in a healthcare setting or due to factors intrinsic to the patient. Healthcare workers can help reduce infection in nursing home residents by frequent hand disinfection and adherence to infection control procedures (2). Reduction in patient risk factors that contribute to the most common infectious syndromes will be discussed later (see also Chapter 50: Infection Control in Nursing Homes).

Patient risk of infection may relate to the presence of intrinsic factors (underlying disease and debility) that frequently lead to the presence of extrinsic factors (use of medications and devices) with their side effects and complications. In the individual patient, prevention of infection should focus on improvement in function and treatment of diseases and their complications so that use of devices and medications can be minimized.

Antimicrobial medications directly inhibit the growth or kill normal flora and allow pathogens to grow. Other medications work indirectly by altering the host environment and providing unfavorable growth conditions for normal flora with subsequent overgrowth of pathogenic flora. Minimizing the use of antibiotics and other unnecessary medications may play a role in the prevention of infection in nursing home residents.

Devices frequently breech normal host defenses and allow pathogenic flora to invade and cause infection. Use of devices can contribute to the development of infections of the urinary tract (urethral catheters), respiratory tract (tracheostomy tubes), and GI tract (feeding tubes and thermometers), and IV catheters can contribute to SSTI and BSI. Devices should be removed as soon as they are no longer necessary to reduce the patient's risk of infection (see also Chapter 40: Prosthetic Device Infections in the Elderly).

2. URINARY TRACT INFECTION (See Also Chapter 34)

2.1. Epidemiology and Clinical Relevance

In general, the urinary tract is the most common source of infection in the nursing home setting. Risk of UTI increases with conditions or diseases that lead to urinary obstruction or stasis, with debility, and with the use of urinary catheters. Increasing age in males is associated with benign prostatic hypertrophy, urinary obstruction, and increased rates of UTI. In females, estrogen deficiency is associated with changes in normally acidic vaginal pH and colonization with gram-positive flora to an environment promotes the growth of pathogenic enteric GNB. Incomplete bladder emptying can ensue as a consequence of cystocoele, cerebrovascular accident, and diabetic neuropathy. Nephrolithiasis and neoplasms can lead to obstruction and urinary stasis. Poor functional status and dependence can lead to potential contamination and colonization of the perineum by pathogenic bacteria from the hands of healthcare personnel during toileting. While urinary catheters relieve urinary stasis, they breech the protective barrier provided by the urinary sphincter and allow pathogens to migrate along the catheter and colonize the bladder. As a result of these factors, a significant proportion of men (15–40%) and women (25–50%) in nursing homes have bacteriuria at any given time and are at risk of UTI (4,5). However, a significant proportion of nursing home residents have asymptomatic bacteriuria (see Diagnosis).

2.2. Etiologic Pathogens

In contrast with healthy women with normal urinary tracts who have recurrent UTIs with *Escherichia coli*, the pathogens causing UTI in nursing home residents are not predictable (Table 1). The bacteria isolated differ with gender. Women in nursing homes are still prone to having UTI regardless of whether they have urinary tract dysfunction or not. Therefore, *E. coli* is most common, followed by other GNB that typically are frequently antibiotic resistant. Men with UTI typically have a urinary tract abnormality or catheter. Bacteriuria in men is more often gram-positive (enterococci), associated with the use of catheters (*Providencia stuartii*, coagulase-negative staphylococci), and antibiotic-resistant GNB (*Pseudomonas*) (4,5).

Table 1 Common Causes of Bacteriuria in Chronic Care Facilities

	Women (%)	Men (%)
E. coli	47	11
Proteus mirabilis	27	30
P. stuartii	7	16
Klebsiella	7	6
Pseudomonas	5	19
Enterococcus	6	5

Source: Adapted from Nicolle LE. Urinary tract infection. In: Yoshikawa TT, Norman DC, eds. Infectious Disease in the Aging. Totowa, NJ: Humana Press, 2001.

2.3. Clinical Manifestations

Typical symptoms of UTI in nursing home residents are symptoms referable to the bladder such as suprapubic pain, dysuria, new or worsening frequency, and urgency. Flank pain and fever also occur in association with pyelonephritis. While fever frequently leads to an evaluation for UTI, UTI only accounts for 10% of fevers in the nursing home setting. As a result, fever associated with change in mental status is rarely a UTI and another cause should be sought. For some older patients with UTI, the clinical findings may be change in functional status (e.g., unable to walk), loss of appetite, acute urinary incontinence, or new-onset delirium. Change in smell or turbidity of the urine can be due to the patient fluid status, the presence of metabolites from food, urinary sediment, or crystals. Neither smell nor cloudiness is a reliable indicator of UTI or the need for treatment (3–5). Again, a large percentage of nursing home residents may have bacteriuria without associated genitourinary complaints.

2.4. Diagnosis

The major dilemma is differentiating UTI from asymptomatic bacteriuria. A significant proportion of nursing home residents will have significant bacteriuria ($>10^5$ colony forming units/mL) without symptoms. Treatment of asymptomatic bacteriuria has demonstrated that no benefit to the patient in terms of improved well-being, relief of chronic symptoms, or survival and antibiotic resistance has emerged.

Pyuria of any degree is not a useful indicator of infection as 30% of asymptomatic residents have chronic inflammation as well. Urinalysis is useful if no pyuria is present. Absence of pyuria strongly correlates with absence of bacteriuria. If urinalysis shows no pyuria or negative leukocyte esterase, then no UTI is present and an alternative diagnosis should be sought (3–5).

Therefore, in the nursing home resident, the diagnosis of UTI traditionally hinges on the presence of new or worsening symptoms and signs referable to the urinary tract. Even in the cognitively impaired nursing home resident, reproducible pain over the bladder or flanks in the presence of significant bacteriuria and pyuria provides presumptive evidence that a UTI is present, particularly if symptoms improve with appropriate antibiotics. As stated earlier, new-onset functional incapacity, anorexia, cognitive impairment, and/or urinary incontinence in the absence of any other causes may be due to UTI. In the absence of such findings, empirical therapy can be tried with the recognition that another source of infection might be present. Failure to improve should lead to evaluation for another source of infection or noninfectious cause (3–5).

2.5. Antibiotic Treatment

Antibiotic therapy should be based on culture results and antimicrobial susceptibilities. Prior culture results rarely predict the causative organism. If the patient is clinically stable, therapy can be withheld until results are known. If the patient has severe dysuria or is unstable then antibiotic choices can be made based on the most likely organism and local susceptibility patterns. If empirical treatment must be started, quinolones, trimethoprim–sulfamethoxazole, or nitrofurantoin can be used to treat most common GNB. However, close follow-up of culture results and antimicrobial susceptibilities is necessary because resistance to all of these drugs is increasing, particularly in *E. coli* worldwide. For patients with bacteriuria and pyuria who have frequent episodes of brief alterations of mental status, some experts have suggested a brief trial of IV fluids to treat dehydration and promote urinary tract flushing before considering antibiotic therapy (3–5).

2.6. Prevention

Prevention of recurrent UTI should focus on the underlying cause. Sources of urinary obstruction or stasis should be sought and corrected surgically or pharmacologically if possible, particularly if the patient has relapse with the same organism. The indication for the use of a urinary catheter should be determined and alternative means of toileting tried if incontinence and convenience are the only indications.

For community-dwelling women, topical estrogen use was associated with normalization of vaginal flora and pH and reduction in UTI episodes. Cranberry juice may inhibit binding of GNB to uroepithelial cells. Once-daily low doses of trimethoprim–sulfamethoxazole, quinolones, or nitrofurantoin have been used in that population with some success. Whether these approaches would be beneficial in nursing homes in women with otherwise normal urinary tracts is not known. Suppressive antibiotics have been effective in reducing the frequency of recurrent UTIs in spinal cord patients with chronic catheters, but resistance rapidly emerges (3–5).

3. PNEUMONIA/LRTI (See Also Chapter 30)

3.1. Epidemiology and Clinical Relevance

Pneumonia is typically the second most common infection in nursing home. Rates of infection vary from 33 to 114 cases per 1000 residents per year or 0.3–2.5 episodes per 1000 days of resident care (6,8). Risk factors for nursing home-acquired pneumonia have included increasing age, increasing debility, poor cough reflex, swallowing disorders, presence of a feeding tube or tracheostomy, alterations in cognition, and chronic lung disease. Silent aspiration of oropharyngeal flora is thought to play a major role in the development of pneumonia in the nursing home.

3.2. Etiologic Pathogens

It is difficult to optimally assess the underlying cause of nursing home-acquired pneumonia due to difficulties in obtaining adequate sputum specimens. In a few carefully performed studies, the bacterial causes of nursing home-acquired pneumonia appear to most closely mirror those seen in older adults in the community rather than in the acute care setting (Table 2). *Streptococcus pneumoniae*, non-typeable *Haemophilus influenzae*, and *Moraxella catarrhalis* are the most common causes of LRTI in nursing home patients. Compared with hospital, pneumonia due to aerobic GNB is uncommon even though colonization with these organisms increases with age, debility, and medications that cause xerostomia. When pneumonia due to GNB occurs, *Klebsiella* is the most common organism.

Atypical pneumonia due to *Legionella*, *Chlamydia pneumoniae*, and *Mycoplasma pneumoniae* has been described in the nursing home setting. Influenza and other viruses are common causes of upper respiratory tract infections (URTI) that can lead to secondary bacterial pneumonia due to pneumococci or *S. aureus*. Primary atypical pneumonia due to viruses such as influenza is uncommon (6–8).

Table 2 Prevalence of Lower Respiratory
Tract Pathogens in Nursing Home Residents

Organism	(%)
Streptococcus pneumoniae	4–30
Klebsiella spp.	4–6
C. pneumoniae	0–18
H. influenzae	0–2
S. aureus	0–4
Moraxella cattarrhalis	0–4
Influenza	0–4
Pseudomonas aeruginosa	0–2
E. coli	0–2
Legionella	0–1

Source: Adapted from Ref. 6.

3.3. Clinical Manifestations

Typical symptoms of bacterial pneumonia are reduced in older nursing home residents. Relatively few residents have symptoms of cough (60%), dyspnea (40%), fever (65%), and altered cognition (50–70%) (8). Only 56% of residents will present with the triad of cough, shortness of breath, or fever (6). Tachypnea and tachycardia are seen in 66% of older adults and may precede other symptoms. Therefore, new and acute onset of nonspecific symptoms associated with pneumonia such as falls, incontinence, or worsening of preexisting comorbid illnesses such as diabetes mellitus, congestive heart failure, or Parkinsonism should prompt evaluation for pneumonia as a cause.

3.4. Diagnosis

In nursing home residents with pneumonia, rales are present on physical examination 55% of the time. Presence of respiratory rates greater than 25 breaths per minute is strongly associated with the presence of pneumonia. This degree of tachypnea and pulse oximetry <90% also herald impending respiratory failure. Chest radiographs can confirm the presence of pneumonia in 90% of nursing residents with LRTI despite technical difficulties or lack of prior films for comparison. Chest radiographs may also provide prognostic information (multilobar disease) or evidence of empyema or mass lesions that might alter treatment (1).

Recommendations regarding the utility of sputum cultures are controversial. Sputum specimens are infrequently obtained and frequently are contaminated with upper airway secretions. Results from cultures of adequate sputum specimens can help guide therapeutic decisions if the patient is not responding appropriately to empiric antibiotic therapy. Sputum specimens also provide important information regarding the presence of antibiotic-resistant bacteria in the facility or uncommon bacteria that might alter infection control procedures.

If rates of URTI and LRTI increase, particularly in winter months, an outbreak of viral infection may be present in the facility. After initiation of appropriate infection control procedures, nasopharyngeal cultures and antigen-based tests for viruses may be useful to confirm that an outbreak of influenza, parainfluenza, respiratory syncitial virus, coronaviruses, adenoviruses, and others are present in the facility. If influenza is detected in the facility, antiviral prophylaxis may be initiated or continued and more intensive infection control measures considered. Unfortunately, one cannot completely rely on current antigen-based tests alone for detection of influenza. If influenza is in the community, clinical symptoms of fever and new respiratory symptoms of <48 hr duration may be just as sensitive a means of diagnosis (16).

3.5. Antibiotic Treatment

Initial empirical therapy of pneumonia in the nursing home should focus on appropriate treatment of *S. pneumoniae*, *H. influenzae*, and *Moraxella*. Rates of multidrug-resistant pneumococci are increased in older adults, particularly in settings where the selective pressure of antibiotic use is high. Currently, it is thought that the levels of penicillin achieved are sufficient to treat most resistant pneumococcal strains. Avoidance of treatment with penicillin or amoxacillin alone has been due primarily to the high prevalence of β-lactamase-producing *H. influenzae*. So for empirical treatment of nursing home pneumonias, use of a penicillin/β-lactamase inhibitor combination (ampicillin plus sulbactam or clavulanic acid or piperacilin plus tazobactam), β-lactamase-resistant cephalosporins (ceftriaxone), ketolides, or quinolones with activity against *S. pneumoniae* (gatifloxacin, moxifloxacin) would be appropriate (6–8,17,18).

Retrospective studies have suggested that patients with community-acquired pneumonia have better outcomes if empirical therapy also includes therapy for *Mycoplasma*, *Chlamydia*, and in endemic areas, *Legionella*. Macrolides, ketolides, and quinolones have activity against these atypical bacteria. Studies have not been done to prove that the outcome of nursing home residents is improved when macrolides are added to penicillins or cephalosporins as outlined earlier or when quinolones are given alone (6–8,17,18).

If pneumonia fails to improve with appropriate empirical antibiotic therapy then further diagnostic studies should be done to exclude the presence of antibiotic resistance, obstruction, or less common causes of respiratory symptoms and pulmonary infiltrates such as tuberculosis (19).

3.6. Prevention

Prevention of pneumonia in nursing home residents should focus on the use of vaccination, prevention of aspiration, and infection control. While, influenza vaccine prevents illness due to the virus itself in only ≈40% nursing home residents, it is highly effective in preventing cardiopulmonary complications including secondary bacterial pneumonia and death. While there is increasing evidence that prophylaxis and treatment of influenza with newer antiviral agents are effective in older adults, these drugs are not a substitute for vaccination. Vaccination of healthcare workers has been associated with a significant reduction in influenza infection in nursing home residents (16).

While the efficacy of the pneumococcal polysaccharide vaccination in nursing home residents remains controversial, its use is recommended (6–8). A large preliminary study by the CDC has confirmed that high influenza and pneumococcal vaccination rates among residents of nursing homes were associated with significant reductions in morbidity and mortality from RTI and its complications (20).

Reduction of aspiration risk may be important in pneumonia prevention. Feeding tubes of any kind actually increase aspiration risk and pneumonia and should be avoided. Feeding techniques and other noninvasive methods designed to reduce aspiration should be tried first. In addition, rates of LRTI may be reduced in nursing home residents with good dentition and intensive oral hygiene programs may be an important preventative measure (6–8).

Elimination of unnecessary medications may also play an important role in pneumonia prevention, and medications that cause sedation should be avoided in nursing home residents if possible. Drugs with anticholinergic activity in particular may also cause dry mouth, promote caries and colonization with pathogens. It has been suggested that drugs that inhibit stomach acid may allow replication of potential pathogens in the stomach that could be aspirated. However, treatment of gastroesophageal reflux with H2-blockers and proton-pump inhibitors has also been reported as a means to reduce aspiration and prevent pneumonia. Further studies need to be done before any specific recommendations can be made with regard to the use of acid-inhibiting drugs (6–8).

4. SKIN AND SOFT TISSUE INFECTIONS (See Also Chapter 35)

4.1. Epidemiology and Clinical Relevance

SSTI are the third most common infectious clinical syndrome in the nursing home. Rates of 1–9% have been reported or a prevalence of 0.9–2.1 per 1000 patient-days (2). Predisposing risk factors for superficial skin infection are common among nursing home residents, such as peripheral vascular disease and conditions that contribute to peripheral edema such as chronic venous insufficiency, lymphedema, and immobility.

In nursing home residents, SSTI primarily result when breaks in skin or mucosa occur as a consequence of physical trauma, maceration, pressure, or use of devices. Wounds may become secondarily infected by pathogens found among the resident's own endogenous flora or exogenously via the hands of personnel, from other residents, or by contact with contaminated environment or fomites.

Primary mucocutaneous infections, conjunctivitis, and secondary infection of pressure ulcers are some of the most common manifestations of SSTI seen among nursing home residents. These less severe primary skin infections are not reportable and whether these infections occur more commonly in nursing home residents than in community-dwelling elderly is not known (9,10,21,22).

Superficial bacterial skin infections found in the nursing home range from common and less severe primary pyodermas to less common and life-threatening deep infection (9,23). Maceration of skin, use of antimicrobials, corticosteroids, and other factors may allow overgrowth of endogenous resident flora, with resulting fungal infection (9). Mucocutanous infection can also occur as ·a consequence of reactivation of latent viral infections with increasing age (23,24). It has been estimated that 10,000 to 20,000 cases of herpes zoster occur in nursing home residents each year (see also Chapter 36: Herpes Zoster). Parasitic infestations can be acquired exogenously from other residents or contamination of the environment (9,23) (see also Chapter 46: Parasites).

Conjunctivitis is another common soft tissue infection that occurs in 0.3–3.4% of nursing home residents or at a rate of 0.1–1.0 cases per 1000 resident-days.

Table 3 Skin and Soft Tissue Infections in Nursing Home Residents

Common pathogens	
Primary infection	
Mucocutaneous	*S. aureus*, β-hemolytic streptococci, herpes simplex and herpes zoster, *C. albicans*, dermatophytes, scabies, and lice
Conjunctivitis	*S. aureus*, β-hemolytic streptococci, *Hemophilus influenzae*, *Moraxella cattarhalis*, and adenovirus (epidemic infection)
Fascia/muscle	*S. aureus* and β-hemolytic streptococci
Secondary infection	
Pressure ulcers	Polymicrobial aerobic and anaerobic GNB and gram-positive cocci

Conjunctivitis has been associated with the presence of chronic eye diseases such as glaucoma, entropion, and ectropion in some studies (21) (see also chapter "Ocular Infections").

The prevalence of pressure ulcers stage II and greater varies widely; rates range from 1% to 11% and rates exceed 20% if stage I ulcers are included (22). Varying prevalences reflect the heterogeneity of resident debility, age, and other risk factors. Risk of development of pressure ulcers increases with the length of stay; ≈20% of nursing home residents will develop an ulcer within 2 years of admission (10,22). Approximately 6% of pressure ulcers in nursing home residents will become infected or 1.4 infections per 1000 resident-days (22).

4.2. Etiologic Pathogens

4.2.1. Primary SSTI

Primary infections of skin and mucosa in nursing home residents may be due to bacteria, viruses, parasites, and fungi (Table 3). Common bacterial causes of primary bacterial SSTI include *S. aureus* and β-hemolytic streptococci, especially group A (9,23). Fungal causes of mucocutaneous infection include *Candida* spp., particularly *albicans*, and dermatophytes (9). Viral etiologies include herpes zoster and herpes simplex (23,24). Parasitic infections are caused primarily by the ectoparasites *Sarcoptes scabiei* and lice (*Pediculus humanus capitus, Pediculus humanus corporis*, and *Phthirus pubis*) (9,23).

4.2.2. Conjunctivitis

Most cases of acute infectious conjunctivitis in nursing home residents are probably due to viruses. Adenovirus has been associated with outbreaks attributed to contaminated ophthalmologic diagnostic equipment or medications. A bacterial cause of acute conjunctivitis has been established in only 38% of cases; most were due to *S. aureus* followed by *M. catarrhalis*, or *Haemophilus* spp. Outbreaks of group A streptococcal conjunctivitis have also been reported (21).

4.2.3. Secondary Infections

Most secondary infections of pressure ulcers are polymicrobial and contain aerobic and anaerobic GNB and gram-positive bacteria commonly found to colonize the perineum and lower extremities. *E. coli, Proteus, Pseudomonas*, staphylococci, and enterococci can be isolated aerobically from tissue while *Peptostreptococcus, Bacteroides*, and *Clostridium perfringens* require anaerobic culture conditions (10,22).

4.3. Clinical Manifestations

The common primary bacterial infections seen in nursing home residents involve skin and subcutaneous tissue such as cellulitis, folliculitis, paronychia, impetigo, and erysipelas. Deep soft tissue infections involving fascia and muscle occur rarely, often as part of an outbreak. If a resident is undergoing appropriate treatment for apparent cellulitis, increasing pain and worsening clinical status out of proportion with the physical examination should prompt immediate evaluation for deep infection or necrotizing process (e.g., necrotizing fasciitis) (9,23).

Mucocutaneuous candidosis may present as thrush, denture stomatitis, chelitis, paronychia, and intertrigo. Skin infections due to dermatophytes infection may manifest as tinea corporis, tinea pedis, tinea cruris, and tinea ungium (onychomycosis) (9).

Herpes simplex infections typically present as mucocutaneous vesicles or ulcerations involving nasolabial, genital, or rectal skin or mucosa. Reactivation of herpes zoster presents as a painful vesicular rash typically in a dermatomal distribution (23,24).

The clinical presentation of scabies infection in nursing home patients can be atypical. Burrows, inflammatory changes in intertrigenous areas, and pruritis may be absent. Debilitated patients may present only with hyperkeratosis or cruster "Norwegian" scabies. Diagnosis of scabies is often made when more typical rash occurs in healthcare workers or visitors. Infectious complications of infected pressure ulcers range from localized involvement of skin, subcutaneous, muscle, and bone to bacteremia and severe systemic infection (9,23).

4.4. Diagnosis

4.4.1. Primary Skin Infection

Causes of superficial skin infection are determined primarily on the basis of typical clinical characteristics. In cases where the presentation is atypical or the patient is not responding to therapy, culture of pus, blister fluid, or scrapings of skin or ulcers can be useful. Gram stain and cultures from abscess material or tissue can be useful to confirm a bacterial cause and, more importantly, its antimicrobial susceptibility. Examination of scrapings with 10% potassium hydroxide can confirm the presence of candida or dermatophytes (9,23).

The presence of giant cells on Tzanck smear is diagnostic of herpetic infection and vesicle fluid for immunofluorescence antigen is sensitive for the detection of herpes zoster. Differentiation between the two viral infections is important because of infection control issues and treatment of postherpetic neuraligia with herpes zoster (23,24).

Examination of deep skin scrapings of atypical rashes under immersion oil can detect mites, ova, and feces typical of scabies. Lice are typically found at the base of hair follicles (nits) or in the seams of clothing (9,23).

4.4.2. Conjunctivitis

Conjunctivitis is primarily a clinical diagnosis. Conjunctivitis has been defined as the presence of purulent exudate or new or worsening redness in one or both eyes for at least 24 hr. Pain or itching may be present, but symptoms should not be attributed to allergy or trauma (21).

4.4.3. Secondary Infection of Pressure Ulcers

Infection of pressure ulcers is diagnosed primarily by the presence of localized clinical symptoms and signs. These local findings may range from nonhealing to overt presence of surrounding erythema, warmth, tenderness, and purulent discharge to presence of necrotic tissue and even crepitus. Signs of systemic inflammation such as fever and leukocytosis may be absent. The criteria of McGeer et al. including the presence of purulent discharge plus four or more of the following are sufficient for the diagnosis of infection of a pressure ulcer: fever $\geq 38°C$ or worsening mental or functional status or warmth or redness or swelling or localized tenderness/pain, or serous drainage (10,22).

All pressure ulcers are colonized by bacteria and only deep tissue biopsy specimens should be taken for culture. Cultures of blood may be useful to determine the infecting organism and provide supporting evidence that the pressure ulcer is infected. Secondary bacteremia can occur and 41% of associated bacterial skin infection will be polymicrobial (1,10,22,25).

Diagnosis of underlying osteomyelitis is made primarily by characteristic histopathology on bone biopsy. Magnetic resonance imaging is a sensitive and specific method to diagnose osteomyelitis and may be useful to choose an optimal site for biopsy. Radiography and radionucleotide scintigraphy are not useful because they cannot reliably differentiate osteomyelitis from pressure-related heterotopic bone formation. Computerized tomography is too insensitive to reliably detect osteomyelitis and its use is limited to evaluation of soft tissues (10,22).

4.5. Antibiotic Treatment

4.5.1. Primary Skin Infection

Empirical treatment should be directed against the most likely cause or based on diagnostic evaluation as described above. For empirical treatment of less severe S. aureus (presumed MSSA) and streptococcal infections, oral treatment with first-generation cephalosporins (cephalexin) and antistaphylococcal penicillins (dicloxacillin, amoxacillin–clavulanate) are appropriate. For penicillin-allergic patients, clindamycin or a quinolone with activity against streptococci (gatifloxacin) can be used. In patients who do not respond to empirical therapy or have known MRSA, trimethoprim–sulfamethoxazole should be considered. For severe bacterial SSTI, IV antibiotics can be considered. Cefazolin and ampicillin–sulbactam can be used if the facility allows three to four doses per day. For severe MRSA infection, vancomycin, daptomycin, or oral linezolid are appropriate choices. As of this writing, the efficacy of treatment of bacterial skin infection with daptomycin or linezolid has not been established (9,14,23).

Most herpes simplex and localized herpes zoster infections can be treated with oral acyclovir, famciclovir, or valcyclovir. Herpes zoster requires higher doses of these agents than does herpes simplex. Patients with disseminated herpes zoster should be treated with IV medications and transferred to a hospital for appropriate treatment and airbone isolation should be considered. Patients with herpes zoster should also receive appropriate management of their acute pain and postherpetic neuralgia (23,24).

Oral candidosis can be treated with topical liquid nystatin, clotrimazole troches, or oral fluconazole. Depending on the severity, infection of intact skin can be treated with topical clotrimazole or oral fluconazole. Dermatophyte infections typically respond to treatment with topical clotrimazole, oral itraconazole, or terbinafine. Onychomycosis typically requires prolonged therapy with an oral agent (9) (see also Chapters 25: Antifungal Drugs and 44: Fungi).

Treatment of scabies in nursing home residents can be difficult. Permethrin 5% cream is the treatment of choice due to its lack of central nervous system toxicity. Nails should be trimmed and cream should be applied from the neck to toes and left in place for up to 12 hr. For residents with crusted scabies, oral ivermectin can be considered. Antipruritic therapy should also be given as needed. For head and pubic lice, permethrin or lindane shampoo is applied with frequent combing to remove nits. For non-hair-bearing areas, lotions may be applied. Residents should be re-examined on a weekly basis to ensure that the scabies and lice have been eradicated (9,23) (see also Chapters 26: Antiparasitic Drugs and 46: Parasites).

4.5.2. Conjunctivitis

Treatment of conjunctivitis should be based primarily on Gram strain, culture, and antibiotic susceptibilities of purulent discharge obtained from the conjunctival sac. Treatment should be directed against *S. aureus* and β-hemolytic streptococci until results of microbiology studies are known. Topical ophthalmic antibiotic drops or ointments, such as erythromycin, quinolones, sulfonamides, and tetracyclines, are appropriate first choices. There is no specific treatment for viral conjunctivitis. Cool compresses, analgesia, and artificial tears may provide symptomatic relief. Residents should be monitored for development of bacterial superinfection (21) (see also Chapter 27: Ocular Infections).

4.5.3. Secondary Infection of Pressure Ulcers

Treatment of infected pressure ulcers should be based on results of deep tissue biopsy culture and antimicrobial susceptibilities, and empirical treatment is directed against both aerobic and anaerobic pathogens. This antibacterial spectrum can be achieved through the use of single IV antibiotic agents such as cefoxitin or cefotetan, broad-spectrum penicillin–β-lactamase combinations such as ticarcillin–clavulanate or piperacillin–tazobactam, or carbapenems (imipenem, meropenem, or ertapenem), or some of the newer quinolones with anaerobic activity and good oral bioavailability such as gatifloxacin. Older antibiotics which do not have anaerobic activity can be combined with clindamycin or metronidazole orally or intravenously. If MRSA is present, vancomycin, daptomycin, or linezolid should be added. Currently, linezolid and daptomycin have not been approved for treatment of osteomyelitis. Debridement of devitalized tissue, appropriate wound care, reduction of pressure, nutritional repletion, and modification of other risk factors are important adjuncts to the treatment of pressure ulcers (10,22).

4.6. Prevention

The primary means of preventing primary skin infection is the use of contact isolation where appropriate. Decolonization therapy has been tried in staphylococcal carriers with recurrent infection, but it is not clear that infection is prevented (14). Herpes zoster is potentially contagious to healthcare workers who have not had primary infection or vaccination and to other compromised residents. At a minimum, residents with herpes zoster should be in a private room with contact precautions until all vesicles have crusted. Some experts recommend airborne isolation in patients with disseminated disease (23,24).

For scabies, clothing, linens, and towels should be laundered in hot water. Nonwashable items can be sealed in plastic for 96 hr. All roommates and persons providing direct care should also be treated even if they are asymptomatic (9,23).

Prevention of pressure ulcers should be directed toward education of health-care workers, identification of residents at risk of developing pressure ulcers, and attention to appropriate use of techniques to reduce pressure and position and turn patients. Treatment of incontinence is essential to reduce skin maceration as well. Prevention of pressure ulcer infection should be directed at use of good infection control techniques when caring for patients, reduction of contamination of wounds by use of sterile instruments, clean dressings, and avoidance of fecal contamination whenever possible (10,22).

5. INFECTIOUS GASTROENTERITIS AND DIARRHEA

5.1. Epidemiology and Clinical Relevance

Older adults are at increased risk of infectious complications of GI conditions that commonly increase with age, such as achlorhydria, diverticulosis, and cholelithiasis. In nursing home residents, GI infection is manifested most commonly as gastroenteritis or diarrhea. Diarrheal pathogens can be readily spread in the closed environment of the nursing home especially when the personal hygiene of residents is less than optimal and toilet facilities are often shared. Use of devices such as feeding tubes or thermometers may also provide an efficient means to directly introduce pathogens into the GI tract (11,26,27).

Causes of gastroenteritis or diarrhea may be bacterial, viral, or, less commonly, parasitic (Table 4). These pathogens may be acquired from environmental sources, direct contact with other infected residents or on the hands of personnel, contamination of common food and water sources, or by pets, and may result in outbreaks. While the exact incidence of these outbreaks in the nursing home is not known, scattered reports of GI infection in numerous facilities suggest that the problem is common (11,12,27,28).

Table 4 Causes of Diarrhea and Gastroenteritis in Nursing Homes

Clinical manifestation	Organism
Invasive disease	
Bacterial	*Salmonella, Shigella,* and *Campylobacter*
Parasitic	*E. histolytica*
Noninvasive disease	
Viral	Rotavirus and norovirus (Norwalk agent)
Parasitic	*Giardia lamblia*
Toxin-mediated disease	
Food-borne	*E. coli* 0157:H7, S. aureus, *C. perfringens,* and *B. cereus*
Non-food-borne	*C. difficile*

Diarrheal infection in older adults is not a trivial matter; most deaths occur in this age group. Greater than 50% of all deaths attributed to diarrhea occur in adults aged 74 and older. One-third of these deaths occur among nursing home residents (11,27,28).

5.2. Etiologic Pathogens

Noninfectious and infectious causes of diarrhea are common in the nursing home setting. For many cases, the cause is frequently not identified, there is no specific therapy beyond symptomatic treatment, and the course is self-limited. Thus, the exact incidence of causes of infectious diarrhea is not known and most information is derived from outbreak investigations (27,28).

C. difficile is the most readily identified cause of infectious diarrhea in the nursing home, probably, in part, because the tests for toxins A and B are easily performed and treatment is available and effective. Sporadic cases and outbreaks of *C. difficile* have been identified in the nursing home setting. In one study, 33% of nursing home residents acquired *C. difficile* within 2 weeks of receiving antibiotic therapy (12).

The GI tracts of older adults are frequently exposed to *C. difficile* spores that readily survive in the healthcare environment and can contaminate the hands of personnel and devices. Asymptomatic colonization of the GI tract can persist in this population because the host response to *C. difficile* is impaired with increasing age and debility. With the selective pressure of broad-spectrum antibiotics so common in the nursing home setting, *C. difficile* can emerge as the dominant flora and diarrhea can ensue (12).

Most other pathogens are identified only after an outbreak of gastroenteritis is identified and viruses or other bacteria are suspected. Most outbreaks have been due to calciviruses such as norovirus (Norwalk virus), rotaviruses, and adenoviruses. Outbreaks of *Salmonella*, *E. coli* 0157:H7, *S. aureus*, and *C. perfringens* have been associated with improper handling of food. Other uncommon bacterial causes of outbreaks in the nursing home have been due to *Shigella*, *Aeromonas*, *Campylobacter*, and *Bacillus* species. Rare outbreaks due to parasitic infections such as *Entamoeba histolytica*, *Giardia lamblia*, and *Cryptosporidium parvum* have also been noted (11,27,28).

5.3. Clinical Manifestations

A typical definition of diarrhea includes the presence of three or more watery, loose, or unformed stools per day for 48 hr or more. Clinical manifestations of toxin-mediated *C. difficile*-associated diarrhea can range from asymptomatic to mild diarrhea, pseudomembranous colitis, and toxic megacolon. Symptoms can vary from fever with mild crampy abdominal pain to ileus and peritonitis. It is not clear that symptoms differ in the elderly, but symptoms are often attributed to other causes and delaying the diagnosis (11,12).

Diarrhea due to noninvasive pathogens such as rotavirus, norovirus, other viruses, and *G. lamblia* is typically watery, nonbloody, and other inflammatory symptoms and signs are absent. Fever is uncommon, and extraintestinal symptoms of nausea and vomiting may be present. In diarrheas due to invasive pathogens such as *Salmonella*, *Shigella*, and *Campylobacter*, bloody stool, fever, and other inflammatory signs can be more prominent (11,12).

Not all bloody stool is due to an invasive pathogen. *E. coli* 0157:H7 and other shiga-toxin-producing strains can cause hemorrhagic colitis and fever is typically absent. Epidemics of nausea and vomiting alone can be seen in nursing homes following the ingestion of food contaminated with toxin-producing strains of *S. aureus*, *Bacillus cereus*, or *C. perfringens* (11,12).

5.4. Diagnosis

In nursing home, diagnosis of *C. difficile* and some invasive diarrheas is important because specific treatment and initiation of infection control procedures is required. The diagnosis of *C. difficile* should strongly be considered if the patient has received antibiotics or chemotherapy in the past 4–6 weeks. Elevated peripheral leukocyte counts and fecal leukocytes may be seen with invasive or toxigenic diarrheas. Very high peripheral leukocyte counts >30,000 cells/mm^3 have been typical of *C. difficile* infection (12).

Some diarrheas are diagnosed by assay of toxin in stool. For *C. difficile*, the diagnosis hinges primarily on the demonstration of toxins A or B in diarrheal stool specimens. Stools should not be sent in patients without diarrhea as asymptomatic carriage of toxin-*producing C. difficile* is common in nursing home residents. The toxin assays are 70–90% sensitive to detect the organism, particularly if multiple specimens are sent. Similarly, stool shiga-toxin can be detected in residents with *E. coli* 0157:H7 infection. Stool culture for *C. difficile* is not useful as non-toxin-producing strains are commonly found in the stool of healthy persons, and many laboratories no longer perform the test. Endoscopy is not a substitute for stool toxin assays as not all cases of *C. difficile* have pseudomembranes and isolated right-sided disease can be missed (11,12).

Invasive diarrheas, such as *Salmonella*, *Shigella*, *Campylobacter*, *Aeromonas*, and other pathogens, can be diagnosed by stool culture. Diagnosis of noninvasive diarrhea and gastroenteritis is generally not warranted unless an outbreak investigation is ongoing. Most new laboratory methods rely on the detection of viral antigens in stool rather than culture (11,12).

5.5. Antibiotic Treatment

In residents with gastroenteritis or diarrhea who are not systemically ill, fluid repletion, treatment of nausea and vomiting, and monitoring and correction of electrolyte imbalances are the primary goals of treatment until results of stool studies are known. For patients with viral gastroenteritis, no treatment is available and symptomatic treatment is sufficient. For *E. coli* 0157:H7, antibiotic treatment is not recommended because of increased risk of development of hemolytic uremic syndrome (11).

For nursing home residents with moderate to severe illness consistent with toxigenic or invasive diarrhea, antecedent antibiotics should be stopped if possible and empirical treatment for *C. difficile*, the most common bacterial pathogen, initiated. For nursing home residents with a functional GI tract and confirmed or presumed *C. difficile*, oral metronidazole 500 thrice daily is as efficacious as oral vancomycin 250 mg four times daily at a lower cost. Treatment should be continued for 10–14 days. Relapses are common and a second course of metronidazole treatment may be necessary. For patients with refractory or recurrent *C. difficile* diarrhea, consultation with a specialist should be sought. Residents found to have *C. difficile* in their stool, but who no longer have diarrhea, should not be treated (12) (see also Chapters 18: Metronidazole in the Elderly and 12: Glycopeptides.

For invasive diarrheas, treatment should be based on the organism identified, the residents's clinical condition, and antibiotic susceptibilities. For empirical therapy, most invasive pathogens are currently susceptible to the quinolones. Older adults are at greater risk of *Shigella* bacteremia and death so treatment should be initiated to eradicate the organism, prevent spread, and potentially reduce the severity of the illness. Treatment of *Salmonella* infection is not recommended in younger adults due to prolongation of shedding. However, metastatic seeding to extraintestinal sites such as vascular and musculoskeletal systems is increased with aging, leading most experts to recommend treatment in the elderly (11).

5.6. Prevention

Fecal–oral spread of infectious gastroenteritis and diarrhea can be prevented by good personal hygiene and hand disinfection on the part of residents, visitors, and healthcare workers. Adherence to appropriate infection control procedures and food preparation guidelines can also prevent spread by contaminated food, water, and other means. To eradicate the environmental reservoir of *C. difficile*, disinfection with a sporocidal agent is recommended. Asymptomatic carriers of *C. difficile* do not have to be isolated (12).

REFERENCES

1. Bentley DW, Bradley S, High K, Schoenbaum S, Taler G, Yoshikawa TT. Practice guideline for evaluation of fever and infection in long-term care facilities. J Am Geriatr Soc 2001; 49:210–222.
2. Nicolle LE. Infection control in long-term care facilities. Clin Infect Dis 2000; 31: 752–756.
3. Yoshikawa TT, Norman DC. Approach to fever and infection in the nursing home. J Am Geriatr Soc 1996; 44:74–82.
4. Nicolle LE. SHEA Long-Term-Care Committee. Urinary tract infections in long-term-care facilities. Infect Control Hosp Epidemiol 2001; 22:167–175.
5. Nicolle LE, Bradley S, Colgan R, Rice JC, Schaeffer A, Hooton TM. Infectious Diseases Society of America guideline for the diagnosis and treatment of asymptomatic bacteriuria in adults. Clin Infect Dis 2005; 40:643–654.
6. Janssens J-P, Krause K-H. Pneumonia in the very old. Lancet Infect Dis 2204; 112–124.
7. Loeb M. Pneumonia in older persons. Clin Infect Dis 2003; 37:1335–1339.
8. Mylotte JM. Nursing home-acquired pneumonia. Clin Infect Dis 2002; 35:1205–1211.
9. Lertzman BH, Gaspari AA. Drug treatment of skin and soft tissue infections in elderly long-term care residents. Drugs Aging 1996; 9:109–121.
10. Smith PW, Black JM, Black SB. Infected pressure ulcers in the long-term-care facility. Infect Control Hosp Epidemiol 1999; 20:358–361.
11. Mishkin DS, Brandt LJ. Management and treatment of infectious diarrhea in the elderly. Clin Geriatr 2003; 11:44–53.
12. Simor AE, Bradley SF, Strausbaugh LJ, Crossley K, Nicolle LE. SHEA Long-Term Care Committee. *Clostridium difficile* in long-term-care facilities for the elderly. Infect Control Hosp Epidemiol 2002; 23:696–703.
13. Bradley SF. Issues in the management of resistant bacteria in long-term care facilities. Infect Control Hosp Epidemiol 1999; 20:362–366.
14. Bradley SF. *Staphylococcus aureus* infections and antibiotic resistance in older adults. Clin Infect Dis 2002; 34:211–216.

15. Loeb M, Bentley DW, Bradley S, Crossley K, Garibaldi R, McGeer A, Muder RR, Mylotte J, Nicolle LE, Nurse B, Paton S, Simor AE, Smith P, Strausbaugh L. Development of minimum criteria for the initiation of antibiotics in residents of long-term-care facilities: results of a consensus conference. Infect Control Hosp Epidemiol 2001; 22: 120–124.

16. Bradley SF, Society for Healthcare Epidemiology of America Committee on Long-Term Care. Prevention of influenza in chronic care facilities: a position statement. Infect Control Hosp Epidemiol 1999; 20:629–637.

17. File TM, Tan JS. International guidelines for the treatment of community-acquired pneumonia in adults: role of macrolides. Drugs 2003; 63:181–205.

18. Mandell LA, Bartlett JG, Dowell SF, File TM, Musher DM, Whitney C. Update of practice guidelines for management of community-acquired pneumonia in immunocompetent adults. Clin Infect Dis 2003; 37:1405–1433.

19. Thrupp L, Bradley S, Smith P, Simor A, Gantz N, The Society for Healthcare Epidemiology of America Committee on Long-Term Care. Tuberculosis prevention and control in long-term-care facilities for the older adult. Infect Control Hosp Epidemiol 2004; 25: 1097–1108.

20. Kazakova SK, Curtis A, Bratzle, Nsa W, McKibben L, Shefer A, Steele L, Richards C, Jernigan JA. Impact of pneumococcal and influenza vaccination on the risk of hospitalization among nursing home residents. 14th Annual Meeting on Society for Healthcare Epidemiology of American Annual Conference, Abstract #61, Philadelphia, PA, Apr 17–20, 2004.

21. Boutstcha E, Nicolle LE. Conjunctivitis in a long-term care facility. Infect Control Hosp Epidemiol 1995; 16:210–216.

22. Livesley NJ, Chow AW. Infected pressure ulcers in elderly individuals. Clin Infect Dis 2002; 35:1390–1396.

23. Schmader K, Twersky J. Herpes zoster, cellulitis, and scabies. In: Yoshikawa TT, Ouslander JG, eds. Infection Management for Geriatrics in Long-Term Care Facilities. New York: Marcel-Dekker. Inc., 2002:283–303.

24. Schmader K. Herpes zoster in older adults. Clin Infect Dis 2001; 32:1481–1486.

25. Muder RR, Brennen C, Wagener MM, Goetz AM. Bacteremia in a long-term care facility: a 5 year prospective study. Clin Infect Dis 1992; 14:647–654.

26. Podnos YD, Jimenez JC, Wilson SE. Intra-abdominal sepsis in elderly persons. Clin Infect Dis 2002; 35:62–68.

27. Strausbaugh LJ, Sukumar SR, Joseph CL. Infectious disease outbreaks in nursing homes. An unappreciated hazard for frail elderly persons. Clin Infect Dis 2003; 36: 870–876.

28. Levine WC, Smart JF, Archer DL, Bean NH, Tauxe RV. Foodborne disease outbreaks in nursing homes, 1975 through 1987. J Am Med Assoc 1991; 266:2105–2109.

SUGGESTED READING

Bentley DW, Bradley S, High K, Schoenbaum S, Taler G, Yoshikawa TT. Practice guideline for evaluation of fever and infection in long-term care facilities. J Am Geriatr Soc 2001; 49:210–222.

Strausbaugh LJ, Sukumar SR, Joseph CL. Infectious disease outbreaks in nursing homes. An unappreciated hazard for frail elderly persons. Clin Infect Dis 2003; 36:870–876.

Yoshikawa TT, Norman DC. Approach to fever and infection in the nursing home. J Am Geriatr Soc 1996; 44:74–82.

Yoshikawa TT, Norman DC. Infectious Disease in the Aging. Totowa, NJ: Humana Press, 2001:1–326.

Yoshikawa TT, Ouslander JG. Infection Management for Geriatrics in Long-Term Care Facilities. New York: Marcel-Dekker Inc., 2002:1–480.

50
Infection Control in Nursing Homes

Lona Mody
*Division of Geriatric Medicine, University of Michigan Medical School and
Veterans Affairs Ann Arbor Healthcare System, Ann Arbor, Michigan, U.S.A.*

Key Points:

- Infections are common in nursing homes and are responsible for significant morbidity and mortality.
- Nursing homes face unique challenges necessitating individualized infection control programs.
- Nursing homes have to comply with Centers for Medicare and Medicaid Services (CMS) and Omnibus Budget Reconciliation Act (OBRA) regulations to establish an infection control program and Occupational Safety and Health Administration (OSHA) regulations for protection of the staff members.
- An infection control practitioner plays a vital role in establishing a comprehensive yet targeted infection control program.
- Infection control programs should address an outbreak control plan for epidemics, surveillance for infections, isolation and precautions, staff education, hand hygiene, employee and resident health programs, and appropriate antibiotic use.

1. INTRODUCTION

The number of people living into old age in the United States is increasing at a steep rate with the most rapid segment being those >85 years old. Although less than 10% of the U.S. population aged ≥65 years reside in nursing homes, it is estimated that of the 2.2 million people who turned 65 in 1990, 43% will spend some time in nursing homes before they die (1). Infections in nursing homes are common and are a major source of morbidity and mortality. Every year approximately 1.5 million infections occur in residents in nursing homes (2); overall rates range from 1.4 to 13.97 infections/1000 resident-days (2–4). Infections are responsible for a substantial proportion of transfers to acute care. Nationally, deaths attributable to nursing home infections are as high as 400,000 each year (5–7). Urinary tract, respiratory, and skin and soft tissue infections are the most common endemic infections among nursing home residents. Epidemic infections most commonly reported are gastroenteritis, influenza, and skin infections (5–7).

2. CONSEQUENCES AND COSTS OF INFECTIONS
    IN NURSING HOMES

Infections are by far the most common cause of acute care hospitalization among nursing home residents, accounting for 27–63% of hospitalization from these facilities (8). Hazards of hospitalization are numerous and include functional decline, delirium, pressure ulcers, and the potential for adverse events. In addition, infections are the most frequent immediate cause of death among nursing home residents transferred to acute care facilities (5,6).

The costs of these infections can be monumental. Direct costs of antibiotics can range from $166 to $967 per month per facility (9). Costs of hospitalizations resulting from transfer of infection can range from $673 million to $2 billion a year (9). Consequences from loss of function and delirium leading to prolongation of hospital stay and antimicrobial resistance may be enormous, both physically and financially. Thus, infection control is considered a vital element in the operation of these facilities. This chapter provides an overview of the regulations governing infection control practices, unique challenges to infection control in nursing homes, and guidelines and resources to establish and sustain efficient infection control programs in nursing homes.

3. REGULATORY ASPECTS OF INFECTION CONTROL
    IN NURSING HOMES

Centers for Medicare and Medicaid Services (CMS) and Omnibus Budget Reconciliation Act (OBRA) regulations require that nursing homes establish prevention and control of infections in accordance with the resident populations they serve. Additionally, nursing homes have to comply with Occupational Safety and Health Administration (OSHA) regulations, which address protection of healthcare workers from blood-borne pathogens such as hepatitis B and human immunodeficiency virus (HIV). Additionally, nursing facilities have to comply with local and state regulations. This information can usually be obtained from the state government website. In addition, nursing homes may choose to make their facility compliant with nursing home requirements of voluntary organizations such as the Joint Commission on Accreditation of Healthcare Organization (JCAHO).

4. UNIQUE CHALLENGES OF INFECTION CONTROL
    IN NURSING HOMES

Older adults, especially in nursing homes, have unique characteristics that create special challenges to implementing an effective infection control program. These include diagnostic uncertainty, time and resource limitations, rapid staff turnover, limited and intermittent physician coverage, increasing acuity of care and frequent care transitions.

These unique concerns may be described in three categories: resident level factors, structural concerns, and process concerns.

4.1. Resident Level Factors

Nursing home residents are particularly susceptible to infections because of the increased prevalence of chronic diseases, increasing severity of illness, medications that affect resistance to infection (such as corticosteroids and frequent antibiotic usage), level of debility, impaired mental status (predisposing to aspiration and pressure ulcers), incontinence and resultant indwelling catheter usage, and the institutional environment in which they live (10,11).

Most infections are thought to be endogenous in nature, resulting from the resident's own flora. They may also serve as reservoirs for certain infectious agents such as methicillin-resistant *Staphylococcus aureus* (MRSA). Additionally, with reducing length of hospital stay, severity of illness among residents of the subacute care nursing unit is increasing with inherent rapid transfers to the hospital and poly-pharmacy. All these factors combined create a vulnerable resident highly prone to infections and morbidity and mortality associated with structural and process concerns facing medical care in nursing homes.

4.2. Structural Concerns

Assessment of structural concerns at a nursing home is an evaluation of the facility's capacity to provide care as opposed to assessment of process of care, which is an eva-luation of the actual service delivery. Structural characteristics of concern in imple-menting an effective infection control program in a nursing home include suboptimal full-time equivalents for registered nurses (RNs), nursing aides, and therapists, high staff turnover, changing case mix, limited availability of information systems, and variable availability of laboratory and radiologic investigations.

The number of staff per resident varies considerably among different types of facilities. Hospital-based nursing homes and skilled nursing homes for residents cov-ered by Medicare have almost twice the nursing staff of other community nursing facilities. The relationship between nursing care intensity and health outcomes for nursing home patients has been examined for years, and associations between increased nursing hours per patient and improved health outcomes have been reported, albeit somewhat inconsistently (12). RN turnover has been associated with increased risk of infection and hospitalization due to infection. The relationship between several structure and process elements of nursing home care and infections, RN turnover was associated with increased risk of infection and a higher risk of hos-pitalization due to infection in a sample of 59 nursing homes in Maryland (13). Potential explanations for this association may include difficulties in establishing and maintaining effective infection control practices, reduced familiarity between staff and resident to detect minor changes in the resident's health status, and incon-sistent supervision and training.

In order to reduce the length of acute hospital stay, nursing homes are now accepting sicker patients with higher severity of illness. This change in case mix has led to increased care transitions between hospitals and nursing homes leading to increased lapses in information exchange. These care transitions also lead to increased risk of transmission of pathogens between the hospital and nursing home.

4.3. Process Concerns

Processes of care in nursing homes pertain to actual healthcare service delivery. Process concerns in nursing homes include variable staff education, availability and utility of diagnostic specimens, use of quality improvement tools such as regional databases, quality indicators, and minimum data sets.

While effectiveness of education alone is controversial, the value of education as a part of a comprehensive quality control program has long been recognized in all healthcare settings. The importance of staff education is further accentuated by the phenomenal turnover in nursing home personnel. Currently, however, there are no standard guidelines regarding curriculum or frequency for staff education in nursing homes including infection control. Nursing aides who are the frontline personnel in recognizing any change in clinical status of nursing home residents may receive little or no formal educational training in various infection control issues such as hand hygiene, antimicrobial resistance, early symptoms and signs of common infection, and infection control measures to reduce infections related to in-dwelling devices. Several nursing homes overcome these barriers by scheduling monthly in-services. However, the content, frequency, and attendance of these in-services may vary among nursing homes.

Diagnostic specimens have limited usefulness in the nursing home population for two reasons: (1) they cannot be or are not obtained and (2) if obtained, the results may not be communicated to the appropriate person in a timely fashion, or in the case of radiological investigations, may not be interpreted accurately. On-site availability of diagnostic or radiologic investigations may be lacking in many nursing homes. In addition, patients may not be able or willing to cooperate in the collection of valid specimens. Diagnostic tests may thus be infrequently requested, resulting in initiation of therapy without having optimal clinical information. In nursing homes, in Rochester, NY, USA, investigations showed that urine culture was obtained for only 57% of episodes that were treated for urinary infection and chest x-rays were obtained for only 24% of treated lower respiratory tract infections (14). While urine specimens are more frequently obtained, prevalence of bacteriuria in 30–50% of urine specimens means that without an assessment of symptoms, a positive culture has a low predictive value for diagnosis of an infection (15). These diagnostic dilemmas can further lead to delay in initiation of care, inappropriate or unnecessary use of antibiotics, and delayed transfers to acute care for sicker patients.

Application of currently available hospital guidelines to nursing homes may be unrealistic and to some extent inappropriate. In view of the unique infection control challenges that exist in nursing homes, infection control must be simple, focused, and practical and must recognize the staffing, budget, and care concerns of older adults.

5. COMPONENTS OF INFECTION CONTROL IN NURSING HOMES (Fig. 1)

5.1. Infection Control Program

An infection control program includes an outbreak control plan for epidemics, a method of surveillance for infections and antimicrobial-resistant pathogens, an employee health program, a resident health program, policy formation and periodic review with audits, employee education and policy to communicate reportable diseases to public health authorities (16).

5.1.1. Outbreak Control

When the number of cases of an illness in a community or region clearly exceeds normal expectancy, it is considered an outbreak. The existence of an outbreak is thus always relative to the number of cases that are expected to occur in a specific population in a specific time period.

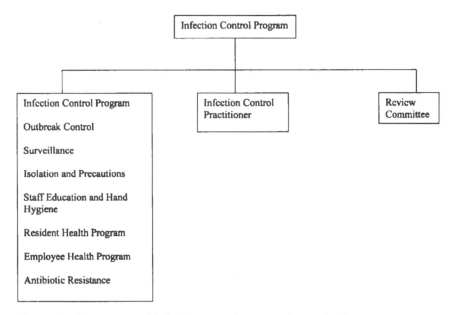

Figure 1 Components of infection control program in nursing homes.

The main objectives of an outbreak investigation are control and elimination of the source, prevention of new cases, prevention of future outbreaks, research to gain additional knowledge about the infectious agent and its mode of transmission, program evaluation and strategies for improvement, and epidemiological training to conduct outbreak investigations. The series of steps shown below provide a framework for a disease outbreak investigation. They highlight the issues that one should consider when conducting an outbreak in any setting: outpatient, acute care, or nursing home.

Since each outbreak varies considerably, the exact order in which one conducts the investigation and the amount of time and resources dedicated to each step will vary. These steps include: (1) establish the existence of an outbreak; (2) identify additional outbreaks; (3) collect preliminary data; (4) characterize the outbreak in terms of time, place, and person; (5) formulate a hypothesis as to the source and mode of transmission; (6) test the hypothesis, reformulate, and retest as needed; and (7) recommend and implement interventions (Table 1).

In order to test the hypothesis in outbreaks, two types of studies may be used: cohort or case–control. In cohort studies, a population that does not have the outcome of interest is identified and members of the cohort are classified based on exposure to the risk factors of interest. The entire cohort is then followed over time and incidences of the outcomes are compared between the exposed and unexposed individuals. Cohort studies can be retrospective or prospective. Cohort studies are particularly useful for rare exposures and in situations where we are interested in more than one outcome. However, cohort studies are generally slow and expensive to conduct. They may also be insufficient for investigating rare outcomes.

In case–control studies, individual cases are identified by the presence or absence of the outcome of interest. Those who do not have the outcome of interest serve as controls. The cases and controls are then compared to assess whether there

Table 1   Steps to Conduct an Outbreak Investigation

1. Establish the existence of an outbreak
   Verify or establish the diagnosis for all reported cases
   Compare the observed number of cases with the expected number of cases
   Consider alternative explanations
2. Identify additional cases
   Actively search for more cases that have not been reported
3. Collect preliminary data
   Identify variables on which to collect data; develop and apply appropriate
      data collection instrument
   Consider collecting data on following broad categories:
      Identifying information
      Demographic information
      Clinical information
      Data on risk factors
      Laboratory results
4. Characterize the outbreak in terms of time, place, and person
   Create an epidemic curve—is the outbreak a common source outbreak or a
      propagated outbreak?
   Plot the location of each case on a spot map
   Characterize the outbreak by person to define the population at risk
5. Formulate hypothesis as to the source and mode of transmission
   Assess all the collected information to formulate a testable hypothesis
6. Test hypothesis, reformulate, and retest as needed
   Formally test the hypothesis using a case–control or cohort study design
7. Recommend and implement interventions
   Implement interventions at various stages of outbreak investigation
   After determining the source of outbreak and its mode of transmission,
      institute control measures to prevent further cases
8. Communicate the findings
   Write up a formal report of the investigation to serve as reference document
      for future outbreaks

were any differences in their past exposure to one or more of the risk factors. The major advantage of case–control studies is that past exposures and outcomes are measured at the same time.

Because of this, studies can be done relatively quickly without the need to wait for an outcome. Case–control studies provide an opportunity to study rare outcomes and outcomes with long incubation periods. Case–control design is also beneficial in studying multiple exposures of the same outcome. [For example, presence of urinary catheter, pressure ulcer, and impaired functional status may all lead to methicillin-resistant *Staphylococcus aureus* (MRSA) colonization.] However, there are several disadvantages to this study design. Case–control studies are prone to selection bias, particularly in the selection of controls, and cannot establish the sequence of events, i.e., exposure may be a consequence of the outcome rather than the cause of it. Additionally, they may not be suitable for studying rare exposures.

It is vital that the infection control practitioner know and understand data collection methods, interpretation of data using simple epidemiologic measures, and these study designs in order to conduct an effective and efficient outbreak investigation and control. It may also be beneficial for the infection control practitioner to have access to a hospital epidemiologist for consultation.

5.1.2. Surveillance

Infection surveillance in nursing homes involves collection of data on nursing home-acquired infections. Collection of data for the purpose of monitoring infections in any setting is considered surveillance. Surveillance can be limited to a particular objective or may be facility-wide. Surveillance is often based on individual patient risk factors, focused on a unit, or based on a particular pathogen or infection type. These varying methods have similar sensitivity and specificity; however, surveillance utilizing laboratory data has the advantage of measuring facility-wide occurrences. Moreover, surveillance can be either passive or active. In passive surveillance, also known as routine surveillance, an infection control professional uses data collected for routine patient care.

While less costly in terms of resources, passive surveillance is inherently biased; in addition, it may underestimate the magnitude of outcome measured and delay the detection of outbreaks. The feasibility of passive surveillance has been demonstrated and has led to continuing education opportunities. However, active surveillance utilizes multiple data sources to detect problems early. It often requires routine patient screening for pathogens. Active surveillance for antimicrobial-resistant pathogens in acute care has created significant debate and has not been proven beneficial in nursing homes. However, it may be very useful in detecting certain highly contagious infections such as tuberculosis and influenza.

For surveillance to be conducted correctly, objective, valid definitions of infections are crucial. Hospital surveillance definitions are based on the National Nosocomial Infection Surveillance (NNIS) criteria, which depend rather extensively on laboratory investigations. Radiology and microbiology data are less available, and if available are delayed; therefore, these criteria may not be applicable in nursing home settings. Modified nursing home-specific criteria have been developed by a Canadian consensus conference, which takes into account the unique characteristics of older adults residing in a nursing home setting (17). They have been used widely, although not uniformly.

Analysis and reporting of infection rates are usually done monthly, quarterly, and annually to detect trends. Since the length of stay at a nursing home is long and thus each resident is at risk of a prolonged duration, analysis of absolute numbers of infections can be misleading. Infection rates (preferably reported as infections/1,000 resident-days) can be calculated by using resident-days or average resident census for the surveillance period as the denominator, using the following formula:

$$\frac{\text{No. of new nosocomial infections} \times 1000}{\text{No. of resident-days in the month}}$$

For example, if there are 30 infections in a month in a nursing home with an average daily census of 300 (resident-days = 300 × 30), then the infection rate is:

$$\frac{30 \times 1000}{9000} = 3.33 \text{ infections/1000 resident days}$$

Critical to the success of any surveillance program is feedback of these rates to the nursing staff, physicians, and appropriate quality control and review committees.

This information should eventually lead to specific, targeted infection control initiatives and follow-up surveillance to evaluate the success of the proposed changes.

5.1.3. Isolation and Precautions

Healthcare Infection Control Practice Advisory Committee/Centers for Disease Control and Prevention (HICPAC/CDC) has proposed two tiers of isolation precautions (18). In the first tier, HICPAC proposes use of standard precautions designed for the care of all patients in hospitals, regardless of their diagnosis, infectious or otherwise. In the second tier are transmission-based precautions designed for the care of patients suspected of or known to have been infected by epidemiologically important pathogens spread by physical contact or airborne or droplet transmission.

Standard precautions apply to blood, all body fluids, secretions and excretions regardless of whether they contain visible blood, non-intact skin, and or mucous membranes. Designed to reduce the risk of transmission of pathogens, both from apparent and ambiguous sources of infection, these precautions include hand hygiene, glove use, masks, eye protection and gowns, as well as avoiding injuries from sharps. Transmission-based precautions are intended for patients who may be infected with highly transmissible or epidemiologically significant pathogens. These include airborne precautions (for example, tuberculosis), droplet precautions (for example, influenza) and contact precautions (for example, *Clostridium difficile*). Although these guidelines were designed for acute care settings, several of them, especially standard precautions, apply to nursing homes as well. These recommendations have to be individualized based on the needs of the facility.

5.1.4. Staff Education and Hand Hygiene

The infection control nurse plays a vital role in educating nursing home personnel on various infection control measures, particularly in view of rapid staff turnover. Informal education during infection control and quality improvement meetings as well as during infection control walking rounds should be complemented with in-services on various topics including hand hygiene, antimicrobial usage and antimicrobial resistance, appropriate and early diagnosis of infections, infection control and prevention measures to prevent these infections, and isolation precautions and policies.

Contamination of the hands of healthcare workers (HCW) has been recognized to play a role in the transmission of pathogenic bacteria to patients since the observations of Holmes, Semmelweis, and others more than 100 years ago (19). Hand antisepsis remains the most effective and least expensive measure to prevent transmission of nosocomial infections. However, compliance with hand-washing recommendations among HCW averages only 30% to 50% and improves only transiently following educational interventions. Reasons frequently reported for poor compliance with hand hygiene include skin irritation from frequent washing, too little time due to a high workload, and simply forgetting (20).

The use of waterless, alcohol-based handrubs as an adjunct to washing with soap and water is becoming increasingly common in acute care facilities. Introduction of alcohol-based handrubs has been shown to significantly improve hand-hygiene compliance among HCW in acute care hospitals and to decrease overall nosocomial infection rates and transmission of MRSA infection in the acute care setting (21,22). Alcohol-based handrubs have been shown to enhance compliance with hand hygiene in the nursing home setting as well and should be used to complement educational initiatives (20).

5.1.5. Resident Health Program

The resident health program should focus on immunizations, tuberculin testing, and infection control policies to prevent specific infections such as skin care, oral hygiene, prevention of aspiration and catheter care to prevent urinary tract infections. Despite proven effectiveness, compliance with vaccinations remains dismally low. Adults age ≥65 should receive pneumococcal vaccination at least once, influenza vaccination every year, and tetanus booster every 10 years. Older adults should also get a two-step tuberculin skin test upon admission, followed by a chest radiograph if the test is positive.

5.1.6. Employee Health Program

The employee health program mainly concerns employees with potentially communicable diseases, policies for sick leave, immunizations, and OSHA regulations to protect them from blood-borne pathogens. It is required that nursing homes bar employees with communicable diseases or infected skin lesions from direct contact with the residents, and prevent employees with infected skin lesions or infectious diarrhea from having direct contact with residents' food. Moreover, on hiring new employees, it is necessary to perform an initial history and physical examination, provide education in infection control, and screen for tuberculosis. Additionally, policies and measures must be in place to address post-exposure prophylaxis for infections such as HIV and hepatitis B. Employees are expected to be up-to-date with their tetanus boosters and receive influenza vaccinations every year. Varicella vaccine should be given to employees not immune to the virus.

5.1.7. Antibiotic Resistance

Infection and colonization with antimicrobial-resistant pathogens are important concerns in nursing homes and develop primarily due to widespread use of empirical antibiotics, functional impairment, use of in-dwelling devices, mediocre adherence to hand hygiene among HCW, and cross-transmission during group activities. A nursing home can reduce infections and colonization with resistant pathogens by emphasizing hand hygiene, developing an antimicrobial utilization program, encouraging evidence-based clinical evaluation and management of infections, and ensuring that the facility has a well-established individualized infection control program. Guidelines to control MRSA and vancomycin-resistant enterococci have been published and should be adapted to develop facility-specific policies (23).

5.2. Infection Control Practitioner

An infection control practitioner (ICP), usually a staff nurse, is assigned the responsibility of directing infection control activities in the nursing home. The ICP is responsible for implementing, monitoring, and evaluating the infection control program. Due to financial constraints, an ICP usually also functions as an assistant director of nursing, or is involved in staff recruitment and education. Whether a full-time infection control practitioner is needed usually depends on the number of beds, the acuity level of residents, and the level of care provided at the facility. Nonetheless, for an infection control program to succeed, the ICP should be guaranteed sufficient time and resources to implement infection control activities. A basic background in infectious disease, microbiology, geriatrics, and educational methods is advisable. The ICP should be familiar with the federal, state, and local regulations on infection control.

The nursing home leadership should be supportive of the mission of infection control. They should encourage educational activities proposed by the ICP and should provide the ICP with internet access in order to keep up-to-date on current literature and nursing home policies and procedures. The administration should also provide adequate financial resources to accomplish these activities. The ICP should have written authority to implement emergency infection control measures. Additionally, an alliance with and access to an infectious disease epidemiologist should be encouraged.

5.3. Review Committee

In the early 1990s, OBRA mandated the formation of a formal infection control committee to evaluate infection rates, implement infection control programs and review policies and procedures. This mandate has been dropped by OBRA at a federal level, although some states may still require them. A small subcommittee or a working group comprised of a physician/medical director, an administrator, and ICP should evaluate the infection rates on a regular basis and present data at quality control meetings, review policies and any research in the area, and make decisions to implement infection control changes. This subcommittee can review and analyze the surveillance data, assure that these data are presented to the nursing and physician staff, and approve targeted recommendations to reduce such infections. Records pertaining to these activities and infection data should be kept and filed for future reference.

5.4. Resources for ICPs

- The Society for Healthcare Epidemiology of America (SHEA) and the Association for Professionals in Infection Control (APIC) both have long term care committees that publish and approve nursing home infection guidelines and publish periodic position papers related to pertinent infection control issues. Their websites have several educational resources for staff education and in-services. In addition, APIC also publishes a quarterly long-term care newsletter.
- Local APIC chapters provide a network for ICPs to socialize, discuss infection control challenges and practical solutions to overcome them, and provide access to educational resources and services. ICPs should become members of APIC at both local and national levels to remain up-to-date with practice guidelines, position statements, information technology resources, and changes in policies and regulations.
- Selected internet websites: CDC, http://www.cdc.gov; SHEA, http://www.shea-online.org/;
- APIC, http://www.apic.org; OSHA, http://www.osha.gov.

REFERENCES

1. Kemper P, Murtaugh CM. Lifetime use of nursing home care. N Eng J Med 1991; 324:595–600.
2. Nicolle LE, Strausbaugh LJ, Garibaldi RA. Infections and antibiotic resistance in nursing homes. Clin Microbiol Rev 1996; 9:1–17.

3. Garibaldi RA. Residential care and the elderly: the burden of infection. J Hosp Infect 1999; 43:S9–S18.
4. Smith PW, Rusnak PG. Infection prevention and control in the long-term-care facility. SHEA long-term-care committee and APIC guidelines committee. Infect Control Hosp Epidemiol 1997; 18:831–849.
5. Federal Interagency Forum on Aging-Related Statistics, Older Americans 2000: Key Indicators of Well-Being. Federal Interagency Forum on Aging-Related Statistics. Washington, DC: U.S. Government Printing Office, 2000.
6. Strausbaugh LJ, Joseph CL. The burden of infections in long-term care. Infect Control Hosp Epidemiol 2000; 21:674–679.
7. Stevenson KB. Regional data set of infection rates for long-term care facilities: Description of a valuable benchmarking tool. Am J Infect Control 1999; 27:20–26.
8. Castle NG, Mor V. Hospitalization of nursing home residents: A review of the literature, 1980–1995. Med Care Res Rev 1996; 53:123–148.
9. Barker WH, Zimmer JG, Hall WJ, Ruff BC, Freundlich CB, Eggert GM. Rates, patterns, causes and costs of hospitalization of nursing home residents: A population-based study. Am J Public Health 1994; 84:1615–1620.
10. Smith PW. Nursing home infection control: a status report. Infect Control Hosp Epidemiol 1998; 19:366–369.
11. Goldrick BA. Infection control programs in skilled nursing long-term care facilities: an assessment. Am J Infect Control 1999; 27:4–9.
12. Cohen-Mansfield J. Turnover among nursing home staff. Nurs Management 1997; 28:59–62.
13. Zimmerman S, Gruber-Baldini AL, Hebel JR, Sloane PD, Magaziner J. Nursing home facility risk factors for infection and hospitalization: importance of registered nurse turnover, administration, and social factors. J Am Geriatr Soc 2002; 50:1987–1989.
14. Montgomery P, Semenchuk M, Nicolle LE. Antimicrobial use in nursing homes in Manitoba. J Geriatr Drug Ther 1995; 9:55–74.
15. Nicolle L. Urinary tract infections in long-term care facilities. Infect Control Hosp Epidemiol 1993; 14:220–225.
16. Smith PW, Rusnak PG. Infection prevention and control in long-term care acility. Am J Infect Control 1997; 25:488–512.
17. McGeer A, Campbell B, Emori TG, Hierholzer WJ, Jackson MM, Nicolle LE, Peppler C, Rivera A, Schollenberger DG, Simor AE. Definitions of infection for surveillance in long-term care facilities. Am J Infect Control 1991; 19:1–7.
18. Garner JS, Simmons BP. Guideline for isolation precautions in hospitals. Infect Control 1983; 4:245–325.
19. Othersen MJ, Othersen HB. A history of hand washing: Seven hundred years at a snail's pace. Pharos 1987; Spring, 23–27.
20. Mody L, McNeil SA, Sun R, Bradley SF, Kauffman CA. Introduction of a waterless alcohol-based hand rub in a long-term care facility. Infect Control Hosp Epidemiol 2003; 24:165–171.
21. Bischoff WE, Reynold TM, Sessler CN, Edmond MB, Wenzel RP. Handwashing compliance by health care workers: The impact of introducing an accessible, alcohol-based hand antiseptic. Arch Intern Med 2000; 160:1017–1021.
22. Pittet D, Hugonnet S, Harbarth S, Mourouga P, Sauvan V, Touveneau S, Perneger TV. Effectiveness of a hospital-wide programme to improve compliance with hand hygiene. Lancet 2000; 356:1307–1312.
23. Strausbaugh LJ, Crossley KB, Nurse BA, Thrupp LD, SHEA long-term care committee. Antimicrobial resistance in long-term care facilities. Infect Control Hosp Epidemiol 1996; 17:119–128.

SUGGESTED READING

Bentley DW, Bradley S, Schoenbaum S, Taler G, Yoshikawa TT. Practice guideline for evaluation of fever and infection in long-term care facilities. Clin Infect Dis 2000; 31:640–653.

McGeer A, Campbell B, Emori TG, Hierholzer WJ, Jackson MM, Nicolle LE, Peppler C, Rivera A, Schollenberger DG, Simor AE. Definitions of infection for surveillance in long-term care facilities. Am J Infect Control 1991; 19:1–7.

Strausbaugh LJ, Joseph CL. The burden of infections in long-term care. Infect Control Hosp Epidemiol 2000; 21:674–679.

Index

T - #0300 - 101024 - C0 - 254/178/41 [43] - CB - 9780824727833 - Gloss Lamination